ERRATUM

Chapter 3
Anterior Cervical Microdiscectomy Without Fusion
by Philip R. Weinstein

page 47, **Algorithm 1**
Delete line below NEGATIVE.
Add arrow line below POSITIVE.

page 52, **Figure 4A**
The dotted line should extend posterolaterally back and out to the uncinate processes of the vertebral body.

page 52, **Figure 4B**
The lines of resection should stop at the posterior longitudinal ligament. The dura and spinal cord are obviously not to be removed.

page 54, **Figure 5B**
The C7 vertebra was inadvertently cropped out of the photo. There was no movement during flexion or extension at C6-7 seen on these postoperative radiographs.

page 55, **Figure 5** legend, line 3
E: delete axial. This is a sagittal section.

Master Techniques in Orthopaedic Surgery, THE SPINE
Chapter 3, pages 47, 52, 54, and 55

MASTER TECHNIQUES IN ORTHOPAEDIC SURGERY

■

THE SPINE

MASTER TECHNIQUES IN ORTHOPAEDIC SURGERY

Series Editor
Roby C. Thompson, Jr., M.D.

Volume Editors

THE FOOT AND ANKLE
Kenneth A. Johnson, M.D.

RECONSTRUCTIVE KNEE SURGERY
Douglas W. Jackson, M.D.

KNEE ARTHROPLASTY
Paul A. Lotke, M.D.

THE HIP
Clement B. Sledge, M.D.

THE SPINE
David S. Bradford, M.D.

THE SHOULDER
Edward V. Craig, M.D.

THE ELBOW
Bernard F. Morrey, M.D.

THE WRIST
Richard H. Gelberman, M.D.

THE HAND
James W. Strickland, M.D.

FRACTURES
Donald A. Wiss, M.D.

THE SPINE

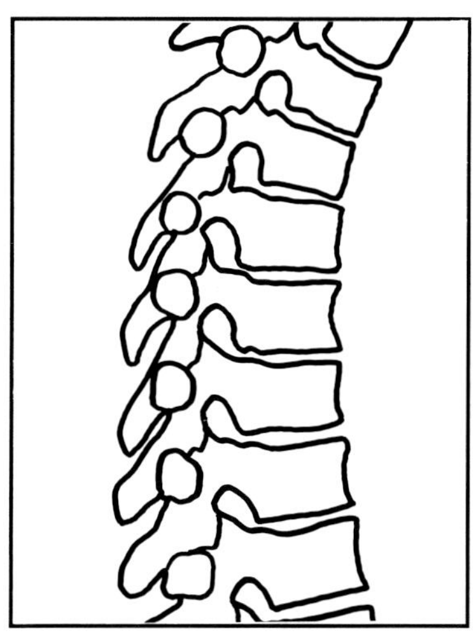

Editor

DAVID S. BRADFORD, M.D.
Professor and Chairman
Department of Orthopaedic Surgery
University of California, San Francisco
School of Medicine
San Francisco, California

Illustrators

Donna Cavi
Baltimore, Maryland

Paul Gross
Nashville, Tennessee

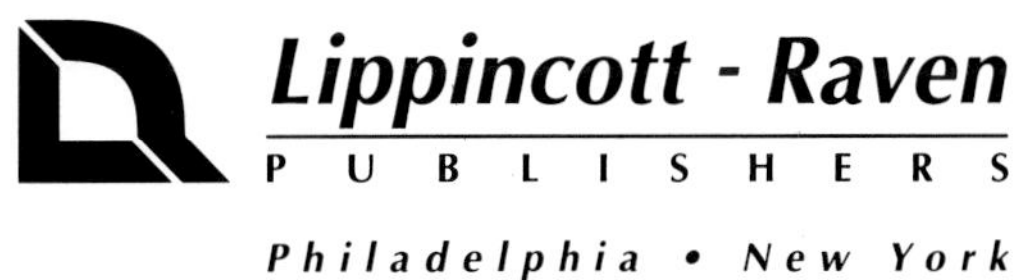

Printed and bound in USA

9 8 7 6 5 4 3 2 1

Library of Congress Cataloging-in-Publication Data

The spine / editor, David S. Bradford ; illustrator, Donna Cavi, Paul Gross.
p. cm.—(Master techniques in orthopaedic surgery ; [v. 7])
Includes bibliographical references and index.
ISBN 0-7817-0033-7
1. Spine—Surgery. I. Bradford, David S., 1936– . II. Series.
[DNLM: 1. Spine—surgery. 2. Surgery, Operative—methods. WE 168 M423 1994 v. 7]
RD768.S672 1995
617.3′75059—dc20
DNLM/DLC
for Library of Congress 97-6252
CIP

Care has been taken to confirm the accuracy of the information presented and to describe generally accepted practices. However, the authors, editors, and publisher are not reponsible for errors or omissions or for any consequences from application of the information in this book and make no warranty, express or implied, with respect to the contents of the publication.

The authors, editors and publisher have exerted every effort to ensure that drug selection and dosage set forth in this text are in accordance with current recommendations and practice at the time of publication. However, in view of ongoing research, changes in government regulations, and the constant flow of information relating to drug therapy and drug reactions, the reader is urged to check the package insert for each drug for any change in indications and dosage and for added warnings and precautions. This is particularly important when the recommended agent is a new or infrequently employed drug.

Some drugs and medical devices presented in this publication have Food and Drug Administration (FDA) clearance for limited use in restricted research settings. It is the responsibility of the health care provider to ascertain the FDA status of each drug or device planned for use in their clinical practice.

To David, Jennifer, and Tyler

■

CONTENTS

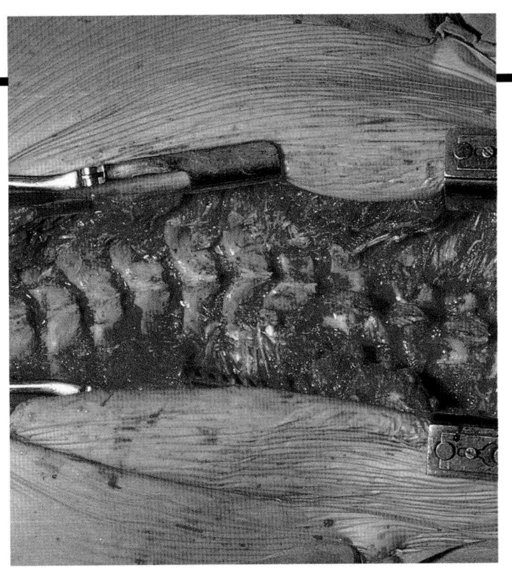

PART III TECHNIQUES—THORACIC/LUMBAR SPINE

CONTRIBUTORS

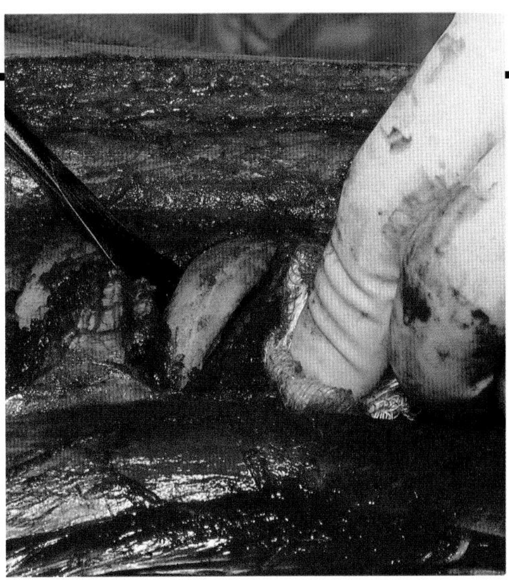

Max Aebi, M.D., F.R.C.S.C.
Professor and Chairman, Division of Orthopaedic Surgery, McGill University, and Orthopaedic Surgeon-in-Charge, Department of Orthopaedic Surgery, Montreal General Hospital and Royal Victoria Hospital, 687 Pine Avenue West, Montreal, Quebec, Canada H3A 1A1

Ben L. Allen Jr., M.D.
Professor, Section of Orthopaedic Surgery, University of South Carolina, Adjunct Professor of Bioengineering, Clemson University; and Chief of Staff, Greenville Unit, Shriners Hospitals for Crippled Children, 950 West Faris Road, Greenville, South Carolina 29605

Marc A. Asher, M.D.
Professor, Section of Orthopedic Surgery, University of Kansas Medical Center, 39th and Rainbow Boulevard, Kansas City, Kansas 66160–7387

Randal R. Betz, M.D.
Assistant Chief of Staff, Shriners Hospitals for Crippled Children, Philadelphia Unit, 8400 Roosevelt Boulevard, Philadelphia, Pennsylvania 19152–1299

Henry H. Bohlman, M.D.
Professor, Department of Orthopaedic Surgery, Case Western Reserve University School of Medicine; and Director, The University Hospitals Spine Institute, 11100 Euclid Avenue, Cleveland, Ohio 44106

David S. Bradford, M.D.
Professor and Chairman, Department of Orthopaedic Surgery, University of California, San Francisco, School of Medicine, 533 Parnassus Avenue, MU320W, San Francisco, California 94143–0728

Samuel J. Chewning, Jr., M.D.
Miller Orthopaedic Clinic, 1001 Blythe Boulevard, Suite 200, Charlotte, North Carolina 28203

Samuel F. Ciricillo, A.B., M.D.
Assistant Clinical Professor, Department of Neurosurgery and Pediatrics, University of California, San Francisco, 533 Parnassus Avenue, San Francisco, California 94143–0112

David H. Clements, M.D.
Assistant Professor, Department of Orthopedic Surgery, Temple University School of Medicine, 3401 North Broad Street, Philadelphia, Pennsylvania 19140

Barbara Dabb, M.D.
Clinical Anesthesiologist, The University Hospitals Spine Institute, 11100 Euclid Avenue, Cleveland, Ohio 44106

Rick B. Delamarter, M.D.
Co-Director, UCLA Comprehensive Spine Center, Associate Clinical Professor, Department of Orthopaedic Surgery, University of California Los Angeles Medical Center, 100 UCLA Medical Plaza, #755, Los Angeles, California 90024

Ronald L. DeWald, M.D.
Professor, Department of Orthopaedic Surgery, Director of Spinal Surgery, Rush Medical College, 1725 W. Harrison Street, #440, Chicago, Illinois 60612

Harold K. Dunn, M.D.
Professor and Chairman, Department of Orthopaedics, University of Utah School of Medicine, 50 North Medical Dr., Salt Lake City, Utah 84132

Michael S. B. Edwards, M.D.
Professor of Neurosurgery and Pediatrics, Director, Division of Pediatric Neurosurgery, Department of Neurosurgery, University of California, San Francisco, 505 Parnassus Avenue, San Francisco, California 94134–0112

Jeffrey S. Fischgrund, M.D.
Department of Orthopaedic Surgery, William Beaumont Hospital, 3535 West Thirteen Mile Road, Suite 604, Royal Oak, Michigan 48073–6705

Steven R. Garfin, M.D.
Professor of Orthopaedic Surgery, University of California San Diego Medical Center, 200 West Arbor Drive, Mail Code 8894, San Diego, California 92103-8894

Charles F. Heinig, M.D.
(Retired) Miller Orthopaedic Clinic of Charlotte North Carolina, 1001 Blythe Boulevard, Suite 200, Charlotte, North Carolina 28203

Harry N. Herkowitz, M.D.
Chairman, Department of Orthopaedic Surgery, and Director, Section of Spine Surgery, William Beaumont Hospital, 3535 West Thirteen Mile Road, Suite 604, Royal Oak, Michigan 48073–6705

John A. Herring, M.D.
Professor, Department of Orthopaedic Surgery, University of Texas Southwestern Medical Center at Dallas, Chief of Staff, Texas Scottish Rite Hospital for Children, 2222 Welborn Street, Dallas, Texas 75219–3993

Serena S. Hu, M.D.
Assistant Professor, Department of Orthopaedic Surgery, University of California San Francisco, School of Medicine, 533 Parnassus Avenue, MU 320 W, San Francisco, California 94143–0728

Kiyoshi Kaneda, M.D., Ph.D.
Professor and Chairman, Department of Orthopaedic Surgery, Hokkaido University School of Medicine, Kita-15, Nishi-7, Kita-ku, Sapporo 060, Japan

John P. Kostuik, M.D., F.R.C.S. (C.)
Professor, Departments of Orthopaedics and Neurosurgery, and Chief, Spine Division Orthopaedics, The Johns Hopkins University Medical Center, 601 North Caroline Street, Baltimore, Maryland 21287–0882

Stephen J. Lipson, M.D.
Associate Professor, Harvard Medical School, and Orthopaedic Surgeon-in-Chief, Department of Orthopedic Surgery, Beth Israel Hospital, 330 Brookline Avenue, Boston, Massachusetts 02215

Hiromi Matsuzaki, M.D.
Associate Professor, Chief of Spinal Division, Department of Orthopedic Surgery, Nihon University School of Medicine, 1-8-13, Kandasurugadai, Chiyoda-ku, Tokyo 101, Japan

Robert F. McLain, M.D.
Associate Professor, and Director of Spine Research, Department of Orthopaedic Surgery, University of California, Davis School of Medicine, 2230 Stockton Boulevard, Sacramento, California 95817

James W. Ogilvie, M.D.
Professor, Department of Orthopaedic Surgery, University of Minnesota, 420 Delaware St. S.E., Box #492, UMHC, Minneapolis, Minnesota 55455

John J. Regan, M.D.
Associate Clinical Professor, Department of Orthopaedic Surgery, University of Texas Southwestern Medical Center; and Texas Back Institute, 6300 West Parker Road, Plano, Texas 75093

Gaetano J. Scuderi, M.D.
Clinical Instructor, Department of Orthopaedics, University of California San Diego Medical Center, 200 West Arbor Drive, Mail Code 8894, San Diego, California 92103-8894

Harry L. Shufflebarger, M.D.
Professor, University of Miami School of Medicine, 1150 Campo Sano Avenue, Coral Gables, Florida 33146

Dan M. Spengler, M.D.
Professor and Chairman, Department of Orthopaedics and Rehabilitation, Vanderbilt University Medical Center, 1161 21st Avenue South, Nashville, Tennessee 37232-2550

Howard H. Steel, M.D.
Emeritus Chief of Staff, Shriners Hospitals for Crippled Children, Philadelphia Unit, 8400 Roosevelt Boulevard, Philadelphia, Pennsylvania 19152–1299

Ensor Transfeldt, M.D.
Twin Cities Scoliosis Spine Center, 2800 Chicago Avenue South, #400, Minneapolis, Minnesota 55407

Philip R. Weinstein, M.D.
Professor and Vice Chairman, Department of Neurosurgery, University of California, San Francisco Medical Center, School of Medicine, 1360 Ninth Avenue, San Francisco, California 94143–0112

ACKNOWLEDGMENTS

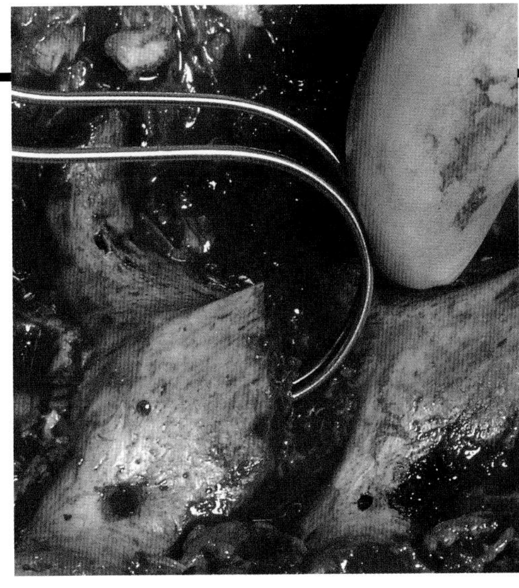

I would like to acknowledge and extend my gratitude to Susan Averbach, research associate, for her immense dedication and diligent work on this project. Particular thanks to my administrative assistant, Janet Jacobsen, who kept this project moving on a timely basis. Kathey Alexander's help and contribution has truly been outstanding. This book would never have been accomplished without her administrative, editorial, and organizational talents, and particularly her patience. Finally, I am indebted to all the authors who contributed their time and energies to make this a truly worthwhile and useful volume for orthopaedic and neurosurgical spinal surgeons.

SERIES PREFACE

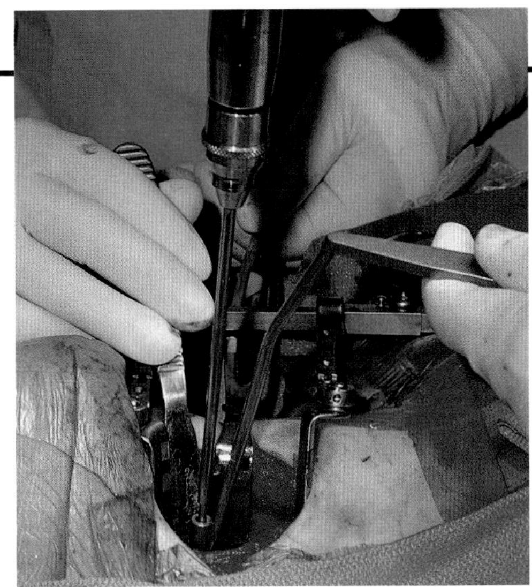

Master Techniques in Orthopaedic Surgery is a ten-volume series of operative atlases designed to provide in-depth descriptions of surgical techniques that are preferred by surgeons recognized by their peers as master surgeons in their area of specialization.

The ten volume editors, all recognized leaders based on their research and educational contributions, have advanced the surgical state of the art in our field. The chapter authors were selected for their experience and skills, and were asked to present their material in a personal manner, highlighting their unique perspectives and observations for the reader.

These atlases are designed to help the practitioner deal with the difficult but common problems encountered in daily practice. Surgical procedures that are in the developmental phase, such as vascularized fibular grafting for osteonecrosis, or procedures largely restricted to referral centers, such as reconstruction for limb salvage following tumor resection, have not been covered since procedures such as these are rarely performed by the orthopaedic practitioner. Likewise, the common, straightforward procedures that offer few complications and little difficulty have also been avoided.

These books take you into the operating room and let you peer over the shoulder of the surgeon at work. The color photographs and accompanying drawings guides the orthopaedist step-by-step through a procedure. The commentary, organized in a standard format throughout the series, offers one specific technical advice, as well as tips and pearls gained through the surgeon's years of experience.

The shared knowledge and expertise found in these pages are presented to enable the surgeon to undertake surgical procedures with greater confidence and improved proficiency.

Roby C. Thompson, Jr., M.D.
Series Editor

PREFACE

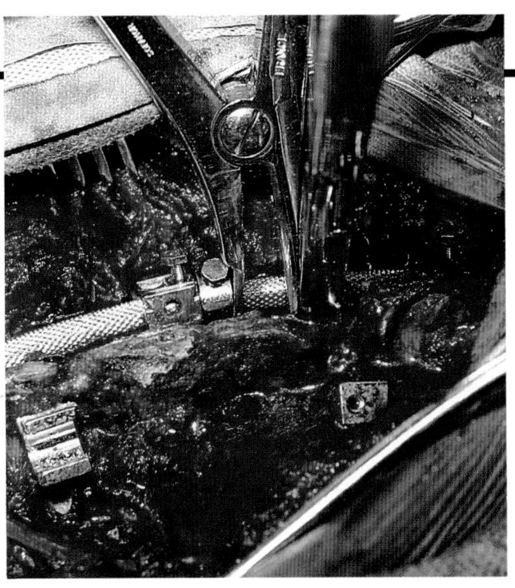

Spinal reconstructive surgery has undergone remarkable advances in the past decade. It is true to state that the technical changes have been so great that there are few operations that we do today that we would have even conceived much less executed a decade ago. Because of these remarkable advances it has become even more expedient that spinal surgeons keep abreast of emerging technologies and improvements in the procedural aspects of their specialty.

This volume was designed not only to provide the reader with an easily useable reference source to review innovative and current technical advances in spinal reconstructive surgery, but also to see first hand what experts in this field are finding most helpful and useful in their own practices. The contributing authors are acknowledged leaders in their subspecialty and well-versed and published in their area of expertise. Fellows, residents, students, and paramedical personnel will find this book a useful reference source.

David S. Bradford, M.D.

MASTER TECHNIQUES IN ORTHOPAEDIC SURGERY

■

THE SPINE

PART I

Surgical Approaches

Master Techniques in Orthopaedic Surgery,
THE SPINE, edited by D. S. Bradford,
Lippincott-Raven Publishers, Philadelphia, © 1997.

1

Anterior Approaches to the Cervical Spine

Gaetano J. Scuderi and Steven R. Garfin

The anterior approach to the cervical spine provides direct access to pathologic processes involving either the vertebral body or intervertebral disc. Under most circumstances, the decision to approach the cervical spine anteriorly or posteriorly should be dictated by the site of primary pathology. A major limitation to anterior exposure is that most fusion techniques do not add spinal stability, and in some cases stability is removed. This is especially true in treating some traumas to the cervical spine.

The cervical spine can be divided into three zones when determining the type of anterior approach. The basi-occiput and first and second cervical vertebrae must be reached directly anteriorly via the pharynx, or, anterolaterally, either anterior or posterior to the carotid sheath. More complicated exposures include tongue-splitting and mandible-splitting approaches. Many of these techniques are facilitated by the assistance of a head and neck surgeon. Likewise, approaches to the lower cervical and upper thoracic segments are numerous. Exposure through the thoracic inlet via sternal splitting and clavicular resection procedures may represent a significant challenge to the spinal surgeon.

Transoral (Pharyngeal) Approach to the Upper Cervical Spine

INDICATIONS/CONTRAINDICATIONS

The transoral approach is relatively straightforward. Specific indications are drainage for upper cervical spine infections, biopsy, debridement/resection of

G. J. Scuderi, M.D. and S. R. Garfin, M.D.: University of California San Diego Medical Center, San Diego, California 92103.

tumor of C1 or C2 anteriorly, and/or excision of the odontoid. It offers direct access to pathology involving the anterior aspect of the second cervical vertebra, which is palpable and "visible" through the mouth. Resection of the odontoid process for nonunions, malunions, or other spinal cord-compromising lesions, as well as excision of pannus secondary to rheumatoid arthritis, may be performed transorally. This approach is also frequently used for drainage of posterior pharyngeal abscesses. The transoral approach can be extended to the basi-occiput superiorly and third cervical vertebra inferiorly. Extension caudally is difficult and may require tongue and mandibular splitting. Considerable retraction may be necessary for visualization cephalically, and division of the soft palate may be considered in order to gain suitable access.

Because of the high rate of infection that has been demonstrated with this method, related to the use of bone graft, we do not routinely recommend fusion using this approach, although occasionally it is necessary.

PREOPERATIVE PLANNING

Because of the significant numbers of normal flora in the oral cavity, broad-spectrum parenteral antibiotics should be used. Antimicrobials can be given based on preoperative nasal-pharyngeal cultures. Penicillin, assuming the patient does not have allergies to it, should also be given to cover anaerobic bacteria. This approach is best used to gain direct anterior visualization of the odontoid. In general, when more extensive and distal resections are necessary, the retropharyngeal approach may be preferable, since it is easier to extend caudally.

SURGERY

Anesthesia should be administered by endotracheal intubation, utilizing a non-collapsible tube and cuff. This cuff prevents the aspiration of blood and other debris into the lungs. A head lamp is recommended for the operating surgeon, if a microscope is not employed. Obtaining bright, consistent lighting in this area is difficult, but essential. A slight Trendelenburg position is also advised so that debris floats superiorly and can be cleared under direct vision prior to extubation. First the uvula is folded back on itself and temporarily sutured. The nasal pharyngeal area is packed with a sponge to prevent pooling of blood in the hypopharynx. Prepping the oral pharynx involves painting the oral cavity with Betadine-soaked sponge sticks. Several landmarks may be palpated before making the incision. The disc between the second and third vertebrae is prominent and can often be felt inferiorly. The anterior tubercle of the arch of the first cervical vertebra may be palpable in the superior hypopharynx. The eustachian tube orifices may be visualized by slight retraction of the soft palate and are found at the level of the basi-occiput. If the surgeon remains unsure of the location for the incision (because of anatomic distortions that occur, for example, with an abscess or large tumor posterior to the pharynx), a spinal needle may be placed through the pharynx into the anterior vertebral column and an intraoperative localizing, lateral radiograph obtained.

A longitudinal incision is made in the midline of the posterior pharynx (Fig. 1). Four thin layers are found at this level: the pharyngeal mucosa, the pharyngeal constrictor muscles, the buccal pharyngeal fascia, and the anterior longitudinal ligament. The incision is carried through all layers to bone. The midline plane of dissection is relatively avascular, and bleeders may be cauterized as necessary. Soft-tissue dissection of bone is performed by using a periosteal elevator to the lateral masses of the axis. Soft-tissue flaps can be held in the retracted position

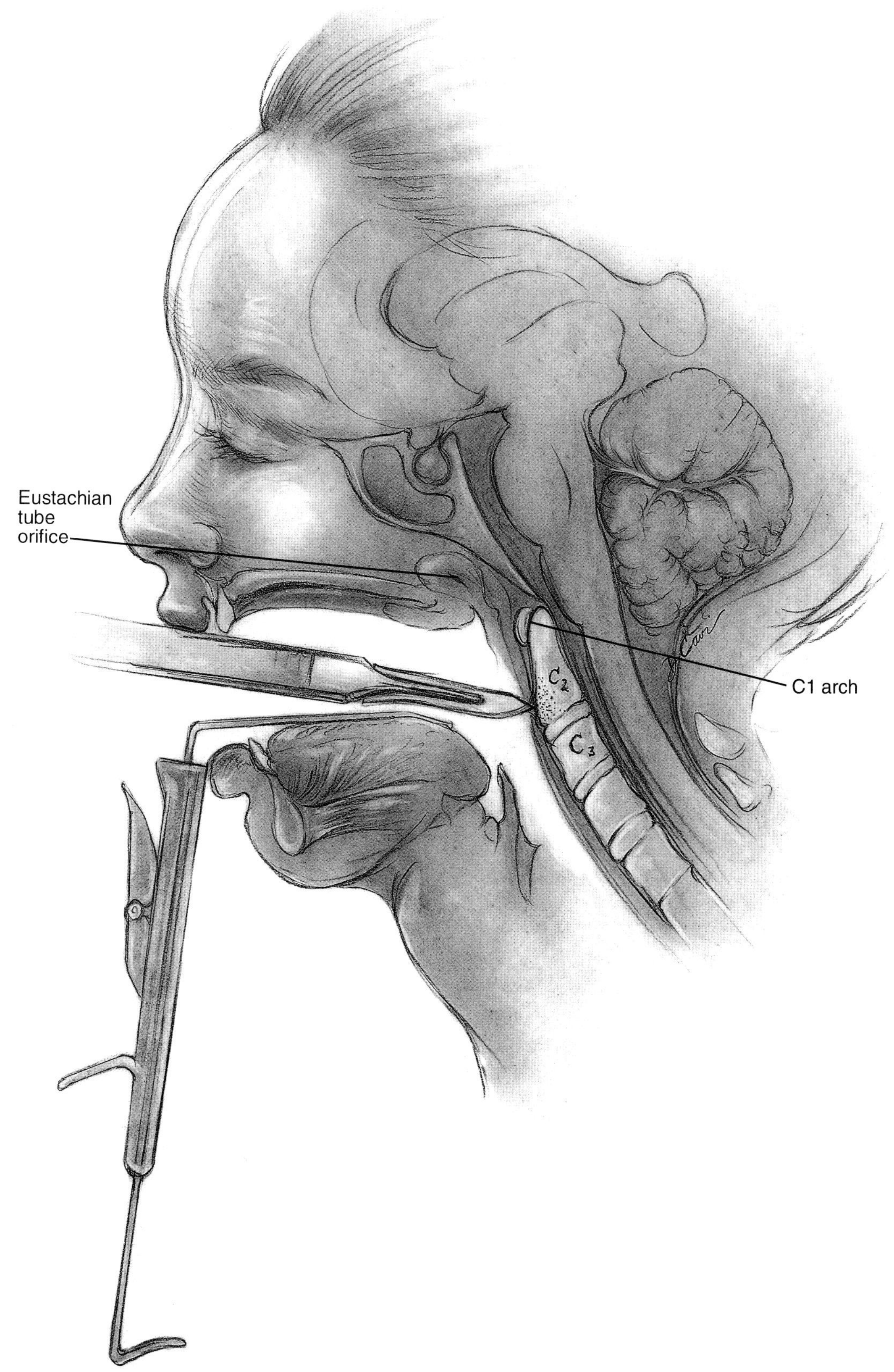

Figure 1. Approach to C1–C2 is through the mouth to the pharynx. A midline incision is made sharply through the mucosa.

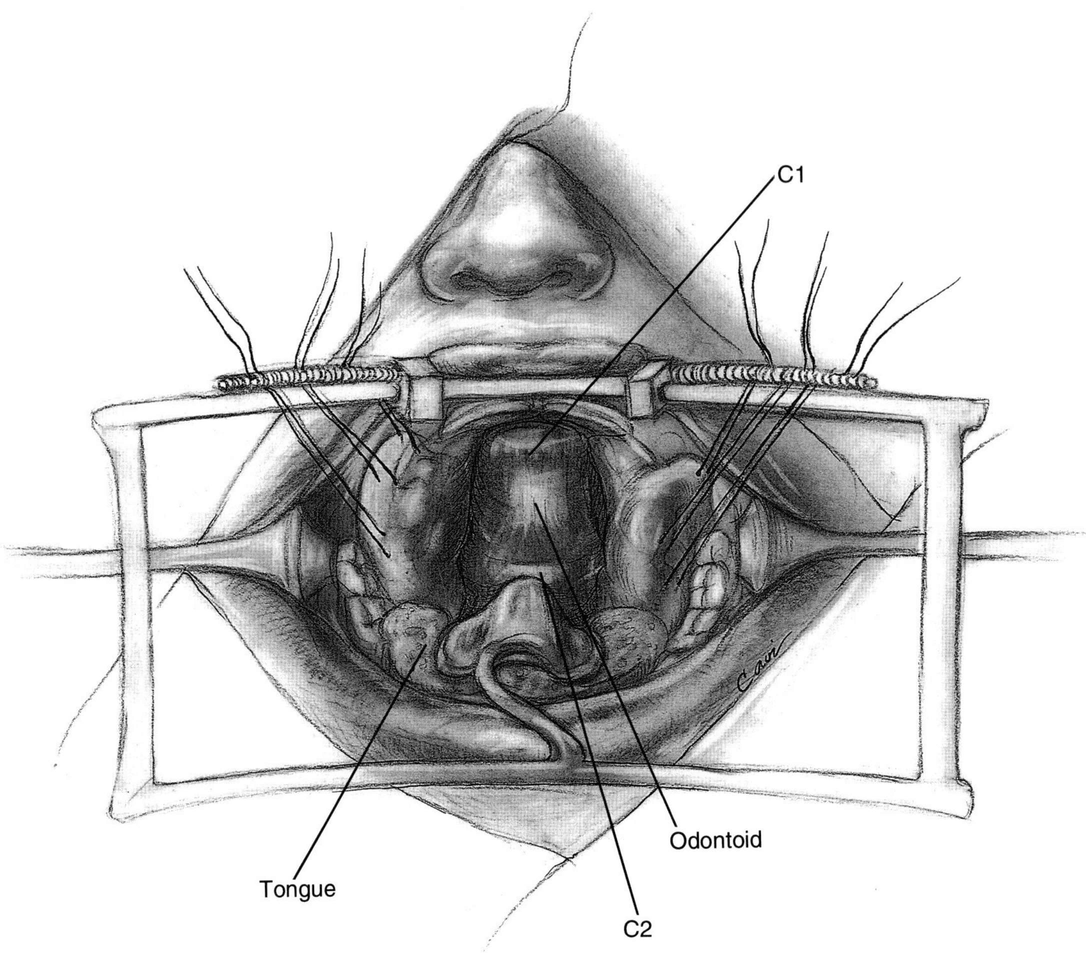

Figure 2. Self-retaining retractors are used to keep the mouth open and allow access to the pharynx and deep structures. After making the midline incision and exposing the anterior aspect of C1–C2, the soft tissue flaps can be held open with long stay sutures tethered to the retractors.

by using long stay sutures (Fig. 2). Long incisions may be necessary for adequate and safe visualization. A tongue retractor attached to a suction apparatus will minimize the need for additional instruments that may obscure the view of the surgeon.

Upon termination of the procedure, the hypopharynx should be carefully irrigated and inspected for debris and clotted blood. The wound may be closed with interrupted absorbable sutures. If drainage is necessary, a rubber drain may be placed through the nasopharynx and into the wound. The authors use antibiotics for 48 to 72 hours. If the surgery is extensive, a tracheostomy may be considered. The airway remains at risk postoperatively due to edema, hemorrhage, and/or continued drainage.

COMPLICATIONS

Complications can be minimized if the surgeon adheres strictly to guidelines. The risk of infection by pharyngeal flora is well recognized and is the primary complication of this approach. A review of the literature reveals that the highest incidence of infection is often related to the addition of bone graft for a fusion through this approach (3, 7). We, therefore, do not routinely recommend fusion through this approach, although many physicians do. We would not add internal fixation. In addition to infection, the one other complication is the limited extensibility of this approach.

Anterior Retropharyngeal Approach to the Upper Cervical Spine: Medial to the Carotid Sheath

INDICATIONS/CONTRAINDICATIONS

If an extrapharyngeal exposure to the basi-occiput is necessary, the approach should be medial to the carotid sheath. The basi-occiput cannot be reached safely through a lateral route. McAfee's approach (described here) is primarily utilized for extensive removal of tumors or infections, as well as bone grafting procedures. It allows access to the C1–C2 joints, as well as C1 and C2 centrally. It is relatively easy to extend this distally, through a more classic Smith-Robinson approach, to access the lower cervical spine, if necessary. Risk of infection is minimized by avoiding the pharyngeal mucosa.

SURGERY

Gardner-Wells tongs or a halo ring are applied preoperatively. The lower strap of a head halter traction device extends too far inferiorly around the mandible and precludes proper surgical preparation and draping of the skin. We routinely use somatosensory and motor evoked potentials to monitor spinal cord function. An awakc intubation utilizing fiberoptic methods may be necessary if concerns exist about upper cervical instability. The mouth should be kept free of all tubes, stethoscopes, and temperature probes, if possible. It is important to keep the mandible closed so as not to limit the operative site.

The approach can be made either from the left or the right side, since the high extrapharyngeal approach is sufficiently superior to the right recurrent laryngeal nerve. A transverse submandibular incision is used, curving toward the midline (Fig. 3). If necessary, the incision can be T-ed to allow inferior exposure. This vertical limb can be extended as inferiorly as necessary. The exposure is a superior extension of the standard anterior-lateral approach to the lower cervical spine, described later. The vertical extension is utilized only for extensive exposure (e.g., tumor resection). The submandibular incision is carried through the platysma and superficial fascia transversely. After mobilizing this layer, the marginal mandibular branch of the facial nerve is found. A nerve stimulator may aid in this. Several retromandibular veins found at this level must be ligated. The common facial vein is continuous with the retromandibular vein, and branches of the mandibular nerve cross the lateral vein superficially and superiorly. By ligating the retromandibular vein as it joins the internal jugular vein, and by keeping the dissection deep and inferior to the vein as the exposure is extended superiorly to the mandible, the superficial branch of the facial nerve is usually protected.

The anterior border of the sternocleidomastoid muscle is identified. It is mobilized by longitudinally transecting the superficial layer of deep cervical fascia. The carotid sheath can then be identified by gentle palpation (Fig. 4). The submandibular salivary gland is then resected in total. Care is taken to identify and ligate the duct to prevent a salivary fistula. Jugular and digastric lymph nodes from the submandibular and carotid triangles can be resected if neoplasm is suspected, or to improve visualization. The posterior belly of the digastric muscle and the stylohyoid muscle are identified, and the digastric tendon is divided and tagged for later repair. It is important to avoid rigorous retraction of the stylohyoid muscle, since this may cause injury to the facial nerve as it exits from the skull.

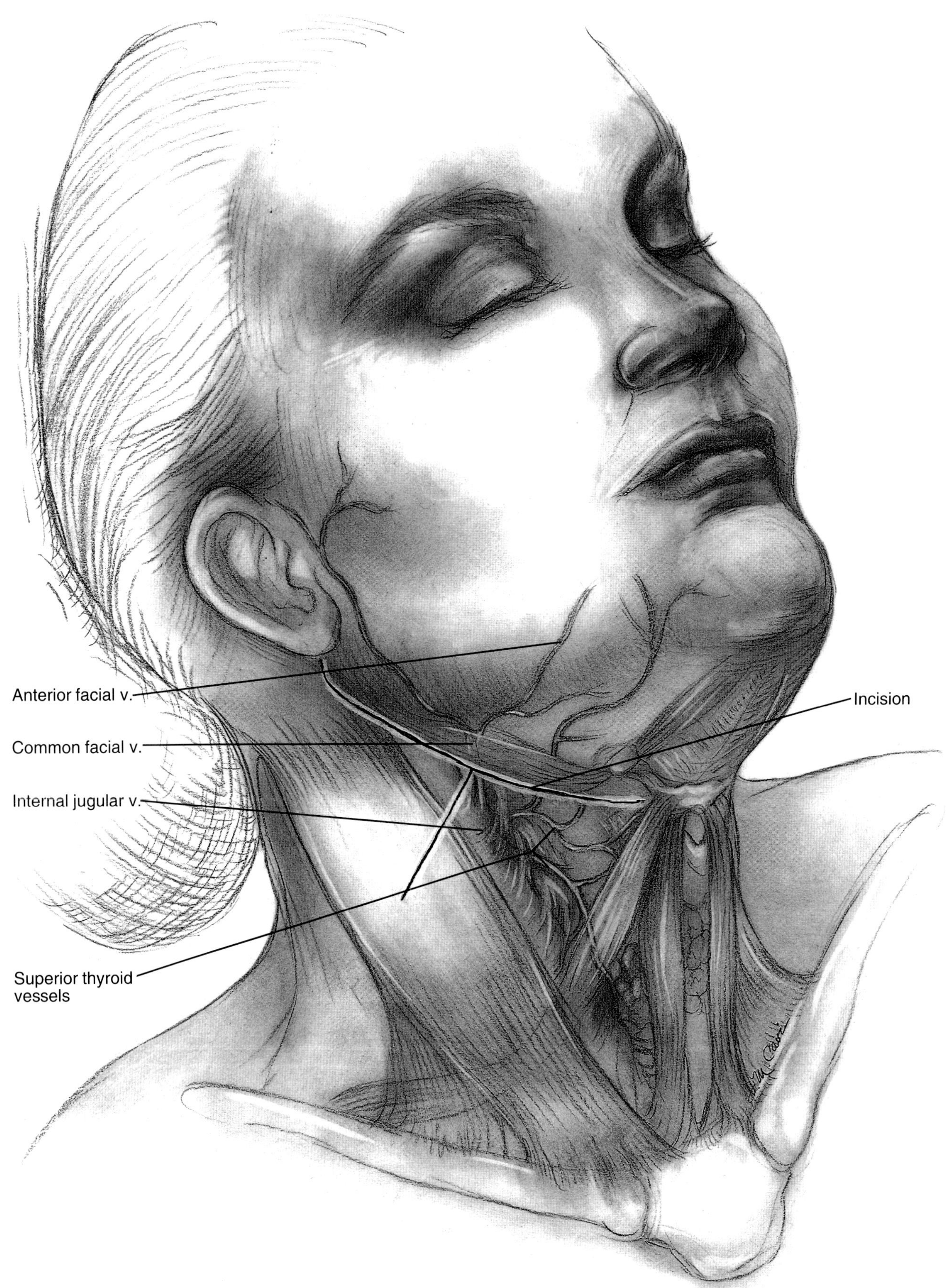

Figure 3. Skin incision for retropharyngeal approach.

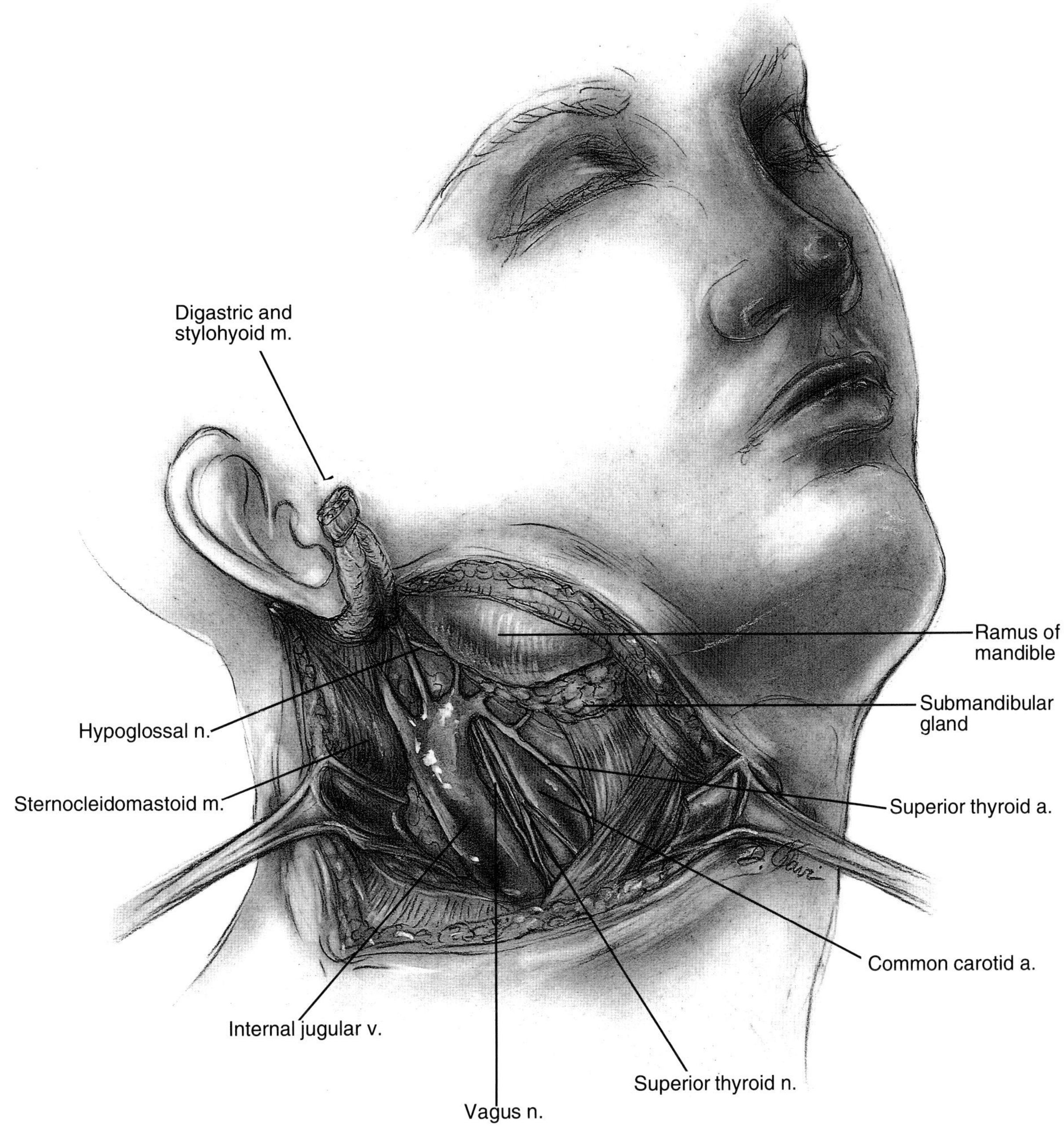

Figure 4. Mobilization of sternocleidomastoid muscle and ligation of the digastric and stylohyoid muscles increase visualization.

Division of the digastric and stylohyoid muscles allows medial retraction of the hyoid bone and hypopharynx. This maneuver helps avoid exposure of the nasopharynx and esophagus, which should be considered contaminated because of their high concentration of anaerobic bacteria.

The hypoglossal nerve is then identified. Again, a nerve stimulator may be useful. It is completely mobilized from its exit from the skull through the neuroforamen to the anterior border of the hypoglossal muscle. It may then be retracted superiorly for the remainder of the exposure. The dissection then enters the retropharyngeal space between the contents of the carotid sheath laterally and the visceral fascia, containing the larynx and pharynx, anteromedially. One can gain additional superior exposure by ligating branches of the carotid artery and internal jugular vein.

Beginning inferiorly and progressing superiorly, the surgeon may ligate the superior thyroid artery and vein, the lingual artery and vein, the ascending pharyngeal artery and vein, and the facial artery and vein. Ligation of these vessels allows mobilization of the carotid sheath laterally. The superior laryngeal nerve is then identified with a nerve stimulator, if necessary. It is mobilized and retracted medially from its origin near the nodose ganglion to its entrance into the larynx (Fig. 5). The alar and prevertebral fascia are then identified and transected longitudinally. This exposes the longus colli muscles, which run longitudinally and insert on the tubercle of the atlas anteriorly. It is important at this point to assess the amount of head rotation. This can be done by noting the orientation of the longus colli muscles. Any rotation of the head is undesirable if the arthrodesis will involve the anterior arch of the atlas. It is also important in assessing the extent of lateral decompression without endangering the vertebral arteries.

The first step in anterior decompression is meticulous removal of the disc between the second and third cervical vertebrae. The body of the second cervical vertebra may then be removed with a high-speed bur. Visualization of the uncovertebral joint helps confirm the orientation of the midline.

After the surgical procedure is completed, the wound is thoroughly irrigated and the digastric tendon reapproximated and sutured. Suction drains are routinely

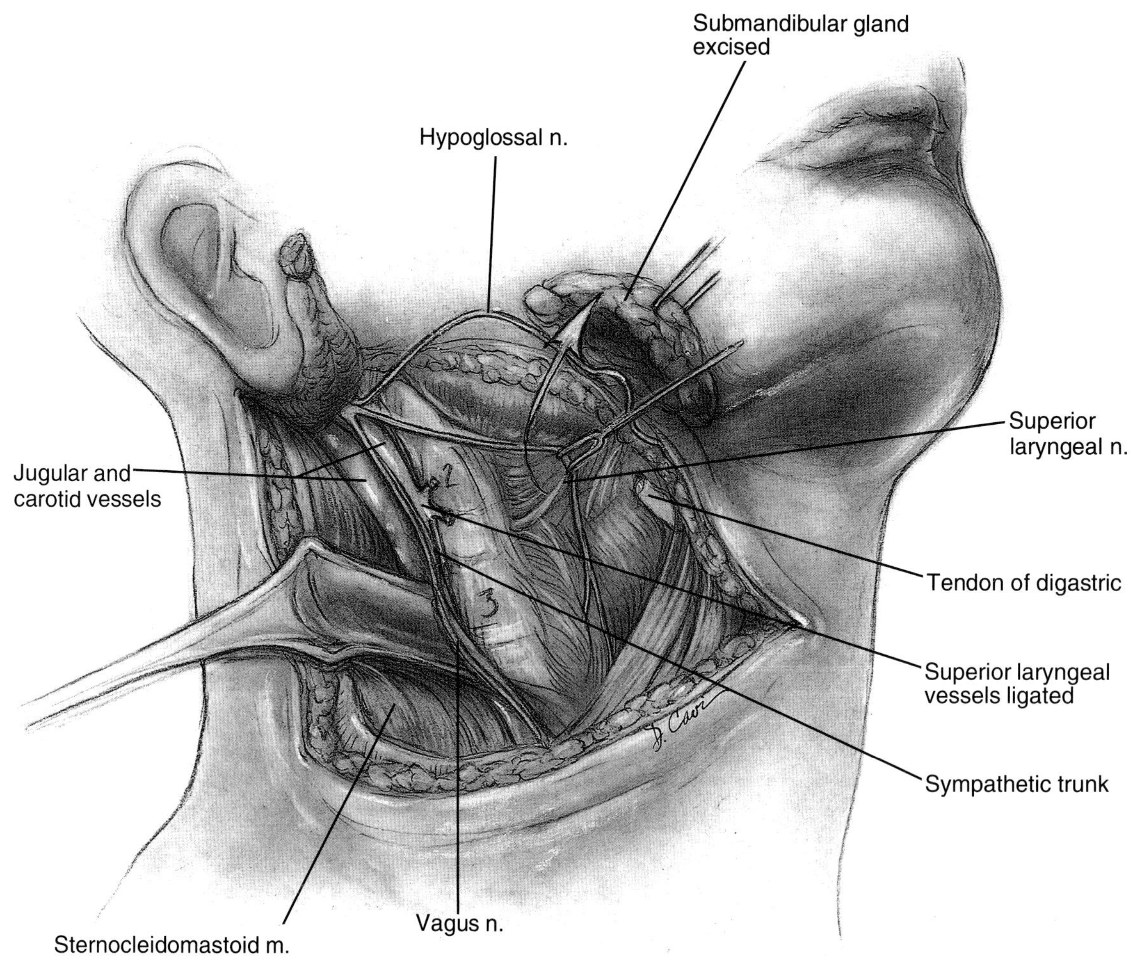

Figure 5. Identification of the superior laryngeal nerve with medial mobilization. The alar and prevertebral fascia have been retracted to expose the vertebral body.

used and placed in the retropharyngeal space and the subcutaneous space. The platysma and skin are sutured in standard fashion. The patient is then awakened and a neurological examination performed. The head of the bed should be elevated 30 degrees to reduce hypopharyngeal edema. Nasal intubation is retained for 24 to 48 hours postoperatively. At the termination of the procedure, if it is anticipated that the degree and duration of retraction of the soft tissue have been such that extubation will not be possible in a reasonable period of time, a tracheostomy should be considered. Gardner-Wells skeletal traction should be continued until a halo vest is placed or an alternative stabilizing procedure is performed.

COMPLICATIONS

Postoperative infection is a rare event. If the hypopharynx has been inadvertently entered, a nasogastric tube should be inserted intraoperatively. The surgeon should observe passage of the nasogastric tube past the hole in the hypopharynx. The laceration is then closed in two layers with absorbable sutures. Parenteral antibiotics, effective against anaerobic bacteria, are added to the regimen of postoperative prophylaxis. We recommend leaving the nasogastric tube in place for approximately 7 to 10 days if a tear occurred and was repaired. This will significantly control secretions, which could lead to mediastinitis.

The hypoglossal, glossopharyngeal, vagus, and accessory nerves, as well as the internal carotid artery and jugular vein, are tethered to the occiput as they leave their foramina. They may be injured by vigorous retraction or dissection. Neuropraxia is a not uncommon complication of this approach. The hypoglossal nerve leaves the occiput from the anterior condyloid foramen just lateral to the midportion of the occipital condyle. The jugular vein and carotid artery enter the skull just lateral to this area, which leaves only approximately 2 cm of working area from the midline to these structures laterally at the base of the skull. The pharyngeal and laryngeal branches of the vagus nerve arise just inferior to this level and may be stretched during anterior retraction of the pharynx.

Airway obstruction secondary to edema, or bone grafting into the posterior pharynx, is the most immediate threat. Tracheostomy may be considered if prolonged intubation is thought to be necessary.

Persistent postoperative hoarseness, laryngeal fatigue, and pharyngeal dysfunction may occur. These are usually secondary to retraction of the laryngeal nerve. Patients should be advised to expect difficulty with phonation and swallowing, especially in the early postoperative course. Similar, but more minor, problems will arise if the external branch of the superior laryngeal nerve has been transected. This nerve courses with the superior thyroid artery, which is often ligated to increase exposure.

Anterior Approach to the Cervical Spine: Medial to the Carotid Sheath

INDICATIONS/CONTRAINDICATIONS

The anterior approach provides direct access to the bodies and discs of the vertebrae from the third cervical through the first thoracic levels. Indications include excision of herniated discs, corpectomies for spondylosis or trauma (fractures), interbody fusion, biopsy and excision of vertebral body tumors, treatment of osteomyelitis and drainage of abscesses, and reconstructive/strut fusion procedures. This is the preferred, if not the only and easiest, approach to the mid and lower cervical spine. Caution should be used if significant carotid vascular disease exists. The risk of infection increases if a tracheotomy is in place.

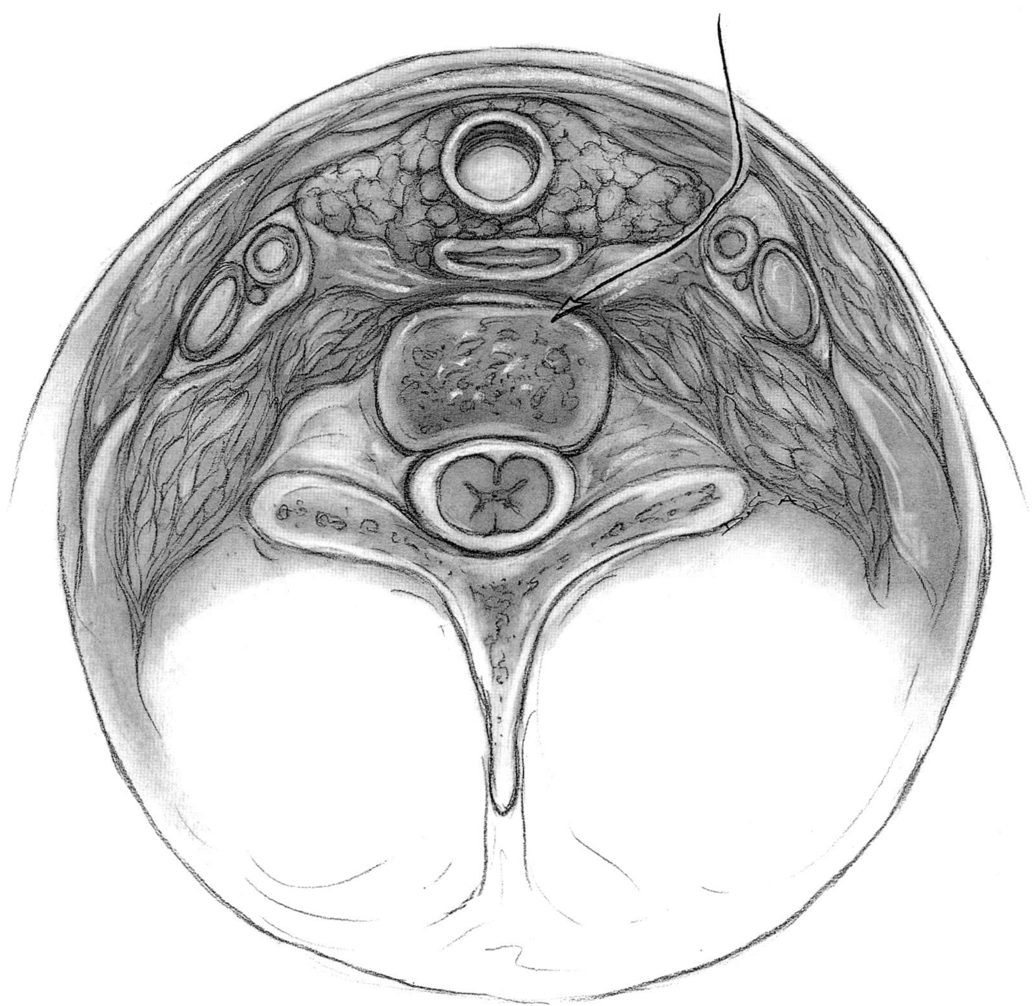

Figure 6. Anterior approach follows a plane medial to the carotid sheath and lateral to the sternocleidomastoid muscle, trachea, and esophagus.

A thorough knowledge of cervical anatomy is vital both to placement of the incision and dissection to the vertebral bodies. One must accurately identify the anterior border of the sternocleidomastoid muscle in order to proceed safely deeply between the carotid sheath laterally and the trachea and esophagus medially (Fig. 6).

SURGERY

The approach can be either from the right or left side of the neck. Right-handed surgeons may prefer a right-sided approach. The major advantage of the left-sided approach is that less risk of injury to the recurrent laryngeal nerve exists, especially when operating at lower cervical levels. The left recurrent laryngeal nerve ascends in the neck between the trachea and the esophagus, having branched off the vagus inferiorly at the level of the arch of the aorta. The right recurrent laryngeal nerve, however, runs along the trachea in the neck after looping around the right subclavian artery. In the inferior aspect of the neck it crosses from lateral to medial to reach the midline trachea; therefore it is slightly more vulnerable than the contralateral nerve during exposure. The surgeon must also be aware of the thoracic duct when approaching from the left side, especially when exposing inferior cervical and upper thoracic segments.

The application of traction may be desired, especially for interbody fusion. Traction may be applied by the use of a head halter or by utilizing Gardner-Wells tongs. Head halter traction may be preferred, as this obviates the necessity of skeletal traction. Ten to 15 pounds is usually helpful/necessary and tolerated. Utilization of higher weight may justify the use of Gardner-Wells tongs. Countertraction can be applied by securing the shoulders with tape to the end of the operating table. When applying countertraction it is important not to pull the

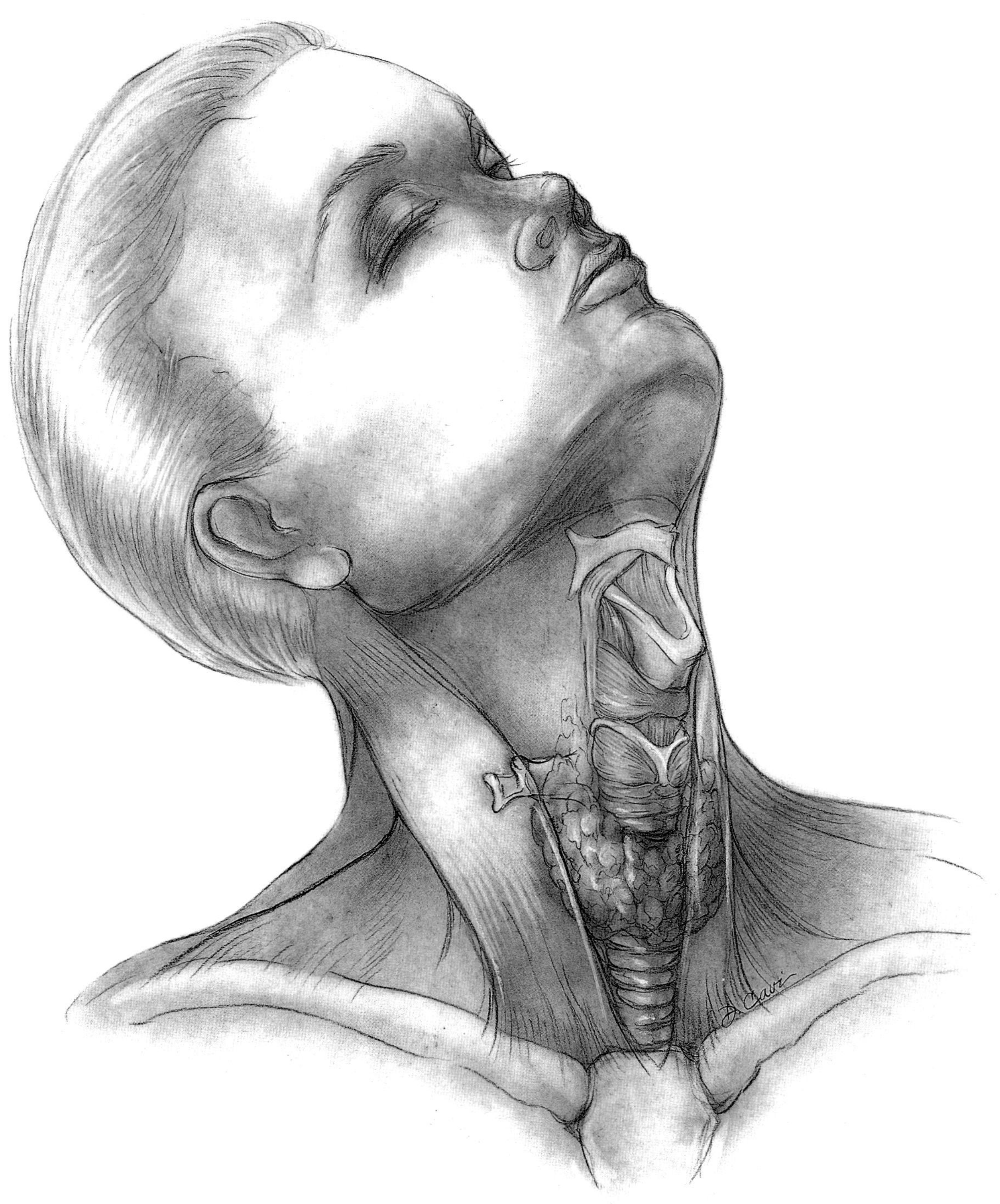

Figure 7. Surface topology of the cervical spine.

shoulders with too much force, as this may result in excess tension to the brachial plexus. For the operation the patient is placed supine on the operating table with a folded towel between the scapulae to position the neck in a slightly extended position. The head should be rotated away from the side of the procedure (i.e., rotated to the right for a left-sided approach). The operating table is then placed in 10 to 20 degrees of reverse Trendelenburg. This will reduce venous pressure and decrease bleeding during the procedure. It is helpful if the endotracheal tube is taped away from the side of the approach with an L connector to the tube, keeping it out of the field.

The area from the mandible to the upper thorax should be surgically prepared and draped. A prophylactic dose of intravenous antibiotics is given, prior to making the incision. A transverse incision is preferred, if possible, as it runs parallel to the cleavage lines of the skin of the neck. This results in a more cosmetically acceptable scar than with oblique incisions. However, if the surgery spans more than two motion segments, an oblique incision, along the medial border of the sternocleidomastoid muscle, is easier to extend (if necessary) to gain access to multiple levels.

Knowledge of surface topology will help with accurate placement of transverse incisions (Fig. 7). Generally, the hyoid bone is at the level of the C3 vertebra. The thyroid cartilage is at C4–C5, and the cricoid cartilage is usually anterior to C6. The carotid tubercle is an enlargement of the anterior tubercle of the transverse process of C6. This may be palpable and of assistance in placement of surgical incisions and/or identifying vertebral levels.

Once through the skin, the superficial fascia that encloses the platysma muscle is encountered. The subcutaneous tissues should be gently elevated off the muscle, if possible. Hemostasis, using electrocoagulation, should be performed at each level, particularly this superficial one. The platysma may be divided transversely or split in-line with its fibers. Flaps should be developed superiorly and inferiorly, superficial to the subjacent deep fascia (Fig. 8). This can be done with Metzenbaum

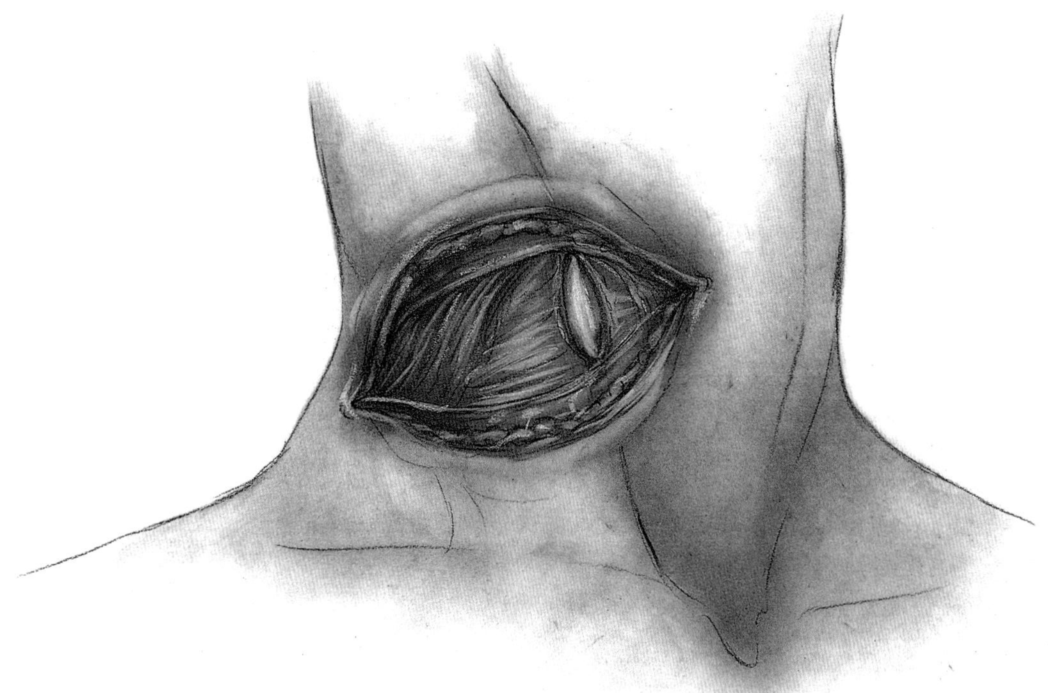

Figure 8. Superficial dissection in anteromedial approach.

scissors and finger dissection. Dissection caudally and cranially at each level markedly extends the exposure obtainable through a transverse skin incision. The plane between the strap muscles of the neck (segmental innervation C1, C2, and C3) and the sternocleidomastoid muscle (innervated by the spinal accessory nerve) more laterally should be identified. The medial edge of the sternocleidomastoid muscle should be clearly identified.

A fascial incision is made just anterior to the border of the sternocleidomastoid. Utilizing blunt and occasional sharp dissection, this interval can be widened in line with the edge of the muscle. An understanding of the fascial planes usually enables the dissection to proceed uneventfully. However, small vessels may traverse the area. They should either be electrocoagulated or ligated and cut. After incising the superficial layer of deep cervical fascia, which encloses the sternocleidomastoid muscle, the pretracheal fascia is identified, usually by finger dissection, medial to the carotid sheath (Fig. 9). The carotid artery should be palpated before any further dissection is performed. If the approach develops within the muscle, rather than medial to it, the dissection tends to be bloody, difficult, and deviated lateral to the carotid sheath. The dissection should proceed between the thyroid medially and the carotid sheath laterally, and then follow between the alar and visceral fascia, behind the esophagus to the anterior aspect of the vertebral bodies. This usually can be performed bluntly, except for an initial incision of the fascia medial to the sheath. This space is entered and widened as much by feel as by direct visualization (Fig. 10). The location of the carotid artery and esophagus must always be clear. Once the carotid artery is palpated, the index finger of the surgeon's nondominant hand is placed on it, and the artery gently rolled laterally under the finger. Dissection should then proceed just off the fingernail, medial to the artery. The tip of the scissors should be curved away from the esophagus, staying on the finger.

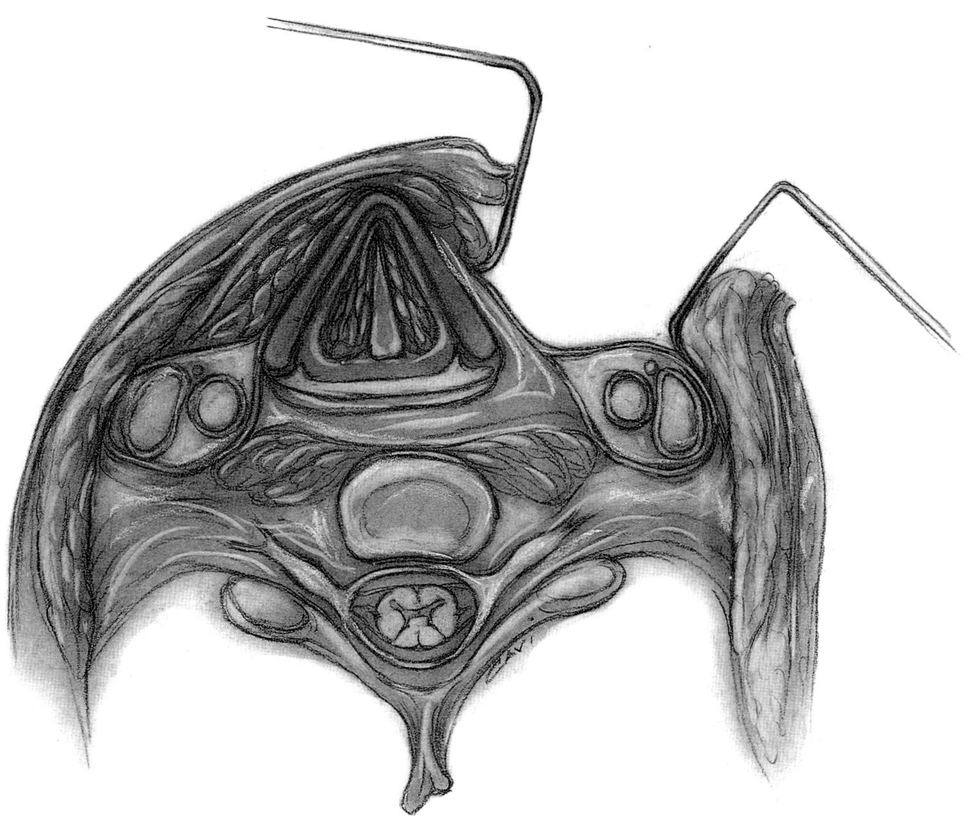

Figure 9. Cervical fascia planes (see text).

The alar fascia surrounds the carotid sheath structures (carotid artery, internal jugular vein, and vagus nerve), whereas the visceral fascia envelopes the esophagus and the recurrent laryngeal nerve. By preserving this fascia, the likelihood of injury to any of the invested structures is significantly diminished. The plane between the alar and visceral fascia should be extended superiorly and inferiorly along the vertebral bodies to allow adequate exposure. Both the superior and inferior thyroid artery connect the carotid sheath with the midline structures. This may limit the extent to which this plane may be opened. Occasionally, it may be necessary to ligate either one or both of these arteries. Deep, blunt, hand-held retractors should be utilized initially to aid in the dissection. Care is required to identify the esophagus properly and protect it during retraction.

The alar fascia is immediately superficial to the prevertebral fascia. The alar fascia spreads like two wings behind the esophagus and surrounds the carotid sheath and enclosed structures laterally. This layer is usually incised simultaneously with the deepest layer, the prevertebral fascia. However, it is distinct and can be separated off the prevertebral fascia. The prevertebral fascia surrounds the anterior portion of the vertebrae and includes the longus colli muscles, as well as the phrenic nerve. A Kitner sponge (small sponge on a stick) can be used to tease the fascia off the vertebral bodies. Staying in the midline is essential to avoid the longus colli muscle and excessive bleeding.

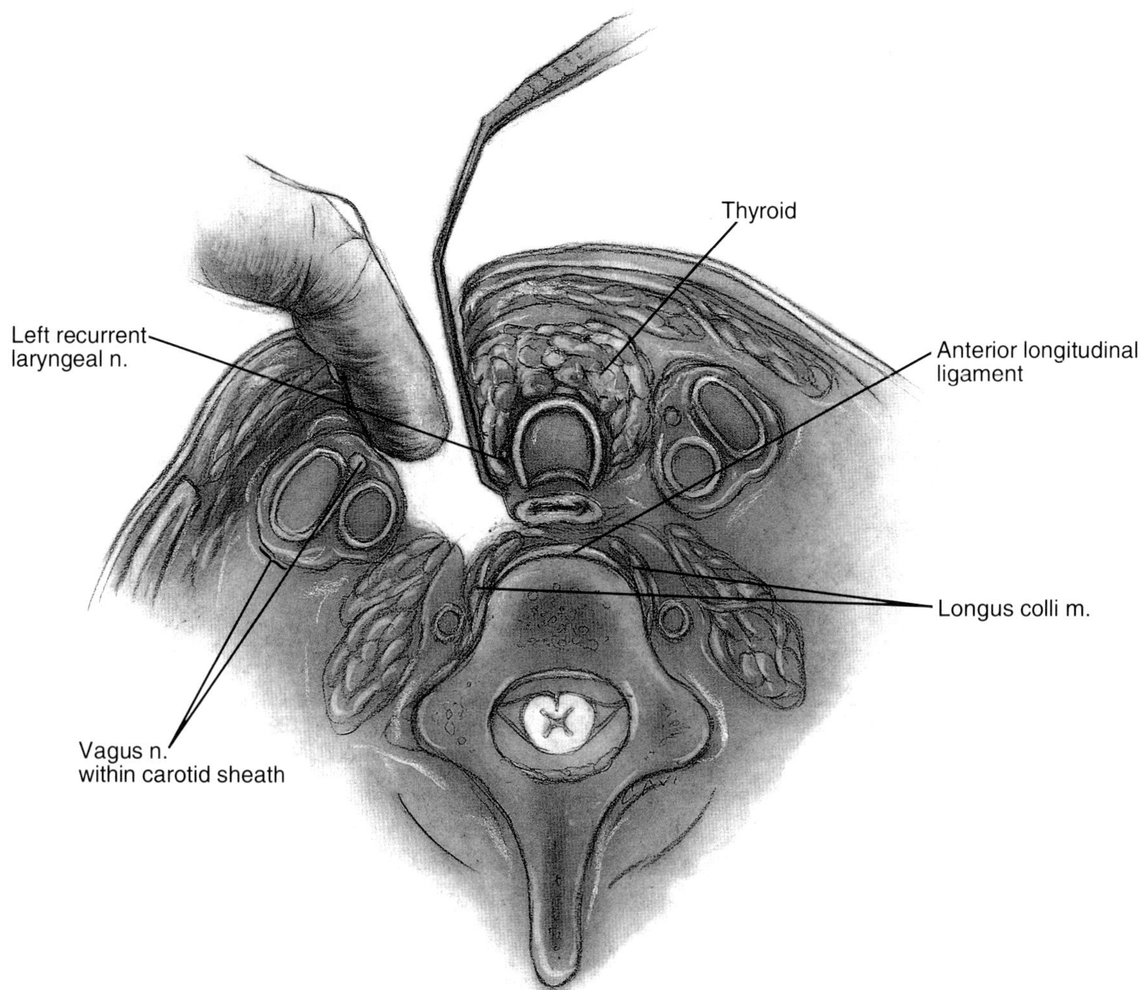

Figure 10. Approach proceeds primarily with blunt, but some sharp, dissection through the prevertebral fascia to the anterior portion of the cervical spine.

The disc spaces can be identified as "hills" and the vertebral bodies as "valleys." After sharp dissection of the deep fascial layers, the translucent anterior longitudinal ligament is visible. The cervical vertebrae are covered laterally by the longus colli muscles. Further laterally, the sympathetic nerves lie over the longus capitis muscles and should not be disturbed. The medial edge of the longus colli muscles should be cauterized and dissected up and laterally, subperiosteally, with an elevator. Perforators are frequent and should be further cauterized as necessary. The medial edges of the longus colli muscles should be retracted approximately at least 3 to 4 mm laterally, to the adjoining transverse process junction, to widen the exposure to the anterior surface of the vertebral bodies. A spinal needle can then be placed in a disc space and an intraoperative, lateral, radiograph obtained to identify the level correctly.

COMPLICATIONS

Several possible complications are associated with this procedure. Postoperative hoarseness is occasionally a problem. This may be secondary to irritation of the trachea or larynx by retraction or endotracheal intubation. It usually resolves and may be minimized by placing the patient in a high-humidity tent for 1 to 2 days postoperatively. Another cause of hoarseness is injury to the recurrent laryngeal nerve. Ordinarily it is protected by the visceral fascia. It may be injured by vigorous dissection or during prolonged retraction. On the right side, the course of the recurrent laryngeal nerve is variable. Occasionally, the recurrent laryngeal nerve may leave the carotid sheath at a higher level, crossing anteriorly behind the thyroid. For this reason, we prefer to approach the cervical spine from the left side. The external laryngeal nerve may also be injured and producc hoarscness. This nerve crosses the neck adjacent to the superior thyroid artery. This nerve innervates the cricothyroid muscle. During dissection of the upper cervical vertebrae, if the superior thyroid artery cannot be spared, it should be dissected out carefully, in an attempt to avoid injury to the nerve while ligating the artery.

Perhaps the most significant potential complication from this approach is injury to the esophagus. These injuries may not always be identified intraoperatively. Early dysphagia associated with an esophageal leak and subsequent mediastinitis carry a high morbidity and mortality. If the location of the esophagus is in doubt, a soft nasogastric tube may be inserted by the anesthetist, thereby allowing identification of the esophagus by "feeling the tube." After localization, the nasogastric tube should be removed, prior to retraction. Hand-held retractors with smooth blades are recommended at this stage. If the esophagus is inadvertently perforated, it should be repaired immediately, usually in two layers. Thorough irrigation should be performed and bone grafting should be delayed, if possible.

It is important to keep dissection of the longus colli muscles subperiosteal. Injury to the sympathetic nerves and, more superiorly, the stellate ganglion, may occur if dissection does not remain directly on bone. A postoperative Horner's syndrome may result from injury to this plexus.

Also, if the dissection strays too far laterally, injury to the vertebral artery may occur. The vertebral artery lies in the transverse foramen in the anterolateral aspect of the transverse processes. Injury may occur by an instrument that enters the transverse foramen between one vertebra and the next. Keeping the dissection medial to the edge of the sternocleidomastoid muscle and the carotid artery, and identifying the anterior border of the cervical spinal column, will help avoid this problem.

The thoracic duct may be injured during dissection in the lower aspect of the cervical spine on the left. The duct ascends from the thorax just lateral to the esophagus, lying in the prevertebral fascia. It then loops over the subclavian artery at the level of the first thoracic vertebral body. It lies anterior to the scalenus anterior and phrenic nerve and enters the subclavian vein. One may consider approaching from the right side if dissection of only the lower cervical and upper thoracic spine is necessary.

Anterior Approach to the Cervical Thoracic Junction

INDICATIONS/CONTRAINDICATIONS

Approaches to the cervical-thoracic junction present a significant challenge to the spinal surgeon. Because of the tremendous forces present at this junction, the tendency, especially with destruction by tumor, is toward kyphosis and collapse. This results in inaccessibility during surgery, due to the kyphosis, combined with the obstruction from the sternum and clavicle. Standard approaches to the lower cervical spine offer good visualization to T1, but the surgical field is limited if more distal dissection is necessary. This approach can be chosen when direct anterior access to the upper thoracic spine is necessary for decompression and reconstruction. It cannot easily be extended distally or proximally.

At the commencement of the procedure, a rolled towel is placed between the scapulae, and the neck is slightly hyperextended and rotated to the contralateral side of the L extension. Gardner-Wells or head halter traction is then applied prior to the surgical incision, in order to provide traction for placement of bone graft after the decompression is completed. Intraoperative monitoring of evoked potentials is optional. For a left-sided approach, an angled incision is made in the skin overlying the anterior aspect of the left side of the neck (Fig. 11). The transverse limb is approximately 2 cm proximal and parallel to the clavicle beginning laterally at the lateral border of the sternocleidomastoid muscle, turning inferiorly at the midline to end at the manubriosternal junction. Skin flaps with underlying subcutaneous tissues should be elevated. Hemostasis should be obtained with electrocoagulation at every level. Dissection is carried through the platysma muscle transversely.

Both the internal and external jugular veins and the medial supraclavicular nerve should be identified and usually can be retracted safely. The sternocleidomastoid muscle is then elevated subperiosteally off its manubrial and clavicular attachments. It should be retracted in the lateral and proximal direction. The strap muscles are then severed just posterior to the clavicle and elevated proximally and medially. The medial third of the clavicle should be carefully subperiosteally stripped. It can then be cut at the junction of its medial and middle thirds with a Gigli saw or small power saw (Fig. 12). It is important to remember the course of the subclavian vein posterior and inferior to the clavicle when placing the Gigli saw into position. The clavicle can then be sharply disarticulated from the manubrium. It can be wrapped in a moist sponge for later use. To increase visualization superiorly, the inferior thyroid vein, which will be crossing transversely, may be ligated. Proximally, blunt dissection is utilized to develop a plane between the carotid sheath laterally and the trachea and esophagus medially. The recurrent laryngeal nerve will be seen in this left-sided approach, ascending between the esophagus and trachea.

This dissection proceeds to the prevertebral fascia. Hand-held Richardson retractors are placed deep into the wound to enlarge the interval (Fig. 13). These broad-faced retractors are useful in retracting small, vital structures as well as vascular tissues. Visualization of the vertebral bodies is aided by the constancy of the distal insertions of the longus colli muscles into the lateral aspects of C7, T1, T2, and T3 vertebral bodies. At this point, a needle is placed into a disc space and an intraoperative radiograph obtained for accurate localization. After reconstruction and stabilization are performed, hemostasis is obtained and a deep

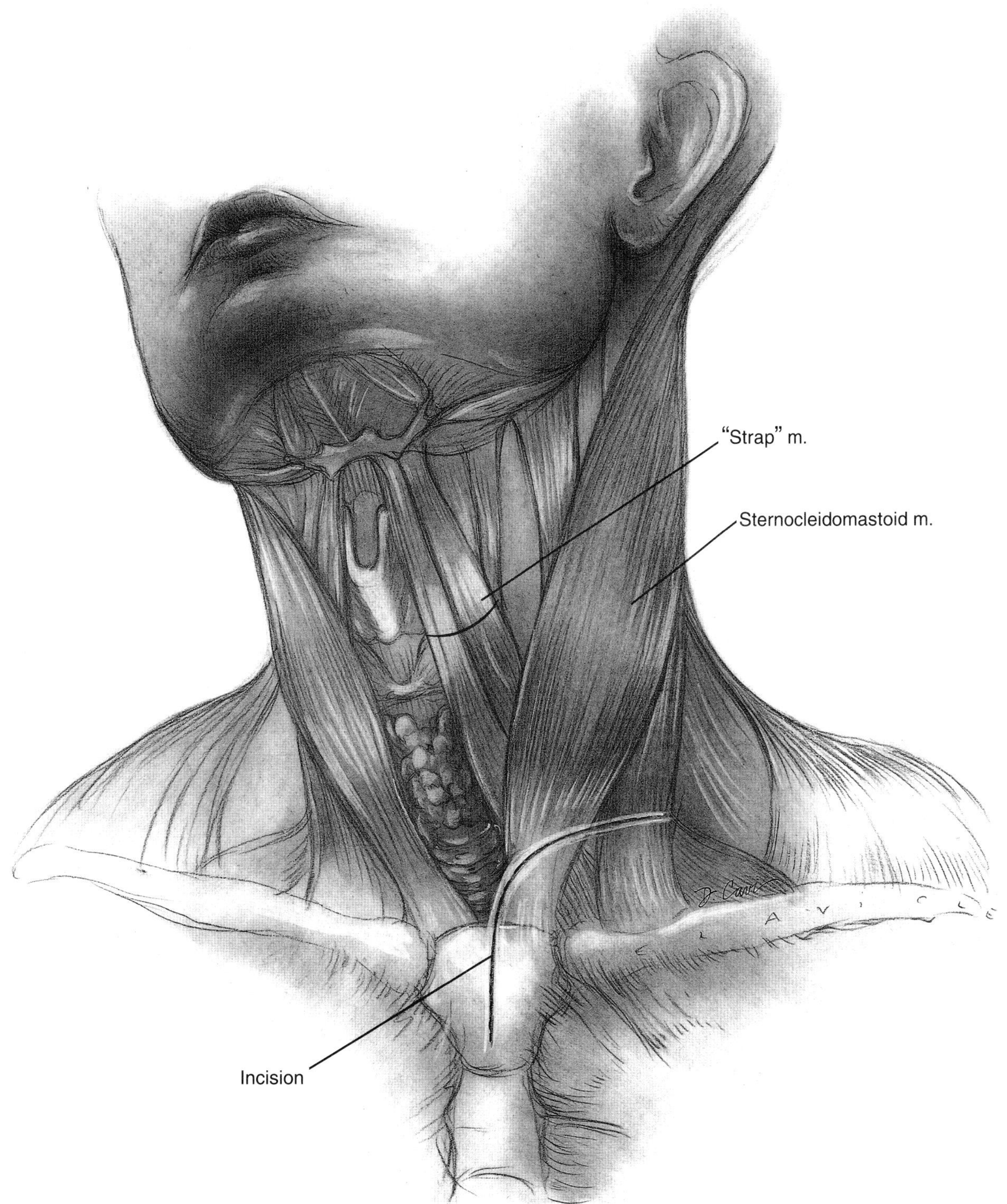

Figure 11. Incision for approach to the cervical thoracic junction.

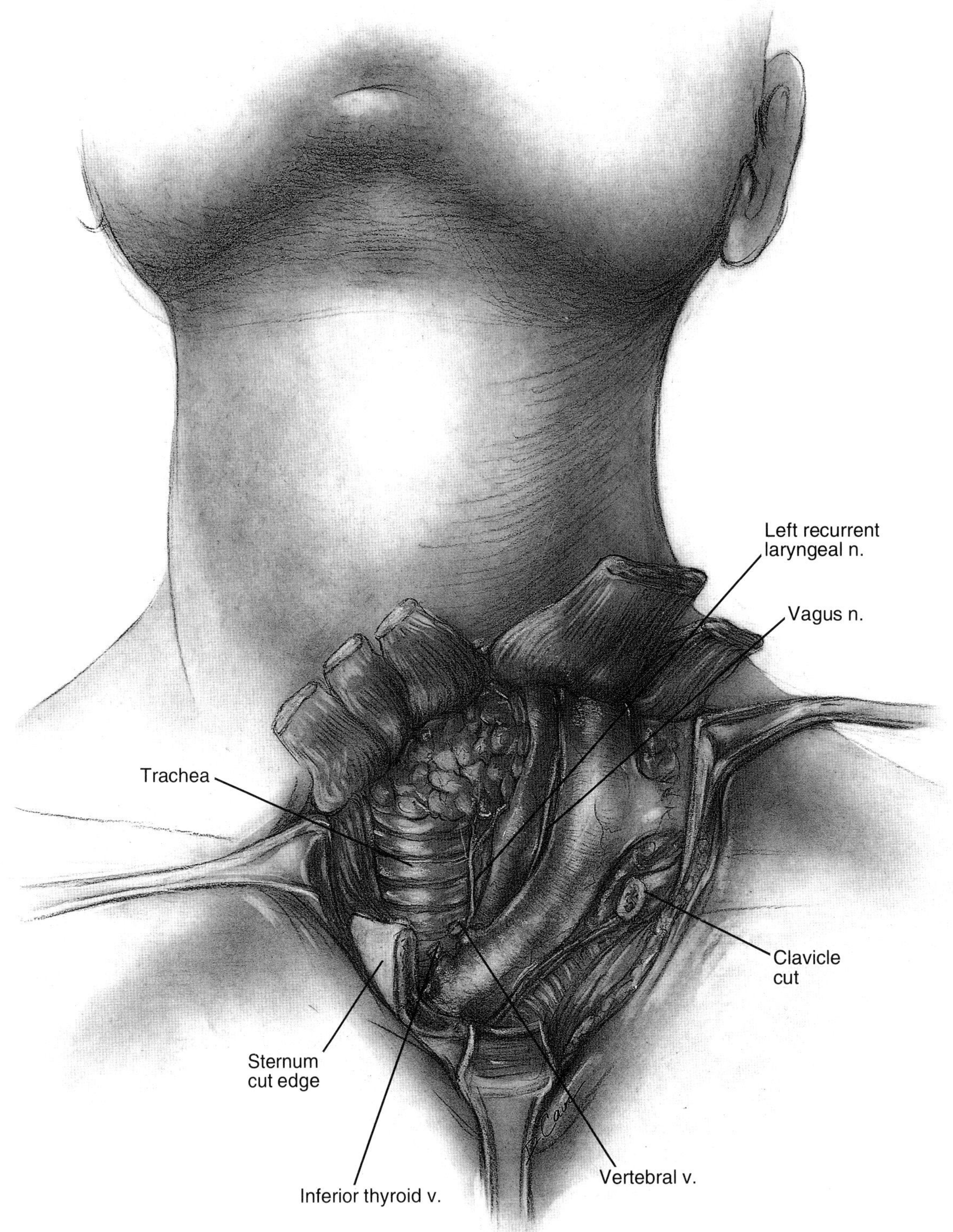

Figure 12. Resection of medial clavicle.

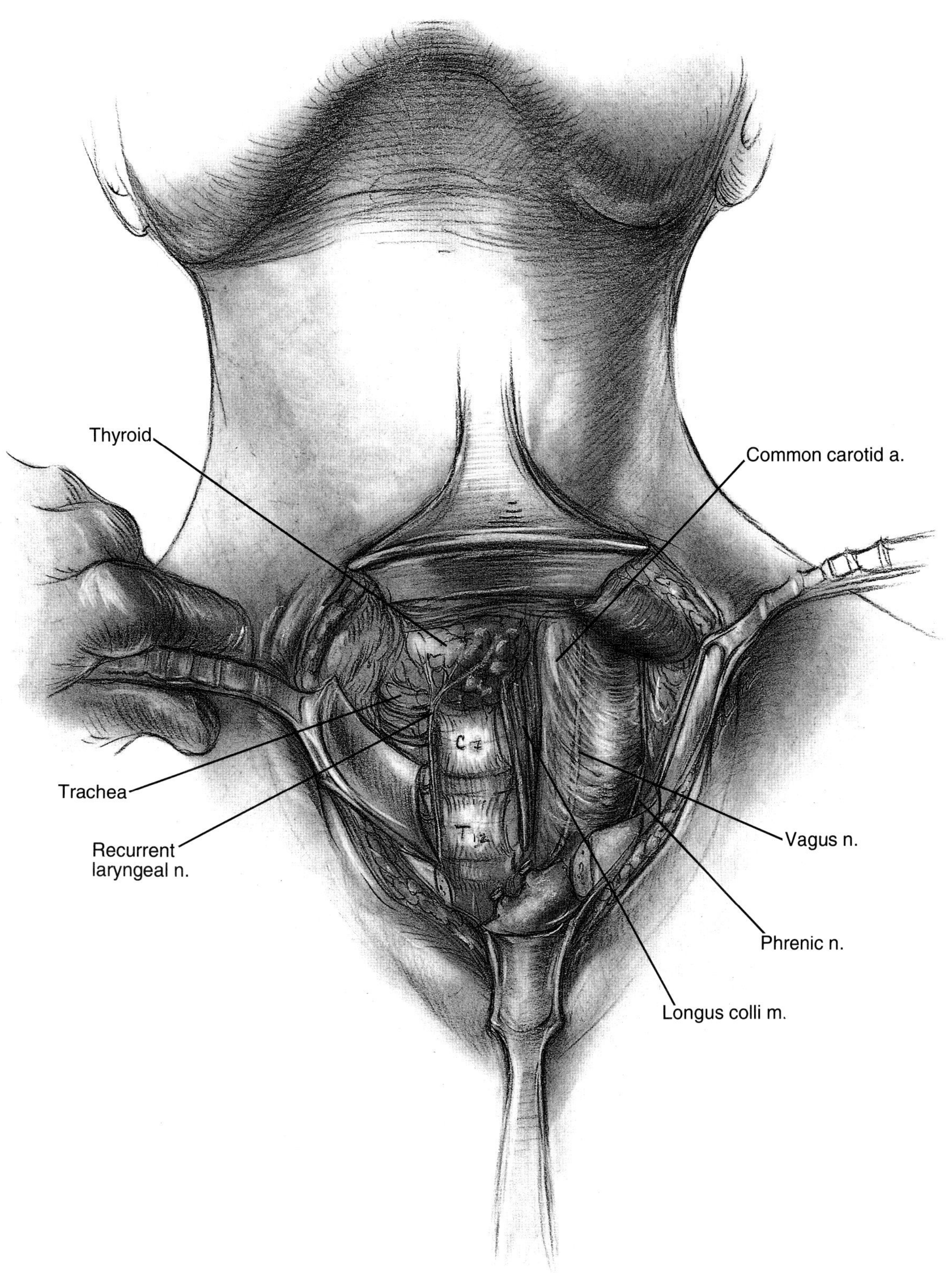

Figure 13. Use of large, blunt retractors increases exposure.

drain is placed. The strap muscles are reapproximated, and the sternocleidomastoid muscle is resutured to the clavicular periosteum. Closure of the subcutaneous tissue and skin is performed in a routine manner.

COMPLICATIONS

The approach can be made from either side of the midline. One may approach from the left side, but identification of the thoracic duct is mandatory. Inadvertent laceration of this duct leads to chylothorax, which may require prolonged chest tube drainage. If the thoracic duct is inadvertently lacerated, and it is identified, it should be ligated with double sutures both proximally and distally. In approaching from the right, the recurrent laryngeal nerve should be identified and protected as it loops beneath the subclavian artery. One must remember that this nerve has a variable course on the right side of the neck.

Vascular drainage can occur. This is usually related to injury when working around the clavicle. Staying subperiosteal until the medial one-third is removed will minimize this risk. A Penrose drain can then be passed around the large vessels to mobilize them gently and move them in and out of the field, always with direct visualization. This approach gives good access from C7 to T3. It is not useful for lower level decompression or grafting.

RECOMMENDED READING

1. Bailey, R. W., and Badgley, C. E.: Stabilization of the cervical spine by anterior fusion. *J. Bone Joint Surg.*, 41A: 565–594, 1960.
2. Bailey, R. W.: Surgical techniques. In: *The Cervical Spine*, Lea & Febiger, Philadelphia, 1974. edited by R. W. Bailey, pp. 146–156.
3. Fang, H. S. Y., and Ong, G. B.: Direct anterior approach to the upper cervical spine. *J. Bone Joint Surg.*, 44A: 1588–1604, 1962.
4. Kurz, L. T., Pursel, S. E., and Herkowitz, H. N.: Modified anterior approach to the cervicothoracic junction. *Spine*, 16S: S542, 1991.
5. McAfee, P. C., Bohlman, H. H., Riley, L. H., et al.: The anterior retropharyngeal approach to the upper part of the cervical spine. *J. Bone Joint Surg.*, 69A: 1371–1383, 1987.
6. Nanson, E. M.: The anterior approach to upper dorsal sympathectomy. *Surg. Gynecol. Obstet.*, 104: 118–120, 1957.
7. Riley, L. H.: Surgical approaches to the anterior structures of the cervical spine. *Clin. Orthop.*, 91: 16–20, 1973.
8. Robinson, R. A., and Southwick, W. O.: Indications and techniques for early stabilization of the neck in some fracture dislocations of the cervical spine. *South Med. J.*, 53: 565–579, 1960.
9. Robinson, R. A., and Southwick, W. O.: *Surgical Approaches to the Cervical Spine*. In: *Instructional Course Lectures. The American Academy of Orthopaedic Surgeons*, Vol. 17. C. V. Mosby, St. Louis, 1960. pp. 299–330.
10. Smith, G. W., and Robinson, R. A.: The treatment of certain cervical spine disorders by anterior removal of the intervertebral disc and interbody fusion. *J. Bone Joint Surg.*, 40A: 607–624, 1958.
11. Southwick, W. O., and Robinson, R. A.: Surgical approaches to the vertebral bodies in the cervical and lumbar regions. *J. Bone Joint Surg.*, 39A: 631–644, 1957.
12. Sundaresan, N., Shah, J., Foley, K. M., and Rosen, G.: An anterior surgical approach to the upper thoracic vertebrae. *J. Neurosurg.*, 61: 686–690, 1984.
13. White, A. A., Johnson, R. M., Panjabi, M. M., and Southwick, W. O.: Biomechanical analysis of clinical stability in the cervical spine. *Clin. Orthop.*, 109: 85–96, 1975.
14. Whiteside, T. E., Jr., and Kelly, R. P.: Lateral approach to the upper cervical spine for anterior fusion. *South. Med. J.*, 59: 879–883, 1966.

Master Techniques in Orthopaedic Surgery,
THE SPINE, edited by D. S. Bradford,
Lippincott-Raven Publishers, Philadelphia, © 1997.

2

Anterior Approaches to the Thoracic/Lumbar Spine

Harold K. Dunn

INDICATIONS/CONTRAINDICATIONS

The indications for a surgical approach to the anterior vertebral elements are numerous. The extent of the surgical exposure needed varies with the individual indication. Often only a single vertebral level needs to be exposed, and the approach can be limited, for example, when biopsy is needed of a vertebral body tumor, or when it is desirable to obtain cultures from (and/or drain) a vertebral abscess or intervertebral disc-space infection. With trauma, more exposure is needed to expose three or four vertebral levels to decompress and/or stabilize burst fractures causing neurologic compromise. When treating deformities of the spine, extensile exposure is often needed to expose 6 to 12 levels of the spine simultaneously. The technique for individual cases varies, but the principles of surgical exposure are constant and will be discussed in detail.

Contraindications to the anterior approach are relatively few. If the pathology is in the posterior elements, it is illogical and therefore contraindicated to approach the spine anteriorly. An anterior approach to an unstable fracture dislocation with locked or jumped facets would require indirect facet reduction. This is often not feasible and results in overmanipulation of the spine with possible damage to the neural elements. A relative contraindication for an anterior approach is poor pulmonary function. In the severely debilitated patient, or in the patient with severely compromised pulmonary function, the anterior approach may not be tolerated. Patients with severe neurologic scoliosis (i.e., from Werdnig-Hoffman syndrome, spinal muscular atrophy, or polio) and others require careful consideration by the surgeon and the anesthesiologist to determine if they have sufficient pulmonary reserve to undergo an anterior spinal approach. This is especially true with the thoracic spine.

H. K. Dunn, M.D.: Department of Orthopaedics, University of Utah School of Medicine, Salt Lake City, Utah 84132.

PREOPERATIVE PLANNING

Anterior thoracolumbar approaches are made through incisions that parallel the neurovascular bundles of the anatomic dermatomes. Each case requires careful preoperative evaluation by the surgeon to determine which levels of the spine need exposure, and the approach is planned accordingly. As a general rule, the approach is made through a dermatomal interval one level above the most superior vertebra to be exposed. That is, if the surgeon is instrumenting or operating from T12 to L2, the incision would be started on the rib of T11. However, if any question or doubt exists as to the superior vertebra, it should be kept in mind that it is extremely easy to extend the exposure caudally by carrying the incision toward the anterior midline and, if necessary, extending caudally at the anterior midline, not crossing any significant portions of the segmental nerves. It is difficult to gain exposure in a cranial direction, because the neurovascular bundles must be crossed proximally as they exit the spinal column, thus denervating significant segments of the torso. Careful consideration of those levels of the spine that require surgical exposure is extremely important.

The spine is actually viewed and worked on anterolaterally when doing the anterior approach. It should be kept in mind that although one can see several vertebrae above the proximal extent of any incision, it is very difficult to work on these vertebrae because of overhang of the torso wall. When in doubt as to which vertebrae will require exposure, always go at least one dermatomal level above the most proximal vertebra that will possibly need exposure. Another way to visualize the approach is to look at an anteroposterior (AP) radiograph of the case and realize that the incision can be carried back along any rib to its anatomic neck, leaving about 1 cm of the rib attached to the spine. A perpendicular line projected laterally from the spine will define the extent of the proximal exposure if the incision is made through that rib bed. The caudal extent of the exposure can be visualized by following the rib anteriorly to the paramedian line. If further exposure is necessary, the incision will need to be extended along the paramedian line.

SURGERY

Anterior thoracic/lumbar approaches are made through incisions that parallel the dermatomal neurovascular bundles. This prevents denervation of muscles and loss of sensation on the torso. The surgeon should decide which levels of the spine

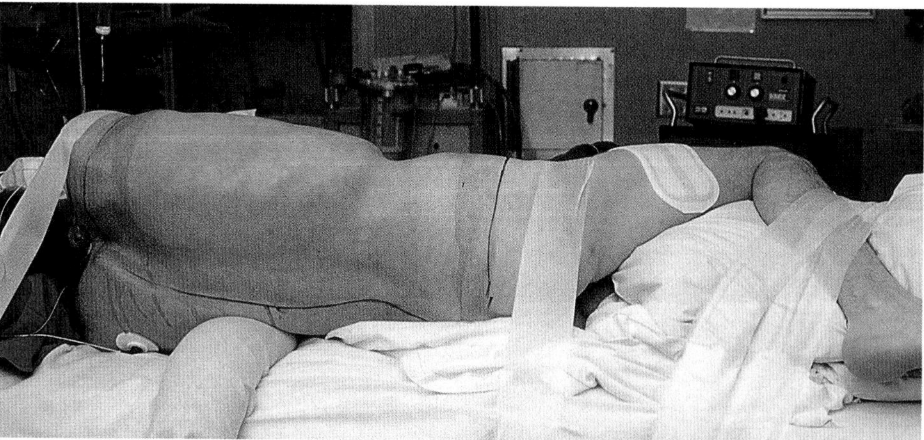

Figure 1. Posterior view of patient positioned for surgery, left side down and right side up.

should be exposed and then decide on the approach. Extension of an anterior approach caudally is relatively easy and has little morbidity. The incision is extended toward the anterior midline and then taken distally, not crossing a significant portion of segmental nerves. Gaining cranial exposure is difficult after the initial approach is made. It necessitates crossing the neurovascular bundles in the posterior aspect of the wound and may denervate a complete dermatomal segment. It is therefore extremely important to plan the approach well. The spine is viewed anterolaterally, not anteriorly, with the anterior approach. Although the surgeon can look up under the chest wall and see several vertebrae above the proximal extent of any incision, it is difficult to work there. When in doubt, make the approach more proximal. A good rule of thumb is to plan the approach one or two levels above the most proximal vertebra that must be addressed surgically. The most cephalad vertebra that can be comfortably instrumented is the one directly across from the proximal part of the incision. In the thorax, this incision can be carried back to within 1 to 1½ inches of the most proximal aspect of the rib. This allows preoperative planning of the incision on an AP radiograph.

Positioning

For all three approaches, the patient is placed in the lateral decubitus position and tilted slightly posteriorly. An axillary roll is positioned to protect the brachial plexus. Exposure is facilitated by positioning the patient's flank over the flexion break in the operating table. Flexion then opens the thoracolumbar and flank area for exposure. This often accentuates scoliotic curves since they are most usually approached from the convex side of the curvature. Spine surgeons most frequently want to manipulate and change the position of the spine with their procedures. For that reason, it is advantageous not to fix the patient rigidly to the operating table. This is a direct departure from the way most chest surgeons position the patient table and should be kept in mind if the spine surgeon is operating in conjunction with a chest surgeon. Spinal correction and wound closure is facilitated by reversing the flex in the operating table. Although it is desirable to allow the patient's spine to have some motion, the patient must be well enough secured that the operating table can be tilted or airplaned for the surgeon's view as well as flexed and extended at the flank. By securing the pelvis and legs to the operating table with tape, safety is ensured (Figs. 1 and 2).

The lower limbs are flexed at the hips and knees. This helps to stabilize the pelvis and relaxes the iliopsoas muscle, aiding exposure of the lumbar spine. The

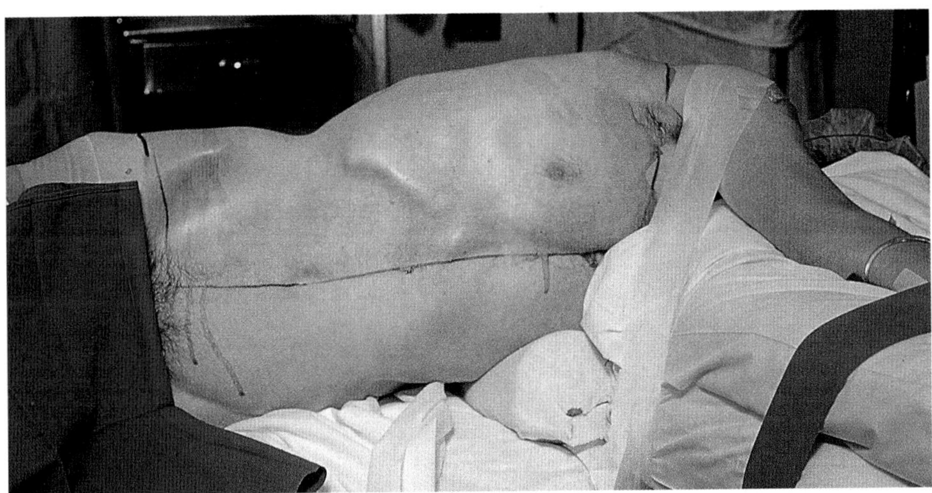

Figure 2. Patient anterior view.

hip is flexed 60 to 70 degrees, and the knee about 90 degrees. Two pillows between the legs both add stability and prevent pressure points. Broad tape extending across the table at about the level of the greater trochanter secures the pelvis. The lower extremities are secured by broad tape, with care taken not to compromise the peroneal nerve. The upper torso can be rotationally stabilized with sandbags on each side of the torso, or a very small bean bag that does not extend to the pelvis. When taping the upper extremity, care must be taken to prevent compromising exposure in the proximal part of the incision. For exposures as high as T4, the shoulder can be secured with tape crossing the table. However, for more proximal exposures, the limb is simply cradled above the patient to allow complete exposure of the torso posteriorly. Again, positioning for the spinal patient is not the customary or routine positioning used by traditional chest surgeons, and this is extremely important to keep in mind for the orthopedic surgeon working in conjunction with a thoracic or general surgeon. If a short surgeon is operating with a taller surgeon, it would be well to discuss this aspect of the case together. Chest surgeons tend to use vacuum bean bags for positioning; these are rigid and preclude position changes during surgery.

When prepping and draping, a tendency exists not to allow sufficient space posteriorly and superiorly. If the general rule is to be followed of prepping 4 cm beyond the extent of draping, and draping 4 cm beyond the extent of any incision, it is necessary to prep and drape well past the midline posteriorly and anteriorly. Inferiorly, one can usually prep to about the level of the greater trochanter. Superiorly, one needs to advance several spinous processes above the level of the dermatomal incision. For exposure above T4, draping the shoulder and upper arm is required. Draping to maintain a sterile surgical field is nicely accomplished by initially using adhesive-edged field drapes overlaid with an iodine-impregnated polymer sheet. The second layer can be a traditional laparotomy sheet modified by enlarging the opening for torso exposure.

After prepping and draping, the suction tubing, power cords, and electrocautery, bipolar and any other cords coming onto the operating table should be brought in and secured over the pelvis. Care should be taken to avoid positioning heavy objects over the upper extremities, so as to prevent brachial plexus injury.

Thoracic Spine

Thoracotomy for exposure of the thoracic spine from T5 to T12 is the easiest of all anterior surgical approaches. The approximate level of the skin incision is made overlying the dermatomal segment to be approached and is determined by palpating the last long rib. This is correlated with the radiograph and the initial skin incision made. This incision is dermal only and is immediately followed by injection into the cutis and subcutaneous layers of 1/500,000 epinephrine in saline. For accuracy in preparation and for ease of use in the operating theater, the solution is best prepared in the pharmacy. Utilization of 1/500,000 epinephrine in saline allows infiltration of the wound safely with up to 200 ml of solution in an average-sized adult patient. Many surgeons dilute premade local injection solutions, such as lidocaine with epinephrine; however, one then has to contend with the introduction of an unnecessary pharmacologic agent into the patient (i.e., the lidocaine or whatever medium contains the local anesthetic). To achieve good cutaneous hemostasis, the epinephrine must react for 2 to 5 minutes before the skin is fully incised. For that reason, surgery can be facilitated by making the initial cutaneous incision and infiltrating the wound immediately after the initial prep and drape but before setting up suction, electrocautery, lights, etc.

The skin and subcutaneous tissue incision is completed, and the anterolateral aspect of the torso is exposed (Figs. 3 and 4). If a question exists as to the exact rib or dermatomal level that is being entered, further verification of level can be

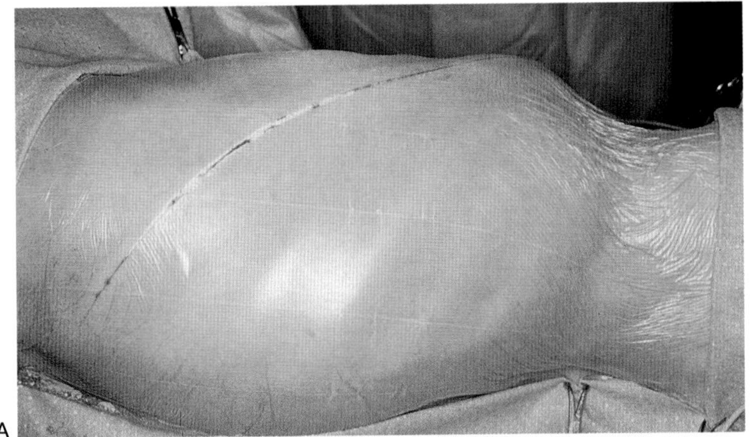

A

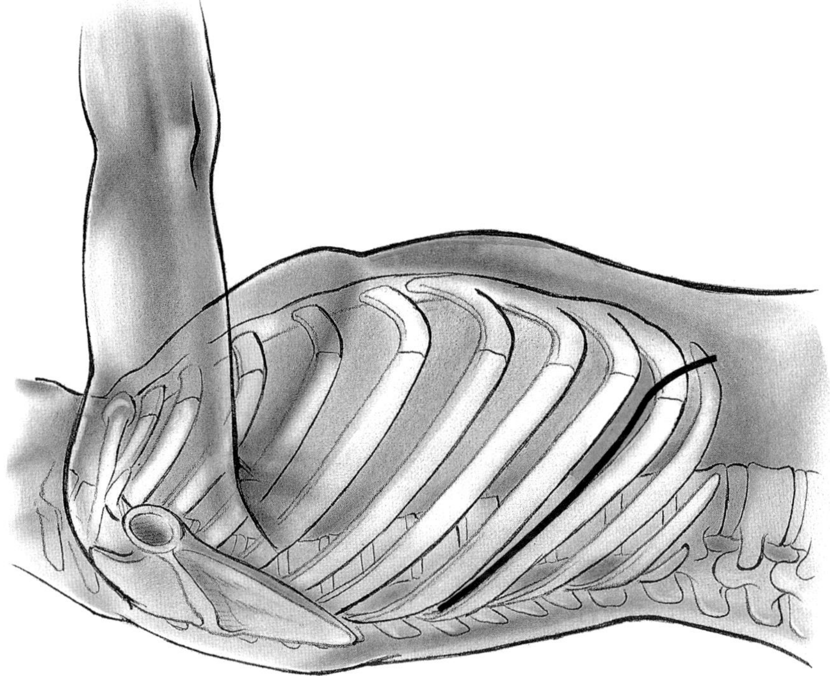

B

Figure 3. **A:** Patient draped. Skin incision from posterior view. **B:** Patient in same position as positioned on table.

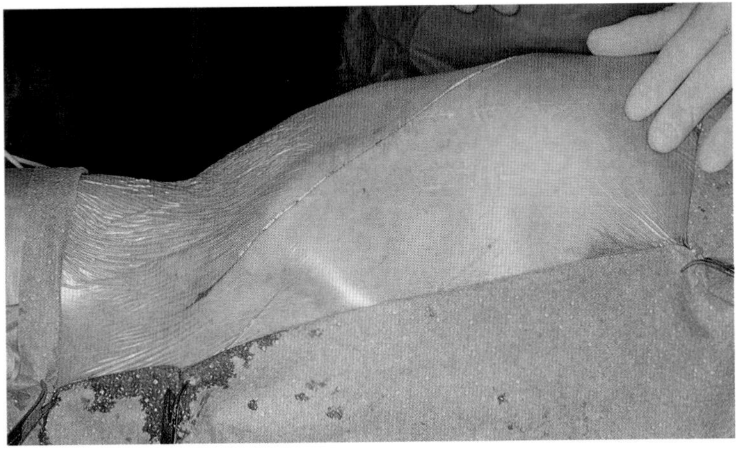

Figure 4. Patient anterior view.

made after incision through the latissimus dorsi. The interval between the shoulder and the chest wall is utilized for a positive rib count from palpation of the T1, T2 interval and counting distally to confirm the level of chest wall incision. The latissimus dorsi is transected as far posteriorly as is necessary to expose the periosteum of the involved rib (Figs. 5 and 6). The rib incision is made with electrocautery for hemostatic purposes (Fig. 7). The incision is initially carried anteriorly to a point about 3 to 5 cm from the midline (Fig. 8). The origin of the external oblique musculature, which is present on the lower eight ribs, is split by the incision (Fig. 9).

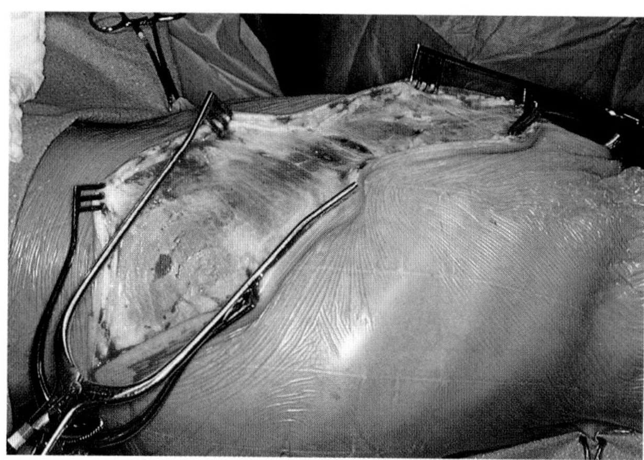

Figure 5. Patient posterior view. Skin incision completed. Latissimus dorsi muscle in view.

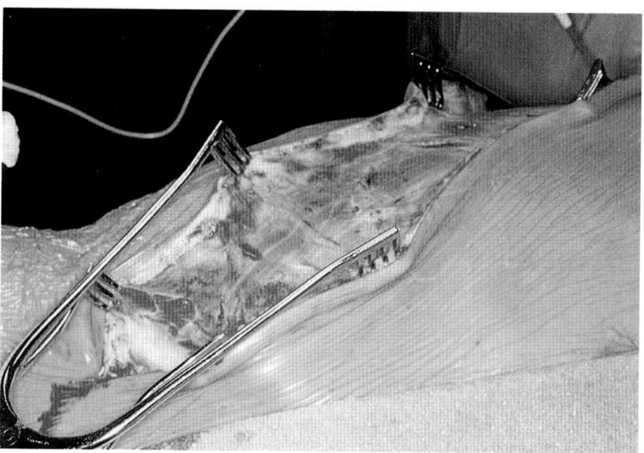

Figure 6. Patient anterior view. External oblique muscle seen.

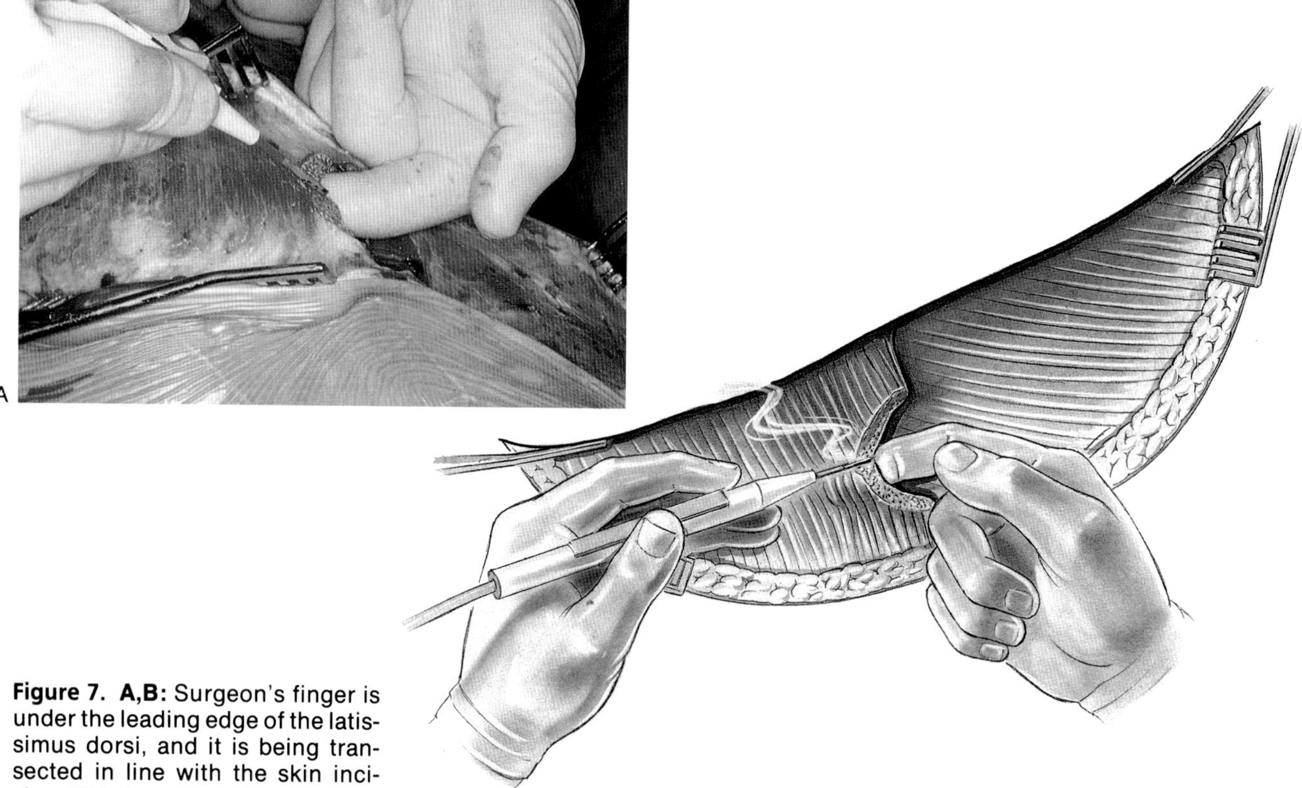

Figure 7. A,B: Surgeon's finger is under the leading edge of the latissimus dorsi, and it is being transected in line with the skin incision. This is a posterior view.

The rib incision is made with electrocautery for hemostatic purposes; the rib is dissected free subperiosteally, and the anterior end of the rib is transected (Fig. 10). The subperiosteal dissection is carried posteriorly to at least the level of the articulation of the rib with the transverse process of the vertebra. At this point, the rib can either be excised or disarticulated from the vertebra (Fig. 11).

It is possible to expose the spine anteriorly without violating the pleura of the chest wall (Fig. 12). After subperiosteal excision of the rib, the inferior periosteum can be sharply incised and the parietal pleura can be dissected free from the chest wall. This is most easily accomplished with blunt dissection utilizing the fingertip, Kitner dissectors, or a sponge on a stick. Subpleural exposure is most easily accomplished in the growing child and is much more difficult in mature adults. Subpleural dissection does have the advantage of preventing adhesions from oc-

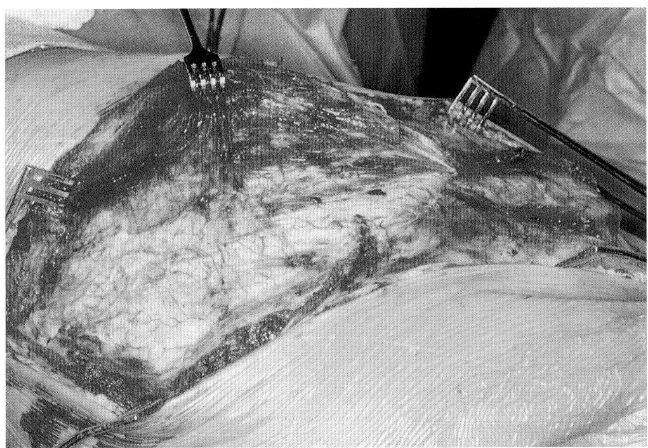

Figure 8. Patient posterior view. Latissimus reflected and bed of rib visible.

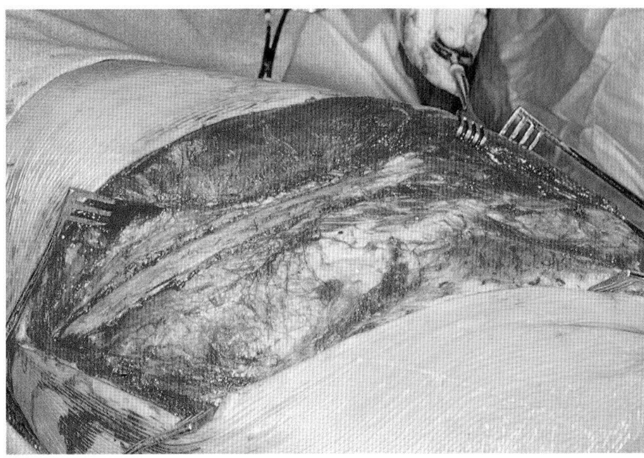

Figure 9. Patient posterior view. Rib exposed by subperiosteal dissection of surface.

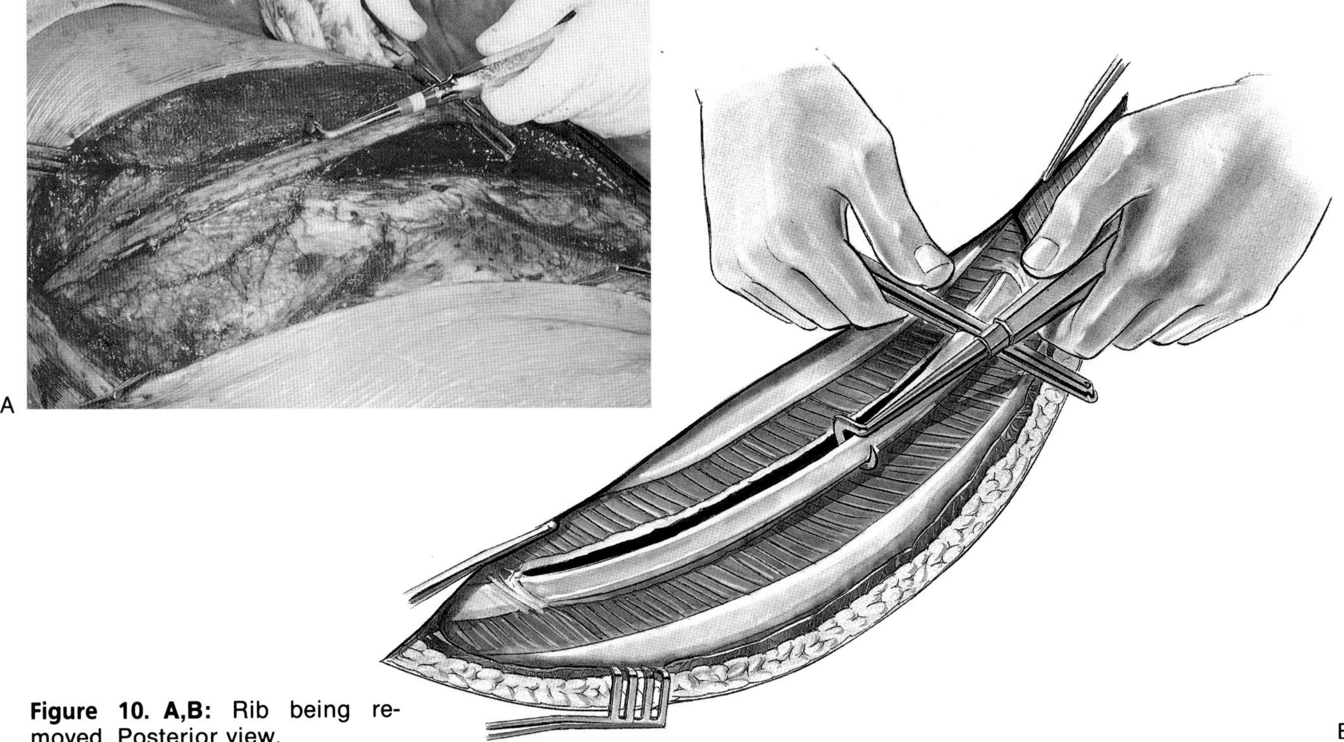

Figure 10. A,B: Rib being removed. Posterior view.

curring between the lung and chest wall and is routinely done in children; in adults, however, because of the difficulty with the dissection and the frequency with which the pleura is inadvertently opened, it is routinely not done unless an indication such as infection exists, in which case subpleural exposure would be desirable.

Usually, immediately following excision of the rib, the incision is carried sharply through the periosteum and pleura, entering the chest cavity. The lung deflates slightly, and is protected by direct visualization. The incision is carried throughout the extent of the rib bed (Figs. 13–15).

The spine is exposed by partially collapsing the lung. The surgeon's field of vision is protected by placing lap pads on the lung and then molding malleable retractors to allow visualization of the spine. The lung on the side of the surgical

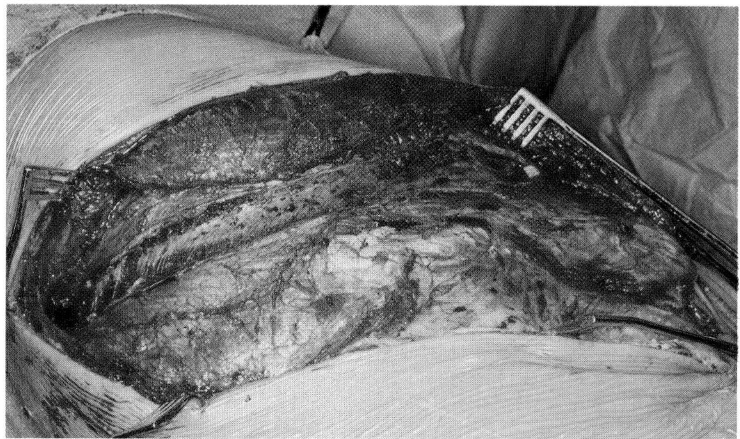

Figure 11. Rib removed.

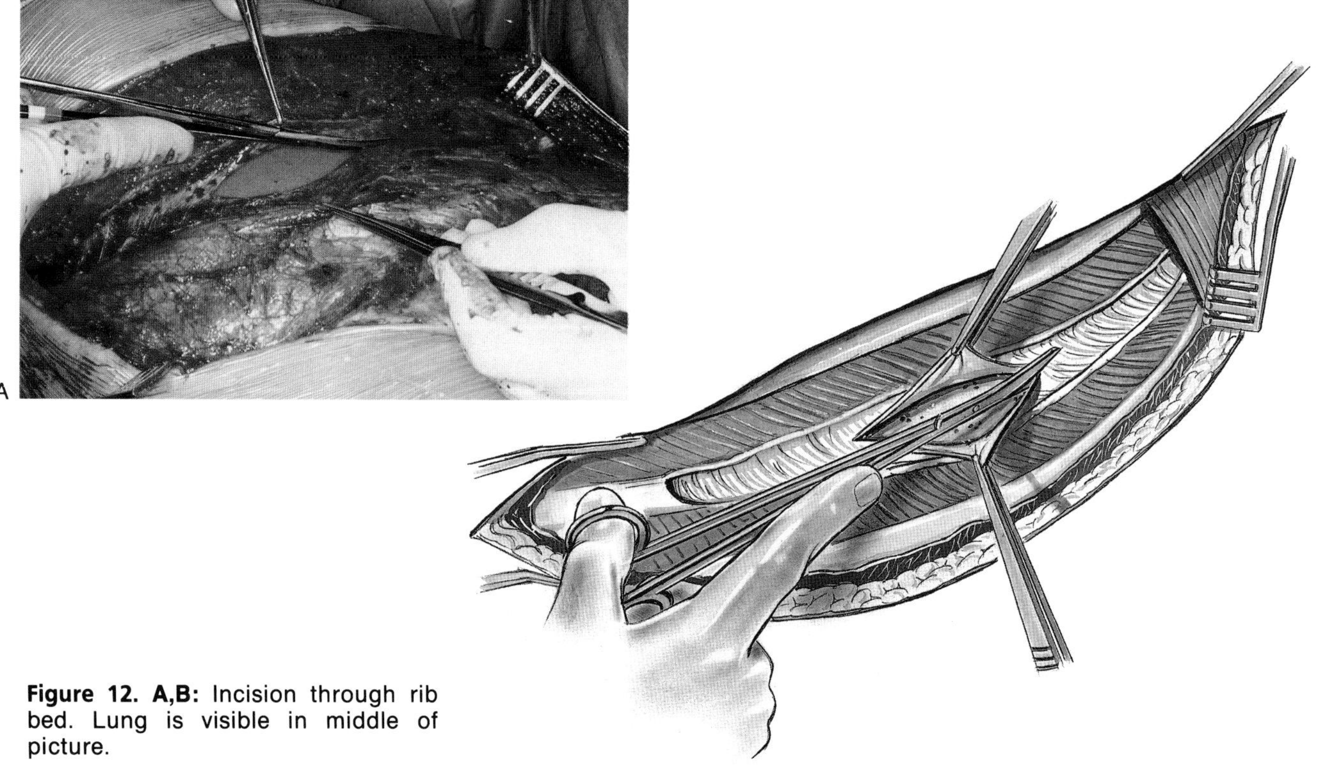

Figure 12. A,B: Incision through rib bed. Lung is visible in middle of picture.

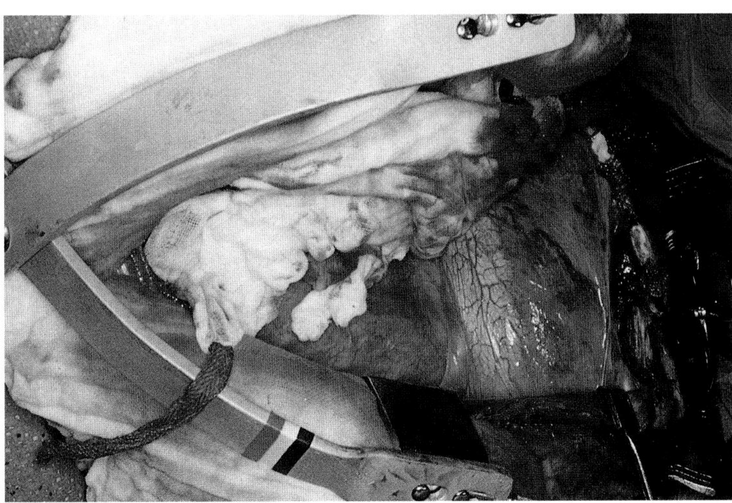

Figure 13. Chest retractor in place and vertebrae visible in back part of wound. Diaphragm to the right.

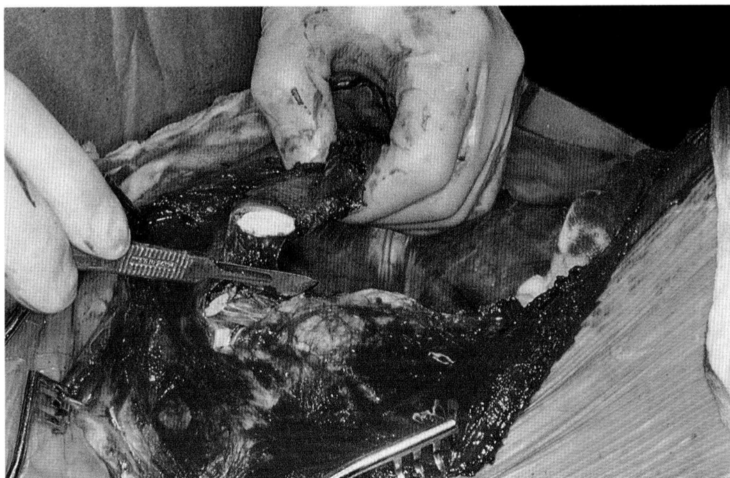

Figure 14. Patient anterior view looking at the extension of the thoracotomy onto the abdominal wall. The external oblique has been split in line with the skin incision. The transsected end of the cartilaginous portion of the rib is seen. Under that is the origin of the diaphragm.

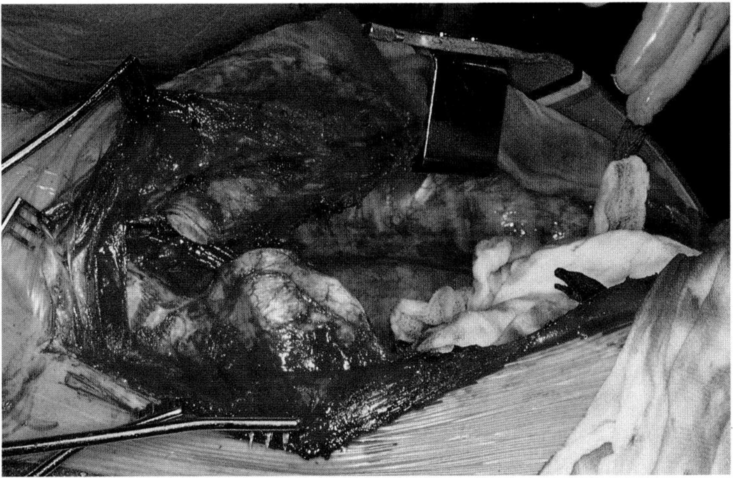

Figure 15. Patient anterior view. Vertebrae visible at about the middle of the picture.

exposure can be completely deflated by doing split bronchial intubation. However, this has a distinct disadvantage of causing profound atelectasis in the involved lung and is unnecessary for exposure of the spine. The spine lies very posterior in the chest cavity, and it is not necessary to collapse the anterior two-thirds of the lung. Less lung collapsed during the operative procedure means less lung atelectasis postoperatively.

A longitudinal incision is made in the pleura overlying the involved vertebra and the pleura is bluntly dissected free to expose the anterior longitudinal ligament, vertebral bodies, discs, and segmental vessels. It is customary to isolate and ligate individually the segmental vessels on each vertebral body. If this is done, it is important that the vessels be ligated well outside the neuroforamina. It has been pointed out by Dommisse that collateral circulation between segmental vessels occurs near the foramina and that ligation of the vessels out on the vertebral bodies does not compromise this circulation (6). Should there be a serious question as to the circulatory status of the cord (i.e., because of prior irradiation, surgery, etc.), many procedures, such as biopsies, disc excision, osteotomies, and others can be done without vessel ligation. However, most of the time, ligation of segmental vessels facilitates bony exposure of the spine for fusion purposes. The usual approach involves subperiosteal exposure of the vertebral bodies and intervertebral discs immediately following ligation of the segmental vessels. This periosteal dissection is facilitated by having angled Cobb periosteal elevators available. Although the vertebral bodies and discs cannot be totally exposed on the side opposite that on which the surgeon is working, they can be safely exposed over about two-thirds of their extent. The operative procedure is accomplished after the spine is adequately exposed.

Wound closure is accomplished after inserting one or two appropriately sized chest tubes. Most spine patients require frequent turning, and it is desirable to position the entry of the chest tube anteriorly, so when the patient is lying on the involved side, they will not be uncomfortable, nor will they kink off their chest tube. The chest tube should be positioned inferiorly and should lie along the posterolateral portion of the chest wall for complete drainage when the patient is in the recumbent position. It is inserted through a small incision and tunneled 6 to 8 cm subcutaneously; then the intercostal space is entered bluntly. The chest tube is secured with an individual strong suture.

It is often not possible to close the pleura over spinal hardware or bone graft. This poses no particular problem, but if the graft material has a tendency to fall away from the spine, it can be held in place by a large Gelfoam pad supplementing the pleural closure. The periosteum of the rib is closed with running nonabsorbable suture. Closure is facilitated by a rib approximator. Care is taken not to impale the inferior neurovascular bundle during this closure. Absorbable retention sutures can be utilized if one has difficulty closing the rib periosteum. Rib closure is facilitated by a rib approximator. The fascia of the latissimus dorsi is approximated with running nonabsorbable suture, as is the external oblique and/or serratus anterior muscle. The skin and subcutaneous tissue can then be closed in a routine manner at the surgeon's discretion.

Lumbar Spine

The lumbar spine can be exposed anterolaterally from either side by an incision placed between the T12–L1 dermatomal intervals. Exposure of the lumbar spine from L2 to L5 is easily accomplished. Exposure above L2 usually requires a thoracolumbar approach. The anterolateral approach below L5 is difficult and requires careful dissection under the iliac vessels. The initial skin incision parallels the 12th rib and is carried downward obliquely and anteriorly parallel to the dermatone. The fascia of the external oblique muscle is divided parallel to the skin incision, and the muscle is split. The internal oblique and transversus abdominis muscles are transected as a unit for later closure as a single layer. The fatty interval between the peritoneum and transversus abdominis muscle is identified. The retroperitoneal space is bluntly dissected free. Exposure of the spine is greatly facilitated by wide retroperitoneal exposure. This is especially true posteriorly and distally. A misconception exists that the lumbar spine is more difficult to approach from the right side because of the presence of the inferior vena cava. This *is* a misconception. The right-sided lumbar approach can be accomplished as easily as the left-sided, and the inferior vena cava is really no more difficult to deal with than is the aorta. The only time that it poses a particular problem is if significant prior irradiation has been performed, which can cause scarring, weakness, and difficulty with dissection. Approaching from the vena cava side often has an advantage if one is planning instrumentation, because hardware can be positioned near a low-pressure venous system without the risk of aneurysm formation, as may occur with the aorta.

The psoas muscle hides the vertebral bodies anterolaterally and must be sharply incised to expose the segmental vessels. The segmental vessels are individually ligated, and these and the psoas muscle are dissected free of the vertebral bodies. The vertebral bodies are exposed subperiosteally. The crus of the diaphragm extends to L3 on the right and to L2 on the left. It can be dissected free for exposure and poses no special problem for closure.

The factor limiting exposure of the spine cranially or superiorly is the overhang of the rib cage. It is extremely difficult to get good exposure above the level of L2 through a strictly lumbar approach.

Caudally or distally, exposure from the body of L5 downward is difficult because the inferior vena cava and aorta are difficult to mobilize. The L5 segmental vessel is large, especially the L5 vein. Care must be taken when ligating this structure not to damage the inferior vena cava if one is on the right side. Furthermore, both the vena cava and the aorta bifurcate at about the midpoint of L4. The common iliacs are difficult to mobilize because the deep iliac vessels plunge into the pelvis, preventing mobilization of these vessels anteriorly. The sacrum can be exposed, along with the other lumbar intervals, through the anterolateral approach retroperitoneally, but it is a very difficult dissection. If just the L5, S1 interspace needs to be exposed, it is easier to accomplish this through a direct anterior approach, going just lateral to the rectus and then proceeding through the abdominal wall in a longitudinal fashion and using a retroperitoneal or transperitoneal exposure. The limitation for this direct anterior approach to L5, S1 is the fact that it cannot be extended superiorly and is only of value for very limited exposure of the spine.

Closure of the lumbar wound is accomplished by approximation of the transversus abdominis and internal oblique muscle with running nonabsorbable suture and similar closure of the external oblique muscle. The skin and subcutaneous layers are closed in a routine fashion at the surgeon's discretion.

Thoracolumbar Junction

Exposure of the thoracolumbar junction requires removal of the diaphragm from its origin on the chest wall. One might think that the morbidity with this approach would be higher than in either a pure thoracotomy or a retroperitoneal lumbar approach; however, it is not. The approach to the thoracolumbar junction is a simple combination of the thoracic and lumbar approaches. The appropriate level or rib incision is selected, in a manner similar to the thoracotomy approach. The skin incision is similar. It is easiest to expose the rib in question and remove it subperiosteally, as described previously. The approach in the chest can then be made subpleurally or transpleurally with the same considerations described for the thoracic approach.

At the point where the diaphragm originates on the rib that has been removed, the interval between the diaphragm origin and the chest wall is identified, and, with an electrocautery, the diaphragm is taken off its origin on the underlying rib bed (Fig. 16). This immediately allows the surgeon to enter the retroperitoneal space of the abdomen. The external oblique muscle will have been split along its origin on the rib during the initial approach. Retroperitoneal dissection under the internal oblique and transversus abdominis muscles allows safe transection of the muscles in line with the skin incision. The surgeon can then extend the excision of the diaphragm from the chest wall. Because the blood supply to the diaphragm is central, the interval between the chest wall and the diaphragm is blood-free. By a combination of blunt dissection in the interval between the ribs and of electrocautery dissection of the diaphragm from its origin on each rib, the diaphragm is removed from the chest wall laterally (Fig. 17). As the incision of the diaphragm

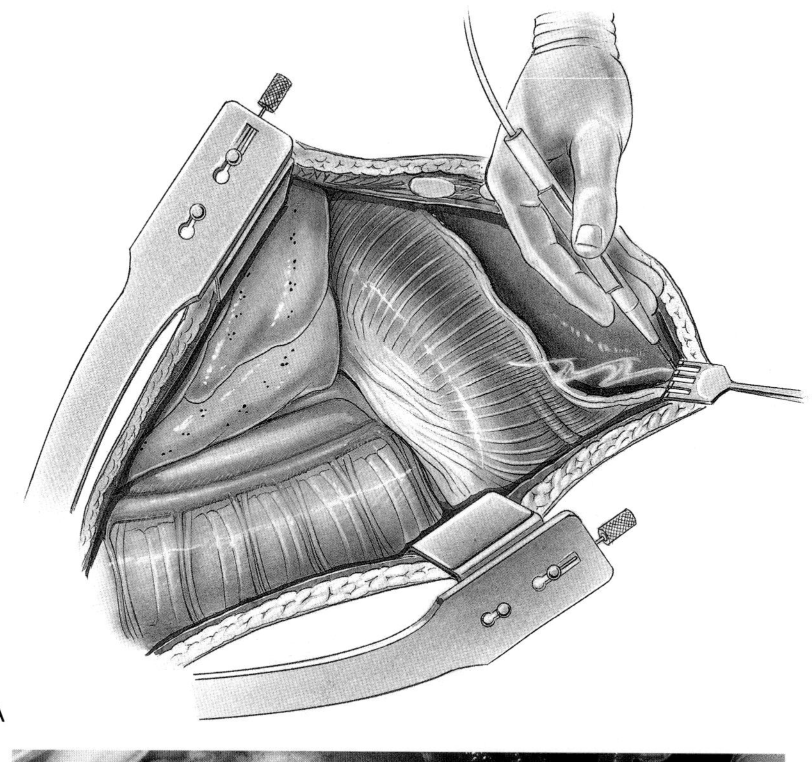

A

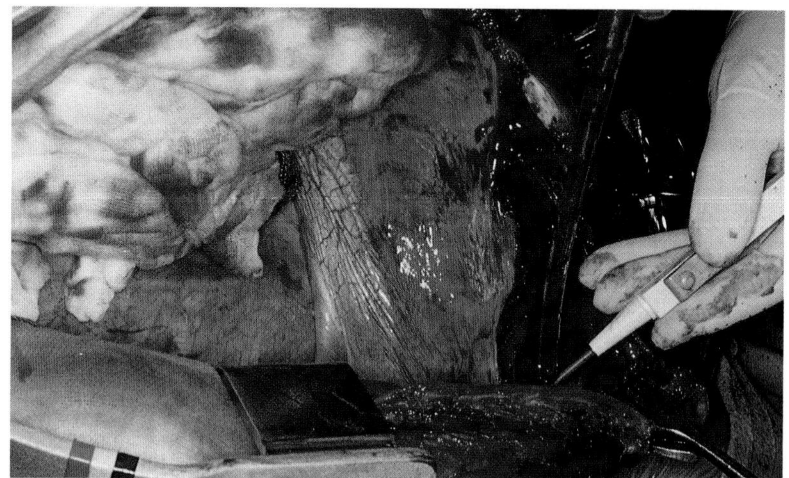

B

Figure 16. A,B: Patient posterior view again. This time the diaphragm is seen, being taken down from its origin on the lower ribs and separated with electrocautery.

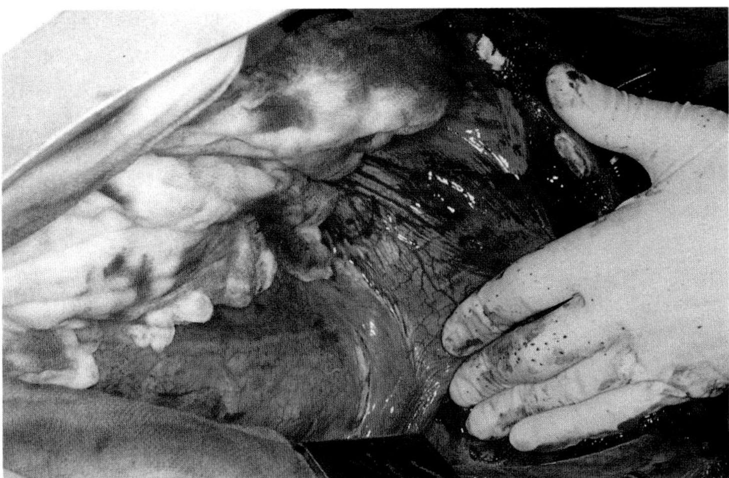

Figure 17. The diaphragm has been removed from the chest wall about three-fourths of the way around. The vertebrae are visible to the left. The crus of the diaphragm is now reflecting back under the surgeon's hand, and the diaphragm is about to be removed from the angle made by the rib and vertebral body.

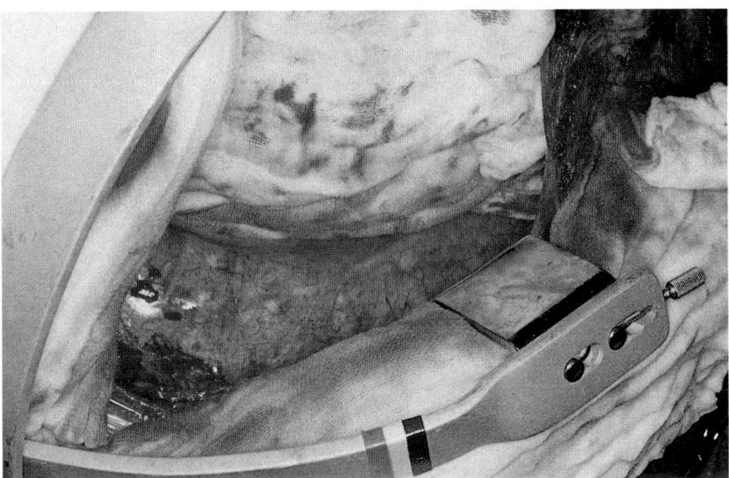

Figure 18. Patient posterior view. Vertebral body covered by pleura.

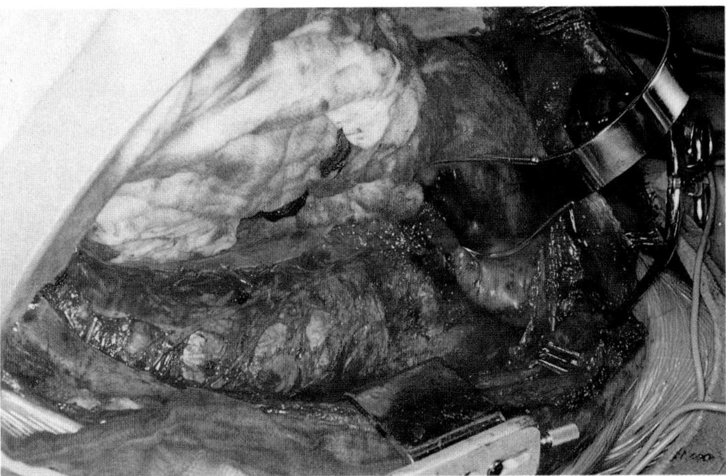

Figure 19. Same view with pleura reflected, showing the intercostal vessels.

approaches the spine, the wound will open to expose the vertebral bodies more adequately (Figs. 18–26). If the approach has been transpleural, the pleura is incised over the lower thoracic vertebrae that are to be involved in the surgical process, and the segmental vessels are ligated as described previously. The crus of the diaphragm lies immediately above the psoas muscle origin, and this interval is entered to expose the lumbar vertebrae. The lumbar vertebrae are then exposed in exactly the same manner as they were during the lumbar approach.

For surgical procedures that require exposure of four to six vertebrae, the entire procedure is usually accomplished through an incision that parallels a single dermatomal interval. However, when one is performing scoliosis and kyphosis surgery and needs to expose the spine over many levels, it is necessary to do a more extensile approach. In a neurologic scoliotic curve, it may be desirable to do an anterior fusion from T5 to the sacrum. If that is the case, the approach would be the skin incision for a T4 thoracotomy as initially described; then at the anterior extent of the incision, approximately 3 to 5 cm from the anterior midline, the

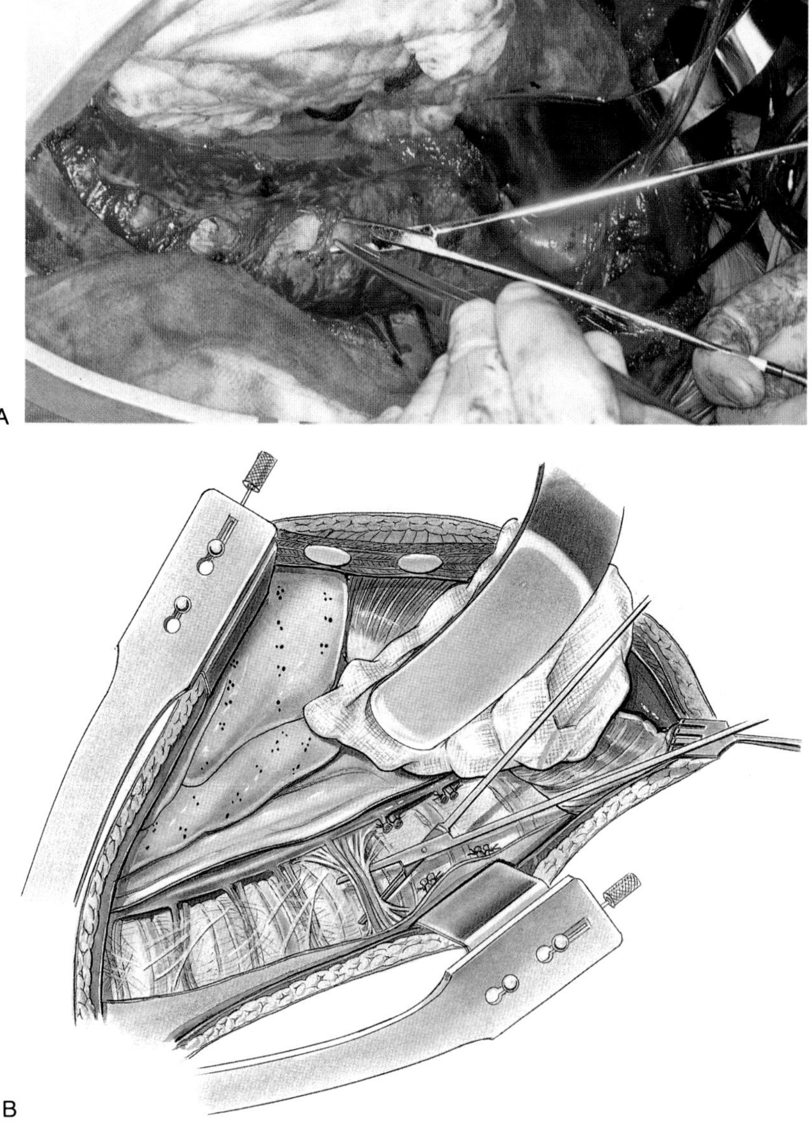

Figure 20. A,B: Intercostal vessels being ligated.

incision is carried distally to below the level of the iliac crest. This incision obviously crosses the segmental neurovascular bundles as far down as L2, but this causes no problem because one is so anterior. This does not seem to denervate the rectus even though it is segmentally innervated. The entire thoracic and abdominal walls can then be reflected laterally and the diaphragm removed from the chest wall at the point at which the incision crossed it anteriorly. The lumbar spine is exposed by retroperitoneal dissection.

Upper Thoracic Spine

Exposure of the upper thoracic spine, that is, T1–L4, requires a more difficult thoracotomy. The upper shoulder must be prepped and draped so an incision can be made parallel to the spinous processes beginning superiorly at about the level of the tip of the seventh cervical vertebra; this incision is carried down to about the tip of the spinous process of T4. It is then carried out over the thorax and around the tip of the scapula. The trapezius is removed from its origin along the spinous processes from about T1–T4 and then split out toward the tip of the scapula. The scapula is mobilized by excising the rhomboid muscles from their

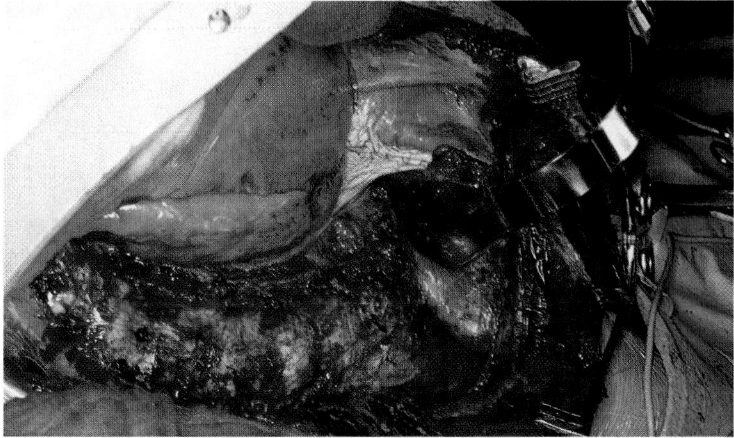

Figure 21. Intercostal vessels ligated showing vertebral bodies and discs.

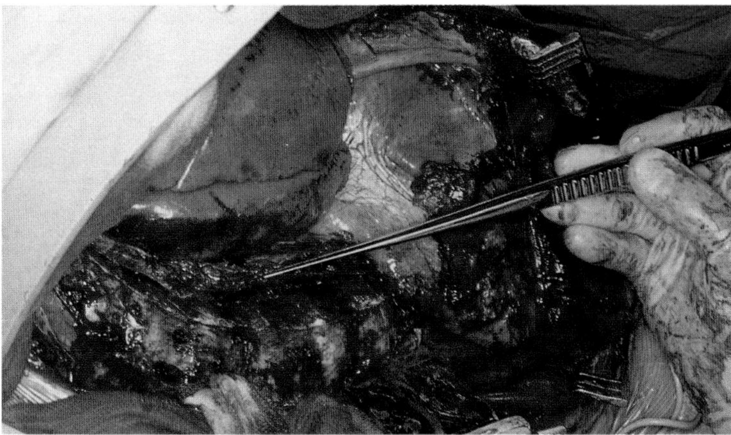

Figure 22. Pleura being reflected away from the vertebral bodies.

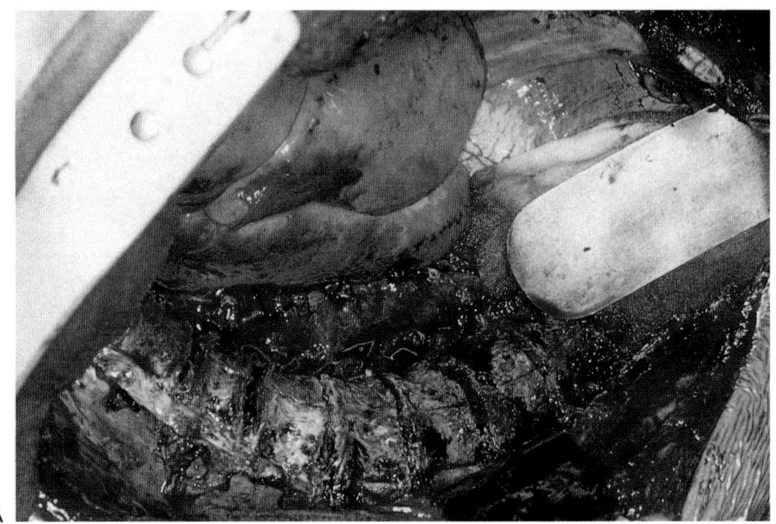

A

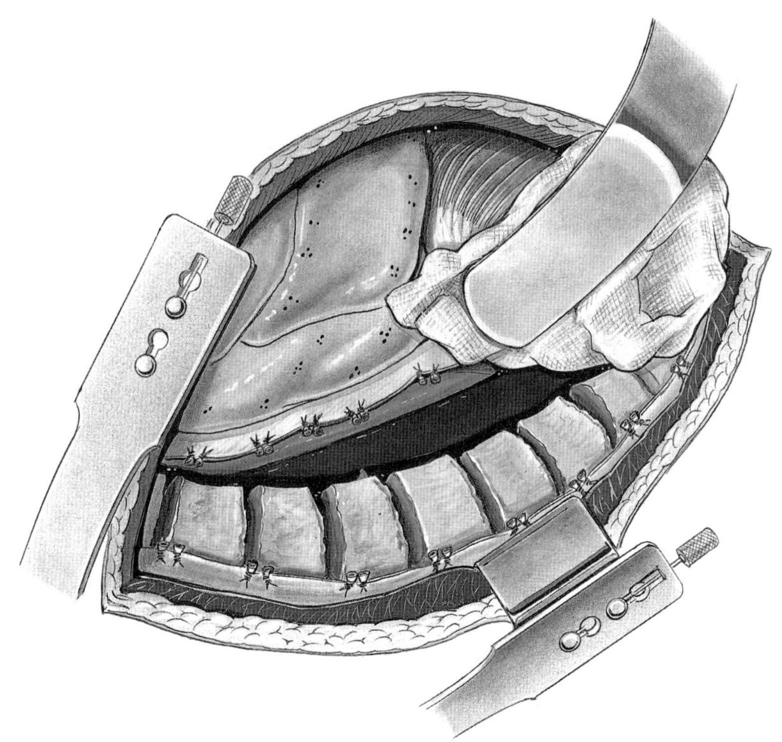

B

Figure 23. A,B: The discs have been removed between the vertebral bodies.

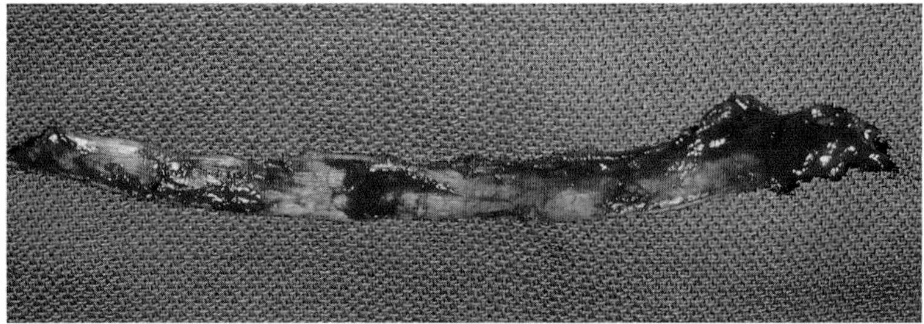

Figure 24. In this particular operation, the anterior longitudinal ligament was excised.

insertion along the medial border of the scapula, and the scapula is retracted with a scapular retractor to expose the T3 rib. A thoracotomy is made through the third rib bed with removal of the entire third rib posteriorly. Through this thoracotomy one can achieve good exposure for the T1–T4 area. Extending this exposure into an extensile exposure for the lower thoracic or lumbar vertebrae is not feasible. If those vertebrae are to be exposed, it is preferable to expose the T1–T4 area with a T3 thoracotomy, then use a T5 thoracotomy to expose the lower thoracic vertebrae and, if necessary, carry that around in an extensile fashion for further exposure.

A

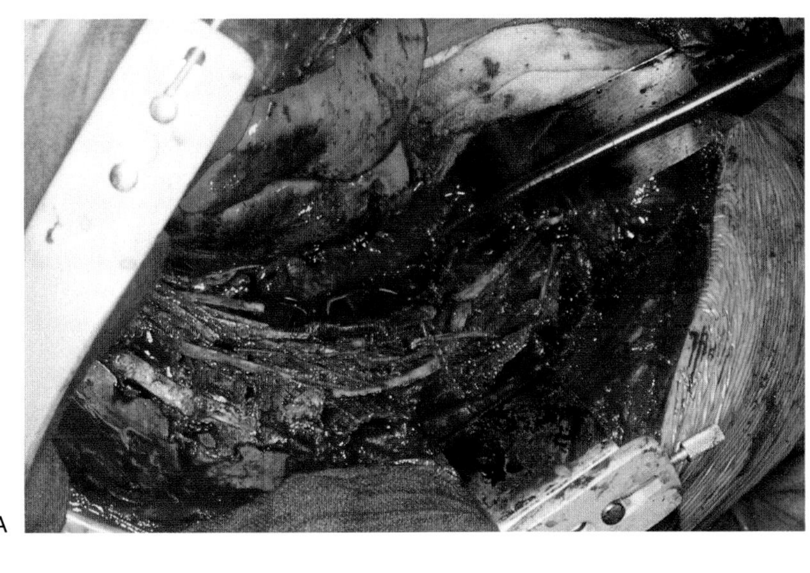

B

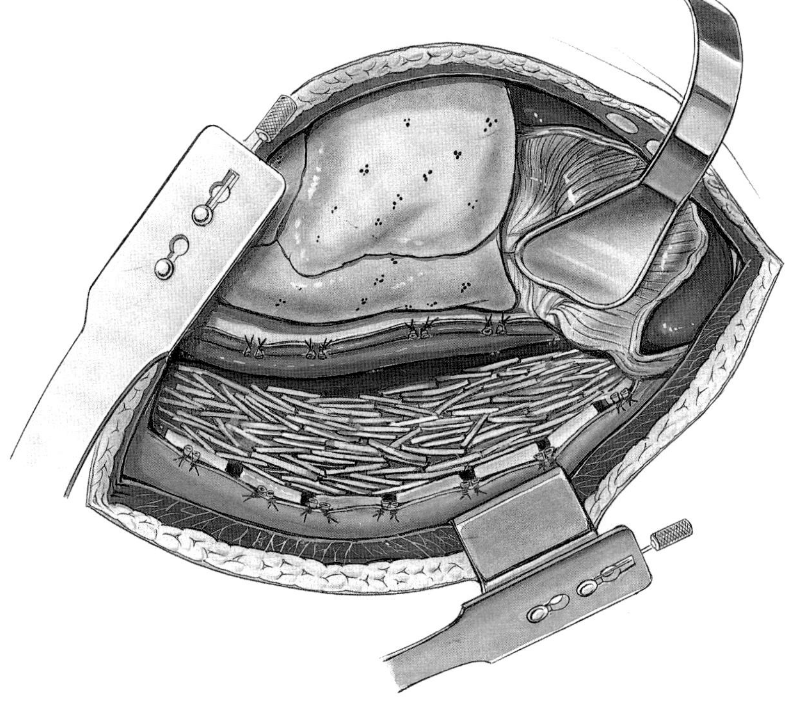

Figure 25. A,B: The fronts of the vertebral bodies have been cut with an osteotome and turned up; loose, match-stick rib grafts have been placed under the osteal and periosteal flaps.

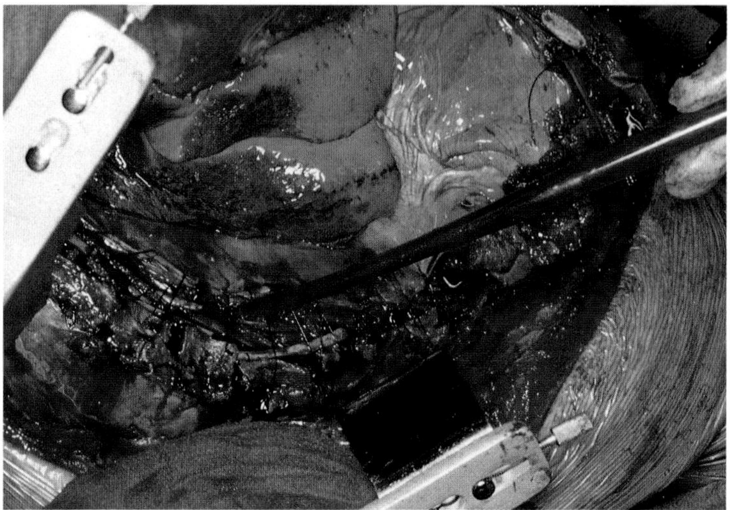

Figure 26. Pleura has been closed over the graft material. Posterior part of the operation will now be done with instrumentation and fusion.

Closure

In general, all three of the anterior approaches to the spine are closed with anatomic layers. The abdominal muscles and the intercostal muscles of the spine can be closed with running sutures. The author prefers nonabsorbable sutures to protect the wound for a long enough period of time to allow for formation of good tensile strength in the healing collagen; however, many surgeons use absorbable sutures and have excellent results.

The diaphragm is traditionally closed by interrupted sutures around its periphery. This is a time-consuming process; for many years the author has routinely closed the diaphragm with a running stitch using a running lock-stitch through the diaphragm musculature. In any of the approaches that involve violation of the pleural cavity, a chest tube of adequate size should be secured in place routinely and placed to water-sealed suction to 15 to 20 mmHg.

POSTOPERATIVE MANAGEMENT

Postoperative management of patients undergoing anterior approaches to the spine will in general be determined by factors other than the approach. The approach will allow the surgeon to accomplish internal fixation and arthrodesis of the spine anteriorly and may or may not be used in conjunction with a posterior procedure. It is the quality of internal fixation that will determine the postoperative rehabilitation course. The better the quality of internal fixation, the less restrictive will be the postoperative management.

The postoperative course can be affected by the approach when the pleural cavity is entered and a chest tube is necessary. The chest tube should be positioned on the posterior medial wall of the thoracic cavity and be of ample size to allow good drainage of the fluids that will collect in the immediate postoperative period. Usually the chest tube will be in place for about 48 to 72 hours. It can be removed when the output has dropped to approximately 100 ml in an 8-hour observation period. Because most anterior approaches are done in conjunction with operative procedures that involve cutting the anterior vertebral bodies and eliciting a fracture response, serum will continue to form in the operative site for a long time following the operative procedure. Unlike cardiac and pulmonary operative procedures, orthopedic procedures on the anterior spine elicit a fracture-healing response in the bone that will result in serous fluid formation, preventing chest-tube output from resolving to zero for a long period. Fortunately, the pleura is capable of absorbing this output, and one does not have to wait until a state of zero output exists before pulling the chest tube.

The other postoperative management concern associated with the anterior approaches relates to extubation of the patient in the immediate postoperative period. It is often desirable to leave the patient intubated for 24 to 48 hours following an anterior procedure. These patients often have compromised pulmonary function because of spinal deformity prior to surgery; also, with the anterior procedure, the mechanics of the chest wall are adversely affected, and splinting secondary to pain results in inadequate respiratory function. This decision is best made cooperatively between the anesthesiologist and the surgeon involved; when in doubt, it is best to leave the patient intubated and evaluate the respiratory effort at intervals following recovery from anesthesia.

It is generally expected that the anterior approach will add morbidity to the postoperative course. I think this reflects the fact that most orthopedic surgeons are more comfortable with posterior approaches, and the unusual nature of anterior approaches may be a factor in this assumption. However, the postoperative course in terms of recovering from ileus, requiring pain medication, getting up and around, and recovering from surgery is no different in anterior than in posterior approaches. If anything, the recovery time following an anterior approach may be a bit quicker, at least as far as ileus is concerned, compared with a posterior procedure.

COMPLICATIONS

Complications associated with thoracolumbar approaches are not frequent. Occasionally the chest tube will have to be reinserted because of excessive pleural collection of serous fluid. Also, an additional tube sometimes has to be inserted because the original tube fails to drain the pleural cavity fully.

Vascular injury can occur during exposure of the vertebral bodies. In my experience, this is extremely rare and has only been associated with previously irradiated patients. Hodgson et al. (3) provided some of the first descriptions of anterior approaches (for tuberculosis). They advocated a left-sided approach to avoid the inferior vena cava in the tuberculous abscess. This concern has been carried forward, and some people feel very uncomfortable with right-sided approaches. I routinely approach the spine from the right side, because anterior implants are much better tolerated by the low-pressure venous system. Mobilization of the vena cava is not difficult nor, is it associated with any particular problems.

In the previously irradiated tumor patient, mobilization of soft tissues in general is a problem around the spine, and a tear in vascular structures can occur, with significant blood loss. These tears are difficult to close and require careful dissection and vascular suture. During the lumbar retroperitoneal approaches, it is possible to dissect behind the psoas muscle and damage lumbar nerve roots or the lumbar plexus. This complication is avoided by continual vigilance regarding tissue planes.

In left-sided approaches at the thoracolumbar junction, one occasionally damages the cisterna chyli. This is noticed when cloudy fluid flows from the soft tissues. These injuries can usually be closed by oversewing the area with fine suture.

RECOMMENDED READING

1. Bridwell, K. H., and DeWald, R. L.: *The Textbook of Spinal Surgery*. JP Lippincott, Philadelphia, 1991.
2. Crock, H. V., and Yoshizawa, H.: *The Blood Supply of the Vertebral Column and Spinal Cord in Man*. Springer-Verlag, New York, 1977.
3. Hodgson, A. R., Stock, F. E., Fang, H. S. Y., and Ong, G. B.: Anterior spinal fusion: the operative approach and pathological findings in 412 patients with Pott's disease of the spine. *Br. J. Surg.*, 48: 172–178, 1960.
4. Riseborough, E. J.: The anterior approach to the spine for the correction of the deformities of the axial skeleton. *Clin. Orthop. Rel. Res.*, 93: 207–214, 1973.
5. Rothman, R. H., and Simeon, F. A., editors: *The Spine*. 3rd ed. WB Saunders, Philadelphia, 1992.
6. Dommisse, G. F.: *Arteries and Veins of the Human Spinal Cord from Birth*. Churchill Livingstone, Edinburgh, London and New York, 1975.

PART II

Techniques—Cervical Spine

Master Techniques in Orthopaedic Surgery,
THE SPINE, edited by D. S. Bradford,
Lippincott-Raven Publishers, Philadelphia, © 1997.

3

Anterior Cervical Microdiscectomy Without Fusion

Philip R. Weinstein

INDICATIONS/CONTRAINDICATIONS

Through an anterior cervical surgical exposure of the vertebral column, microsurgical techniques can be used to perform partial or complete discectomy and osteophyte resection to decompress the neural canal and foramen. Use of the operating microscope provides magnification, improves illumination, and reduces the amount of vertebral body resection required to expose the herniated disc or osteophyte. Because the circumferential and longitudinal resection of ligament, anulus, and vertebral bone is limited, radiculopathy and myelopathy can be relieved without interbody bone graft fusion. The anatomical rationale for anterior decompression is to provide direct access through the disc space to remove the lesion from anterior to the cord without further displacing or disturbing the neural elements. The physiological rationale is to relieve compression directly of the anterior spinal artery and its branches, to reverse the major ischemic component of discogenic or spondylotic myelopathy.

Anterior cervical discectomy (ACD) without autogenous bone graft fusion eliminates the risk of donor site complications, including postoperative pain, infection, and hemorrhage. It also reduces the length of the operation and prevents problems related to graft displacement or collapse and pseudarthrosis. Furthermore, spontaneous intervertebral osseous fusion rates of 70% to 80% have been reported after ACD without fusion. Thus placement of bone grafts—even allografts, which avoid donor site but not implant site complications—is not necessary to obtain satisfac-

P. R. Weinstein, M.D.: Department of Neurosurgery, University of California San Francisco, San Francisco, California 94143-0112.

tory results. Recurrent disc herniation at other levels above or below the affected level may be less likely after simple discectomy than after discectomy with bone graft fusion.

The disadvantages and complications of ACD without fusion include temporary persistence or increase in cervical and brachial pain (4% to 60%), which usually resolves within 1 week, and persistence or worsening of neurological deficit due to retained disc or osteophyte (2% to 4%). Postoperative spinal instability characterized by anterior angulation at a single operated level or kyphotic deformity due to anterior collapse at multiple levels may be more common after ACD without fusion, but it also occurs even when bone grafts have been placed. Instability requiring reoperation is rare.

ACD without fusion is used to treat intractable, progressive, or repeatedly disabling unilateral or bilateral radiculopathy or progressive myelopathy caused by traumatic or degenerative disc disease in patients whose radiographic images show a focal mass lesion anterior to the compressed neural structures that correlates anatomically with the distribution of clinical symptoms and signs. Lesions at multiple levels may also be treated by ACD without fusion. Simple discectomy may be effective in some cases when cervical rather than brachial symptoms are the major complaint, but in such patients we prefer to use bone graft fusion to immobilize the painful joint.

In our experience, ACD without fusion is indicated for soft disc herniation or spondylosis causing primarily appendicular rather than axial pain. Other indications include painless radiculomyelopathy; spondylosis or disc herniation with a collapsed intervertebral space and absent or minimal translational motion on lateral flexion-extension radiographs; multilevel spondylosis with stable motion segments or spontaneous fusion and well-preserved cervical lordosis; and disc herniation or spondylosis in patients with severe osteoporosis or other systemic skeletal disorders, in whom interbody fusion often fails.

ACD without fusion may be contraindicated in patients with severe axial pain and either occipital or interscapular radiation; degenerative spondylolisthesis or hypermobility on flexion-extension radiographs; fracture or posttraumatic ligamentous instability; and instability or hypermobility during intraoperative testing after discectomy in a well-preserved or widely debrided intervertebral space and preoperative kyphotic deformity or, in multilevel cases, straightening of the cervical lordosis. Other contraindications include severe, surgically inaccessible stenosis of the lateral foramen requiring distraction of the intervertebral space by a bone graft; congenital midbody stenosis, bridging posterior osteophytes due to severe spondylosis, or ossification of the posterior longitudinal ligament (PLL) requiring median corpectomy for adequate spinal cord decompression; and severe segmental posterior indentation of the thecal sac due to buckling of a thickened ligamentum flavum slackened from disc collapse that requires distraction by placement of an intervertebral bone graft.

PREOPERATIVE PLANNING

Preoperative planning for ACD without fusion consists primarily of selecting appropriate cases based on neurological and radiological criteria (Algorithm 1). Lateral flexion-extension radiographs of the cervical spine should be obtained along with cervical spine radiographs in all patients. The initial diagnostic procedure of choice is high-resolution, 1.5-Tesla magnetic resonance imaging (MRI) of the cervical spine. When images are inadequate because of patient motion or if the results are equivocal with respect to diagnosis of foramen stenosis, a thin-section, high-resolution computed tomography (CT) scan of the cervical spine with sagittal and coronal reformatted images should be obtained. In complex cases where neurological correlation is lacking or osseous anatomy is distorted by ossifi-

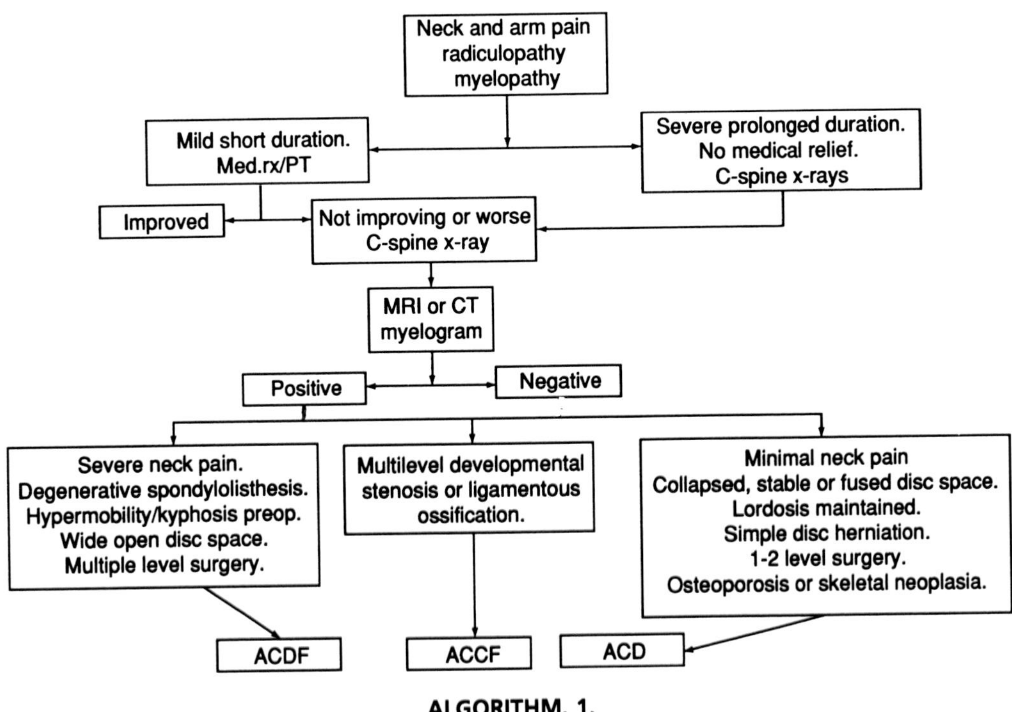

ALGORITHM. 1.

cation of the PLL, developmental deformity, trauma, or previous surgery, a CT scan or myelogram should be obtained after intrathecal injection of contrast material. Such studies permit more accurate estimation of the relative size of the spinal cord and surrounding subarachnoid space as well as the extent of cord atrophy or cavitation caused by syringomyelia.

Preparations for possible bone grafting are made and operative consent for fusion is obtained in case hypermobility or instability is unexpectedly encountered. Patients with a carotid bruit or a history of stroke symptoms should undergo preoperative ultrasound, MRI, or angiographic studies to rule out an unstable carotid stenosis or ulceration that requires treatment before carotid artery retraction during ACD.

SURGERY

The operation is performed with the patient in the supine position. Care is taken to avoid manipulating the neck during endotracheal intubation. Before anesthesia is induced, the anesthesiologist should check the maximum degree of cervical flexion or extension tolerated by the patient. The head and neck are extended slightly and placed in a sponge cradle; a flat gel pad is placed across the shoulders to elevate the upper thorax, and a rolled sheet is placed behind the neck. Because intraoperative observations will be considered in determining whether autograft fusion will be required, the iliac crest is also prepared and draped.

The surgical approach is most comfortable from the patient's right side for a right-handed surgeon and from the left side for a left-handed surgeon. Steps in the surgical exposure are illustrated in Fig. 1. A transverse incision is made at the appropriate level, as determined from the lateral radiograph by the relationship of the target disc to a palpable landmark such as the cricoid or thyroid cartilage. Magnifying loupes and a headlight are used during the initial exposure. The incision is centered over the medial edge of the sternomastoid muscle. The platysma

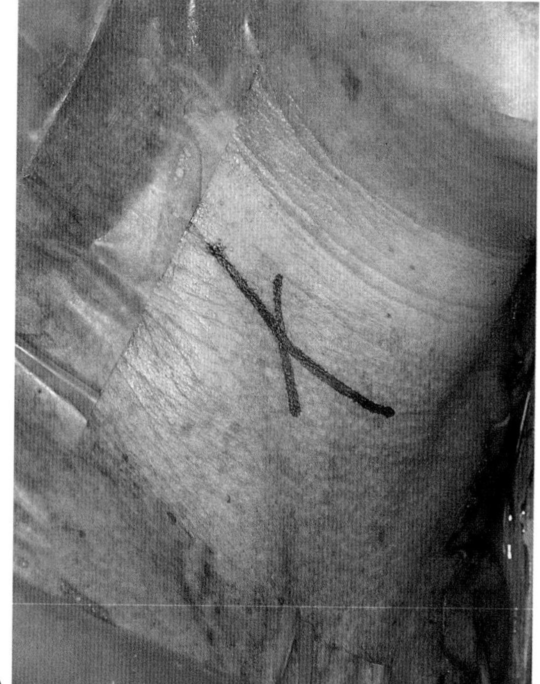

A

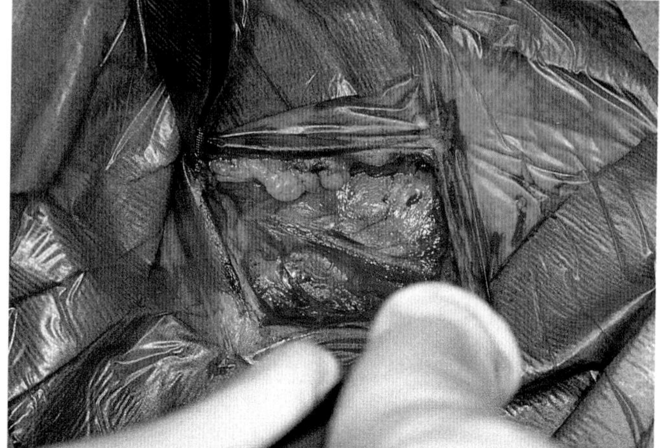

B

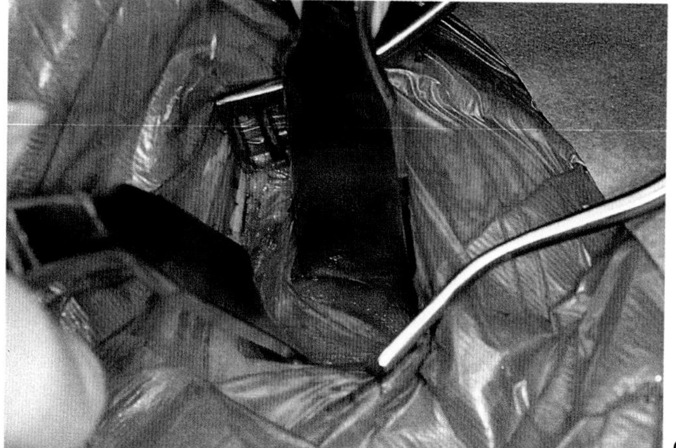

C

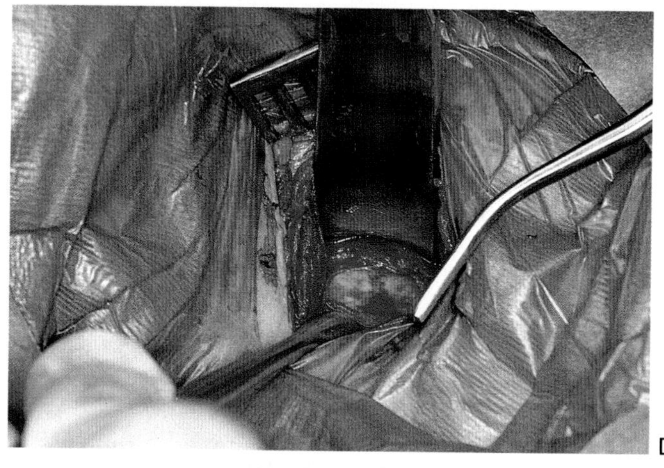

D

Figure 1. Sequential steps for surgical exposure during anterior cervical discectomy. **A:** A transverse midcervical incision is outlined at the level of the cricoid cartilage for exposure of the C5–C6 and C6–C7 discs. The vertical line marks the border of the medial sternomastoid muscle. **B:** The incision is deepened through the platysma layer to expose the external jugular vein on the surface of the sternohyoid muscle. **C:** The anterior and middle cervical fascia layers are incised. Angled, flat, back retractors deflect the sternomastoid muscle laterally and the tracheoesophageal complex medially. **D:** The carotid artery is identified, exposed, and retracted laterally. **E:** The anterior longitudinal ligament is exposed through a longitudinal incision in the deep cervical (prevertebral) fascia. The longus colli muscles have been detached from the anterior longitudinal ligament and elevated. **F:** The transverse and longitudinal self-retaining retractor system has been placed and secured to complete the exposure before the disc is excised and the operating microscope is brought into position for discectomy and foraminotomy.

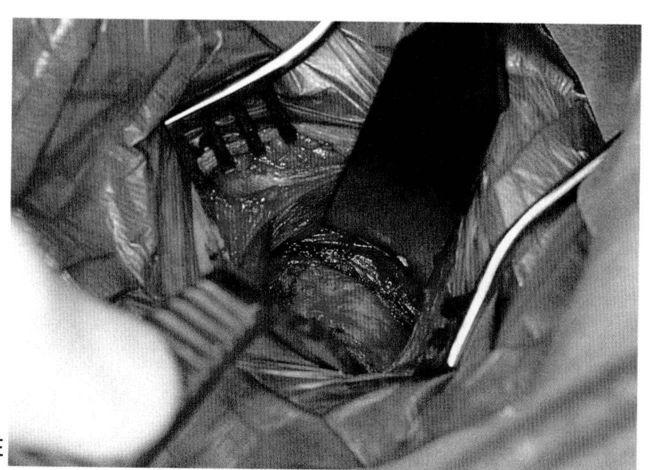

E

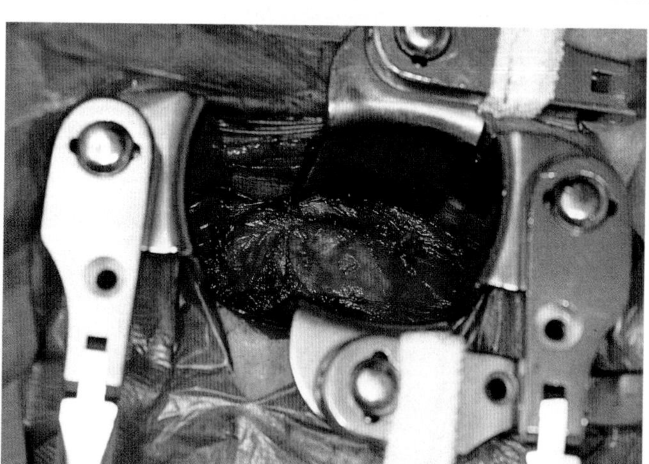

F

muscle is divided transversely, and the anterior cervical fascia and underlying adipose tissue are incised obliquely along the medial sternomastoid border for several segments above and below the target disc level. Difficulties with deeper exposure most often result from inadequate superficial layer dissection. The carotid artery is retracted laterally with the sternomastoid muscle, and the sternothyroid muscle is retracted medially along with the trachea and esophagus. The inferior thyroid veins and artery are divided if necessary, and the recurrent laryngeal nerve is carefully isolated and retracted medially if encountered. The superior laryngeal nerve may be seen during exposure of the C3–C4 or C4–C5 levels, and it must also be protected. A lateral radiograph of the cervical spine is then obtained with a needle marker in place to identify the disc levels.

After the longus colli muscles are separated and elevated from their attachment to the anterior longitudinal ligament, a Caspar or Cloward self-retaining retractor system is placed (Fig. 2). The transverse retractor blades are inserted under the longus colli fascia and muscle if possible, and "tie downs" are inserted by looping strip gauze around the retractor and securing it to the operating table rail to keep

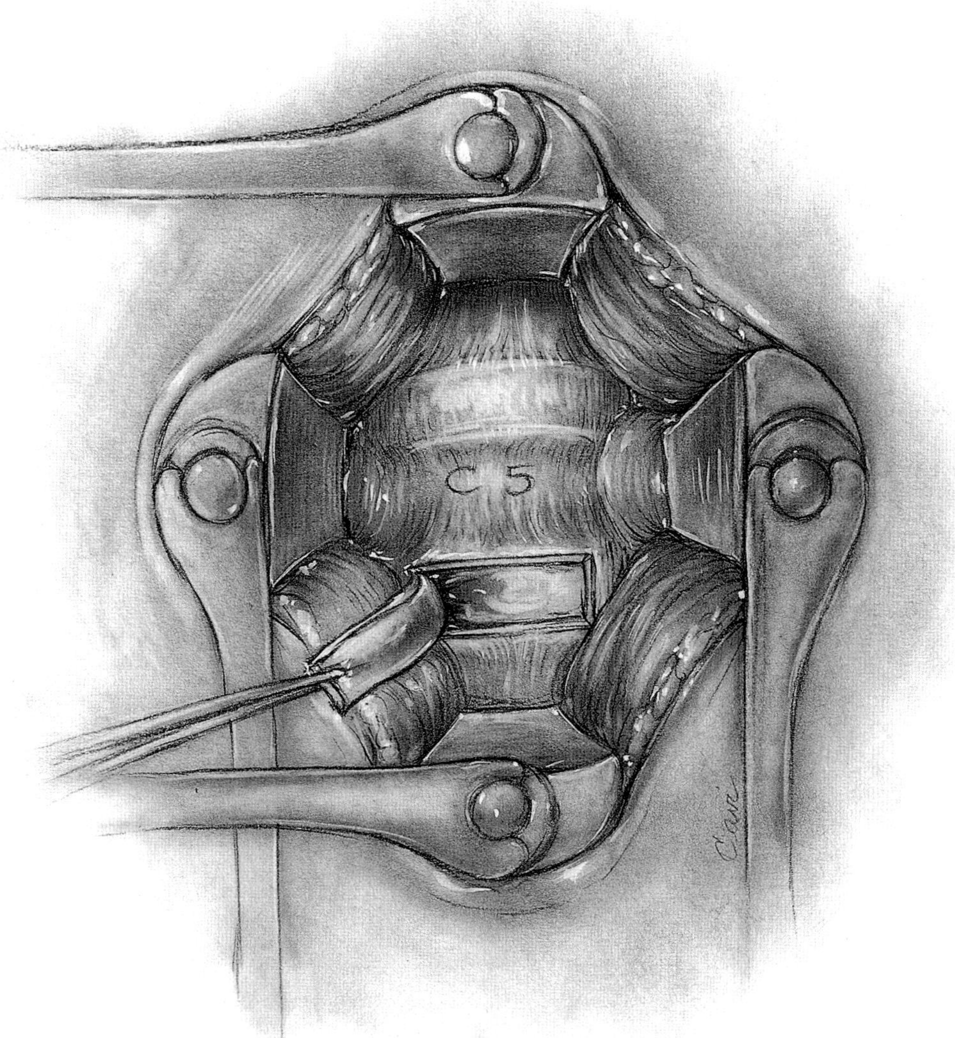

Figure 2. Diagram showing surgical exposure with Caspar retractors in place after initial incision through the anterior longitudinal ligament and excision of the anterior anulus to a distance of 6 mm on either side of the midline. The right carotid artery is retracted laterally with the sternomastoid muscle, and the trachea, esophagus, and sternothyroid muscle are retracted medially.

the retractor vertical. The longitudinal retractor is then inserted to expose one, two, or three disc levels as needed.

A transverse incision is then made extending approximately 6 mm on either side of the midline through the anterior longitudinal ligament and anulus (Fig. 2). If the midline is difficult to identify because of anterior osteophyte formation and spondylotic vertebral deformity, an anteroposterior (AP) radiograph may be obtained. To enhance postoperative stability, care is taken to preserve the lateral ligament and anulus as well as any lateral bridging osteophytes. In cases of soft disc herniation, the intervertebral space may be sufficiently open anteriorly that the vertebral edges need not be resected. To avoid postoperative collapse, excessive anterior wedging, and subsequent kyphotic deformity, at most only a 4 to 5-mm space between adjacent vertebrae should be opened. In some cases of spondylosis, large anterior midline osteophytes must be removed with a curette, osteotome, or drill to gain access to the intervertebral space. After the anterior disc space is opened, a rectangular fenestration is made through the anulus, and all accessible disc material is removed with curettes and discectomy rongeurs. This procedure is repeated at additional levels if necessary. The operating microscope is then brought into the surgical field to complete the discectomy (Fig. 3A).

A variable-speed, foot-pedal–controlled high-speed power drill with a 30 degree angled handpiece and a 4-mm cutting bur is used to debride, but not necessarily resect, the cartilaginous plates above and below the disc space. Residual disc material is detached and removed. Bayonet-handled straight and forward-angled or back-angled Karlin microcurettes are used to complete the discectomy and osteophyte resection.

First the drill is used to open or widen the posterior intervertebral space by resecting the marginal osteophyte or vertebral body lip (Fig. 3B). Degenerative collapse of the space may have occurred after disc herniation or extrusion followed by formation of an osteophyte that bridges the intervertebral space with bone. The herniated disc will be encountered only after the ossified anulus has been removed. For the same reason an extruded disc may be sequestered in the epidural space behind the thickened or ossified PLL, especially in chronic cases. Thus the surgical anatomy may be far more complex than the more typical finding of a herniated or protruding segment of "soft" fibrocartilage penetrating through or detaching the anulus. The posterior intervertebral space must be opened widely and all intervening soft tissue and bone must be removed so that the dura and both nerve roots can be seen clearly to verify adequacy of the decompression (Fig. 3C).

Before the PLL is opened, the upper and lower margins of the vertebral body are undercut 2 to 4 mm with the drill, and uncinate process or medial foraminal osteophytes are debrided if present. As long as the PLL remains intact to protect the dura, the cutting bur can be used. Once the dura has been exposed adjacent to a drilling site, the diamond bur is preferable to avoid dural perforation. Soft disc herniations or extruded fragments are then removed with microcurettes and rongeurs.

After the PLL has been divided or removed, the drill with a diamond bur should be used if needed to resect bone that cannot be removed with curettes. To avoid spinal cord or nerve root injury, angled curettes no larger than 3–0 should be used for undercutting in the neural canal and foramina. At this stage of the procedure, the anesthesiologist should reverse muscle paralysis so that inadvertent motor stimulation due to neural compression or displacement caused by surgical manipulation can be identified immediately.

When all osteophytes have been resected, or debrided in spondylosis cases, any residual soft tissue becomes pliable. The PLL, if intact, is then perforated with a blunt 45- or 90-degree angled dissector, elevated, and transected with a scalpel, taking care to protect the dura beneath. After resection of disc, osteophyte, and ligament is complete, the pulsating ventral dura should bulge into the decompression site. If the dura remains tented away from the surgical opening in the posterior intervertebral space, a search should be made for residual disc or osteophyte. Foraminotomies are completed and nerve roots are examined by angling the microscope and, if necessary, rotating the operating table to provide a better line of sight (Fig. 3D). An intervertebral distractor may be used to enhance surgical exposure. In cases of spondylosis, the intervertebral distractor is not used during ACD without fusion in order to avoid fracturing lateral bridging osteophytes

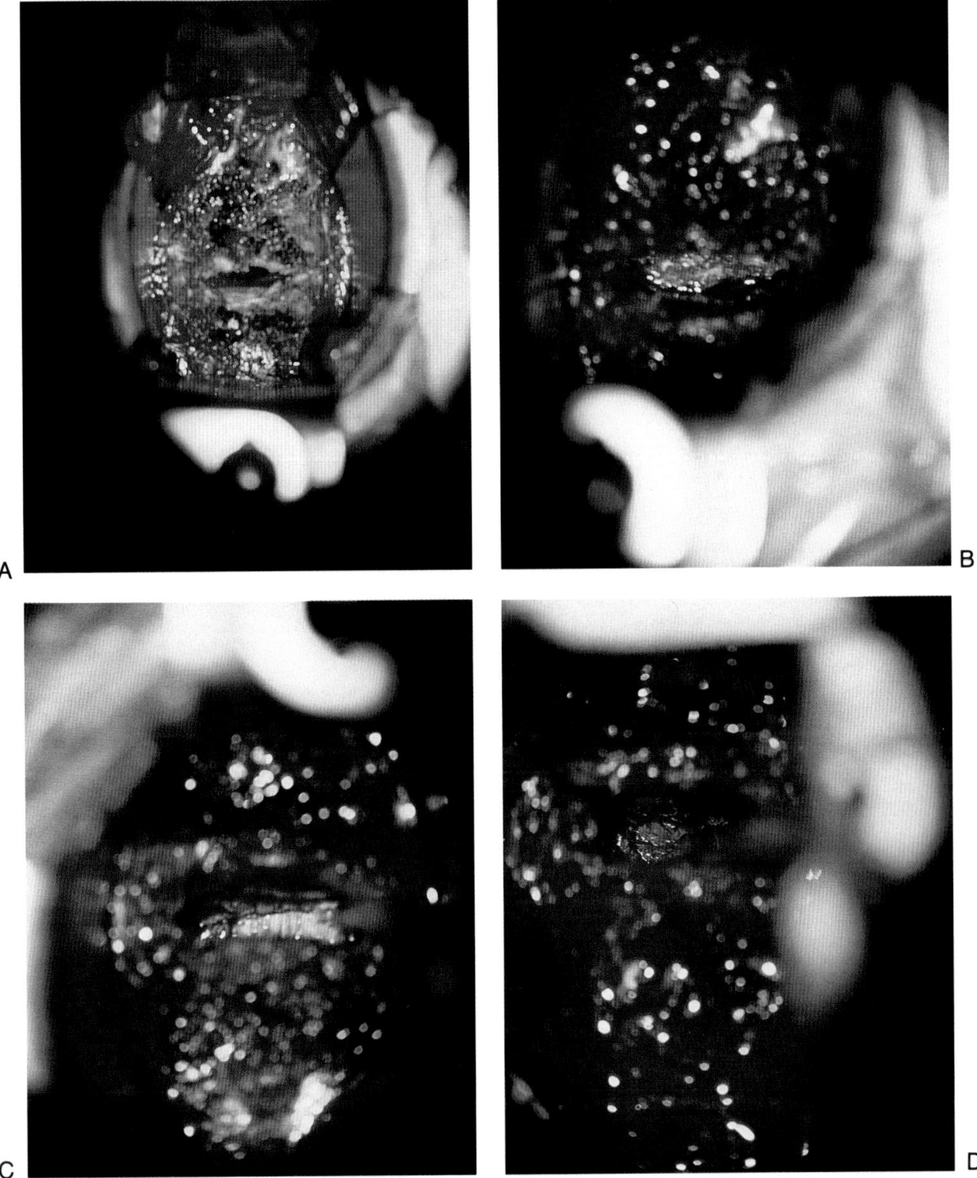

Figure 3. A: Surgical photo at low-power magnification taken through the operating microscope shows incision through ligament and anulus before total discectomy and debridement of rostral and caudal cartilaginous plates. Osteophytes remain where vertebral end plates touch anteriorly and posteriorly. **B:** The discectomy cavity, shown at higher magnification, has been deepened by resection of the marginal osteophytes and calcified anulus with the high-speed drill and curettes to expose the thickened and usually ossified posterior longitudinal ligament (*PLL*). **C:** After incision of the PLL, the ventral dura expands into the surgical defect. **D:** After decompression by lateral discectomy and resection of the PLL, osteophyte, and uncinate process, a clear view of the foramen is provided by rotating the operating table away from the surgeon and adjusting the microscope incline. Patency of the foramen is verified by visual inspection and palpation.

that might contribute to postoperative stability. To prevent postoperative pain due to stretching of the facet capsule during soft disc removal, distraction is limited to a few millimeters. Intervertebral distraction during decompression may provide the surgeon with a temporary and false sense of accomplishment, especially with respect to foramen patency. Therefore the neural canal and foramina should be palpated again after the distractor has been removed.

The neural canal and foraminal decompression are checked by palpation with the angled dissector. The rostral-caudal extent of neural canal decompression should be 10 to 12 mm, and the transverse diameter of decompression should be 16 to 24 mm (Fig. 4), depending on the transverse interpedicular distance and on the length and horizontal angle of the foramina. Estimates may be obtained from axial CT scans or MRI. In complex cases, an AP radiograph obtained after placement of contrast material or a metallic marker in the epidural space may help to verify the transverse extent and midline position of the decompression.

Several problems and potential pitfalls may arise during the course of microsurgical ACD, owing to the relatively limited intervertebral exposure needed to preserve spinal stability when a bone graft is not to be implanted. The angle of intradiscal exposure varies from 10 to 20 degrees caudad to the vertical plane. Thus the microscope must be aimed rostrally and the plane of dissection must be slanted. This may present a problem with deeper exposures in a patient with a large neck, especially at the C6–C7 level. Lowering the head of the operating table to place the patient in the Trendelenburg position may help by adjusting the disc space more toward the vertical plane. Tension on the transverse retractor by the trachea and esophagus or asymmetrical dissection and elevation of the longus colli muscles may displace the retractor off a midline or vertical orientation. This can result in a line of sight and dissection that slants from the patient's right anteriorly toward

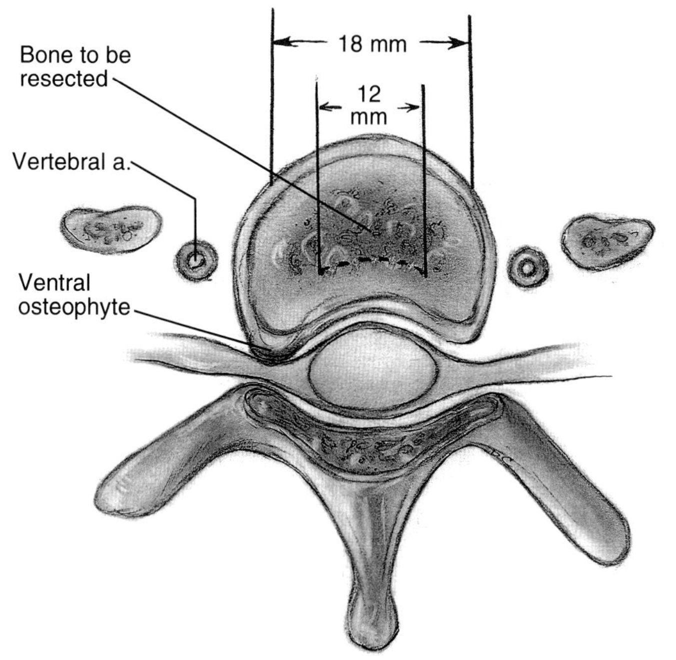

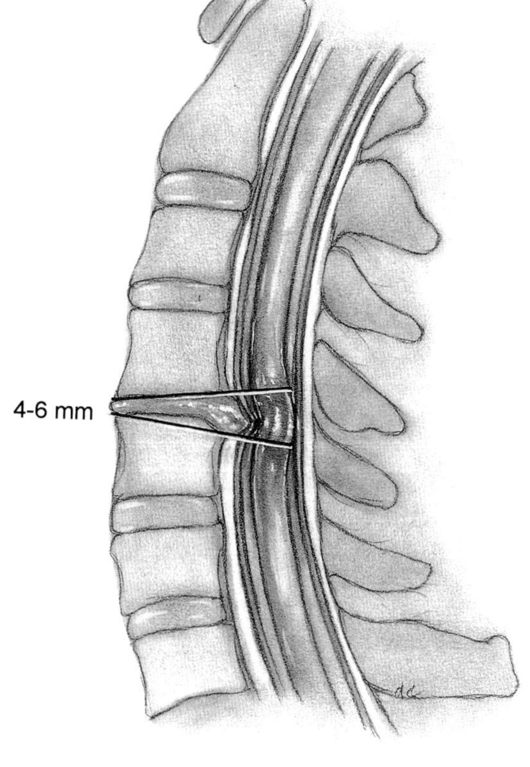

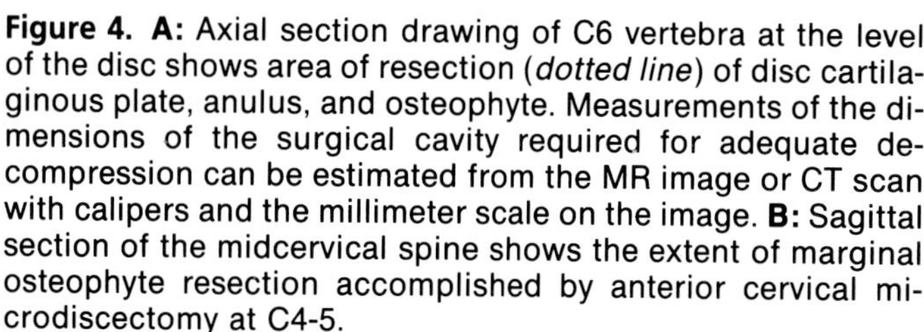
Figure 4. A: Axial section drawing of C6 vertebra at the level of the disc shows area of resection (*dotted line*) of disc cartilaginous plate, anulus, and osteophyte. Measurements of the dimensions of the surgical cavity required for adequate decompression can be estimated from the MR image or CT scan with calipers and the millimeter scale on the image. **B:** Sagittal section of the midcervical spine shows the extent of marginal osteophyte resection accomplished by anterior cervical microdiscectomy at C4-5.

the left posteriorly when the operation is performed from the right side. Inadequate or incomplete discectomy and foraminotomy on the right can be prevented in difficult cases by rotating the microscope binocular to the opposite side of the table or by using a diploscope to complete the right-side decompression from the patient's left side.

Excessive bleeding from bone can usually be controlled by applying thrombin-soaked Gelfoam, Avitene or, as a last resort, because it inhibits arthrodesis, bone wax. Venous bleeding from the PLL or epidural venous plexus can be controlled by bipolar cautery with microbayonet forceps at low current levels under irrigation. Arterial bleeding from the foramen is usually caused by avulsion of an osseous or radicular branch of the vertebral artery, which must be controlled with bipolar cautery or by gentle tamponade with Gelfoam packed loosely to avoid nerve root injury. Massive hemorrhage from a vertebral artery injury can occur, usually as a result of arteriosclerotic ectasia of the artery or an anatomical variation that results in medial displacement of the foramen transversarium. Both of these conditions can be anticipated and avoided by careful review of the axial CT scans or MR images.

Cerebrospinal fluid (CSF) leakage from a meningeal laceration usually ceases spontaneously after the subarachnoid space has collapsed. The opening can be covered with a piece of muscle or fat and sealed with a collagen sponge that serves as a tissue adhesive or with a Gelfoam pledget. Suture repair is rarely feasible. A lumbar subarachnoid drainage catheter may then be placed for 2 to 3 days postoperatively to avoid CSF fistula, especially in older patients with large CSF volumes or when the dural defect is large.

Finally, a narrow intervertebral exposure may render complete resection of large osteophytes difficult or impossible. Under such circumstances, the intervertebral space should be opened until adequate decompression is feasible, even if the plan to avoid bone graft fusion must then be abandoned to prevent postoperative spinal instability.

POSTOPERATIVE MANAGEMENT

Postoperative care includes routine observation for airway obstruction due to edema or hemorrhage. Upper airway problems, such as dryness or obstruction from secretions, may be alleviated with vaporized oxygen or a mist air mask. Regular neurological observation is necessary to detect new neurological deficit that could reflect epidural hematoma. If dysphagia is present after surgery, the diet is advanced slowly from liquids to soft foods. For comfort and to prevent excessive mobility and facilitate spontaneous intervertebral fusion, a hard collar is used for 4 to 6 weeks after surgery.

Patients are routinely discharged from the hospital on the first to third postoperative day, the hospital course having been shortened by the absence of iliac incision pain at the bone graft donor site. Return to sedentary occupational activity is expected within 10 to 14 days after surgery; return to strenuous physical labor or recreational and athletic activity ranges from 6 weeks to 3 months.

Routine postoperative follow-up visits are scheduled at 7 to 10 days, 6 weeks, and 3 months. Lateral cervical spine flexion-extension radiographs are obtained at 6 to 12 weeks to determine if fibrous union or spontaneous arthrodesis is complete.

In rare cases, a new pattern of segmental cervical and shoulder or upper brachial pain is present for 1 to 3 weeks after surgery. This may be due to ligamentous or capsular inflammation that results from collapse of the intervertebral space after discectomy.

Good or excellent results can be expected in 80% to 100% of operated cases (1,4,10). Patients with preoperative neurological deficit usually recover from radiculopathy within several hours or weeks, depending on the severity and duration of the preoperative deficit. Myelopathy may resolve more slowly, over 3 to 12 months after surgery. In some cases, progression of preoperative deterioration is arrested without measurable neurological improvement.

COMPLICATIONS

Complications of anterior cervical surgery include carotid artery, recurrent laryngeal nerve, and esophageal injury. The most troublesome neurological compli-

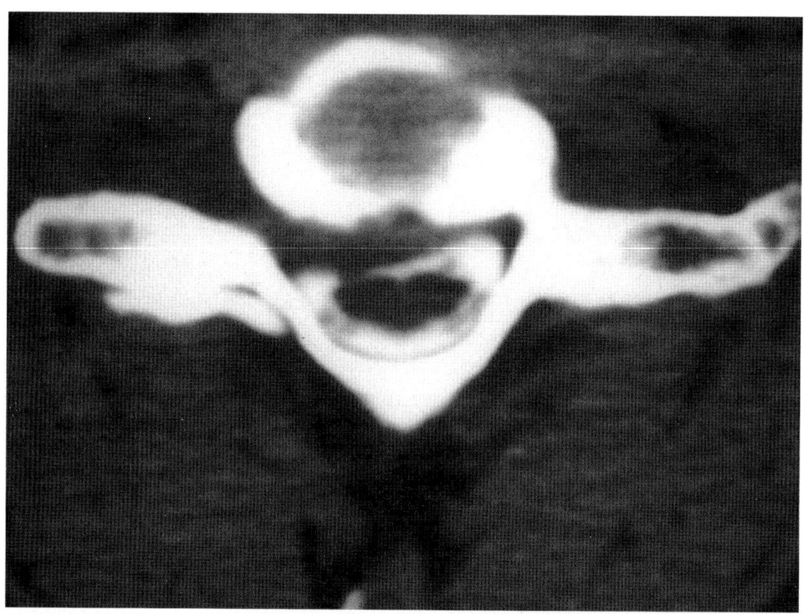

A

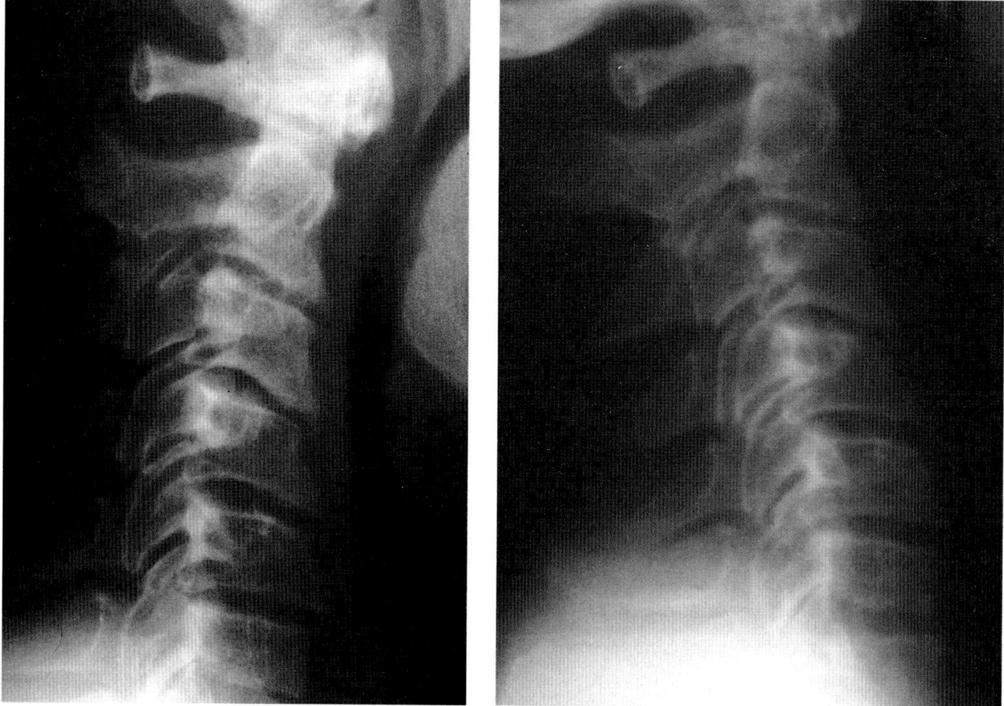

B C

Figure 5. A: Axial section from preoperative CT myelogram shows disc herniation at the C6–C7 level. **B,C:** Lateral flexion-extension radiographs of the cervical spine obtained 8 weeks after C6–C7 anterior cervical microdiscectomy without fusion demonstrate a stable motion segment after spontaneous arthrodesis. No evidence is seen of further disc space collapse or kyphotic angulation.

cation is radiculopathy or myelopathy due to surgical injury to the nerve root or spinal cord. This can usually be avoided by meticulous microsurgical technique. For example, drill bits must be irrigated constantly to prevent heating and thermal injury to adjacent neural structures. Rongeurs larger than the 2-mm Kerrison or angled curettes larger than size 3–0 should never be inserted into the foramen or neural canal unless a space large enough to accommodate the instrument has already been cleared.

Complications specifically related to discectomy without fusion include delayed onset of new neurological deficit or pain due to collapse or instability causing spondylolisthesis or kyphosis. Symptomatic postoperative foramen stenosis usually occurs on the side opposite the predominant preoperative lesion. Therefore even if only one side is symptomatic preoperatively, bilateral foraminotomies are necessary, as some settling will occur after discectomy. Reoperation for additional

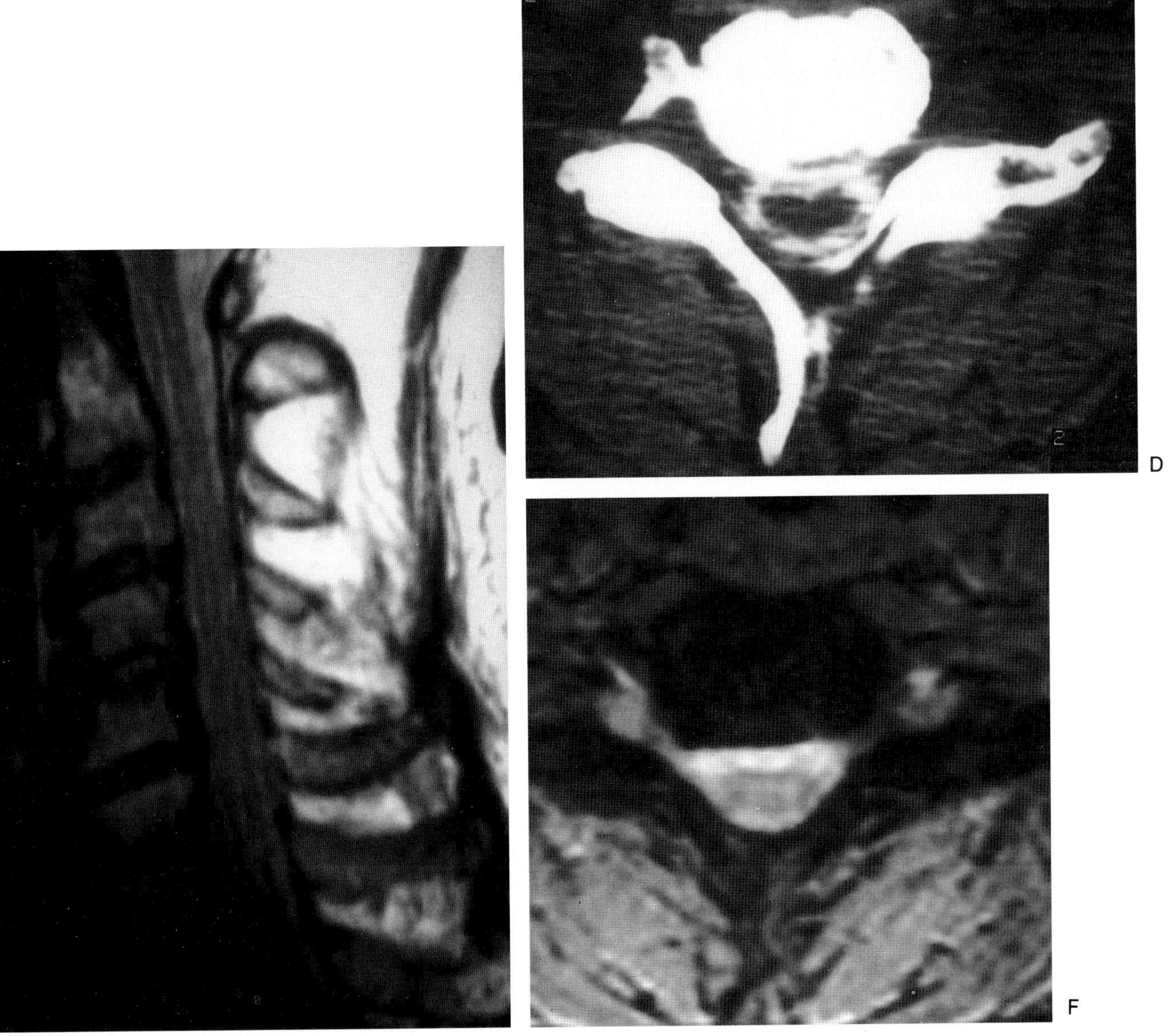

Figure 5. (*Continued.*) **D:** Axial CT myelogram in the same patient 2 years after discectomy shows no evidence of residual or recurrent disc herniation or spondylosis at C6–C7. **E,F:** However, axial sections from sagittal (E) and axial (F) MR images demonstrate uncinate hypertrophy and a broad-based osteophyte at C4–C5.

decompression and distraction by fusion may be required in severe cases of persistent radiculopathy.

Infection may occur, causing intervertebral, epidural, or retropharyngeal abscess. In such cases, an esophagogram may be indicated to rule out esophageal fistula. Reoperation is usually required to debride and drain the abscess, although patients without evidence of progressive neurological deficit may be managed by needle aspiration, culture, and antibiotic therapy.

ILLUSTRATIVE CASE FOR TECHNIQUE

A 42-year-old man presented with intractable right arm pain and C7 sensory radiculopathy without motor deficit (Fig. 5A) Computed tomography myelography showed a disc herniation at the C6–C7 level. ACD without fusion was performed. Radiography obtained 8 weeks after surgery demonstrated stable motion segments after spontaneous arthrodesis (Fig. 5B,C). The patient returned 2 years after discectomy with recurrent symptoms of neck and arm pain with numbness. Axial CT scans showed no evidence of residual or recurrent disc herniation or spondylosis at C6–C7 (Fig. 5D). Although new discogenic spondylosis was found at C4–C5 to explain recurrent symptoms, no abnormalities were demonstrated at C5–C6 or C7–T1, immediately above and below the previously operated level. Axial sections at C4–C5 from sagittal and axial MR images (Fig. 5E,F) showed hypertrophy of the uncinate process and a broad-based osteophyte consistent with a history of progressive recurrence of neck and positional upper arm pain as well as bilateral numbness in the C5 distribution. ACD without fusion at C4–C5 relieved all symptoms and signs.

RECOMMENDED READING

1. Bertalanffy, H., and Eggert, H. R.: Clinical long-term results of anterior discectomy without fusion for treatment of cervical radiculopathy and myelopathy. A follow-up of 164 cases. *Acta Neurochir. (Wien)*, 90: 127–135, 1988.
2. Bollati, A., Galli, G., Gandolfini, M., Marini, G., and Gatta, G.: Microsurgical anterior cervical disk removal without interbody infusion. *Surg. Neurol.*, 19: 329–333, 1983.
3. Cuatico, W.: Anterior cervical discectomy without interbody fusion: an analysis of 81 cases. *Acta Neurochir. (Wien)*, 57: 269–274, 1981.
4. Grisoli, F., Graziani, N., Fabrizi, A. P., Peragut J. C., Vincentelli, F., and Diaz-Vasquez, P.: Anterior discectomy without fusion for treatment of cervical lateral soft disc extrusion: a follow-up of 120 cases. *Neurosurgery*, 24: 853–859, 1989.
5. Hankinson, H. L., and Wilson, C. B.: Use of the operating microscope in anterior cervical discectomy without fusion. *J. Neurosurg.*, 43: 452–456, 1975.
6. Robertson, J. T., and Johnson, S. D.: Anterior cervical discectomy without fusion: long-term results. *Clin. Neurosurg.*, 27: 440–449, 1980.
7. Rosenörn, J., Hansen, E. B., and Rosenörn, M. -A.: Anterior cervical discectomy with and without fusion. *J. Neurosurg.*, 59: 252–255, 1983.
8. Van de Kelft, E., van Vyve, M., and Selosse, P.: Postsurgical follow-up by MRI of anterior cervical discectomy without fusion. *Eur. J. Radiol.*, 15: 196–199, 1992.
9. Wilson, D. H., and Campbell, D. D.: Anterior cervical discectomy without bone graft. Report of 71 cases. *J. Neurosurg.*, 47: 551–555, 1977.
10. Yamamoto, I., Ikeda, A., Shibuya, N., Tsugane, R., and Sato, O.: Clinical long-term results of anterior discectomy without interbody fusion for cervical disc disease. *Spine*, 16: 272–279, 1991.

Master Techniques in Orthopaedic Surgery,
THE SPINE, edited by D. S. Bradford,
Lippincott-Raven Publishers, Philadelphia, © 1997.

4

Cervical Vertebrectomy

Rick B. Delamarter

INDICATIONS/CONTRAINDICATIONS

The primary indication for cervical vertebrectomy is spinal cord and cervical nerve root compression. Spinal cord or nerve root compression can be caused by degenerative disc disease (including herniated disc and osteophyte formation), ossification of the posterior longitudinal ligament (OPLL), fracture/subluxation leading to bony or disc compression on the neural structures, tumors (including benign, malignant, and metastatic types), infections with bony involvement or epidural abscess formation, and cervical deformity (usually kyphosis) leading to cord compression. Contraindications include tracheal-esophageal trauma that would not allow safe exposure of the anterior cervical spine and severe osteoporosis that could lead to kyphotic and/or graft collapse.

PREOPERATIVE PLANNING

Patients considered for cervical vertebrectomy require careful preoperative evaluation, including a detailed physical examination with a careful neurologic assessment, noting radicular signs and symptoms or myelopathy. Evaluation of head position on the thorax is important, particularly with cervical deformity, and assessment of range of motion is critical, especially neck extension, since this maneuver may increase spinal cord compression during intubation and during the intraoperative period. Radiographic evaluation must include plain roentgenograms, including flexion-extension views, and may require a long spine film, including the head and thorax, particularly in patients with kyphotic deformity.

Assessment of neural compression may include magnetic resonance imaging (MRI) and a computed tomography (CT) scan with myelographic enhancement.

R. B. Delamarter, M.D.: UCLA Comprehensive Spine Center; and Department of Orthopaedic Surgery, University of California Los Angeles Medical Center, Los Angeles, California 90024.

Magnetic resonance imaging provides excellent evaluation of the neural structures and the soft tissues, including soft disc herniations, but is limited in bony visualization, particularly with osteophytic formation and OPLL. Computed tomography scanning following a myelogram provides excellent visualization of the bony structures, as well as nerve root and spinal cord impingement.

Evaluation of the vascular structures, primarily the vertebral arteries, in cases of tumor involvement of the vertebral bodies or spinal cord, may require a preoperative angiogram. In some cervical tumors requiring anterior vertebrectomy, preoperative embolization of a vascular tumor and/or preoperative occlusion of the vertebral artery may be utilized. Occasionally electrical studies may prove valuable in neurologic assessment, including electromyograms, nerve conduction velocities, and somatosensory evoked potential evaluation. Preoperative traction via Gardner-Wells tongs or a halo ring may be necessary for reduction of cervical fracture subluxations and cervical kyphotic deformities (postlaminectomy kyphosis). Preoperative planning for cervical vertebrectomy always requires determination of the appropriate type and size of bone graft for vertebral body replacement. In general, I utilize autologous iliac crest for one- and two-level vertebrectomies; if more than two vertebral bodies must be removed, a fibular strut is recommended. As a rule of thumb, I always utilize the patient's own bone, either iliac crest or fibular graft; with careful surgical technique, bone donor site problems are minimal. Many surgeons use allograft fibular strut or iliac crest grafts for anterior cervical surgery. The literature suggests that allograft bone in anterior cervical surgery has an acceptable rate of fusion, although the time for bony incorporation is longer, the infection rate is slightly higher, and several reports exist of human immunodeficiency virus transmission from allograft bone. The final item in preoperative planning is fitting the patient for a postoperative orthosis (i.e., soft collar, Philadelphia collar, Minerva orthosis, and/or halo apparatus).

SURGERY

Positioning

Patients are positioned in the prone position, with the arms tucked to the sides. Positioning of the neck and head during intubation and operation is of paramount importance in any cervical decompressive surgery. When a patient is under anesthesia or under the influence of muscular relaxing agents, the inherent protective mechanisms are absent, and neck extension or excessive traction may cause permanent spinal cord and/or nerve root damage. Awake nasotracheal intubation or fiberoptic intubation is utilized in many patients.

Patients require some type of intraoperative traction. For single-level vertebrectomies, a head halter traction may be satisfactory. With multilevel vertebrectomies, I utilize Gardner-Wells tongs. If the patient will require a halo apparatus postoperatively, the halo may be placed following intubation and used for intraoperative traction; the halo vest may be placed at the conclusion of the case. Intraoperative traction of 7 to 10 pounds helps to stabilize the head and spine, and traction can be easily increased intraoperatively for slight distraction during placement of the strut graft. The shoulders may be taped down with mild caudad traction to allow radiographic evaluation using either plain films or fluoroscopy (of the C6, C7, and T1 levels).

If iliac crest graft is to be utilized, a small bump is placed underneath the iliac crest. If fibular strut graft is to be utilized, the lower leg is prepped in the usual fashion, with placement of a thigh-high tourniquet. Both the neck and bone graft site are prepped and draped in the usual fashion. A surgical microscope is placed on either the right or left upper corner of the table. The high-speed air drill utilized for bony removal is placed at the foot end of the table, on the side opposite the scrub nurse.

Surgical Approach

A transverse incision is generally preferred because of superior cosmetic results (Fig. 1). With adequate fascial release, one can easily expose up to four vertebral bodies. A longitudinal incision may be useful when more than four cervical verte-

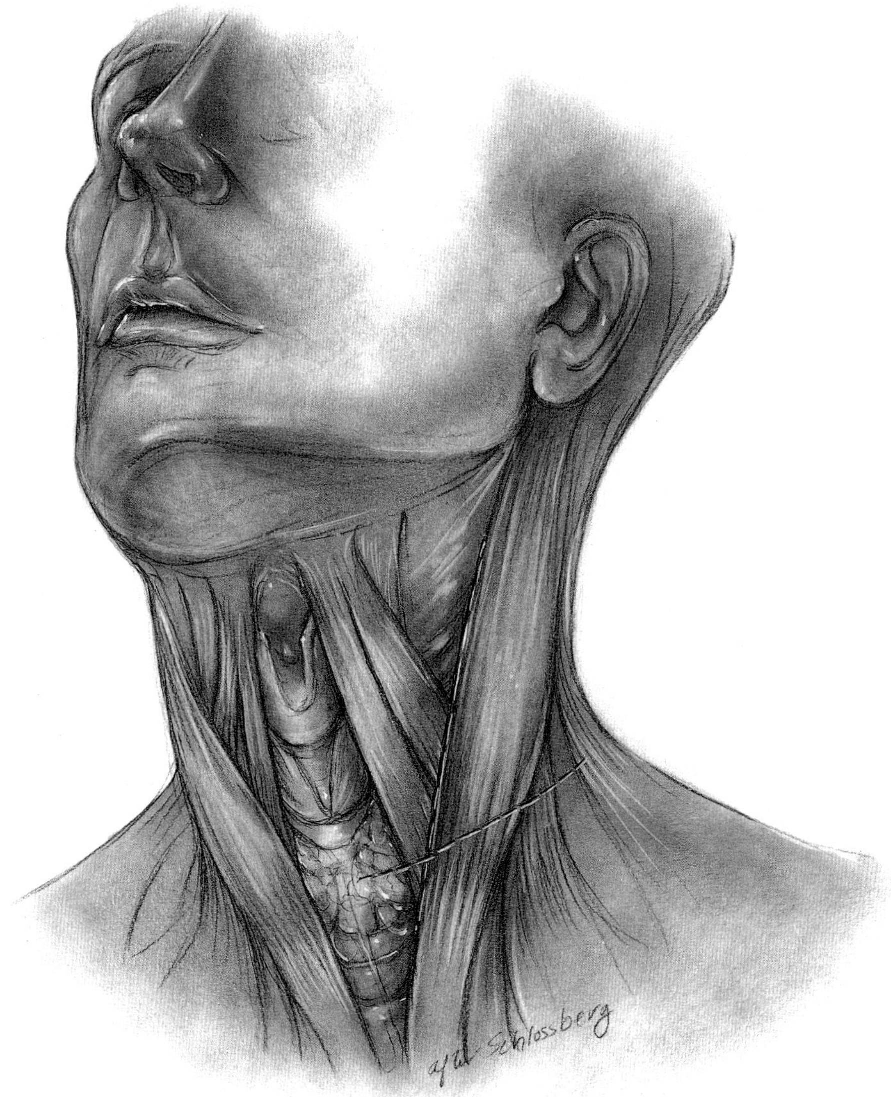

A

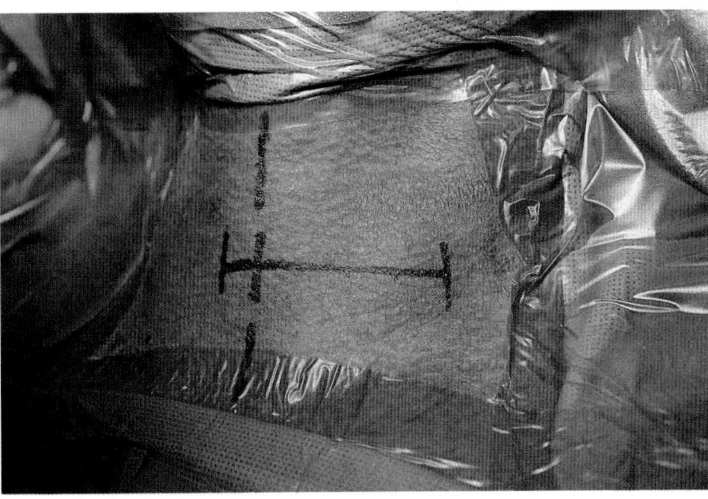

B

Figure 1. **A:** Transverse skin incision used for anterior cervical exposure for cervical vertebrectomy. The *dotted line* shows the midline of the cervical spine; the transverse incision begins about 1 cm right of midline and extends over to the left sternocleidomastoid musculature. **B:** Transverse skin incision (*solid line*) as well as the alternative vertical incision along the medial border of the sternocleidomastoid muscle (*dotted line*).

bral bodies need to be exposed. I prefer to expose the anterior cervical structures through an incision based on the left side of the neck because of the more consistent position of the recurrent laryngeal nerve on the left than on the right. After exposure of the cervical spine from the left side, one can easily work from either the right or left sides.

For a single level vertebrectomy, a 4- to 5-cm incision is made, beginning at the midline and extending over toward the sternocleidomastoid muscle (Fig. 2). For a two-, three-, or four-level vertebrectomy, the skin incision is extended across the midline and to the lateral border of the sternocleidomastoid muscle. The level of the transverse position may be determined by a preoperative lateral roentgenogram of the neck, determining the distance of the vertebrectomy segment superior to the clavicle. In general, the cricoid cartilage represents the C5–C6 level and the thyroid cartilage the C4–C5 level. I more commonly utilize the distance above the sternal notch (i.e., two fingerbreadths above the sternal notch C6–C7, three fingerbreadths above the sternal notch C5–C6, four fingerbreadths above the sternal notch C4–C5, etc.).

Following skin incision and sharp dissection through the subcutaneous fat, the platysma muscle, which may be only a whisper of muscular fibers (especially in females), is sharply incised in the line of the transverse incision. The medial border of the sternocleidomastoid muscle should be visible at this point (Fig. 3). The thin fascial fibers below the platysma are then grasped with forceps and separated with the Metzenbaum scissors. The large anterior jugular vein generally is found below this fascia and can be tied off at this point. The fascia enveloping the sternocleidomastoid muscle is then released with the Metzenbaum scissors, both cephalad and caudad. This release of sternocleidomastoid fascia is the critical maneuver allowing extensile exposure of the cervical spine. The carotid sheath is then palpated with the index finger, and in the interval medial to the carotid sheath, the spine is easily palpated. A hand-held Cloward or Army-Navy retractor is then inserted to hold the medial structures, including the trachea, esophagus, and thyroid. The pretracheal fascia is split bluntly with a Kidner dissector, and the anterior surface of the spine is easily visualized. The prevertebral fascia can be split with the Kidner dissector or sharply with Metzenbaum scissors. The vertebral bodies, anterior longitudinal ligament, and longus colli muscles are at this point clearly visible.

At this point, I generally take a radiograph with a spinal needle in a particular disc space. Once the level is identified, the appropriate level or levels can be

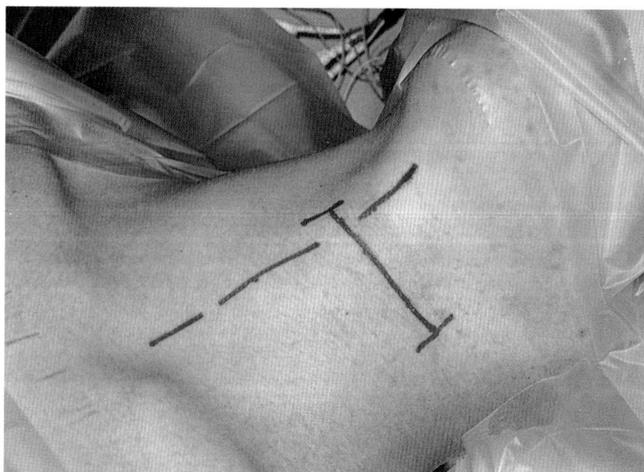

Figure 2. A second photo of the transverse cervical incision, beginning 1 cm right of midline and extending over to the sternocleidomastoid musculature. The dotted line shows the midline of the cervical spine.

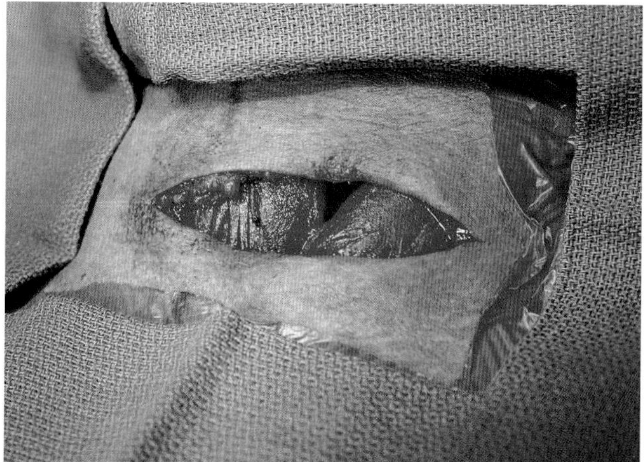

Figure 3. An anterior cervical incision exposes the sternocleidomastoid musculature and the strap muscles and also reveals the interval between these two structures. The skin and the platysma have been cut.

mobilized with elevation of the longus colli muscle on both sides of the spine out to the lateral borders of the vertebral bodies; even part of the transverse processes can be exposed. Elevation of the longus colli muscle can be easily accomplished with a small Freer dissector and bipolar cautery. Care is taken to remain under the longus colli muscle, since aggressive retraction on top of it may jeopardize the sympathetic chain. When obtaining exposure of the sixth and seventh cervical vertebral bodies, the superior thyroid artery and vein will cross the vertebral bodies and may be ligated and divided; simple retraction will often allow adequate exposure. The digastric and stylohyoid muscles generally may be simply retracted but occasionally may need division, particularly for exposure in the upper cervical spine. When exposing the second and third cervical segments, the hypoglossal and superior laryngeal nerves cross the plane of dissection and care must be taken in gentle retraction of these structures.

Once the longus colli muscles have been elevated, the deep retractors may be placed, first placing the mediolateral retractors directly underneath the longus colli muscles (Figs. 4 and 5). In general, I use smooth-tipped retractors, both medially and laterally, since sharp-toothed retractors can perforate the esophagus medially and the carotid sheath laterally. The cephalad caudad retractor deep blades are then placed, again utilizing the smooth-tipped blades. If at this point the exposure does not allow adequate visualization of all the cervical segments that require decompression, the retractors may be removed, further fascia released, particularly the fascia around the sternocleidomastoid muscle, and the surgically exposed soft tissue spread bluntly. One will also find that the retractors, over time, will be able to expand the area of visualization as they stretch the soft tissue. With this exposure, one can easily perform vertebrectomies from the C2 cervical segment to the first thoracic segment. At this time I bring in the microscope for thc decompressive procedure.

Before removing any disc or bone, it is of paramount importance to locate the lateral borders of the vertebral bodies to help understand the anatomy of the vertebral artery. In the degenerative arthritic spine, the lateral vertebral bodies may be palpated and visualized with a small Freer, Penfield, or curette in the middle aspect of the vertebral body. The surgeon may be misled by the anterior osteophytic lipping and significant osteophytic changes on the lateral aspect of the disc spaces. Mistaking a lateral vertebral osteophyte for the lateral vertebral body wall may result in removal of too much bone laterally and possible injury to the vertebral artery (4).

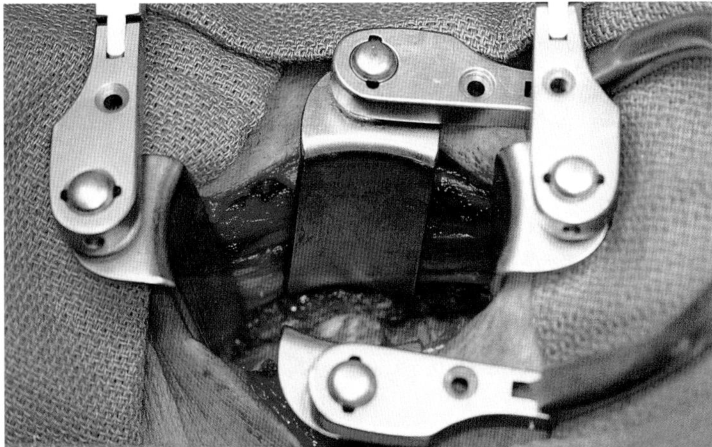

Figure 4. Retractor placement underneath the longus colli muscles in the mediolateral direction.

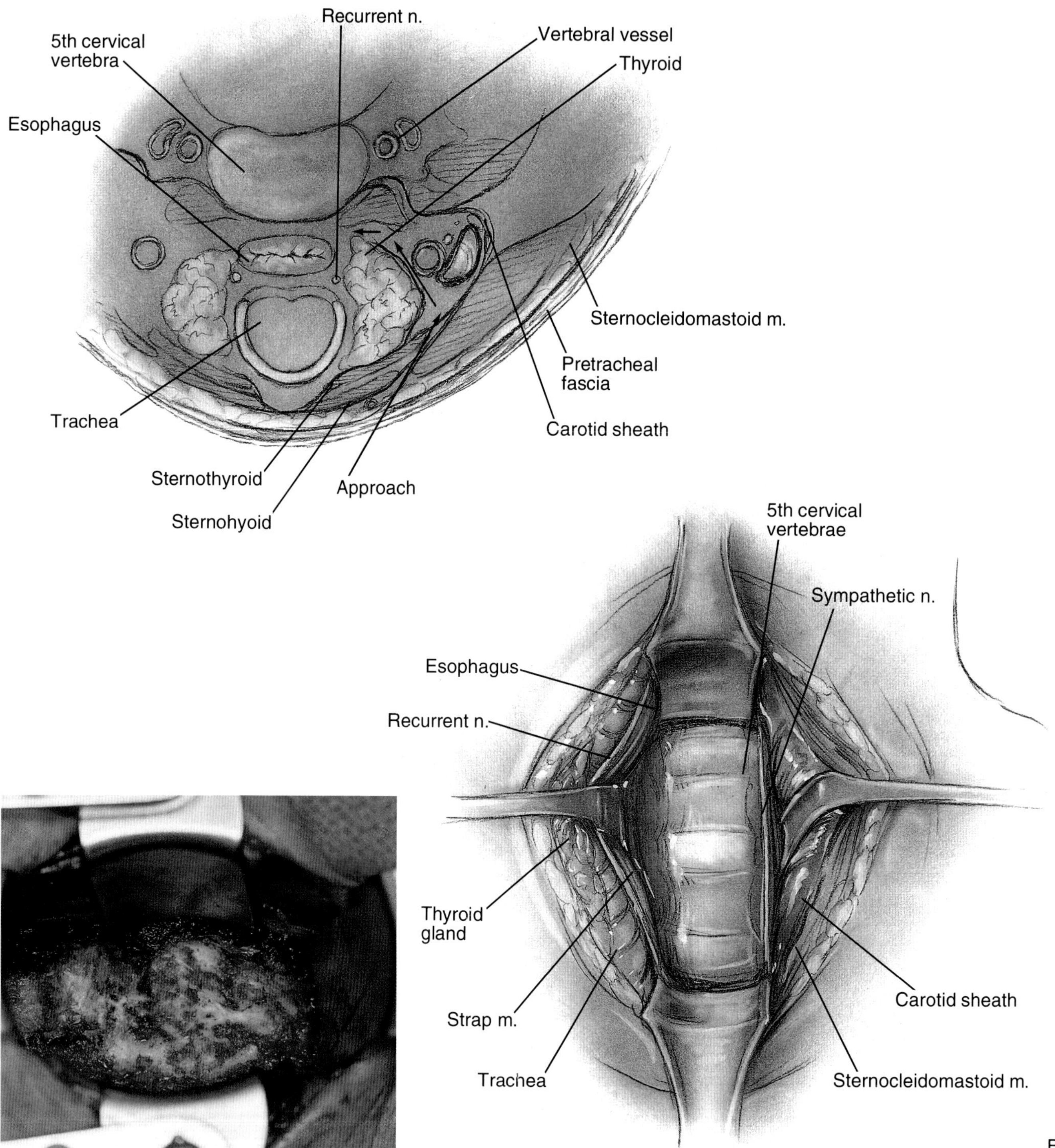

Figure 5. A: Retractors in position and the anterior cervical spine exposed. **B, Top:** Transverse view of the cervical spine through the fifth cervical vertebra. The *arrows* denote the anterior approach through the platysma, medial to the carotid sheath and lateral to the trachea, esophagus, and thyroid. **Bottom:** The view is similar to that of A and shows the complete exposure of the cervical spine with the retractors underneath the longus colli musculature.

For a single-level vertebrectomy, I begin by excising the discs above and below the vertebral body to be removed, as well as the posterior vertebral osteophytes at the interdiscal space, which allows one to find the back of the vertebral body. This allows visualization of the uncovertebral joints, helping the surgeon understand the lateral boundaries of decompression. Resection of the vertebral body is best accomplished with a high-speed bur (Fig. 6A). I prefer the Midas Rex AM-8 bur for outlining the lateral borders of decompression, and removing the cortical end plates and interdiscal osteophytes (Fig. 6B). Following disc and osteophyte removal, one may switch to a 1-cm bur, which allows safe and quick removal of the vertebral body back to the posterior vertebral body cortex. As one begins the vertebrectomy, bleeding in cancellous bone can be controlled with small amounts of bone wax on a Penfield or Freer elevator. Once the cancellous bone has been removed back to the posterior vertebral body cortex, this thin posterior cortex may be removed with a small forward-angled curette, or, if the spinal canal is large enough, a 1- or 2-mm Kerrison rongeur may be used to bite away the remaining posterior vertebral body wall (Fig. 7A). The lateral vertebral body wall should be left intact, with a minimum of 5 mm and up to 10 mm of bone remaining of the vertebral body. The 1- or 2-mm Kerrison rongeur can be utilized to remove the lateral recess back to the pedicle. OPLL requires removal of the posterior ligament; the dura should be freed from the PPL with a small forward-angled

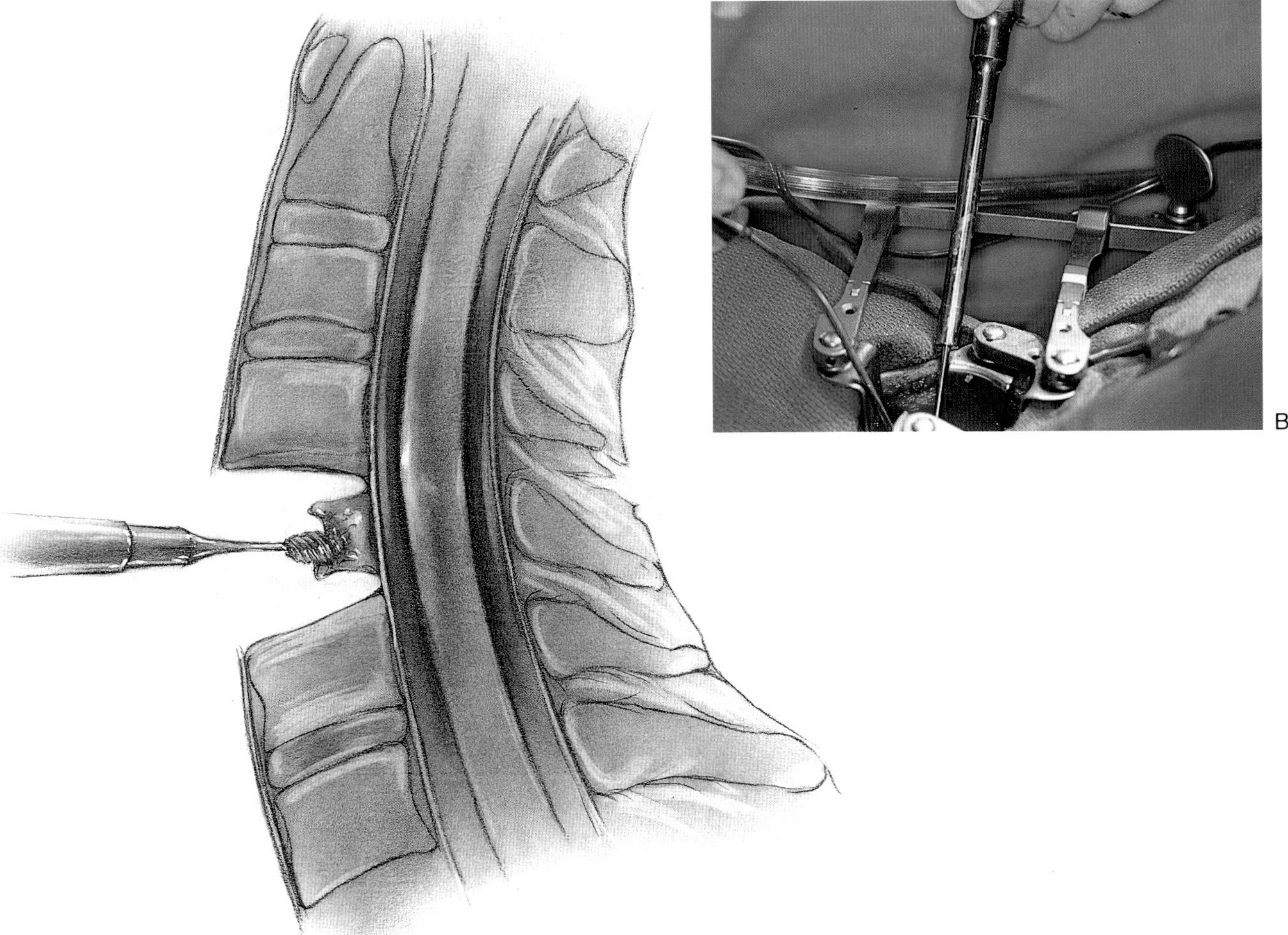

Figure 6. A: The vertebrectomy being completed by a high-speed bur. The discs above and below this vertebra have already been removed. **B:** Midas Rex drill used to accomplish bony removal for the vertebrectomy.

curette, since the dura may be adherent to the calcified PPL. I frequently use a small micro-skin hook to help retract the OPLL away from the spinal cord while freeing the adherent dura. The calcified ligament can then be removed with the small Kerrison rongeur.

Once the vertebrectomy has been completed and the spinal canal decompressed, simple anteroposterior (AP) and lateral radiographs with contrast agent in the vertebrectomy hole will help ensure adequacy of bony removal and appropriate alignment of the decompressive site (Fig. 8). After adequate decompression, the reconstruction is begun with creation in the upper and lower vertebral bodies of a small area of end-plate and vertebral body removal, from 2 to 4 mm in depth, leaving the cortical outer rim. One should be able to place the tip of the little finger in this indentation in the cortical ridge. A 4-mm ledge of bone is left posteriorly to protect the bone graft from migrating into the spinal canal. Determination of the size of the bone graft is done with either #18-gauge wire or microsurgical calipers, which are used to determine the distance between the two vertebral bodies, as well as the depth from the anterior cortical rim to the posterior cortical rim. This appropriately sized graft is then taken from the anterior iliac crest with the oscillating saw in a tricortical fashion (Fig. 9). The bone graft is then trimmed to the appropriate dimensions of the vertebrectomy site. This trimming of the bone graft can be done with the AM-8 bur or a small rongeur. The graft is held with a Kocher, additional traction up to 30 to 40 pounds is placed on the neck, and the graft is

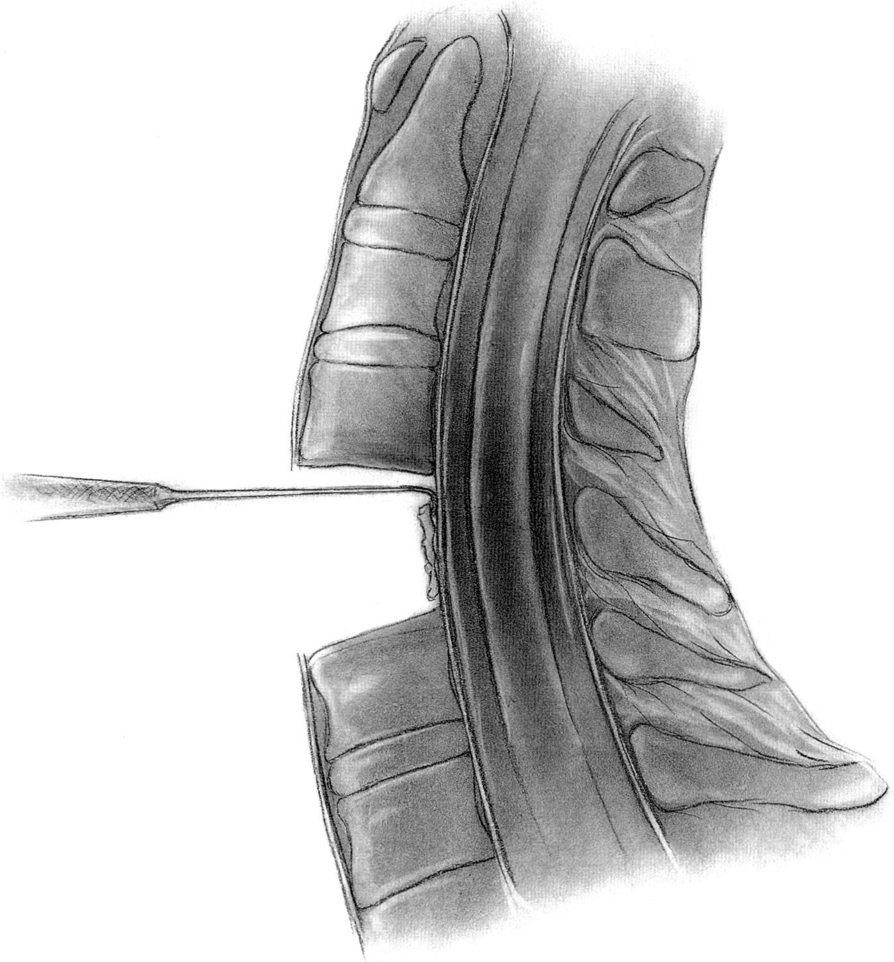

Figure 7. Vertebrectomy being completed: the last thin layer of vertebral body is removed with a small forward-angled curette. A 1- to 2-mm Kerrison rongeur may be used.

tapped into the upper vertebral body. With gentle tapping on the caudad part of the graft, it is countersunk into the concavity of the bottom vertebra and traction is released. The graft should be stable at this point (Fig. 10).

If all the posterior elements are intact and no preoperative instability was present, in many single-level vertebrectomies no further stabilization is necessary and the vertebral reconstruction may heal in a simple rigid neck brace. In many in-

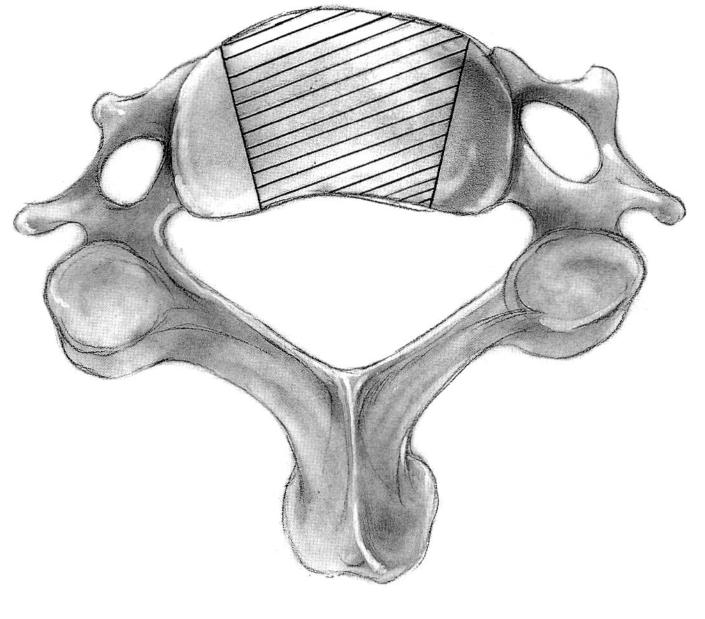

A

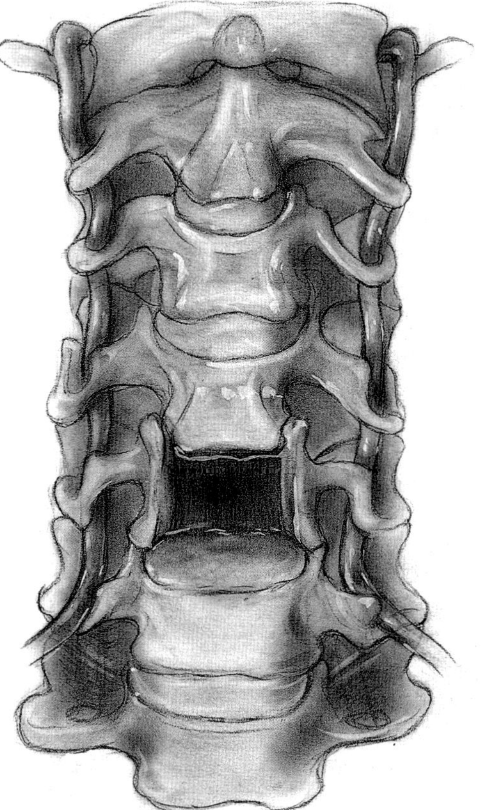

B

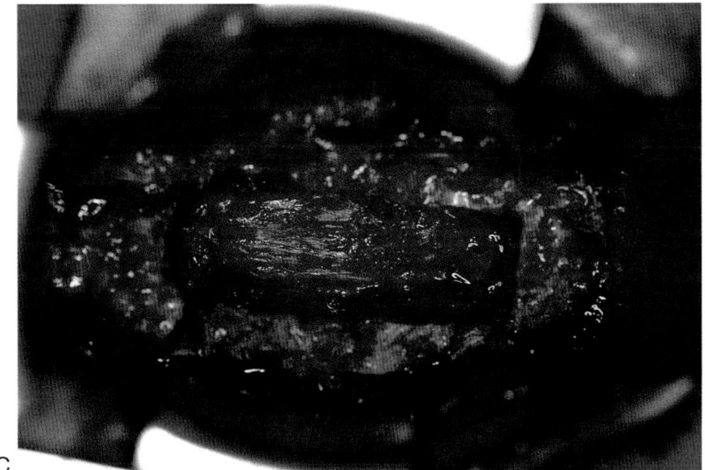

C

Figure 8. A: Transverse view of the C5 vertebral body showing the area to be removed (*shaded area*) in a standard vertebrectomy. Care is taken to leave a small wafer of bone medial to the vertebral artery. **B:** Anterior view of the C5 completed vertebrectomy. **C:** Intraoperative view of completed vertebrectomy. Note the remaining size of the vertebral body as well as the exposed spinal cord in the depth of the incision.

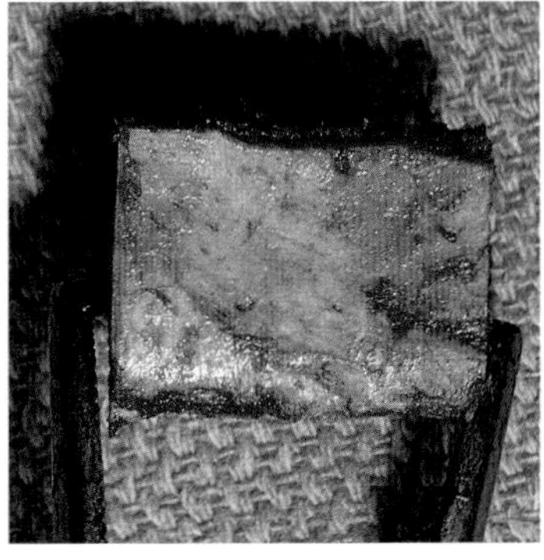

Figure 9. Tricortical strut graft taken from the iliac crest.

stances, when preoperative instability exists from fracture-subluxations, posttraumatic kyphosis, or posterior element instability, I use an anterior plate for further stabilization (Fig. 11). A variety of plates have been designed for improved stability and anterior fixation, but I presently prefer the AO titanium locking screw plate system (1,2,6,7). This allows rigid fixation and does not require the purchase of the posterior wall of the vertebra (3,5).

Anterior Cervical Plate Fixation

Following placement of the vertebral body strut graft, the appropriately sized plate is selected and placed on the cervical spine, primarily to determine the upper

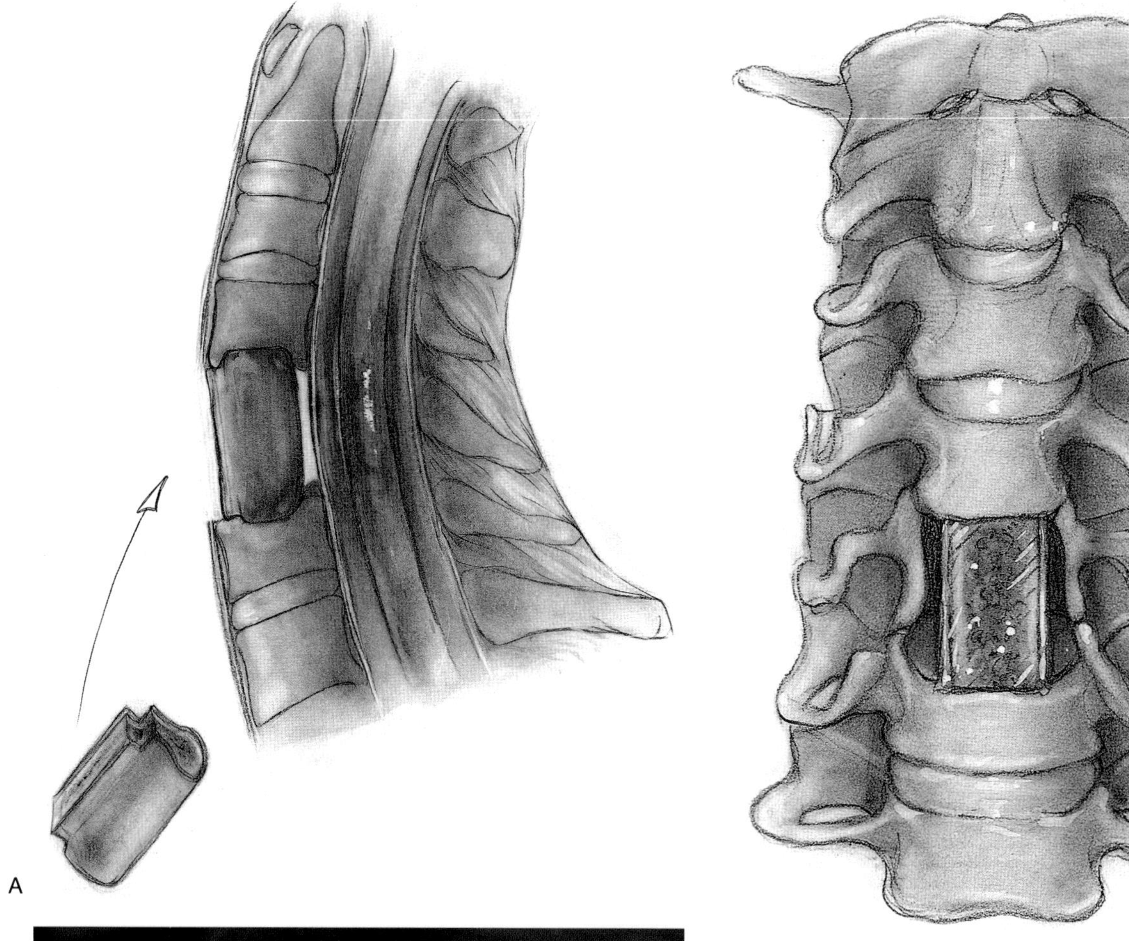

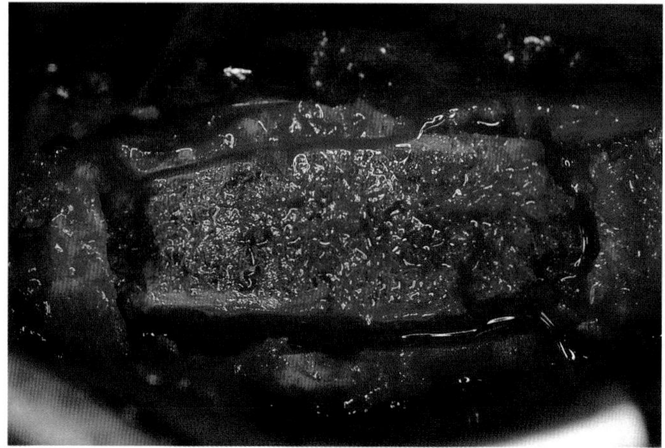

Figure 10. A: Tricortical strut graft from the iliac crest locked into position in the upper and lower vertebra. Note the beveling at both ends of the iliac crest graft, which allows the graft to be locked into the upper and lower vertebrae. **B:** Anterior view of the completed vertebrectomy with the iliac crest strut graft locked into position. **C:** Iliac crest strut graft in place, locked into position in the upper and lower vertebral bodies.

and lower aspects of the plate, since they should not interfere with the disc space above and below the construct. In cases of significant osteophyte formation at the discs above and below the construct, a radiograph should be taken to visualize the extent of the plate. The plate must be kept directly in midline. This is easily accomplished by visualizing the lateral edges of the middle aspect of the vertebral body and not utilizing the lateral disc space area, since the osteophytes at the disc space level may mislead the surgeon as to orientation of the plate. The plate is then held in proper position and the power drill is used to drill the two holes in the upper vertebral body with the stop guide to avoid penetration of the spinal canal (Fig. 12). The screw holes are then tapped and the solid titanium screws tightened into position and countersunk under the anterior lip of the plate (Fig. 13). The two screws at the bottom of the plate are then drilled with the power

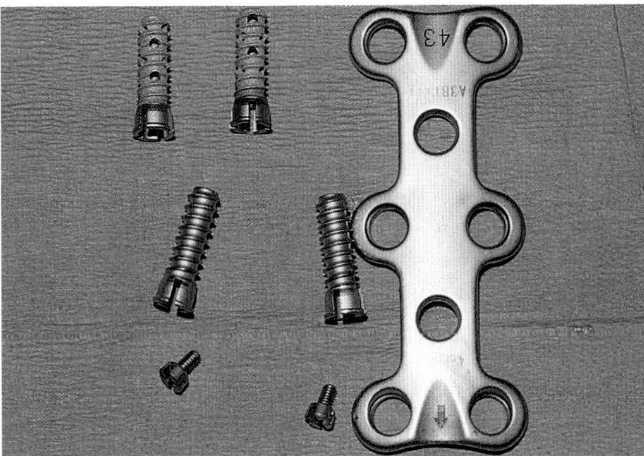

Figure 11. AO anterior cervical plate and screws. The bottom screws are fenestrated titanium (which are no longer used due to breakage through the fenestrations). The middle screws are the most commonly used 14-mm titanium screws. The top small set screws interlock and lock the screws into the plate.

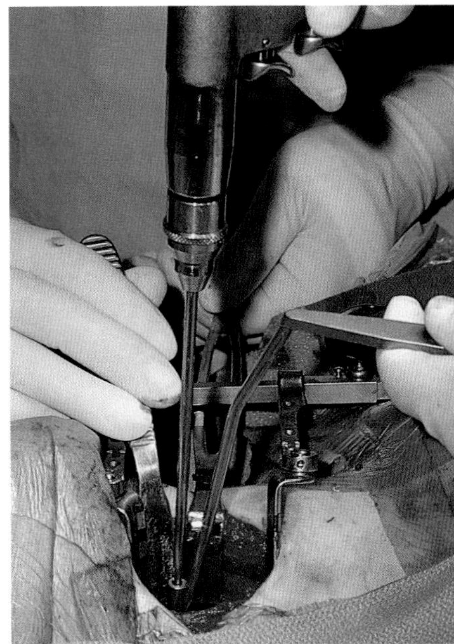

Figure 12. Intraoperative photograph of the drill used to drill through the plate into the vertebral bodies.

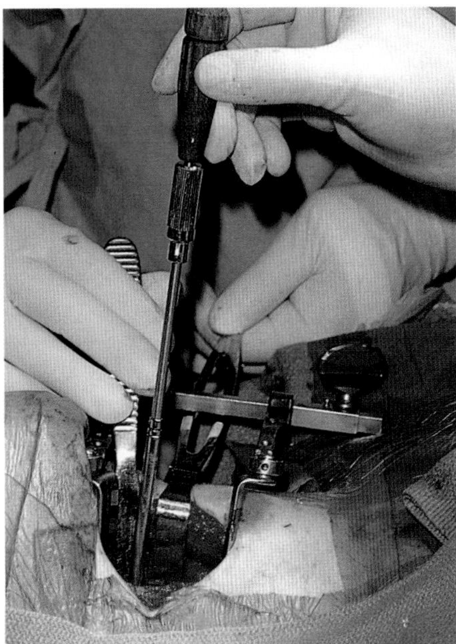

Figure 13. Intraoperative photograph of the tap. All screw holes are tapped following drilling.

drill and tapped in an identical fashion, and solid titanium screws are placed and countersunk (Fig. 14). A radiograph is taken and if alignment and position of the vertebral body reconstruction plate and screws are satisfactory, the small locking set screws are inserted into the larger vertebral body screws. The top locking set of screws actually expands the head of the large screw and locks it into the plate in an attempt to avoid screw loosening and migration. One or two screws may be placed in an identical fashion into the strut graft to secure its position (Fig. 15).

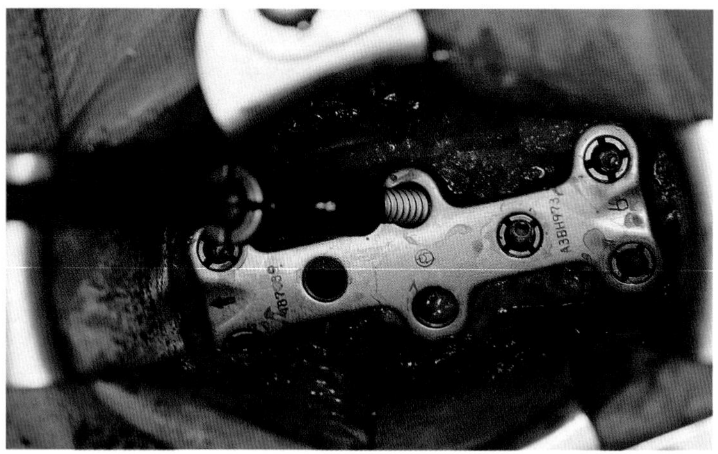

Figure 14. Intraoperative photograph of the screw in position and placement of a screw.

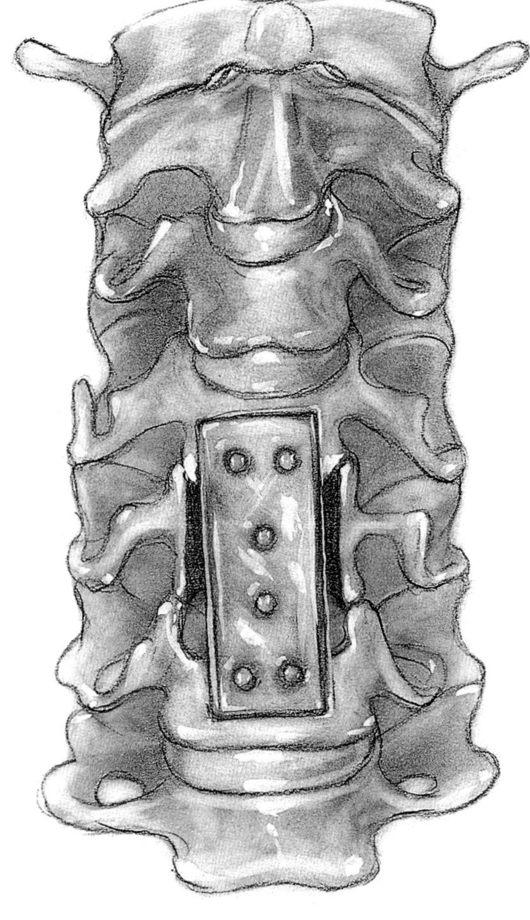

A

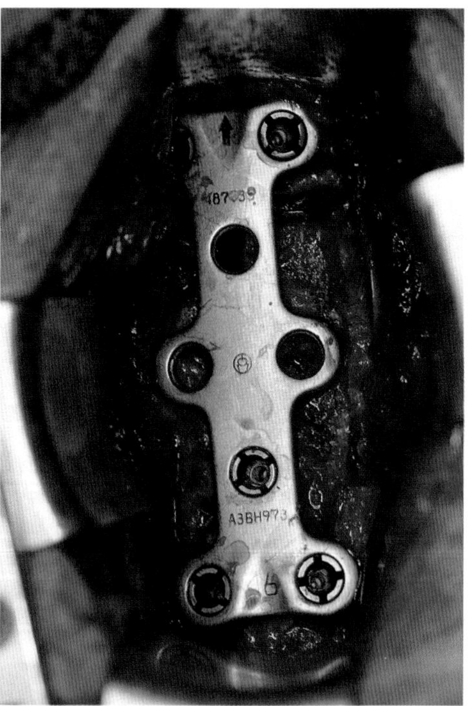

B

Figure 15. A: Anterior view of the completed cervical plating. The surgeon must be careful to keep the plate in midline because lateral placement of the plate and screws may jeopardize important structures such as the vertebral artery or exiting nerve root. **B:** Plate in position, all screws in place.

After thorough irrigation of the surgical area, the retractors are removed. The anterior structures of the neck, including the trachea, esophagus, thyroid, and carotid sheath, are inspected, and the closure is begun over a small Silastic drain brought out through the incision.

The anterior neck closure can be accomplished by closure of the platysma and fascia with 3–0 Vicryl suture in an interrupted fashion, closure of the subcutaneous tissue with 4–0 Vicryl in an interrupted fashion, and then simple Steri-stripping of the skin.

Iliac Crest Versus Fibular Strut Graft

When doing a one- or two-level vertebrectomy, I routinely use iliac crest. When more than two vertebral bodies are removed, the iliac crest curvature makes it quite difficult to fashion the iliac crest in the appropriate vertebral body dimensions. Thus, when more than two vertebral bodies are removed, I utilize fibular strut grafting, which is taken from the middle third of the fibula. After harvesting the fibula, the ends are beveled accordingly to allow easy countersinking into the remaining vertebral bodies proximally and distally. The fibula is tapped into position in an identical fashion as the iliac crest graft with one of the flat triangular portions of the fibula placed directly posteriorly, recreating the normal posterior vertebral body wall anatomy.

When utilizing the iliac crest, the solid anterior cortex of the iliac crest tricortical graft is used as the posterior vertebral body wall; this may need to be fashioned with the AM-8 bur into a flat rather than curvilinear dimension. The anterior cervical plating can be accomplished with the fibular strut graft in a manner identical to that mentioned above, with the iliac crest graft.

POSTOPERATIVE MANAGEMENT

All patients who have a cervical vertebrectomy require some type of postoperative immobilization, in general from 8 to 12 weeks, depending on the length of the reconstruction. Following an anterior cervical plating of a cervical vertebrectomy, I place all patients in a semirigid Philadelphia collar for a minimum of 6 weeks, although one may consider using a halo apparatus if gross instability or severely osteoporotic bone exist. If a patient has had a subsequent posterior fusion following anterior cervical vertebrectomy, a semirigid Philadelphia collar is all that is necessary. If posterior surgery has not been performed or an anterior plate is not utilized and the patient remains unstable or has grossly osteoporotic bone following the cervical vertebrectomy, a halo apparatus may be utilized for up to 12 weeks and in multilevel vertebrectomies for up to 12 to 16 weeks. Elderly individuals with osteoporotic bone require additional protection.

The average cervical vertebrectomy patient requires 3 to 5 days of hospitalization, with removal of the drains as well as a clear liquid diet on the first postoperative day. Ambulation is started on the first postoperative day, although if a fibular strut graft is utilized, crutch ambulation may be beneficial during the first week. In the immediate postoperative period (postoperative days 1 through 3, careful neurologic follow-up is advisable as well as evaluation for a wound hematoma, which has the potential of obstructing breathing and swallowing. Swallowing can be difficult for the first 2 to 3 days following retraction of the esophagus and is generally due to inflammation and edema. Severe swallowing symptomatology due to edema may be treated with a short course of steroids. Cervical wound hematomas are rare, but if breathing difficulties occur, a simple procedure of opening the incision and draining the hematoma provides rapid relief of symptoms.

The iliac crest bone graft site is injected prior to closure with 0.5% Marcaine, and an ice pack is placed on the iliac crest beginning in the recovery room and continuing for 48 hours. Iliac crest bone graft symptoms are kept to a minimum by careful surgical exposure (avoiding cutting of muscle and remaining in the intramuscular planes), careful subperiosteal elevation, control of bleeding with bone wax and cautery, and tight closure of the muscular fascia over the iliac crest bone site. After discharge from the hospital (usually after 2 to 5 days), patients are seen in follow-up at 10 days, at 4, 8, 12, and 24 weeks, and at 1 year postoperatively. A patient's neurologic recovery may begin immediately postoperatively, with relief of pain and sensory and motor dysfunction. Myelopathic findings may take considerable time (weeks to months) to stabilize.

REHABILITATION

Rehabilitation of a patient following cervical vertebrectomy during the time of postoperative bracing is somewhat limited; the patient is only able to do ambulation and some lower extremity strength training. I allow patients to ambulate the day following surgery, and 1 to 2 weeks following surgery a progressive walking program can be employed. All types of overhead lifting activities are avoided until a solid fusion is obtained. Once the cervical vertebrectomy has solidly fused and neck bracing is removed, a physical therapy program with neck strengthening and range of motion (ROM) may be utilized. In general, it is not important to stress ROM immediately following brace removal, as extremes of motion may exacerbate some of the neck symptomatology, and ROM will expand over the subsequent weeks and months. As a rule of thumb, a patient can expect to lose around 20% of neck ROM following a single-level vertebrectomy and 35% to 40% of ROM with a two-level vertebrectomy.

Common Problems

The most common problems of this procedure are as follows: (a) inadequate exposure of the vertebral bodies; (b) malalignment with removal of too much lateral vertebral body on one side, occasionally encountering the vertebral artery; (c) inadequate decompression of the lateral spinal canal; (d) extrusion of the strut graft; and (e) loosening or migration of the anterior plate and screws.

Inadequate exposure can be remedied by further release of the fascial layers of the neck, primarily the enveloping fascia of the sternocleidomastoid muscle, release of the digastric or stylohyoid muscles, and/or repositioning of the retractors midway through the procedure.

Malalignment of the decompression comes solely from misorientation of the surgeon. Significant osteophytosis around the intervertebral disc space with collapsed kyphotic vertebral bodies can be particularly disorienting. This situation can be remedied by concentrating on the lateral border of the vertebral body at the middle aspect of the body at each level. The hard osteophytes at the intervertebral disc space frequently extend several millimeters from the disc space and can cause a surgeon to resect too much lateral bone and inadvertently get into the vertebral artery. If a surgeon is unsure of the extent of his lateral decompression, AP and lateral radiographs with contrast in the vertebrectomy site will clearly show the mediolateral extent of decompression and the cephalad-caudad decompression. Following evaluation of these radiographs, one can easily extend the decompression, either medial or lateral, or cephalad or caudad.

A loose bone graft strut generally comes from taking too small a bone graft and measuring the vertebrectomy site without traction on the spine. I generally take a bone graft that is 2 to 3 mm longer than I have measured; this can be easily trimmed with a rongeur or the high-speed air drill immediately prior to insertion. Extrusion of the bone strut also commonly occurs when the anterior and posterior vertebral body edges are not left intact, providing a supporting rim around the strut graft. Use of anterior plate fixation will also eliminate extrusion of the strut graft.

Loosening and/or migration of the plate and screws occur most frequently when the screws have not been locked into the plate. One must angle the screws into the vertebral body 10 to 15 degrees to allow countersinking of the head of the screws underneath the plate. If the head of the screw is not countersunk, the locking inner set screw will not expand the head to lock into the plate. We have found it difficult to angle the screw with all the cervical retractors in place and have occasionally found it beneficial to remove the mediolateral and cephalad-caudal retractors and use hand-held retractors, which will easily allow the appropriate angulation of the drill and tap. The other common reason for loosening or migration of plate and screws is inadequate postoperative bracing and/or severe AP instability requiring additional posterior fixation.

COMPLICATIONS

A large number of vital structures, including neural, vascular, intestinal, and respiratory organs, traverse the cervical spine in the region of anterior cervical surgery. A complete understanding of the cervical anatomy and meticulous surgical exposure will help avoid complications during cervical vertebrectomy surgery.

The most common complication following anterior cervical vertebrectomy surgery is that of temporary dysphasia and hoarseness, generally due to edema, secondary to retraction against an in situ endotracheal tube. Hoarseness following anterior cervical surgery may occur in 15% to 20% of cases and is usually temporary. This complication is usually mild and generally resolves within 2 to 4 days. If these complaints are severe, early recognition is necessary to guard against tracheal obstruction. Such complaints can easily be controlled with a short course of steroids to reduce the tracheal esophageal edema. Perforation of the pharynx, trachea, and esophagus is unusual and should be avoided by careful retraction of these structures and careful placement of cervical retractors, avoiding sharp retractors and placement of the tips of the blade underneath the longus colli musculature.

Recurrent laryngeal nerve palsy causing temporary or permanent vocal cord paresis has been commonly described and is most likely the result of nerve injury due to prolonged pressure against the trachea. Permanent injury to the recurrent laryngeal nerve can be avoided by staying in the fascial planes and avoiding sharp dissection. The nerve is less likely to be injured with a left-sided approach because of its more consistent protected position in the tracheal-esophageal groove.

Horner's syndrome is the result of injury to the cervical sympathetic chain, which lies lateral and ventral to longus colli musculature. Injury to the cervical sympathetic chain is avoidable by avoiding lateral dissection of the longus colli musculature and keeping the retractors underneath the musculature.

Wound hematomas are generally avoidable by placement of a drain, either a small Silastic or small Penrose, which is brought out through the incision and generally removed the morning after surgery. A progressive hematoma may cause increasing swallowing and breathing difficulties and must be recognized to guard against tracheal obstruction. Simple opening of the incision will evacuate a wound hematoma.

Cerebrospinal fluid leaks are uncommon but are most likely to occur in patients with OPLL, which may erode the dura; removing the OPLL may reveal no remaining dura. The dura may also be torn by the high-speed air drill, and the use of a diamond-tipped bur may decrease the incidence of dural penetration. A dural tear in the anterior cervical spine may be difficult or impossible to close, and the use of a fascial graft or fibrin glue may be of benefit.

The surgeon must be constantly aware of the possibility of neural tissue damage (i.e., spinal cord or nerve root injury). Patients most at risk for neural tissue damage are those with a very narrow spinal canal and severe neural compression, since the neural tissue physiologic reserve has already been compromised and may be injured by minor indirect trauma or vascular compromise. Any anterior operation in which instrumentation enters the spinal canal, such as a Cloward's drill or dowel technique, entails an increased risk of spinal cord or nerve injury, particularly if the spinal canal is narrow. The neurologic injury may be indirect via injury to the anterior spinal artery system and is not always the result of direct trauma. Clearly, patients with narrow spinal canals, especially with OPLL, are at increased risk for neurologic deterioration following anterior decompressive surgery; if the spinal canal measures less than 6 or 7 mm, one can consider a posterior laminoplasty to enlarge the spinal canal prior to anterior decompression. The C5 nerve root is particularly vulnerable to motor and sensory deficits following cervical vertebrectomy surgery.

Bone graft complications (i.e., graft dislodgement and graft collapse) are generally technique-related problems and are more frequent in osteoporotic bone. These problems can be avoided by careful placement of strong strut grafts, use of anterior cervical plate fixation, and postoperative bracing.

ILLUSTRATIVE CASE FOR TECHNIQUE

A 61-year-old woman developed progressive cervical myelopathy over a 2-year period. She was referred after losing the ability to ambulate and severe loss of hand function. She had severe OPLL with severe spinal cord compression (Fig. 16). A C5 vertebrectomy and C4–C6 fusion with anterior cervical plating was accomplished. The surgeon avoided the upper and lower disc spaces of the uninvolved levels. Twenty-two months postoperatively the patient had solid fusion with excellent cervical alignment (Figs. 17 and 18). This patient had excellent neurologic recovery with a return to fairly normal ambulation as well as a return of hand coordination.

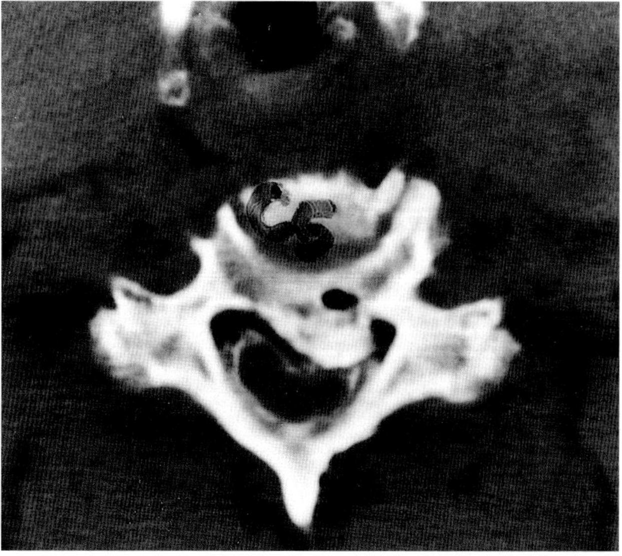

Figure 16. CT scan showing severe ossification of posterior longitudinal ligament with severe spinal cord compression.

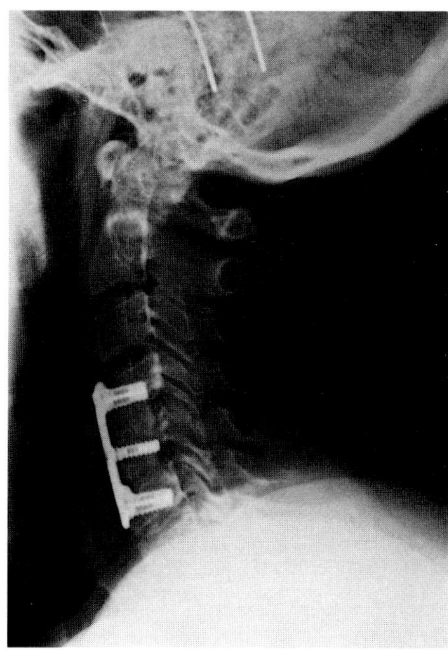

Figure 17. Lateral cervical radiograph, 22 months postoperatively, reveals solid fusion with excellent cervical alignment.

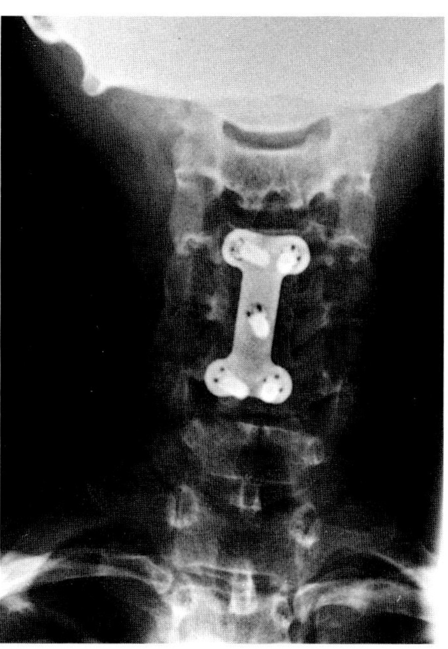

Figure 18. AP radiograph showing placement of the anterior plate and screws.

RECOMMENDED READING

1. Coe, J. D., Warden, K. E., Sutterlin, C. E., 3d, and McAfee, P. C.: Biomechanical evaluation of cervical spinal stabilization methods in a human cadaveric model. *Spine*, 14: 1122–1131, 1989.
2. Garvey, T. A., Eismont, F. J., and Roberti, L. J.: Anterior decompression, structural bone grafting, and Caspar plate stabilization for unstable cervical spine fractures and/or dislocations. *Spine*, 17[suppl 10]: S431–435, 1992.
3. Kostuik, J. P., Connolly, P. J., Esses, S. I., and Suh, P.: Anterior cervical plate fixation with the titanium hollow screw plate system. *Spine*, 18: 1273–1278, 1993.
4. Smith, M. D., Emery, S. E., Dudley, A., Murray, K. J., and Leventhal, M: Vertebral artery injury during anterior decompression of the cervical spine. A retrospective review of ten patients. *J. Bone Joint Surg.*, 75B: 410–415, 1993.
5. Suh, P. B., Kostuik, J. P., and Esses, S. I.: Anterior cervical plate fixation with the titanium hollow screw plate system. *Spine*, 15: 1079–1081, 1990.
6. Tippets, R. H., and Apfelbaum, R. I.: Anterior cervical fusion with the Caspar instrumentation system. *Neurosurgery*, 22(6 Pt 1): 1008–1013, 1988.
7. Traynelis, V. C., Donaher, P. A., Roach, R. M., Kojimoto, H., and Goel, V. K.: Biomechanical comparison of anterior Caspar plate and three-level posterior fixation techniques in a human cadaveric model. *J. Neurosurg.*, 79: 96–103, 1993.

Master Techniques in Orthopaedic Surgery,
THE SPINE, edited by D. S. Bradford,
Lippincott-Raven Publishers, Philadelphia, © 1997.

5

Anterior and Posterior Cervical Osteotomy

Henry H. Bohlman and Barbara Dabb

POSTERIOR APPROACH

Indications/Contraindications

Posterior cervical osteotomy is most commonly indicated in the patient with long-standing ankylosing spondylitis, who has developed a painful and disabling cervical kyphotic deformity. This may occur at any age and may be associated with kyphotic deformities of the thoracic and lumbar spine. The kyphosis may result from an occult fracture of the base of the cervical spine in a minor fall or traumatic episode; the patient may then develop a progressive and severe cervical kyphosis with ankylosis in the fixed kyphotic position. On the other hand, the patient with ankylosing spondylitis may develop severe kyphotic deformity without any trauma or fractures. In this situation the bone, which is a living organ, continues to remodel. As the deformity increases to 50 to 60 degrees of kyphosis, the bone continues to remodel under the weight of the head, and the deformity becomes increasingly severe over a period of years. In the worst situation, the patient may develop a chin-on-chest deformity and be unable to eat solid foods. The major indications for surgical correction are chronic neck pain as well as increasing deformity. In most situations the patient is unable to drink out of a glass or look ahead without flexing the hips and knees to compensate.

Posterior cervical osteotomy is contraindicated when the major deformity is in the thoracolumbar spine or hips and when a cervical kyphosis of less than 45 degrees has been stable on serial radiographs. Other general contraindications include severe cardiovascular or pulmonary disease, bleeding diathesis, and impaired mental status that would prohibit normal recovery and rehabilitation.

The posterior procedure alone is primarily indicated for patients with ankylosing spondylitis in whom full correction can be obtained by laminectomy followed by corrective osteotomy, and whose ossified spine fractures anteriorly without the necessity of an anterior release.

H. H. Bohlman, M.D. and B. Dabb, M.D.: Department of Orthopaedic Surgery, Case Western Reserve University School of Medicine, The University Hospitals Spine Institute, 11100 Evelid Avenue, Cleveland, Ohio 44106

Preoperative Planning

It is extremely important for these patients to have a thorough medical workup as well as pulmonary function and blood gas studies since they have restrictive lung disease and in some situations are smokers. The entire operative procedure is explained to the patient in great detail, including the potential hazards of malunion, nonunion, neurologic deficit, and death, as well as the benefits of correction of deformity and restoration of much more normal activities with relief of pain. Preoperative anteroposterior (AP) and lateral radiographs of the entire spine including the cervical, thoracic, and lumbar areas should be obtained. The degree of correction to be obtained depends on the angle of the cervical deformity or the chin-brow to vertical angle. The degrees of kyphosis are measured in all three areas of the spine. One must not overcorrect the deformity so that the patient cannot look down. Therefore, the patient does have to have some slight residual (15-degree) kyphosis. Preoperative cervical to upper thoracic magnetic resonance imaging (MRI) is carried out to be certain that there is no intraspinal pathology that would compromise the spinal cord as the deformity is corrected. In addition, AP and lateral tomograms are very helpful when conventional radiographs do not define the bony anatomy or when ruling out occult fractures, which may or may not be healed, especially at the thoracolumbar junction. We do not believe that computed tomography scan with myelography is necessary. If there is a severe kyphosis of both the cervical and lumbar spine, we recommend doing the cervical osteotomy first so that intubation can be performed for the lumbar procedure. If hip flexion contractures are present, we carry out the lumbar osteotomy first so that lying and sleeping can be done prone, which ordinarily corrects these.

The patient is brought into the hospital 1 day prior to surgery for application of a halo ring and a molded rubber body cast under local anesthesia. Care is taken to prep and sterilize the scalp thoroughly after it is shaved to minimize the chance of pin tract infection since the halo is worn for 3 months. A molded Risser cast is applied with an abdominal hole for breathing since the patients have no chest expansion and are abdominal breathers. The cast is allowed to set and dry over night. The halo will be attached to the cast after the osteotomy. A halo vest does not give adequate fixation around the pelvis and torso.

Surgery

Anesthesia. The patient is lightly premedicated with midazolam (0.5 to 2.0 mg) before being taken to the operating room. An arterial catheter is inserted and the patient is seated on the operating room table as comfortably as possible before the procedure begins. An action pad (''jelly roll'' silicone mattress) is placed under the patient, a pillow is placed under the flexed knees, and pillows are placed in the patient's lap for arm supports. Once the patient is positioned, the other monitors are then placed (electrocardiogram, noninvasive blood pressure cuff, pulse oximeter, and precordial Doppler probe for detection of air embolus). As the patient is prepared, additional midazolam and either fentanyl or sufentanil in small increments are given. The nasal airway is inserted after spraying the nares with a 3% xylocaine/0.25% phenylephrine solution, and a clear light-weight plastic mask with a catheter attached for capnography is placed on the patient's face.

During the initial portions of the procedure, either ketamine or propofol is administered by continuous infusion for sedation and titrated to allow the patient to remain conscious and able to follow commands. Ketamine also provides excellent analgesia, and jaw muscle tone is maintained. When using ketamine, it is important to administer midazolam 10 to 15 minutes before starting the ketamine infusion to avoid the excessive cardiostimulatory effect. The usual dose range of ketamine is 0.5 to 1.0 mg/kg/hr. When using propofol, intermittent doses of fentanyl (25 to

30 μg) or sufentanil (2.5 to 5.0 μg) are usually needed for analgesia. The usual dose range of propofol is 30 to 70 μg/kg/min. Constant communication and verbal reassurance is required.

At the time of performing the corrective osteotomy, brief general anesthesia is used. When ketamine has been used for the sedative/analgesic, the infusion is stopped and a methohexital bolus is given (0.75 to 1.0 mg/kg) to produce unconsciousness. If propofol has been used for sedation, a propofol bolus is given (beginning with 0.5 mg/kg). Usually a 7- to 12-minute period of unconsciousness is required, and additional methohexital or propofol boluses are given if needed.

The final part of the procedure takes about 40 to 60 minutes, and the patient is again conscious and able to follow commands. During this period, additional midazolam, propofol, or fentanyl is given as needed.

Technique. The patient is in the sitting position on the operating table, so that the head and neck are in a vertical position, and suspended with 10 pounds of traction from an overhead pulley attached to the halo ring. The patient must be strapped into the seated position so that during the corrective osteotomy the torso does not slide forward and off the operating table when the posteriorly directed correcting forces on the head and neck are applied. Therefore, a seat belt is placed around the waist of the cast. It is important to make sure that the cast is cut out low enough dorsally to allow for draping and operative exposure (Fig. 1).

We utilize a small Luque rectangle bent to the estimated corrected deformity and fixed with Drummond wires and buttons to the intact spinous processes superiorly and inferior to the laminectomy. This allows for relatively rigid internal fixation and should be available on the set. The patient's posterior neck and lower scalp are shaved and prepared and draped off, utilizing intravenous poles to hold the drapes to either side. The operative procedure is initiated under a local anesthetic with the operative surgeon and assistants standing behind the patient. The local anesthetic is ordinarily a solution of 0.75% marcaine with epinephrine diluted in 1:2 with saline, which allows for enough volume of anesthetic to be effective through the procedure. The anesthetic is injected subcutaneously from the spinous

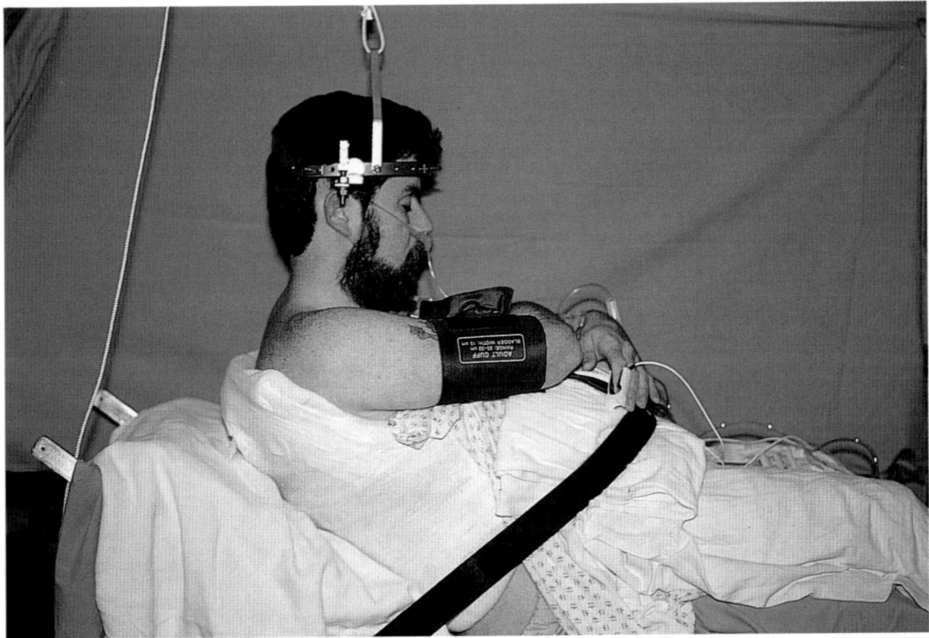

Figure 1. Lateral view of patient in case 1 in the operating room in his halo cast and traction. The patient is strapped onto the operating table in the sitting position with the head and neck vertical. The operating surgeon stands behind the patient to carry out the surgery.

processes of C4 down to T2 and then infiltrated down to the periosteum on both sides of the cervical and upper thoracic spine.

Once the local anesthetic has had its effect, a midline incision is made from approximately C4 to T2. Subcutaneous bleeders are clamped and cauterized, and dissection is carried down to the spinous processes with a knife; the erector spinae muscles are then elevated off the spinous processes and calcified interspinous ligaments utilizing a periosteal elevator. Once the spine is exposed, self-retaining retractors are placed and a check radiograph is obtained to identify the correct level. The osteotomy site is carried out at C7–T1, below the entrance of the vertebral arteries at the sixth cervical vertebra (Figs. 2 and 3). Using a bone cutter, the spinous processes of C6 and C7 are removed. One must be certain that the lateral dissection at C7–T1 is well beyond the lateral facet joint so that total exposure of the foramen can be obtained. Using the Leksell rongeur, the bases of the spinous processes are removed as well as the laminae of C6 and C7 and the upper portion of the T1 lamina (Fig. 4). Once the spinal canal is entered, a Penfield #3 elevator is utilized to break up any adhesions of the dura to the inner laminar surface, and a small Kerrison punch is then used to carry out the laminectomy. Epidural bleeders are controlled with Gelfoam and coagulated with a bipolar coagulator.

Once the laminectomy has been performed and the dura is well exposed, the surgeon can explore the lateral margins of the spinal canal and palpate the pedicles of the C7 and T1 vertebrae on both sides. By this method the eighth nerve root is identified in the C7–T1 foramina. The Leksell rongeur is utilized to remove the lateral portions of the facet joints at C7–T1, and then a Penfield #4 elevator is used to elevate the adhesions away from the dural sac and C8 nerve root sleeves. An open wedge foraminotomy is completed by using a small Kerrison punch and also a diamond bur. At this point there are small epidural vessels and veins that have to be coagulated, and the patient may feel paresthesias in the C8 nerve distribution. If this is painful, a small cotton patty can be utilized, soaked with 2% xylocaine, over the nerve root. The patty should not be placed over the dural sac more centrally, which would be dangerous and could possibly anesthetize the

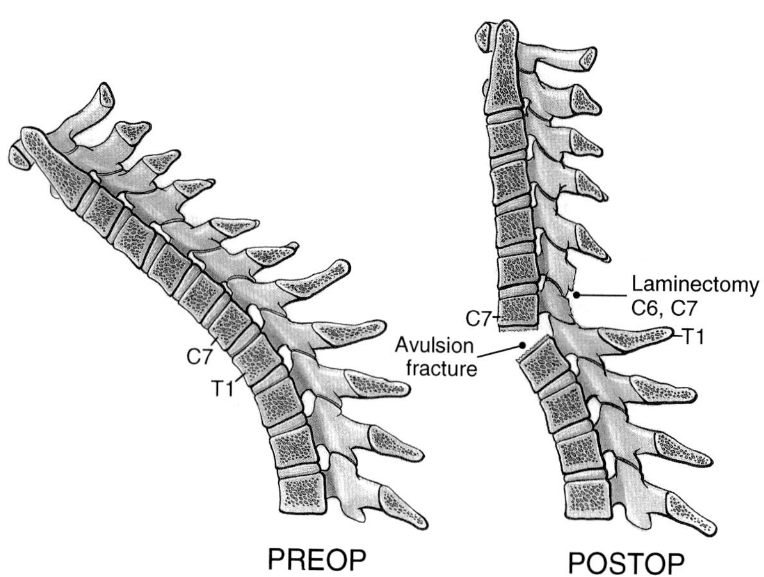

Figure 2. Illustration demonstrating the level of the osteotomy at C7–T1 and the amount of correction obtained.

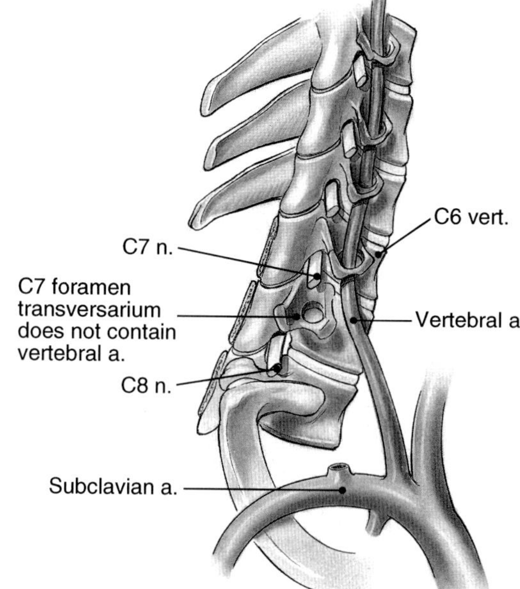

Figure 3. Illustration demonstrating the entrance of the vertebral artery at the C6 vertebral level, which is the indication for carrying out the osteotomy at C7–T1 so as not to damage the arterial structures.

cord. The foraminotomy must be carried all the way laterally into the soft tissue so that there is no bony bridge left posteriorly at the facet joint. At this point the bone edges are bone waxed to control bleeding. The dura is kept moist with wet cotton pledgets soaked with saline. The inferior half of the pedicle of C7 is then burred away with a diamond bur until there is adequate room for the C8 nerve root during the osteotomy and correction (Fig. 5). On occasion, some of the superior portion of the T1 pedicles must be removed to provide enough room for the C8 nerve roots during the osteotomy if a severe deformity is to be corrected.

Throughout the procedure the anesthesiologist and surgeon talk to the patient and make sure that the patient is moving all four extremities. All the bone that was removed is collected into a small pan for placement into the lateral gutters of the osteotomy.

Sixteen-gauge Drummond wires are placed through drill holes and buttons in the base of the spinous processes of C4 or C5 and T1 or T2. The Luque rectangle, which has been prebent for the correction, is then slid down on either side of the Drummond wires and placed over the spine prior to the osteotomy being performed. Deep stay sutures are placed for closure of the muscle layers prior to the osteotomy because the wound becomes markedly deformed from the previously vertical orientation to a horizontal orientation and is quite difficult to close unless the sutures are placed beforehand.

At this point the entire anesthesia, surgical, and technical teams are prepared and coordinated to carry out the osteotomy (closed anterior osteoclasis). The surgeon who is the assistant goes to the front of the table and firmly grasps the halo ring for control during the osteotomy. The operating surgeon then asks the

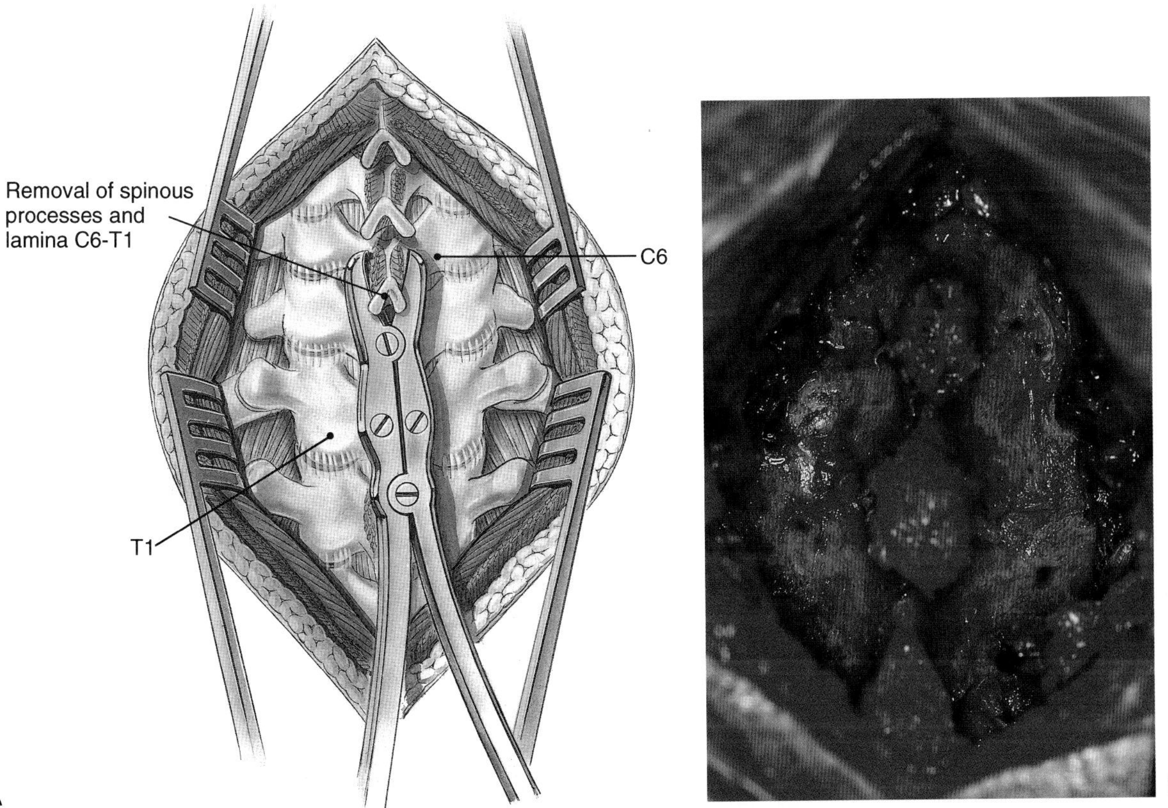

Figure 4. A: Illustration demonstrating the exposure of the spinous processes and placement of self-retaining retractor. A Leksell rongeur is utilized to remove the spinous processes and initiate the cervical laminectomy. **B:** Operative photograph of the exposed posterior cervical spine with self-retaining retractors placed. One can visualize the C6, C7, and T1 processes.

anesthesiologist to begin the brief general anesthetic. Once the patient is asleep the operative team is organized so that the surgical assistant in the front can maintain stability of the halo and the operative surgeon can begin slow posterior traction on the halo ring until the correction begins to occur.

It is quite easy to see the dura begin to wrinkle in the corrected position (Fig. 6). If the patient has a preoperative rotary deformity as well as kyphosis, more bone has to be removed on one side in order to correct the rotational deformity. That can be gauged during the procedure. As the osteotomy is completed, the operating surgeon can walk around to the front of the table and easily visualize the correction by seeing the alignment of the brow and the chin in relationship to the chest. The corrected position is then maintained with vertical traction and the assistant at the front of the patient.

Gelfoam is placed over the dura and C8 nerve root sleeves. The posterolateral aspect of the osteotomy should show close approximation of bone as the opening lateral wedges have been closed down. The bone that was removed is now placed as bone graft over the lateral masses and the slightly decorticated laminae above and below. The Drummond wires are utilized to attach the Luque rectangle in the corrected position and twisted down, following which a suction drain is placed. The wound is closed with the previously applied sutures. The skin is closed, the

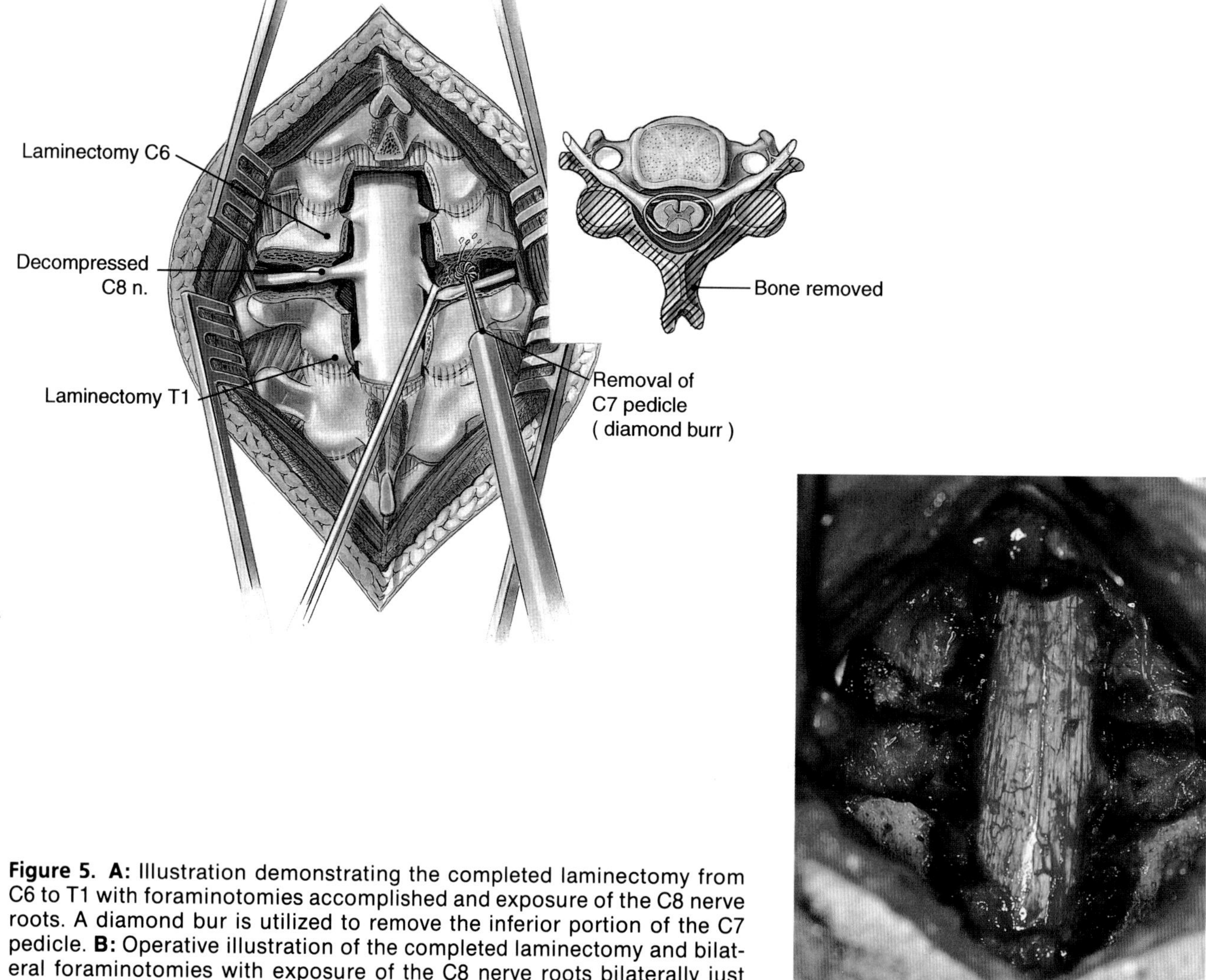

Figure 5. A: Illustration demonstrating the completed laminectomy from C6 to T1 with foraminotomies accomplished and exposure of the C8 nerve roots. A diamond bur is utilized to remove the inferior portion of the C7 pedicle. **B:** Operative illustration of the completed laminectomy and bilateral foraminotomies with exposure of the C8 nerve roots bilaterally just prior to the osteotomy procedure.

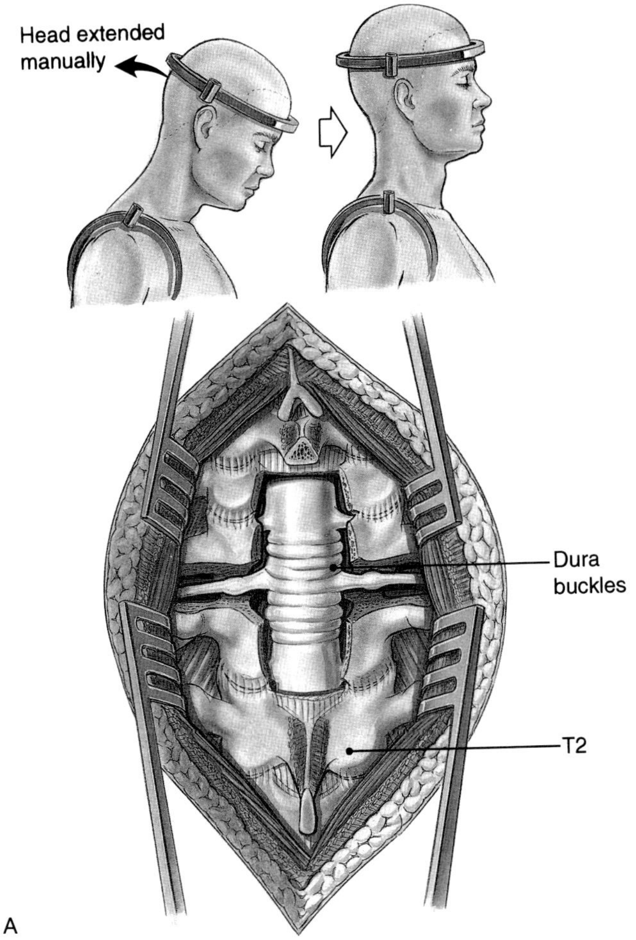

Head extended manually
Dura buckles
T2

A

Figure 6. A: Operative illustration of the osteotomy being performed. Note the correction of the head and neck position and the buckling of the dura as the head and neck are brought back into extension. **B:** Illustration demonstrating the completed laminectomy and osteotomy. Gelfoam is placed over the dura. The bone chips removed from the laminectomy are placed in the lateral gutters. A wire loop has been inserted with Drummond buttons to attach to the spinous processes, and a suction drain is placed prior to closure.

Bone chips
Decompressed C8 n.
Gel-foam
Luque rectangle

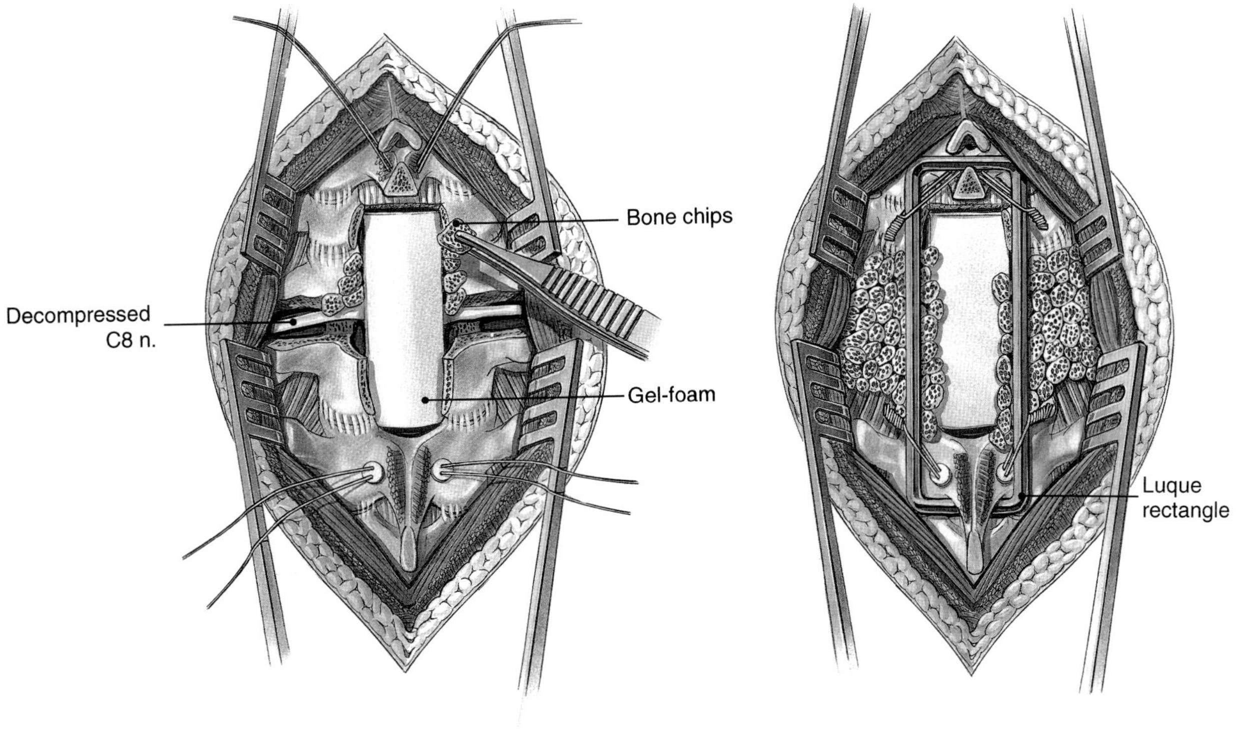

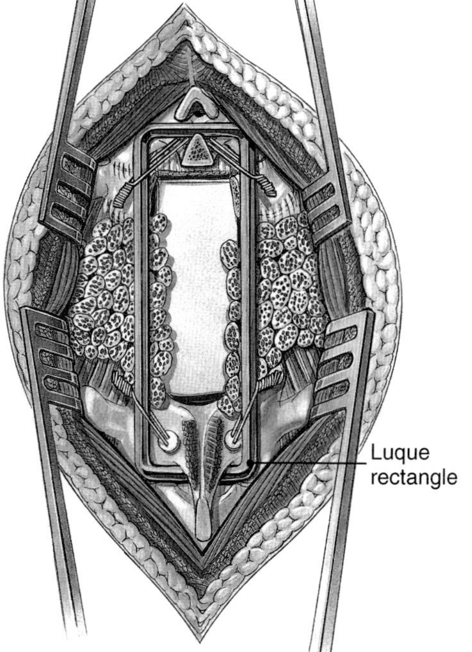

B

dressing is applied, and the patient is awakened to make sure that all four extremities are moving and there is no paralysis. The halo is now attached to the plaster jacket with the vertical struts and the patient is taken out of cervical traction, placed in bed, and taken to the recovery room for observation until the patient appears to be perfectly stable and awake (Fig. 7).

Postoperative Management

The patient is kept on intravenous fluids until the following day and then allowed to take oral liquids. A regular diet is then introduced. Occasionally, in the more severe deformity corrections, the patient will have dysphasia because of the angulation the esophagus takes around the anterior C7–T1 osteotomy site. This ordinarily resolves uneventfully. The patient is allowed to ambulate in a walker the day following surgery. The drain is removed on the second postoperative day. We utilize a prophylactic broad-spectrum antibiotic intraoperatively and for 3 days postoperatively. Radiographs, including swimmer's view, are taken before discharge; lateral tomograms may also be used to ascertain that the osteotomy site is in correct position. The family and patient are instructed in pin care.

The patient is discharged when nutrition is adequate, oral medications are sufficient for pain control, and ambulation is independent. The halo cast is worn for 3 months postoperatively, at which point the patient returns to the hospital as an outpatient; the halo cast is removed and a rigid two-poster orthosis is applied for an additional 3 months (Fig. 8). At that point AP and lateral tomograms are performed to judge the healing of the fusion and the osteotomy. At 6 months the patient is taken out of all orthotic devices and repeat radiographs are performed to ascertain complete healing.

By and large we have been extremely gratified with the results utilizing the above technique, and the patients are extraordinarily grateful when their deformity is corrected, since it totally changes their life style and their ability to perform activities of daily living. We do not expect absolutely natural sagittal balance but

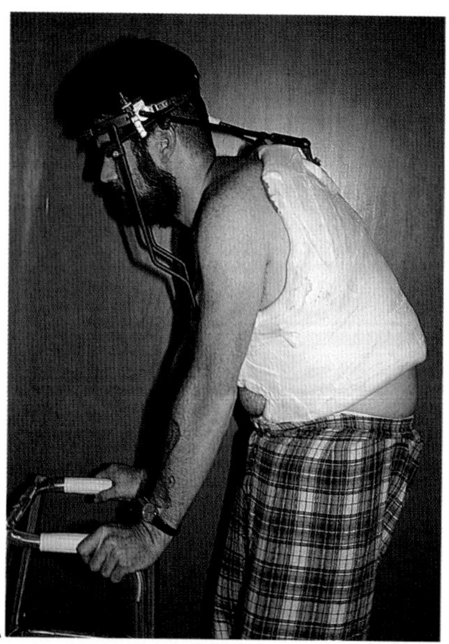

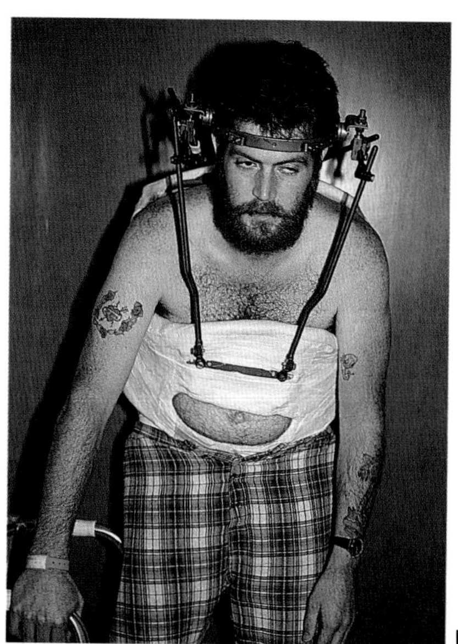

Figure 7. A: Lateral postoperative view of the patient in the halo cast. Note the cervical correction but persistence of lumbar kyphosis frontal. **B:** Frontal view. Note that the patient can look ahead rather than down at the floor.

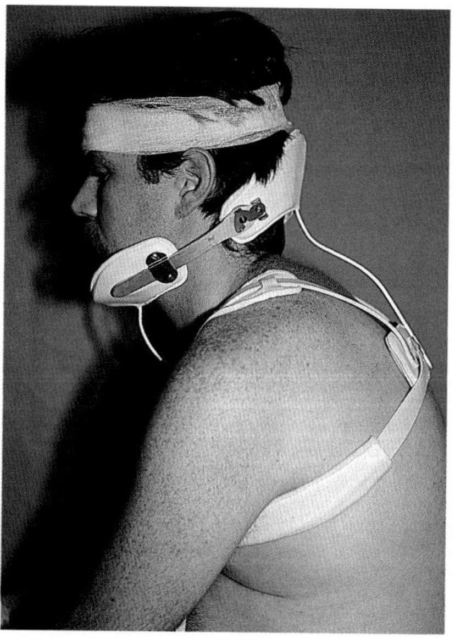

Figure 8. Postoperative photograph of patient at 3 months. The halo was removed and a rigid two-poster brace was placed for a subsequent 3 months.

hope for slight (20-degree) positive sagittal balance so the patient can look down. Once the deformity is corrected, relief of pain in the cervical and shoulder region is almost universal. Of the 26 patients corrected since 1976, all living patients healed, and correction has been maintained. We recently had one cardiac arrest and death 6 weeks after a lumbar osteotomy in a patient on whom we had performed a cervical correction 1 year previously.

Complications

The most serious complication, obviously, is paralysis and death secondary to pulmonary complications. Of the 26 patients we have operated on in 20 years, one patient died; the fixed chin-on-chest deformity had been present for 5 years, and a 90-degree corrective osteotomy was required. Paralysis ensued in the operating room after the corrective osteotomy because the anterior cervical musculature became so taut that it pulled the superior portion of the cervical spine forward on the thoracic spine at C7–T1 and compressed the spinal cord. This was relieved by readjusting the halo, and the paralysis resolved over a 3-day period, but recurred when the same forces were applied at the osteotomy site. Unfortunately, at that time we had no internal fixation devices to control the osteotomy. The patient became completely quadriplegic in the halo cast and ultimately died of pulmonary dysfunction and pneumonia. Retrospectively, anterior tenotomies of the sternomastoid muscles would have aided maintenance of the spinal correction.

Paralysis of the C8 nerve roots may occur if inadequate bone is removed in the neural foramen to allow for the corrective osteotomy. If paralysis is mild postoperatively, it almost always resolves. Postoperative epidural hematoma, producing compression of the spinal cord, has been noted, but this has not occurred in our experience. We have had no infections and no pseudoarthroses, with the exception of one patient who developed a recurring deformity and telescoping of C7 in front of T1 2 months postoperatively after being involved in a truck accident in which his vehicle struck a tree while he was in the halo. This patient developed recurring intrinsic weakness of the C8 nerve root but was corrected 9 months later with skeletal traction for 1 week, repeat posterior fusion with a Luque rectangle fixation, and anterior decompression and fusion. We have had no patients with vertebral artery thromboses. Pseudarthrosis can occur, but it can be repaired with an anterior or repeat posterior fusion.

COMBINED ANTERIOR AND POSTERIOR APPROACH

Indications/Contraindications

Patients with severe degenerative osteoarthritis of the cervical spine who develop severe kyphotic deformities with rather fixed kyphosis secondary to spontaneous fusions may require a cervical osteotomy. In addition, we have had experience with iatrogenic cervical kyphoses secondary to malunions of anterior and posterior fusions; a posterior approach or an anterior approach alone will not suffice to correct the deformity. In these patients we carry out a posterior decompression, that is, laminectomy and foraminotomies as described above, and then apply an onlay sliding iliac graft followed by an anterior osteotomy and fusion.

A cervical laminectomy with and without facetectomy may result in progressive cervical kyphosis and require a combined anterior and posterior procedure. Contraindications for the combined approach are similar to those with the posterior osteotomy.

Preoperative Planning

The patient is completely informed of the seriousness of this combined procedure, the potential risks of paralysis and nonunion, and the potential benefits of correction of the deformity and relief of pain. Preoperatively routine cervical spine radiographs, AP and lateral tomograms, cervical myelography with CT scanning, and MRI of the cervical spine and cord are taken. This allows assessment of any intraspinal pathology that may be present.

Surgery

For this combined procedure a general anesthetic is utilized with fiberoptic intubation. The patient is placed on a regular operating table in the supine position. The scalp is shaved, prepped, and draped, and a halo ring is applied. The anterior halo vest with struts is then attached. The patient is turned prone on the operating table and the posterior neck and scalp are prepped and draped in the usual manner. A solution of saline with 1:500,000 epinephrine is injected subcutaneously and down to the cervical laminae.

A midline incision is made from C5 to T2. Subcutaneous bleeders are clamped and cauterized. Further dissection is carried out with a knife to strip away the erector spinae muscle attachments. Using a periosteal elevator, the remaining attachments are removed from the laminae, and self-retaining retractors are placed. The spinous processes of C7 and T1 are then removed and the interlaminar space is entered with a small Kerrison punch. The ligamentum flavum is detached and, using a Kerrison punch, a laminectomy of C7 and T1 is performed. A wide foraminotomy is then carried out to decompress the C8 nerve roots totally, and an opening wedge of bone is burred away with a diamond bur to gutter the foramen completely out to the soft tissue laterally, much the same as in the cervical osteotomy for ankylosing spondylitis. Once the eighth nerve roots are completely decompressed, Gelfoam is placed over them, epidural bleeders are controlled with bipolar coagulation, a gelatin sponge is placed over the dura, and a thick strut of cortical cancellous iliac graft is taken approximately 2 inches in length and cut in two strips. These are then laid onto the posterior cervical spine as an onlay graft bilaterally.

The wound is closed over a suction drain. The posterior part of the halo vest is applied, and the vertical struts are attached. The patient is then turned supine. The struts are detached and the patient is placed in skeletal traction utilizing the halo ring and approximately 15 pounds of cervical traction.

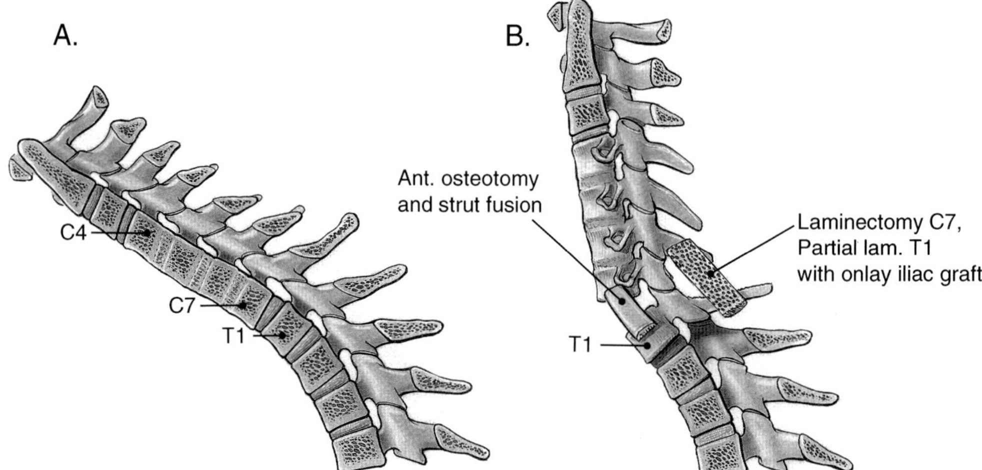

Figure 9. A: Illustration of an iatrogenic rigid, postoperative cervical kyphosis. **B:** Illustration of the kyphosis following correction by laminectomy, posterior-only graft, and anterior discectomy with strut fusion C7–T1.

The anterior neck is prepped and draped in the usual manner, as is the iliac crest. An anterior approach is made to the cervical spine through the left side of the neck. Dissection is carried down through the transverse incision to the platysma, which is split transversely. The external layer of deep cervical fascia is split transversely. Further dissection is carried down medial to the carotid sheath, which is retracted laterally, and the fascia is split once again. The fascia surrounding the carotid sheath is split medial to the sheath and the pretracheal and prevertebral fascia are split longitudinally, exposing the anterior vertebral body surfaces. Either a discectomy is performed at the C7–T1 level or a corpectomy of C7—whichever is necessary. This is carried out in the usual fashion utilizing power burs back to the posterior longitudinal ligament. At this point the patient's head and neck are extended gradually with radiographic control. Performing the correction at the C7–T1 level avoids vertebral artery injury. Once the kyphosis has been corrected satisfactorily, an anterior iliac bone graft is inserted and the wound is closed over a mastoid drain. The wound is dressed and the anterior portion of the halo vest and struts are attached; the patient is awakened and returned to the recovery room (Fig. 9).

Postoperative Management

Postoperatively the patient is kept in the halo vest for 3 months until the anterior and posterior grafts are consolidated. This is usually confirmed by plain radiographs as well as AP and lateral tomograms. The halo vest is then removed and the patient is allowed to regain as much cervical motion as possible.

Complications

Potential complications are pseudarthrosis of the bone grafts, although this is extraordinarily rare; it can be corrected by regrafting. Inadequate correction of kyphosis may occur, but ordinarily with the double approach excellent correction

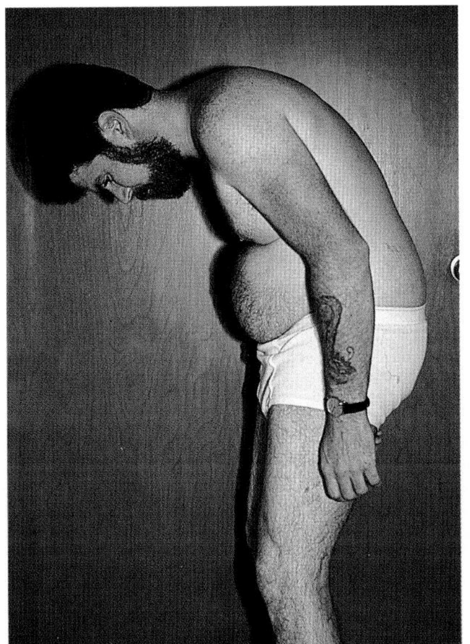

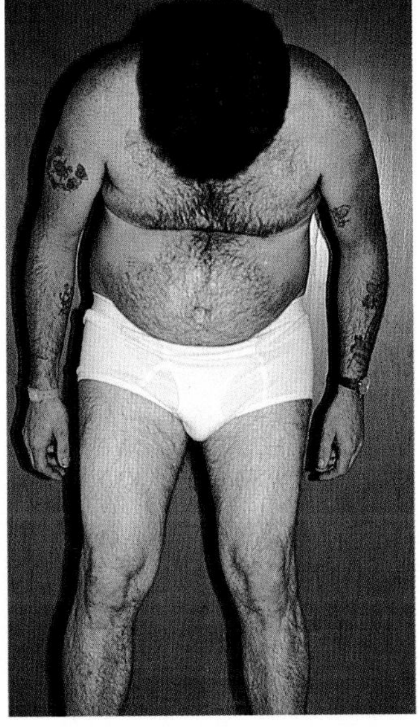

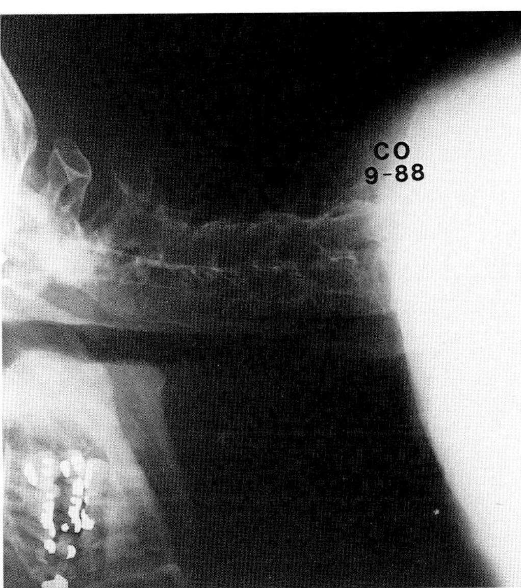

C

Figure 10. A: Lateral view of the patient in case 1, a 35-year-old man with severe cervical as well as lumbar kyphosis. Note the chin-brow to vertical angle in 90 degrees in the lateral view. **B:** Frontal view of the patient who cannot look ahead but sees the floor secondary to the severe cervical, thoracic, and lumbar kyphotic deformity. **C:** Lateral radiograph of the patient shows ankylosing spondylitis with severe cervical kyphotic deformity.

can be obtained and maintained. Postoperative soft-tissue swelling can occur from the anterior procedure if a more extensive corpectomy is performed. We have not had any neurologic complications with this technique, and the end results have been quite satisfactory.

ILLUSTRATIVE CASES FOR TECHNIQUE

Case 1

A 35-year-old man with long-standing ankylosing spondylitis and severe, progressive cervical and lumbar kyphosis had been unable to see straight ahead or lie flat in bed for 8 years (Fig. 10). A cervical osteotomy was performed, and the results were successful (Fig. 11).

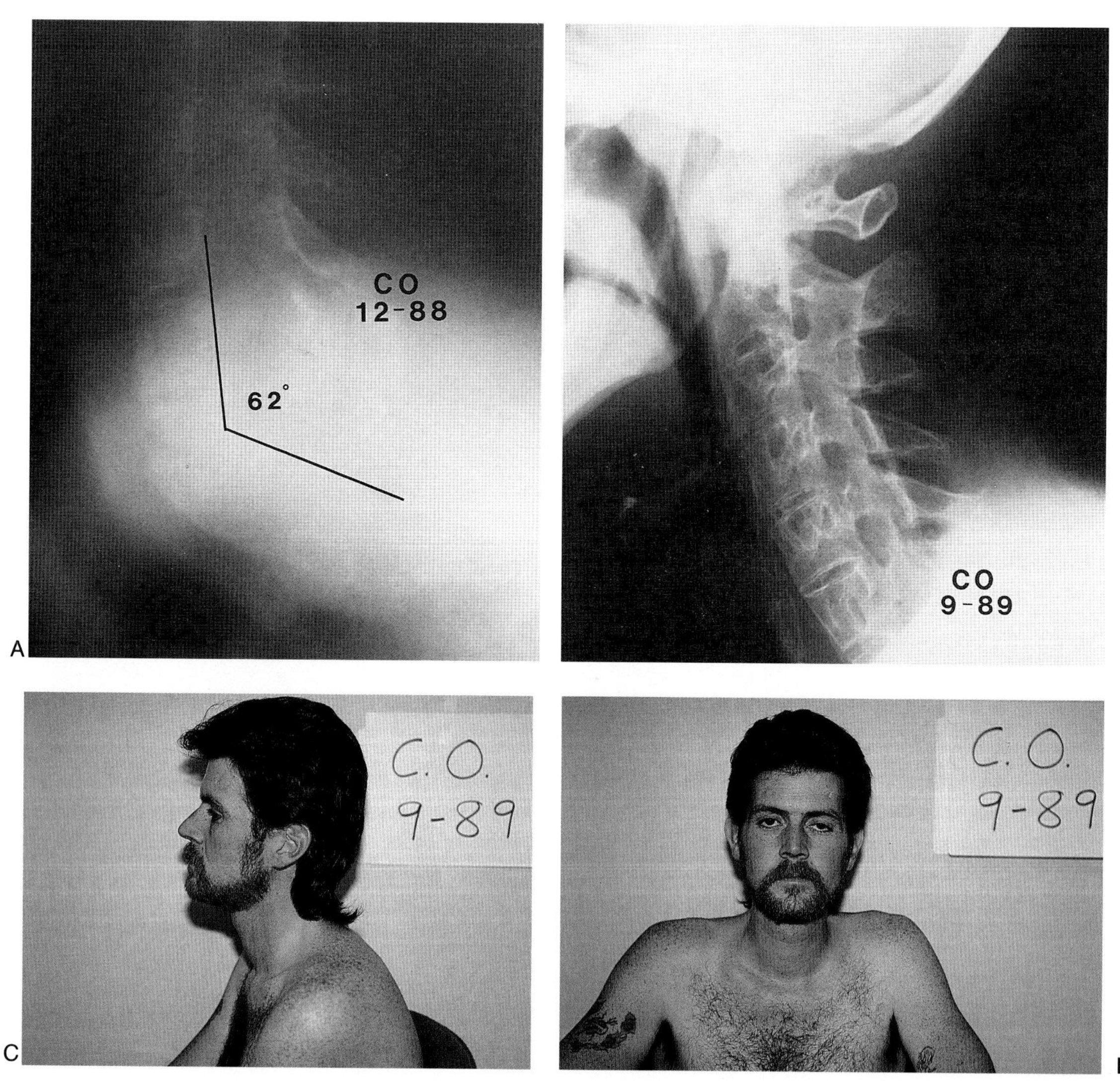

Figure 11. A: Postoperative tomogram at 3 months following cervical osteotomy, revealing a 62-degree correction of the kyphosis and complete bony union of the osteotomy site anteriorly as well as posteriorly. **B:** Lateral radiograph of the cervical spine at 1-year follow-up, revealing an excellent correction of his cervical kyphosis. Lateral **(C)** and frontal **(D)** view of the patient 1 year postoperatively demonstrating the corrected cervical kyphosis. At this point he is able to look straight ahead.

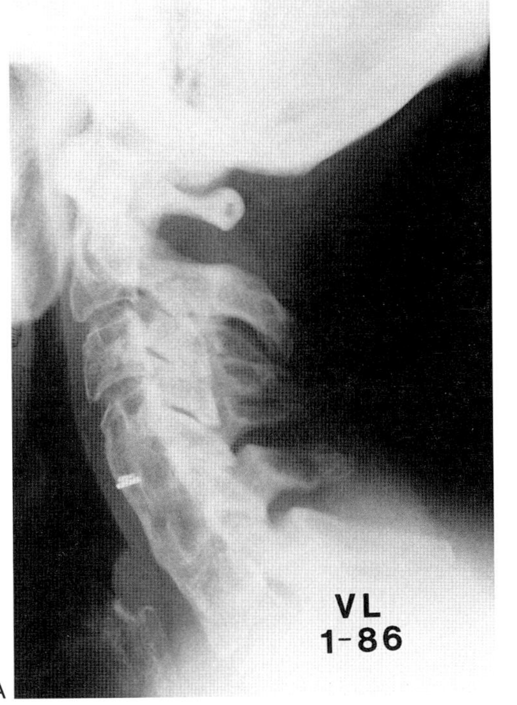

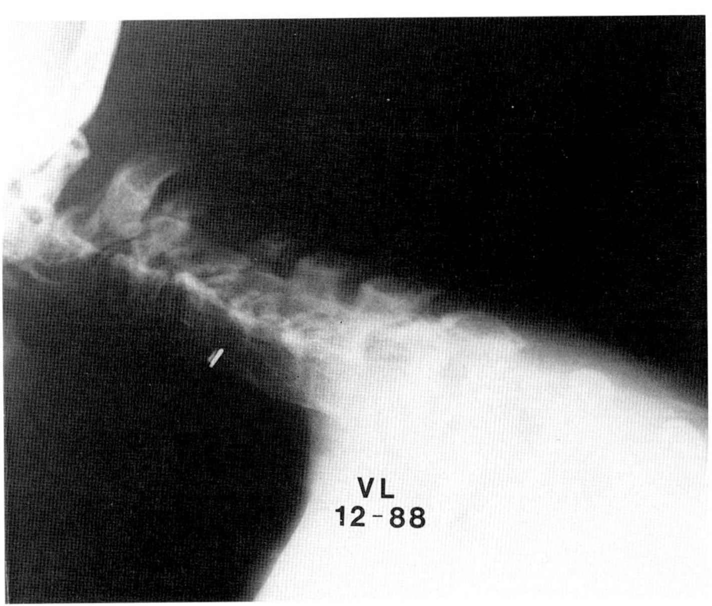

A B

Figure 12. A: Lateral radiograph of a 56-year-old woman who had undergone two previous anterior cervical discectomies and fusions for cervical radiculopathy. Note the solid fusions at C4–C5, C5–C6, and C6–C7. **B:** Lateral radiograph approximately 3 years later, at which time the patient had undergone a cervical laminoplasty with disruption of the posterior laminae and muscular attachments and developed a severe 70-degree cervical thoracic kyphosis. She was unable to hold her head up, look forward, or drink out of a glass. She had constant neck and shoulder pain and some recurring radiculopathy.

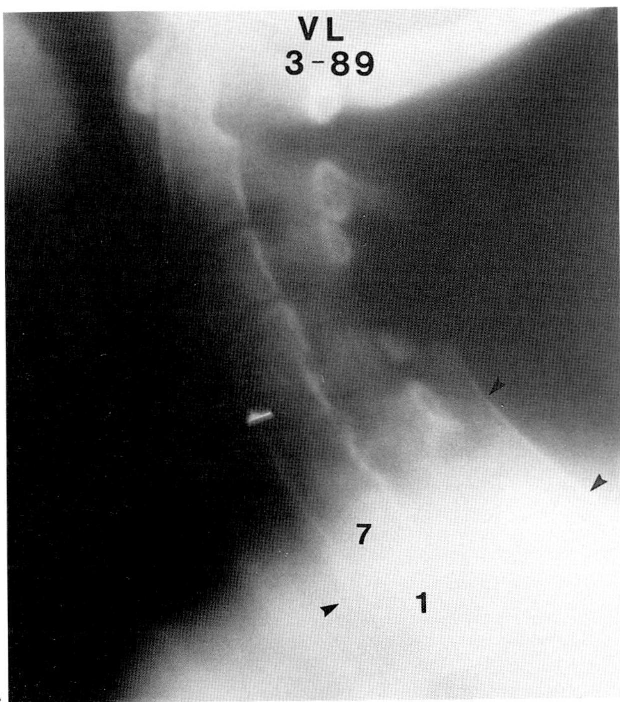

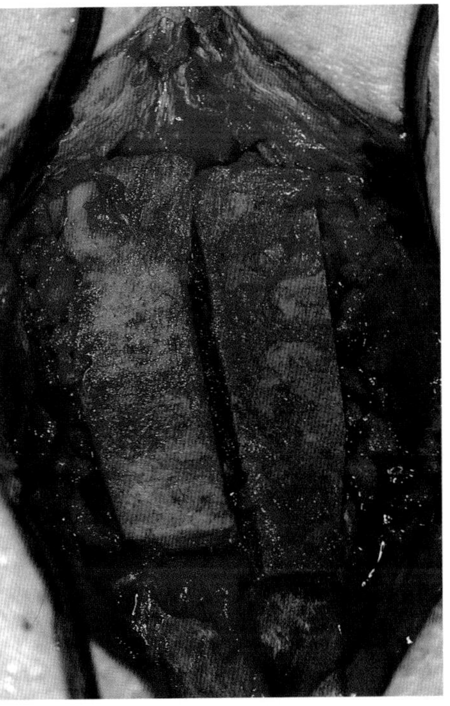

A B

Figure 13. A: Lateral tomogram of the cervical spine postoperatively after a cervical laminectomy, foraminotomy, osteotomy, and onlay iliac bone graft followed by an anterior cervical fusion at C7–T1. Note the correction of the cervical kyphosis and complete arthrodesis of the bone grafts. **B:** Operative photograph of the onlay cortico-cancellous iliac grafts posteriorly. The medullary portion of the graft is placed against the laminae.

Case 2

A 56-year-old housewife had multiple operative procedures, including previous anterior discectomies and fusions, followed by a cervical laminoplasty; she then developed cervical kyphosis with fixed deformity (Fig. 12). A combined anterior and posterior approach was necessary to correct her deformity (Fig. 13).

RECOMMENDED READING

1. Adams, J. C.: Technique, dangers and safeguards in osteotomy of the spine. *J. Bone Joint Surg. [Br.]*, 34: 226–232, 1952.
2. Briggs, H., Keats, S., and Schlesinger, P. T.: Wedge osteotomy of the spine with bilateral intervertebral foraminotomy: Correction of flexion deformity in five cases of ankylosing arthritis of the spine. *J. Bone Joint Surg.* 29: 1075–1082, 1947.
3. Graham, B., and Van Peteghem, P. K.: Fractures of the spine in ankylosing spondylitis. Diagnosis, treatment and complications. *Spine*, 14: 803–807, 1989.
4. Kostuik, J. P.: Ankylosing spondylitis. Surgical treatment. In: *The Adult Spine, Principles and Practice*, Vol. I, edited by J. W. Frymoyer, pp. 719–743. Raven Press, New York, 1991.
5. Simmons, E. H.: The surgical correction of flexion deformity of the cervical spine in ankylosing spondylitis. *Clin. Orthop.*, 86: 132–143, 1972.
6. Simmons, E. H.: Kyphotic deformity of the spine in ankylosing spondylitis. *Clin. Orthop.*, 128: 65–77, 1977.
7. Simmons, E. H., and Duncan, C. P.: Fracture of the cervical spine in ankylosing spondylitis—an analysis of its influence on severe deformity presenting for spinal osteotomy. *Clin. Orthop.* 133: 277, 1978.
8. Urist, M. R.: Osteotomy of the cervical spine: Report of a case of ankylosing rheumatoid spondylitis. *J. Bone Joint Surg. [Am.]*, 40: 833–843, 1958.

Master Techniques in Orthopaedic Surgery,
THE SPINE, edited by D. S. Bradford,
Lippincott-Raven Publishers, Philadelphia, © 1997.

6

Anterior Cervical Discectomy and Spine Fusion

Jeffrey S. Fischgrund and Harry N. Herkowitz

INDICATIONS/CONTRAINDICATIONS

Anterior cervical discectomy and fusion has been widely performed since the initial description of the procedure by Smith and Robinson in the late 1950s. Currently, we recommend anterior cervical discectomy and fusion for the treatment of single- and multiple-level radiculopathy in patients who have failed nonoperative treatment.

The current indications for surgery in cervical radiculopathy are as follows: (a) persistent or recurrent arm pain not responsive to a trial of conservative treatment (3 months), (b) progressive neurologic deficit, (c) static neurologic deficit associated with radicular pain, (d) confirmatory imaging study consistent with clinical findings [computed tomography (CT)/myelogram or magnetic resonance imaging (MRI)].

We currently recommend anterior cervical discectomy and fusion for the surgical management of cervical posterior lateral or central soft disc herniations. Anterior cervical discectomy/fusion is also the procedure of choice for multiple-level spondylitic radiculopathy. Posterior laminotomy/foraminotomy may be considered in the following situations: (a) technical limitations of the anterior approach, or (b) prior anterior surgery restricting access to the surgical level. The laminoplasty procedure is preferred for patients with developmental canal stenosis, failure of multiple-level anterior fusion, or prior anterior neck surgery preventing access to the surgical site. Cervical laminectomy may be considered for patients with failed laminoplasty or patients with anterior bony ankylosis due to degenerative or inflammatory disorders.

J. S. Fischgrund, M.D., and H. N. Herkowitz, M.D.: Department of Orthopaedic Surgery, William Beaumont Hospital, Royal Oak, Michigan 48073-6705.

PREOPERATIVE PLANNING

The preoperative physical examination can usually localize the level of nerve root or cord compression. C3 radiculopathy is due to pathology at the C2–C3 interspace and is very rare, with no detectable motor involvement. C4 radiculopathy also has no obvious motor deformity but is usually accompanied by pain radiating to the shoulder or midscapular region. Spondylosis or disc herniation at the C4–C5 level will affect the C5 nerve root and cause pain midway down the lateral aspect of the arm. The patient will usually complain of difficulty elevating the arm and clinically will have deltoid weakness on examination. C6 radiculopathy is the second most commonly involved nerve root. The patients often complain of radiating pain to the index finger and thumb. Additionally, they will have a decreased biceps reflex and weak wrist extension. The most common level of cervical disc herniation is at the C6–C7 level. The resultant C7 radiculopathy will cause radiating pain to the middle finger, a decreased triceps reflex, and weakness of the triceps muscle. A C8 radiculopathy can cause numbness on the ulnar half of the hand and weakness of hand grip.

The patient should also be examined for signs of myelopathy. These signs include hyper-reflexia below the level of the anatomic lesion and pathologic reflexes such as a positive Babinski sign in the lower extremity and a positive Hoffman reflex in the upper extremities. Clonus may be present in the lower extremities and a myelopathic hand sign characterized by loss of power of adduction and extension of the ulnar two or three fingers may be present in the upper extremities.

Preoperative radiographic studies should include a lateral radiograph of all seven cervical vertebrae. Oblique radiographs are helpful for evaluating foramen size. Flexion-extension views should be obtained to rule out occult instability. Imaging of the spinal cord and nerve roots must be performed prior to surgical intervention. Myelography followed by CT provides an accurate and often specific evaluation of extradural, intradural, and intermedullary lesions. Magnetic resonance imaging, when available, is an excellent test to evaluate the intervertebral disc, nerve roots, and spinal cord. In addition to the excellent visualization of the root and cord compression, it is noninvasive and does not expose the patient to radiation.

SURGERY

After the induction of general anesthesia, the patient is positioned supine on the operating room table (Fig. 1). A small, rolled towel should be placed under the buttocks to assist in exposing the anterior crest for graft harvesting. A second rolled towel is then placed between the scapula to extend the neck slightly. If possible, the head section of the operating room table should be lowered to increase neck extension further. The endotracheal tube should be taped to the right corner of the mouth by the anesthesiologist so that the left side of the neck can be adequately prepped and draped. Wide adhesive tape is used to lower the shoulders bilaterally. We prefer a left-sided approach in order to decrease the risk to the recurrent laryngeal nerve. On the left, the nerve enters the thorax within the carotid sheath. It then loops under the aortic arch and ascends into the neck beside the trachea and esophagus. On the right side, however, it may leave the carotid sheath at a higher level and course anteriorly behind the thyroid, thus leaving itself more susceptible to injury if the incision is on the right.

The incision may be transverse or longitudinal, following the anterior border of the sternocleidomastoid muscle. Knowledge of the anatomic landmarks is helpful in placement of the skin incision (Fig. 2). Generally, the hyoid bone is at the level of C3, the thyroid cartilage is at C4–C5, and the cricoid cartilage lies at the level of C6. The transverse incision is preferred for a one- or two-level fusion, while the longitudinal approach is best for three or more levels. At the cervicothor-

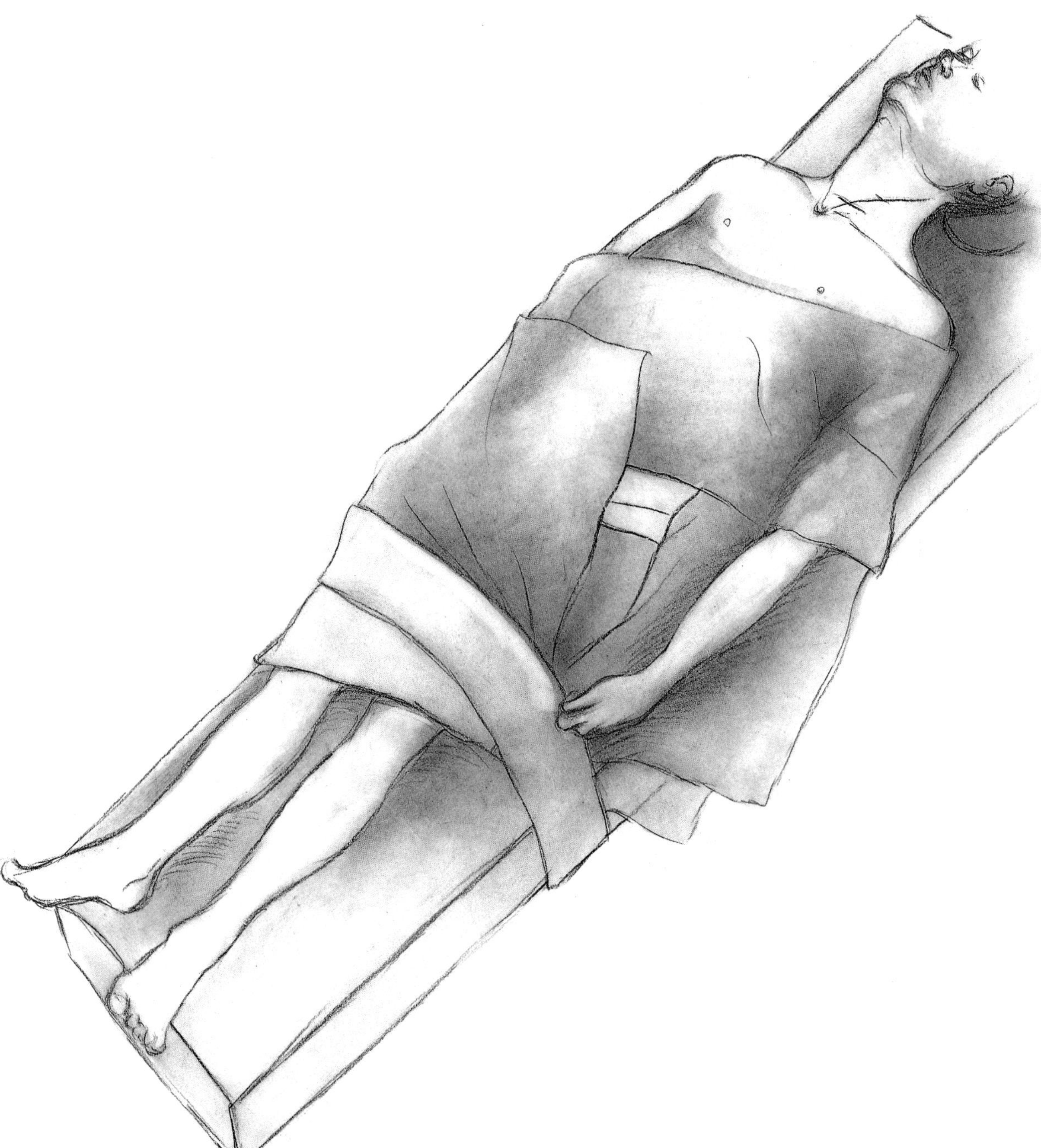

Figure 1. Positioning for a left-sided anterior approach to the cervical spine. Wide tape can be used to depress and secure the shoulders.

acic junction, the longitudinal incision may be preferred since inadvertent injury to the inferior thyroid vessels can be managed more readily through a longitudinal approach. Once the incision is made, the superficial platysma muscle is easily identified and should be incised transversely with electrocautery (Fig. 3). The approach should then proceed medial to the sternocleidomastoid muscle (Fig. 4). The carotid sheath is then retracted laterally and the esophagus and trachea are retracted medially using hand-held blunt retractors (Fig. 5). The superior and inferior thyroid vessels, which traverse from the carotid artery and thyrocervical trunk to the midline structures, may limit the extent to which this plane can be opened and may have to be divided. The vertebral bodies and disc can then be identified by palpation in the midline. A subperiosteal dissection of the preverte-

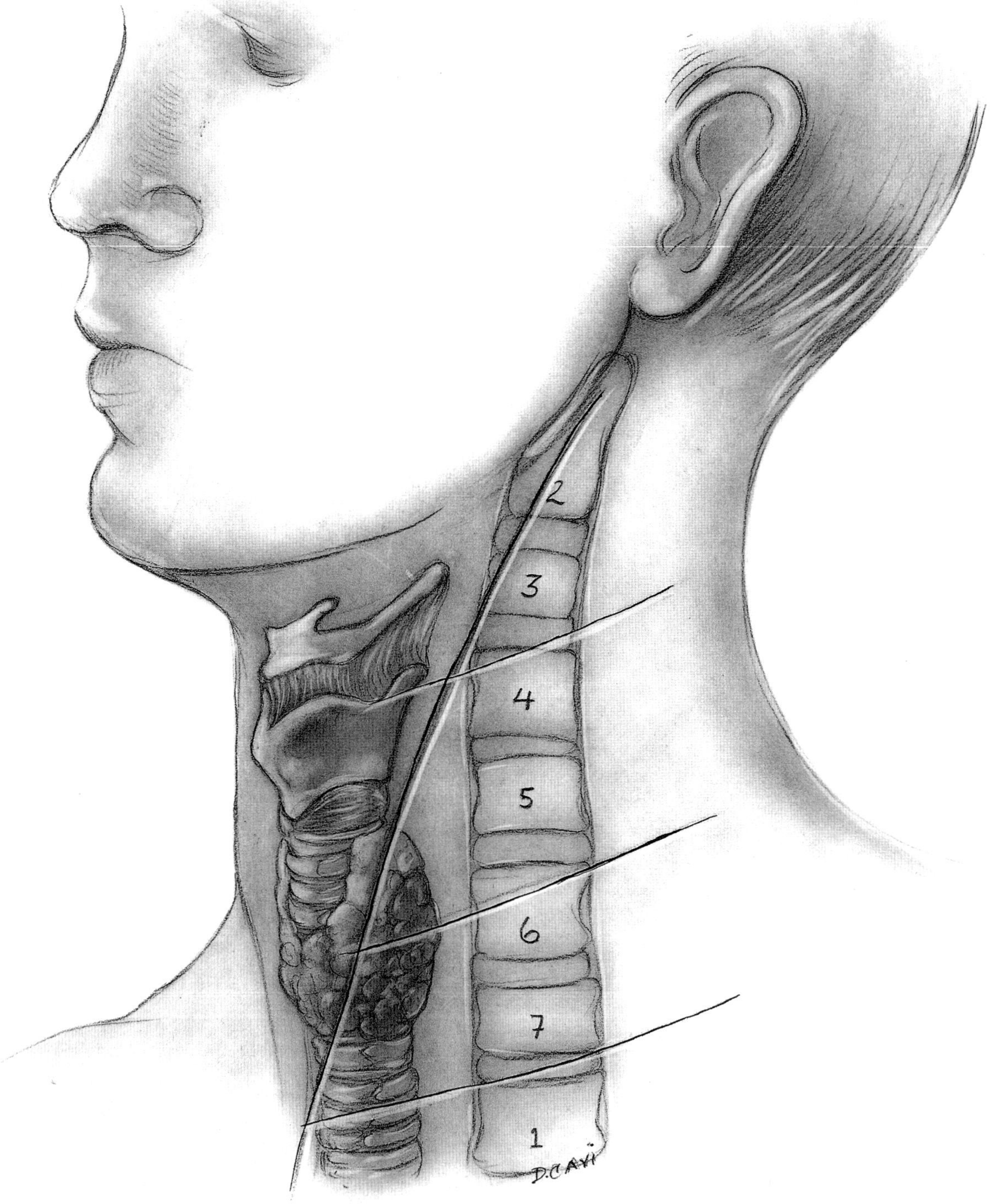

Figure 2. Superficial landmarks are helpful in placing the skin incision. The hyoid bone is at the level of C3, the thyroid cartilage is at C4–C5, and the cricoid is opposite C6.

bral fascia and longus colli muscles using an elevator should then be performed over the disc space only. At this point, we usually place a spinal needle in either one or two levels and obtain a lateral radiograph to confirm the correct level of surgery (Fig. 6).

With exposure of the disc space complete, we then perform an anterior discectomy. Using a #15 scalpel blade on a long handle, we make a rectangular incision

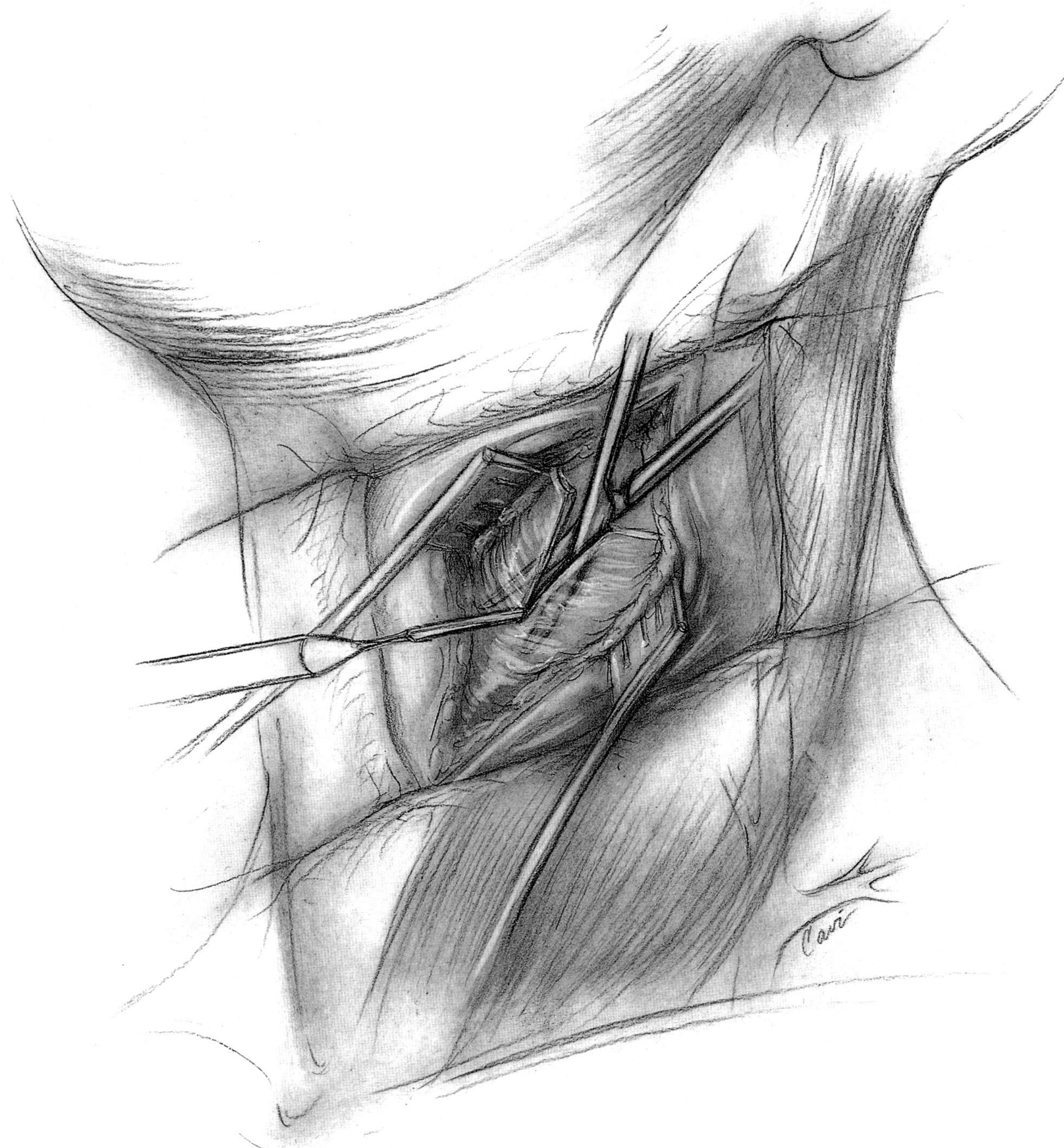

Figure 3. Transverse skin incision exposing the platysma muscle, which is incised transversely with electrocautery.

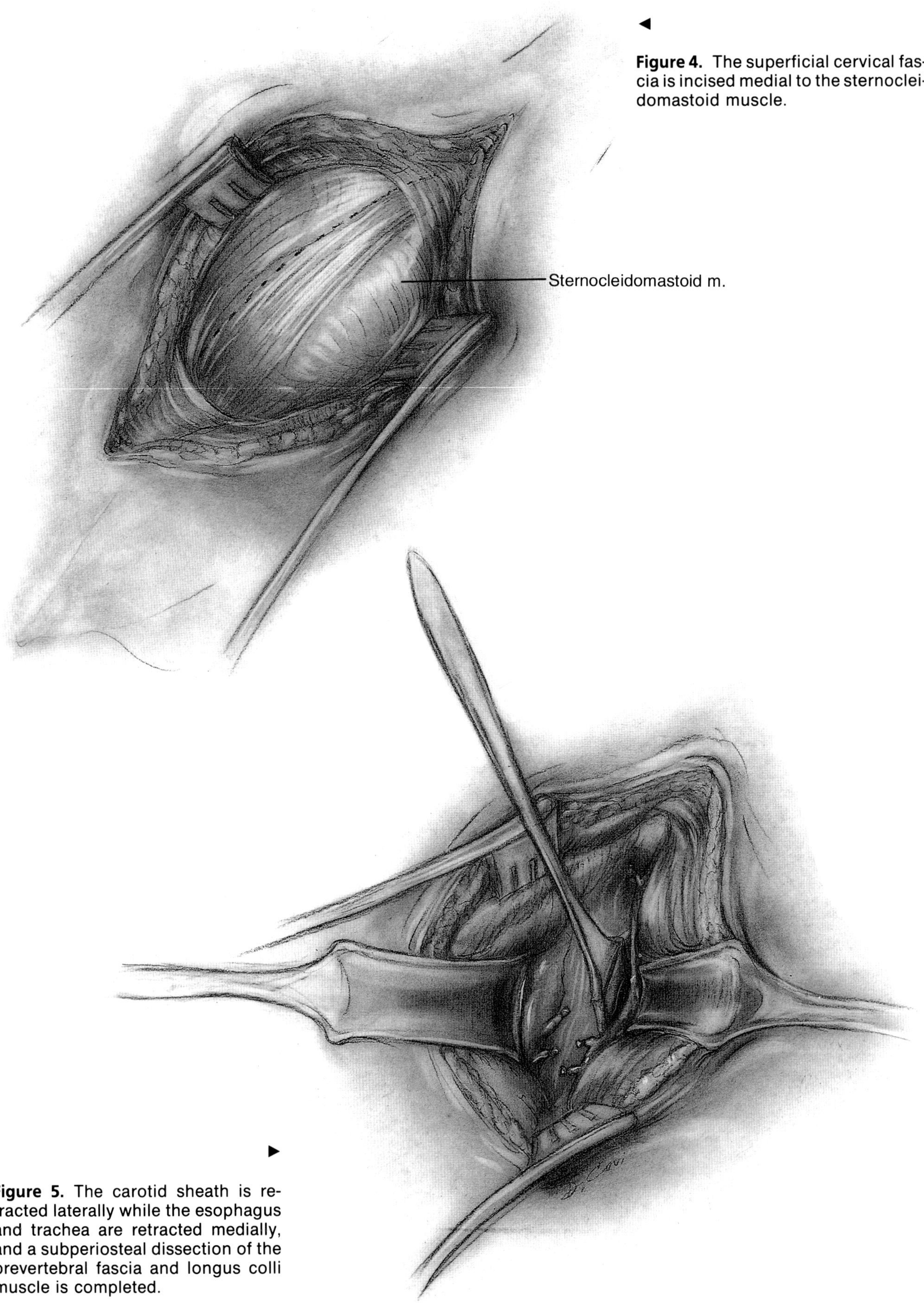

◀

Figure 4. The superficial cervical fascia is incised medial to the sternocleidomastoid muscle.

▶

Figure 5. The carotid sheath is retracted laterally while the esophagus and trachea are retracted medially, and a subperiosteal dissection of the prevertebral fascia and longus colli muscle is completed.

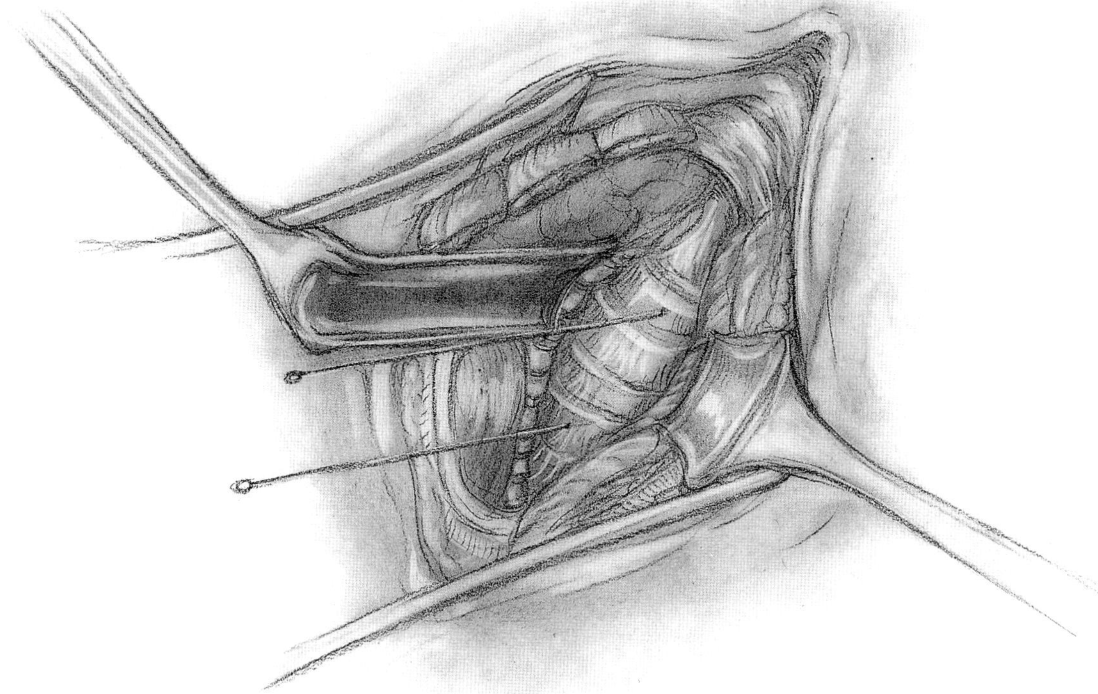

A

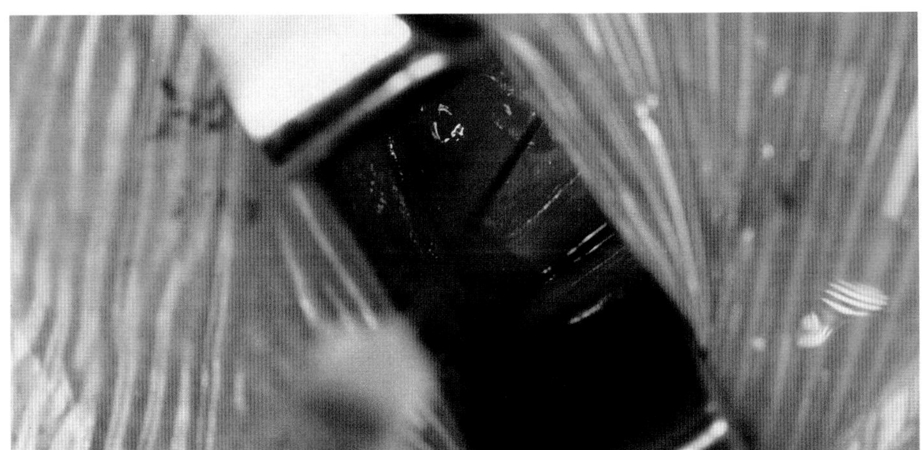

B

Figure 6. A,B: A spinal needle is placed in the disc space and a lateral radiograph (*not shown*) is obtained to confirm the correct level of surgery.

through the anterior longitudinal ligament and outer anulus (Fig. 7). Through this opening, the intervertebral disc, including the degenerated nucleus pulposus, is removed with a pituitary rongeur. After a significant amount of disc material is removed, a small intervertebral body spreader is placed lateral to the midline to allow careful distraction of the disc space. The remainder of the disc and the cartilage end plates are then removed with a combination of pituitary rongeurs and curettes (Figures 8 and 9). The intervertebral spreader should then be removed and replaced along the contralateral side of the disc space in order to allow complete removal of all disc material. Occasionally, large overhanging osteophytes may need to be partially removed in order to improve the exposure of the disc space and define the anterior vertebral body border. However, care should be taken to preserve the anterior cortical edges of the adjacent vertebral bodies. All cartilage should be removed, but the bony end plates should not be resected. The posterior longitudinal ligament should be visualized but not incised if the ligament is intact. If a tear is seen in the ligament, then resection of the ligament can be performed with a 1-mm Kerrison rongeur. After complete resection, a micronerve hook should be used to probe the posterior border of the superior and inferior vertebrae for any sequestered disc fragments. Removal of the posterior osteophytes is not routinely recommended, since resorption of the osteophytes often occurs with a solid fusion. When compression by an osteophyte is thought to cause significant neurologic problems, a more generous resection of the vertebral body should be carried out, allowing direct visualization of the osteophyte so that excessive manipulation of the spinal cord can be minimized.

After complete discectomy, both posterior joints of Luschka should be visualized. The disc space is next prepared for insertion of the graft. The disc space height and depth is then measured. The depth is then measured by placing a wire into the back of the disc space and measuring the length. The space can usually accept a block of bone up to 10 mm high, 10 to 15 mm wide, and 12 to 17 mm deep. To avoid resorption, the graft should measure a minimum of 5 mm high.

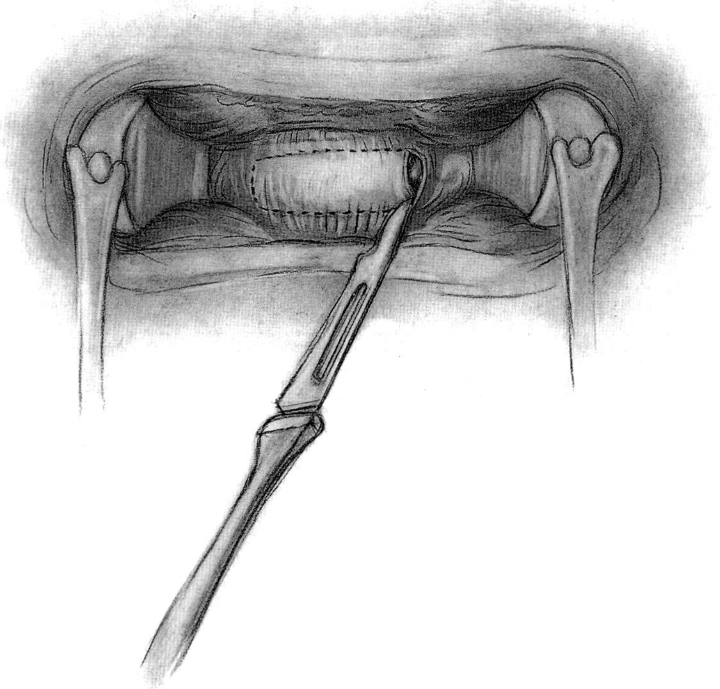

Figure 7. Exposure of the disc space is complete, and a scalpel is used to initiate disc removal.

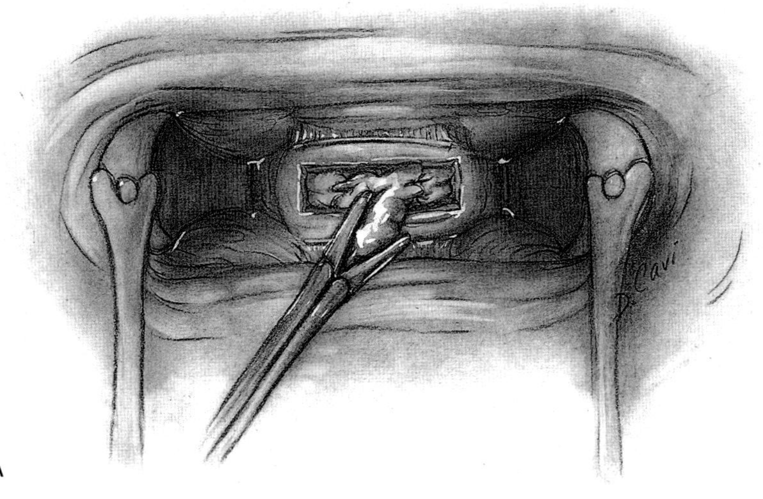

A

Figure 8. A–C: The disc and cartilaginous end plates are removed with a combination of pituitary rongeurs and curettes. A small lamina spreader improves the exposure.

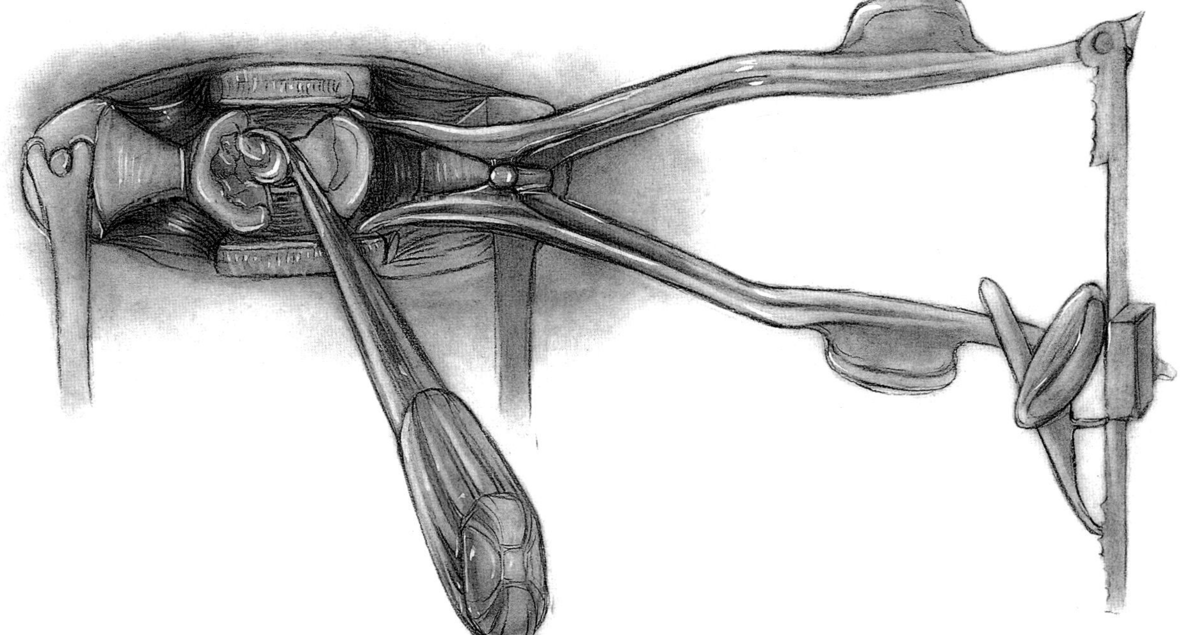

B

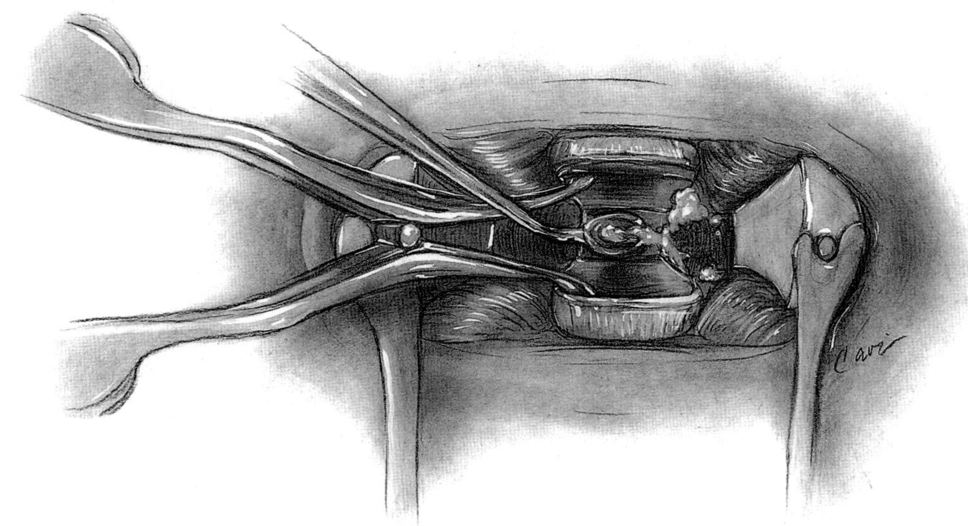

C

A small incision is then made over the crest of the ilium at least 2 cm behind the anterior superior iliac spine in order to avoid the lateral femoral cutaneous nerve. The size of the initial bone plug should be greater than the size of the final trimmed graft. After subperiosteal exposure of both the inner and outer tables of the crest, two vertical cuts are made using a power oscillating saw (Fig. 10). These parallel cuts are usually 2 cm deep and are made approximately 10 to 15 mm apart along the top of the iliac crest. The tricortical graft is then removed from the crest, and all soft tissue should be removed with a rongeur. The graft is then trimmed with either a rongeur or bur. We usually bevel the graft so that the anterior height is approximately 2 mm larger than the posterior height (Fig. 11). This beveling of the graft increases the ease of insertion of the horseshoe-shaped tricortical graft into the appropriate disc space.

The prepared disc space is then distracted after holes are made in the bony end plates superiorly and inferiorly with curettes. The distraction can be accomplished by the addition of weights to either a previously placed head halter or tong traction. We prefer distraction of the disc space to be done manually by the anesthesiologist. The bone graft is then placed in position and tapped into the disc space with a bone tamp and mallet (Fig. 12). The graft should be countersunk 1 to 2 mm in relation to the anterior cortical edges of the adjacent vertebral bodies. At this point, we routinely obtain a second lateral radiograph of the cervical spine in order to confirm adequate placement of the graft.

We normally place a soft Jackson-Pratt drain in the neck wound. The fascia over the platysma is usually reapproximated with 2–0 Vicryl sutures. We normally close the skin with a running absorbable subcuticular stitch.

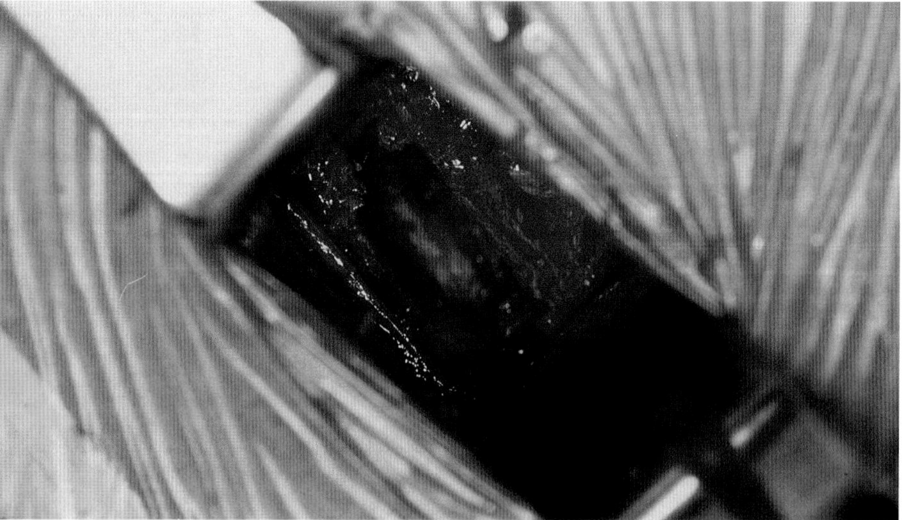

Figure 9. Surgical view of Fig. 8.

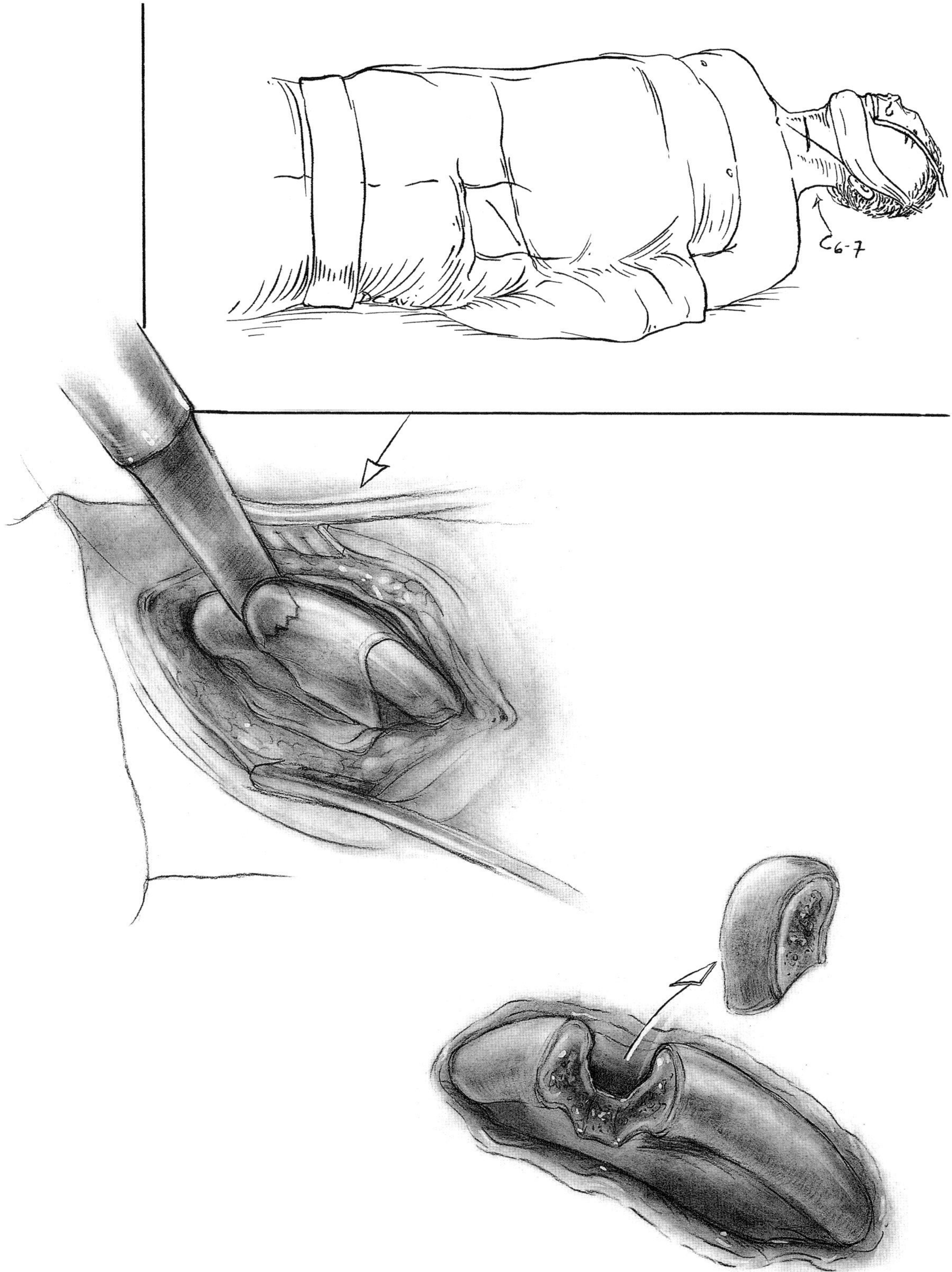

Figure 10. A tricortical iliac crest bone graft. The graft is harvested at least 2 cm behind the anterior superior iliac spine.

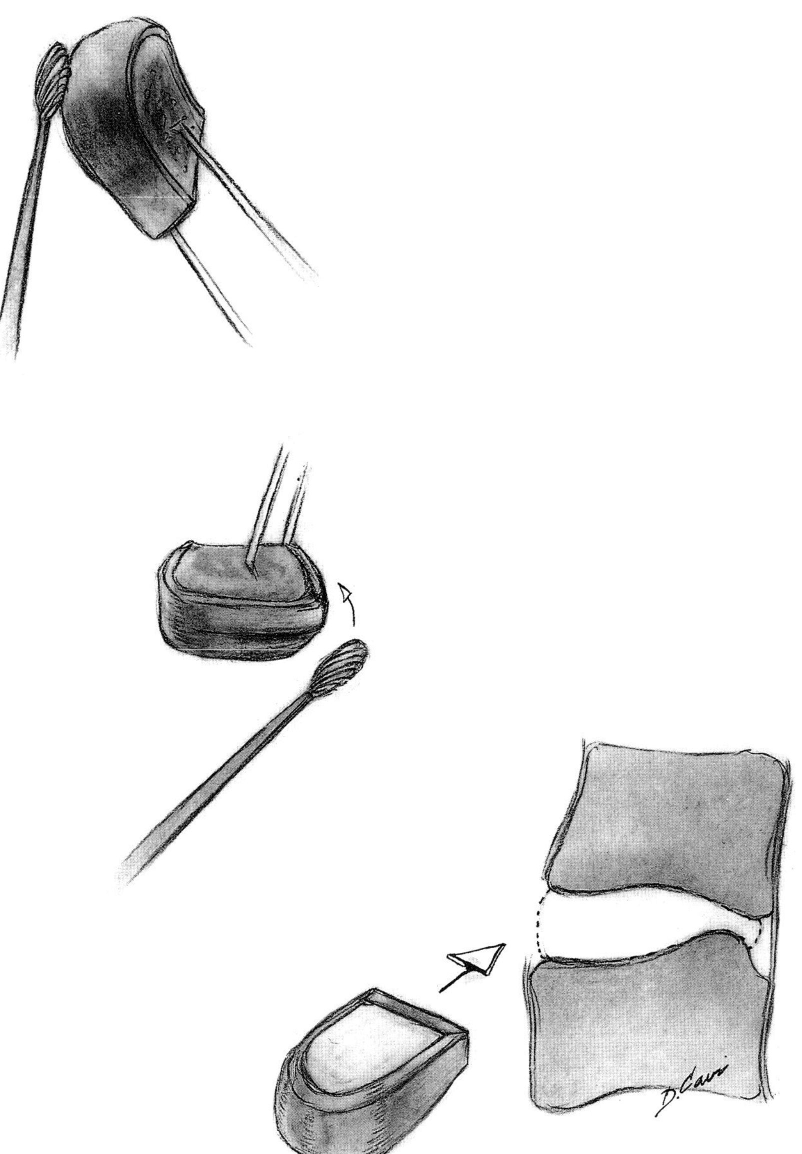

Figure 11. The graft is bevelled with a bur so that the anterior height is 2 mm larger than the posterior height.

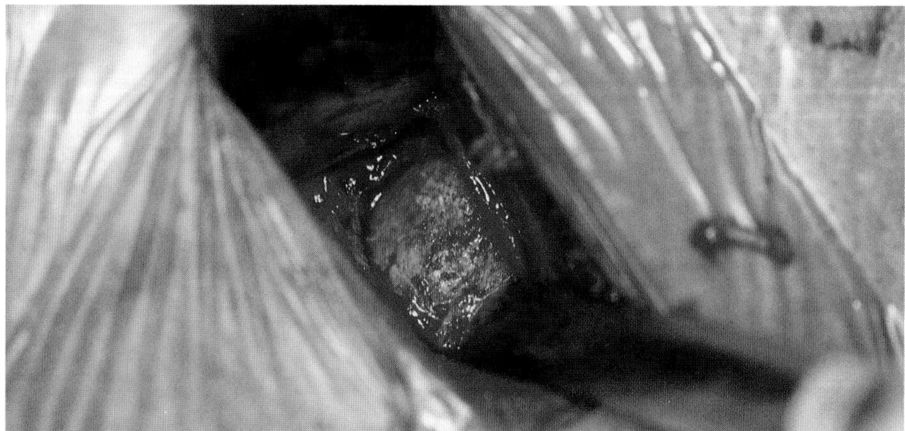

Figure 12. The tricortical graft is inserted into the disc space with the intact iliac crest cortex anterior in the disc space.

POSTOPERATIVE MANAGEMENT

As soon as both wounds are closed, the patient is immediately placed in a rigid Philadelphia cervical collar. We routinely leave drains in the neck and the iliac crest graft site for 24 to 48 hours. All patients are encouraged to be ambulatory on hospital day 1 or 2. Most patients are discharged from the hospital 2 or 3 days after the operative procedure in either a rigid Philadelphia cervical collar or other similar orthosis. The orthosis can usually be discontinued by 6 weeks; however, a longer period may be necessary if fusion has not been demonstrated radiographically at follow-up. After this time period, patients are instructed to begin isometric neck exercises while wearing a soft collar for comfort only. Most patients can expect to return to full activity 3 months after surgery.

Preoperatively, most patients are told that the procedure has a 90% chance of significantly reducing their arm pain. We specifically tell all patients that this procedure will not reduce their neck pain. Additionally, patients are instructed that usually no significant loss of neck motion occurs postoperatively after a one- or two-level fusion.

COMPLICATIONS

Complications can be divided into those occurring at the graft site and those occurring at the neck. Robinson's initial report describes no complications in 48 of 56 patients. Four patients had temporary unilateral paralysis of the vocal cords, two patients had marked dysphagia, and two patients had a transient Horner's syndrome. The most common problem seen postoperatively in the neck is transient sore throat or difficulty in swallowing. The risk of this injury can be decreased by using dull retractors. Perforating injuries to the esophagus are rarely reported but can be life-threatening. Neurologic complications were reported by Flynn (7), who compiled the replies of 704 neurosurgeons describing over 36,000 anterior cervical interbody fusions. The single largest neurologic complication was recurrent laryngeal nerve palsies. As stated previously, the risk to the recurrent laryngeal nerve can be decreased by using a left-sided approach. The most feared neurologic complication is that of spinal cord injury. In his large series, Flynn (7) reported 100 cases of significant permanent myelopathy or myeloradiculopathy. Seventy-five percent of these patients had an immediate deficit postoperatively, while 25% of the patients developed a neurologic deficit during the postoperative recovery period. Analysis of the data led Flynn to conclude that regardless of the etiology of the myelopathy, reoperation had little effect on the ultimate status of the neurologic deficit. In addition, most surgeons were unable to determine the etiology of the neurologic deterioration.

Graft extrusion may still occur despite meticulous grafting techniques. If the graft completely extrudes, it should be replaced to avoid esophageal damage. The occurrence of a pseudarthrosis has been found to be inversely proportional to the number of levels fused. However, many authors have found that the presence of a pseudarthrosis fails to affect the quality of the result statistically. The lack of correlation between a successful fusion and a patient outcome can be explained by the fact that even though bone union does not occur, a stable fibrous union does. Second, removal of the degenerative disc alleviates some of the mechanical pressure on the nerve root. Finally, distraction of the disc space and neuroforamen occurs even though much of the initial height of the interspace gained by the bone graft is lost.

Complications occurring commonly at the donor site include hematoma, infection, lateral femoral cutaneous nerve injury, muscle herniation, and persistent pain over the iliac crest. Although frequently reported, these complications usually do not cause a permanent disability. Careful attention to placement of the incision and meticulous hemostasis with placement of drains prior to closure will minimize some of the risks.

ILLUSTRATIVE CASE FOR TECHNIQUE

E. M. is a 35-year-old man who presented with bilateral arm numbness and right arm and leg weakness. Approximately 6 months previously, he suffered a hyperextension injury while playing volleyball. At that time, he noted an acute transient episode of numbness of all four extremities. Since the initial injury he has had several transient episodes of lower extremity numbness that occurred with hyperextension. Additionally, he has noted the gradual onset of bilateral

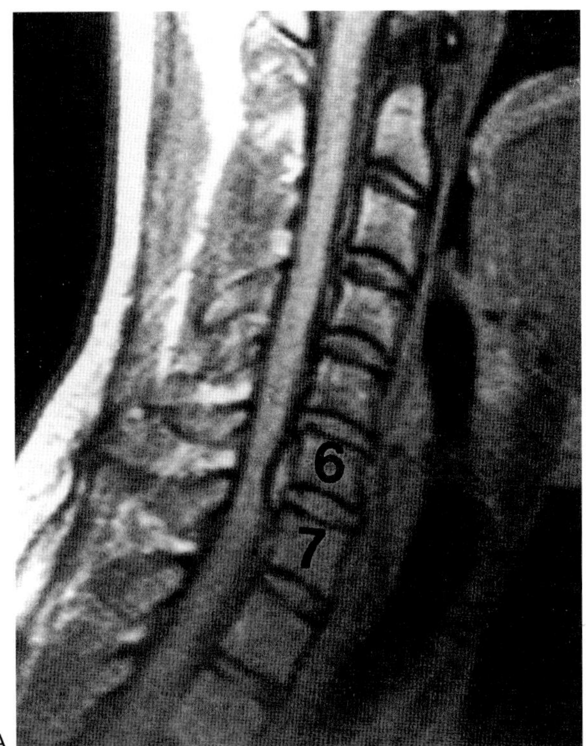

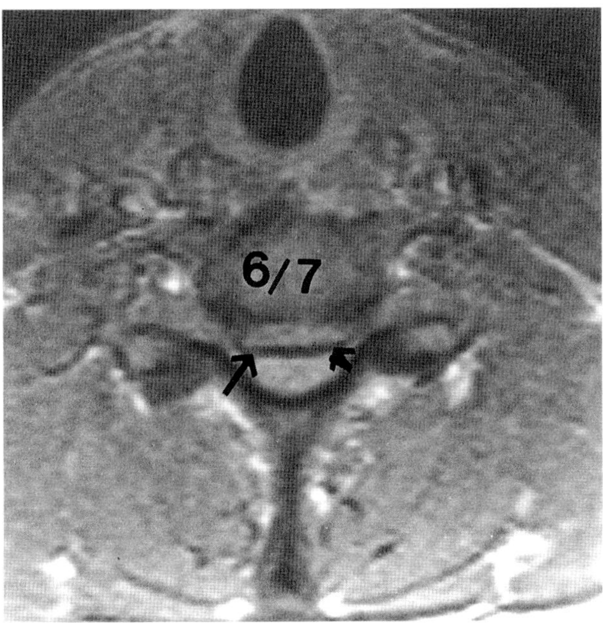

Figure 13. A,B: MRI scans demonstrating a large central herniated disc at C6–C7.

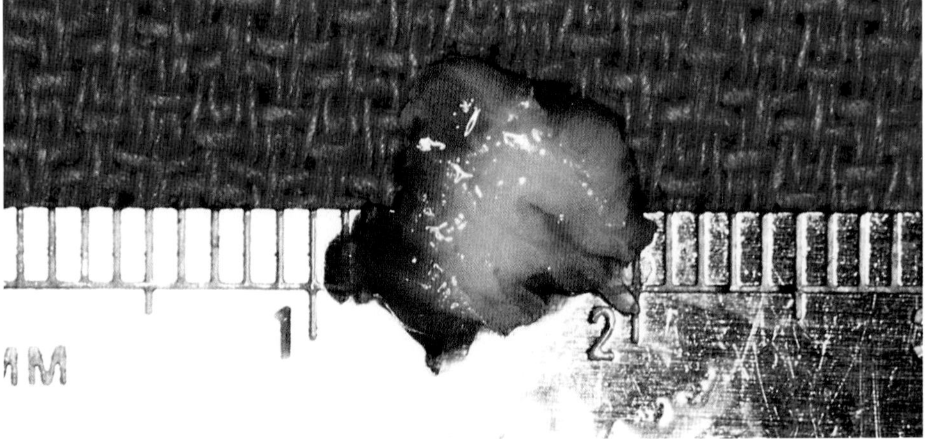

Figure 14. A sequestered disc fragment was removed posterior to the posterior longitudinal ligament.

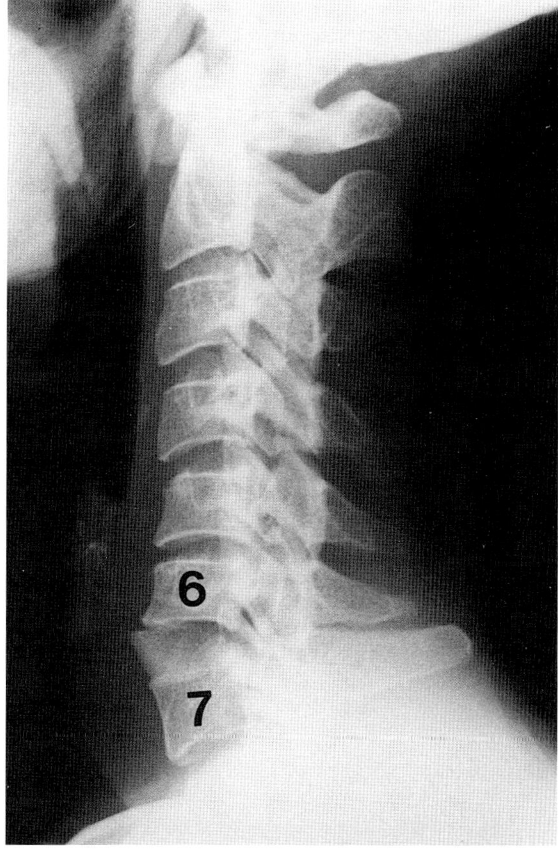

Figure 15. Postoperative lateral radiograph demonstrating slight protrusion of the C6–C7 graft.

numbness in the ulnar digits of both hands. Most recently, he complained of right-hand clumsiness and right-leg weakness.

Physical examination was significant for grade 4 or 5 weakness in the right triceps muscle. The patient ambulated with a slightly wide-based gait and had a positive Babinski sign and positive Hoffman sign on the right; MRI revealed a large central herniated disc at the C6–C7 level (Fig. 13).

The patient was recommended for a C6–C7 anterior cervical discectomy and fusion. Intraoperatively, a tear was noted in the posterior longitudinal ligament. Exploration of the space behind this ligament revealed a large sequestered disc fragment, which was removed (Fig. 14). A tricortical graft measuring 11 mm in height was then placed in the C6–C7 interspace. Postoperatively, the patient noted relief of the upper extremity numbness, although the pathologic reflexes persisted (Fig. 15).

RECOMMENDED READING

1. Nurick, S.: The natural history and the results of surgical treatment of the spinal cord disorder associated with cervical spondylosis. *Brain*, 95: 101–108, 1972.
2. Robinson, R., Walker, A., and Ferlic, D.: The results of anterior interbody fusion of the cervical spine. *J. Bone Joint Surg.*, 44A: 1569–1587, 1962.
3. Herkowitz, H., Kurz, L., and Overholt, D.: Surgical management of cervical soft disc herniation: a comparison between the anterior and posterior approach. *Spine*, 15: 1026–1030, 1990.
4. Herkowitz, H.: A comparison of anterior cervical fusion, cervical laminectomy, and cervical laminoplasty for the surgical management of multiple level spondylotic radiculopathy. *Spine*, 113: 774–780, 1988.

5. Hukuda, S., Mochizuki, T., Ogata, M., Shichikawa, K., and Shimomura, Y.: Operations for cervical spondylotic myelopathy. *J. Bone Joint Surg.*, 67B: 609–615, 1985.
6. Crandall, P., and Gregorius, F.: Long term follow-up of surgical treatment of cervical spondylotic myelopathy. *Spine*, 2: 139–146, 1977.
7. Flynn, T.: Neurologic complications of anterior cervical interbody fusion. *Spine*, 7: 536–539, 1982.
8. Yamamoto, I., et al.: Clinical long term results of anterior discectomy without interbody fusion for cervical disc disease. *Spine*, 16: 272–279, 1991.
9. Fernyhough, J., White, J., and LaRocca, H.: Fusion rates in multilevel cervical spondylosis comparing allograft fibula with autograft fibula in 126 patients. *Spine*, 16: 5561–5564, 1991.
10. Zdeblick, T., and Ducker, T.: The use of freeze-dried allograft bone for anterior cervical fusions. *Spine*, 16: 726–729, 1991.

Master Techniques in Orthopaedic Surgery,
THE SPINE, edited by D. S. Bradford,
Lippincott-Raven Publishers, Philadelphia, © 1997.

7

Posterior Arthrodesis of the Cervical Spine

Stephen J. Lipson

INDICATIONS/CONTRAINDICATIONS

Posterior arthrodesis is indicated in patients with rheumatoid arthritic subluxations for reversal or stabilization of cervical myelopathy and for treatment of pain unresponsive to nonoperative measures. Subluxations include atlantoaxial impaction, atlantoaxial subluxation (commonly anterior, but not exclusively, since posterior and lateral subluxations are found), and subaxial subluxation. Successful posterior arthrodesis of the cervical spine is dependent on many factors, including the patient's debilitation, skin condition, airway, cervical instability, susceptibility to infection, and wound-healing abilities. The technical preparation of the patient for cervical spine surgery, meticulous preparation of the host area to be arthrodesed, and adequacy of the bone graft as a structural biomaterial are of paramount importance. Because patients with severe rheumatoid arthritis and cervical spine subluxation have all the obstacles mentioned and present a challenge to the spine surgeon before the patient is ever taken to the operating room, I will consider the entire perioperative management of these patients (5). The principles are applicable to arthrodesis in nonrheumatoid patients but are confounded in rheumatoid arthritics by all of the issues raised. In particular, the autogenous bone graft, which is typically osteopenic and mechanically weak as a biomaterial, is fragile and difficult to incorporate into a fusion mass for a successful arthrodesis. These problems call for the addition of an implant to allow stabilization and permit the patient to tolerate the rehabilitative setting by avoiding external immobilization with a halo vest.

S. J. Lipson, M.D.: Beth Israel Hospital, Harvard Medical School, Boston, Massachusetts 02215.

No absolute contraindications to surgery exist, except for those such as severe cardiopulmonary conditions, in which the patient's likelihood of survival of any anesthetic course is questionable.

PREOPERATIVE PLANNING

Preoperative planning starts with a history to elicit the presence of pain and neurologic symptoms of paresthesias, numbness, weakness, and vertebrobasilar complaints. Physical examination will determine postural deformity of the neck and neurologic conditions of radicular deficits and cervical myelopathy with upper motor neuron findings. Patients with severe postural deformity, usually a head tilt (Fig. 1), and those with significant neurologic deficits, characterized as Ranawat IIIA and IIIB, may require preoperative traction for correction. The neurologic deficit is more responsive to intervention when the condition has lasted for no more than months. Plain radiographs with flexion-extension lateral views are essential in characterizing the subluxations present and their reducibility in traction. It is essential to know whether a subluxation can be reduced by simple positioning or whether preoperative traction is necessary to reduce the subluxation. Magnetic resonance imaging (MRI) has been invaluable in the examination of spinal cord compression in these patients and is used routinely to determine whether cord compression can be reduced by traction versus the need for decompression.

Radiologic parameters demonstrating the need for surgical intervention include the presence of atlantoaxial impaction with a cervicomedullary angle of less than 135 degrees on MRI, anterior atlantodental intervals of 9 mm or more, posterior atlantodental intervals of 14 mm or less, and the presence of subaxial subluxation of more than 3 to 5 mm (1,5). Even in the absence of neurologic symptoms and signs, these parameters suggest that the patient is at risk for the development or progression of neurologic loss, indicating impending neurologic deficit (2). In the subaxial spine, a measurement called the cervical height index, indicating the components of postural deformity in the subaxial spine, has been described as a very strong marker of the need for subaxial correction (3).

The next decision is whether to utilize preoperative traction. Patients who require this maneuver are those with Ranawat IIIA and IIIB deficits, irreducible subluxations, and severe head tilt (Fig. 1). It is better to reverse a neurologic deficit before surgery, since the patient becomes stronger and can appreciate the results of surgery, which is designed to stabilize the corrected position. Once the deficit has been corrected in traction, the surgery can proceed on an elective basis.

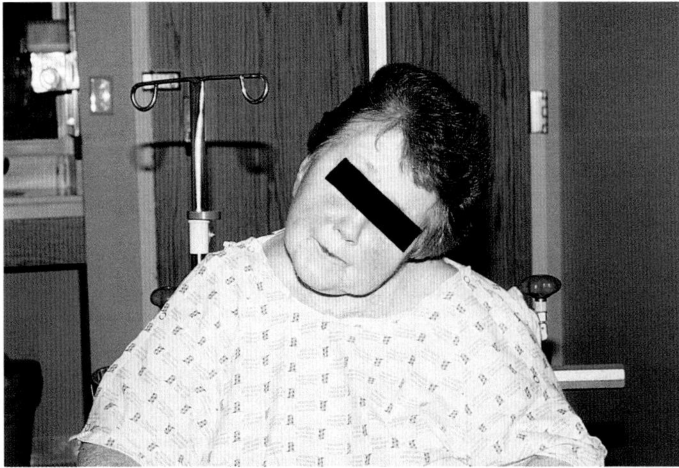

Figure 1. A rheumatoid arthritic with severe head tilt.

Correcting subluxation prior to surgery not only improves posture but permits an easier operation, since a spine in a more anatomic position is technically easier to visualize (Fig. 2) and stabilize operatively, making the surgery safer for both patient and surgeon. Additionally, anesthetic management is easier since some of the postural deformity of the airway reduces, making intubation easier (7).

Preoperative traction is undertaken in a halo wheelchair (Fig. 3), which has a

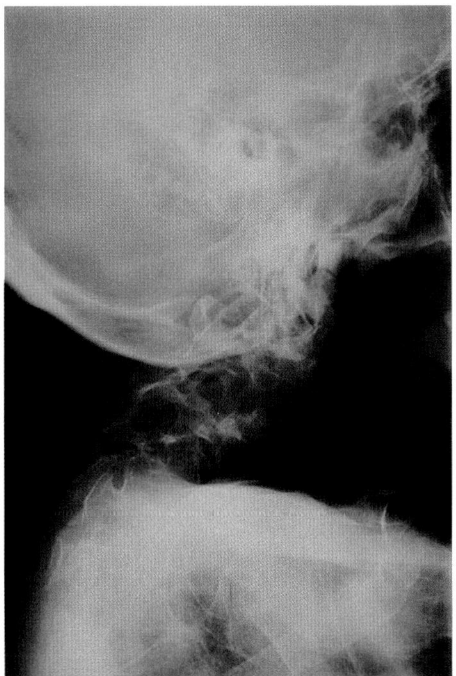

A

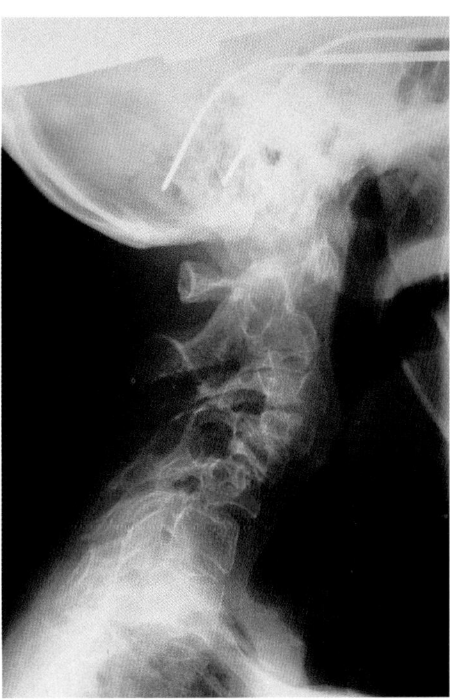

B

Figure 2. Severe subluxations of atlantoaxial impaction, anterior atlantoaxial subluxation, and subaxial subluxations before preoperative halo traction **(A)** and after traction **(B)** with marked correction of deformities on lateral radiographs.

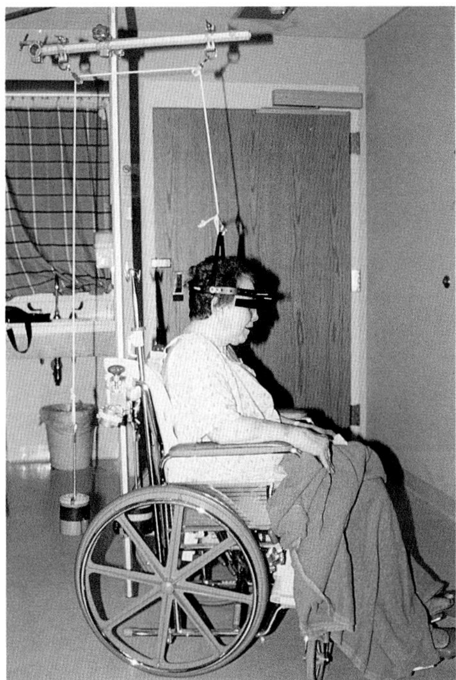

A

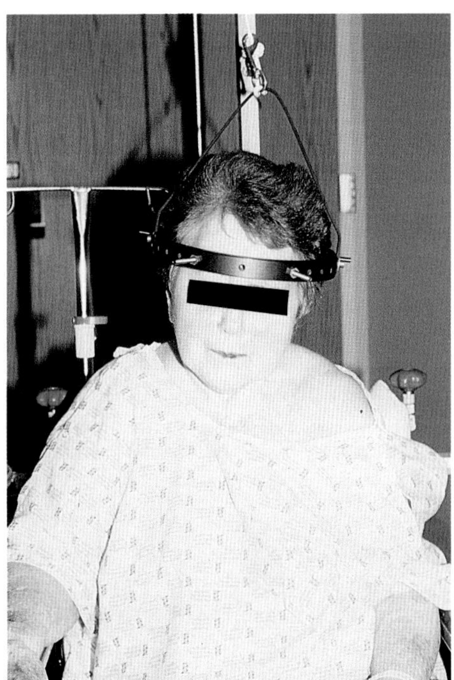

B

Figure 3. The patient in Fig. 1 in a halo wheelchair from the lateral aspect **(A)** and a frontal view **(B)** with marked correction of her deformity.

Balkan frame attached firmly to an overhead pulley. Weights are attached in the front portion of the chair to counterbalance the traction weight so that the chair does not topple backward. Halo traction is also maintained in bed. The patient is transferred from bed to chair with the assistance of a nurse. This traction allows the patient to sit up, change positions, decrease skin pressure, toilet in an upright position, eat upright, increase pulmonary ventilation, converse upright, and leave the room; thus the patient usually feels better emotionally, compared with bed confinement in limited positions. Reduction of subluxations and neurologic reversal can usually be accomplished within 2 days of traction. Cervical spine radiographs in traction document the correction or lack of correction to the subluxations, so that intraoperative decompression can be planned out preoperatively.

SURGERY

Anesthetic considerations are of paramount importance in beginning a posterior arthrodesis in patients with rheumatoid arthritis. The patient is brought to the operating room in traction if it has already been used. All preparations are done with the patient awake so as to protect the spinal cord. Adequate intravenous lines are placed along with appropriate monitoring (e.g., central venous pressure, arterial line, pulse oximeter) preoperatively, since the arms will not be accessible during surgery. An awake fiberoptic intubation is very important to protect the cervical spinal cord and because when this procedure is not performed a 13% incidence of postoperative airway obstruction is seen (7). If halo traction has not been used preoperatively, general anesthesia is induced once the patient is intubated, and Trippe-Wells tongs are applied for intraoperative traction. The eyes are protected to avoid drying and corneal abrasion.

I place the patient prone on the operating table on rolls and use a cerebellar (horseshoe) headrest with a pulley for traction. I believe it is prudent for the surgeon, not the anesthesiologist, to take control of the head for the transfer to the operating room (OR) table. Once the patient is positioned, the eyes are again carefully inspected to be sure there is no pressure on them; otherwise central retinal artery occlusion and blindness as well as corneal abrasion may result. It is prudent for both the surgeon and anesthesiologist to inspect the eyes. A lateral cervical spine radiograph is taken to make sure the cervical spine is reduced to the surgeon's satisfaction. If a position change is needed, it is best done before the neck is prepped. A position change is done by at least two people, with the surgeon taking control of the head. Most anterior subluxations are corrected by posteriorly translating, not extending, the headrest.

Once the head position is satisfactory by visual and radiographic inspection, the operation may begin. The arms are tucked at the side in a comfortable position with sponge cushions over the cubital ulnar canals, the hands, and the lines (Fig. 4). The intravenous lines must be checked to make certain they are free-flowing. The shoulders are taped down to the body to smooth out skin wrinkles. This assists in opening and closing the skin wound (Fig. 5). I do not like taping to the OR table since if the patient had to be rapidly removed from the table such taping would delay the transfer. I keep a stretcher in the OR room at all times during prone procedures since the emergency need to remove the patient from the prone to supine position for an event such as loss of airway requires utmost speed and the presence of a stretcher. The anesthesiologist must check the ventilation on transfers and secure the endotracheal tube to prevent displacement. Antibiotic prophylaxis is used. The posterior neck to the level of the occipital tuberosity is prepped. An iliac crest bone graft site is prepped out and draping performed. A midline incision is used over the appropriate extent. The incision must be adequate to visualize all the structures to be included in the construct.

Occipitocervical Arthrodesis

For occipitocervical arthrodesis, the incision is usually just caudad to the occipital tuberosity and to C2. Cutting cautery is used. The ligamentum nuchae is identified and the midline preserved so as to avoid excessive bleeding. Splenius capitis muscles are divided in the midline to avoid bleeding. For an occiput-to-C2 arthrodesis, the extensor muscles inserting onto the bifid C2 spinous processes are preserved along with the C2–C3 interspinous ligament. Small elevators and cautery are useful to strip the musculature off the occiput, C1 posterior arch, and C2 laminae. The occipitoatlantal and atlantoaxial membranes are preserved. They are often fragile. Dissection laterally on the arch of C1 is done carefully, particularly beyond 1 cm from the midline, so as to avoid the vertebral artery. A venous plexus is often apparent before the artery is found further laterally. Bipolar cautery is used to control bleeding in this region as well as gentle Gelfoam pledgets if needed.

Once the area is adequately exposed, the anterior portion of the posterior arch of C1 is dissected out using a variety of small elevators to release the membranes and avoid pressure on the spinal cord. A doubled #19 gauge wire is then passed by making a loop under the arch. It is grasped by a nerve hook and then a needle holder. The wire is fed under the arch gently so as to not pull on the arch. Defects from synovitic destruction adjacent to the lateral masses of C1 can weaken the bone, and strong traction may fracture the arch of C1. The wire is then bent to the side of the wound and held with a clamp. At the base of the spinous process of C2, a small hole is burred on each side through the bony cortex and the hole completed with a towel clip. The hole is inspected for cerebrospinal fluid (CSF). If CSF appears, the hole must be remade more dorsally. Then a #19 gauge wire on a swadged-on needle is passed through the hole. The wire is passed caudad to the spinous process of C2 under the muscles attached to the spinous process tips and the interspinous ligament of C2–C3. A second wire is passed in the same manner but from the opposite direction. At the occiput, paired full-thickness bur holes are made on each side about 1 cm off the midline and 1 to 2 cm above the foramen magnum. An air-powered bur is used to reach the dura. A small curette is used to enlarge the holes. A small elevator is used to dissect the dura off the inner table of the skull and a curved elevator to permit connection of the holes. In each pair of anchor bur holes, a double #19 gauge wire is passed and gently pulled through. The wires are shown in Fig. 6.

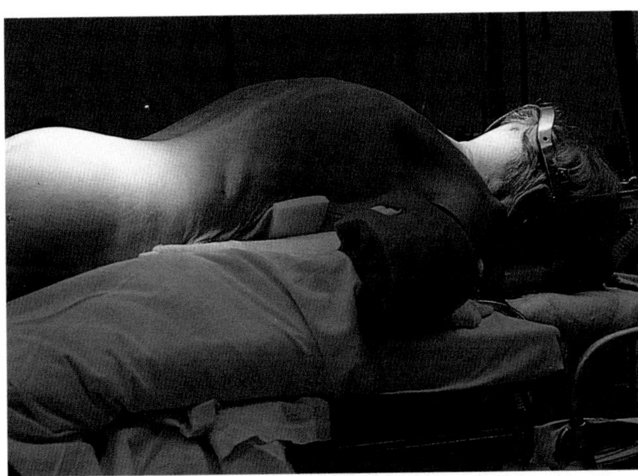

Figure 4. A patient in position for surgery on rolls, in halo traction, on a cerebellar headrest, and with the upper extremities protected.

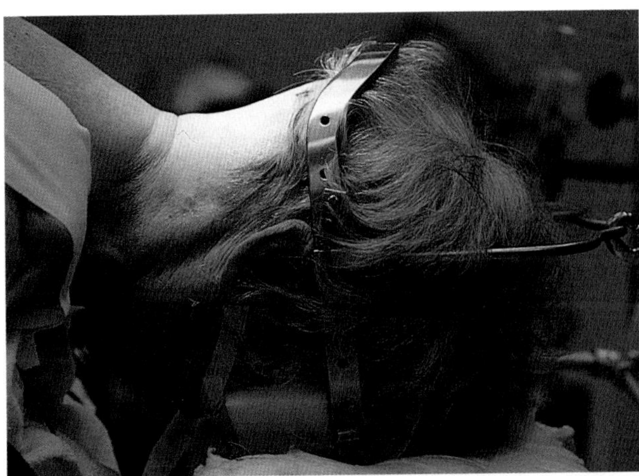

Figure 5. The patient's eyes are protected, the shoulders taped down to decrease the skin folds, and the endotracheal tube secured.

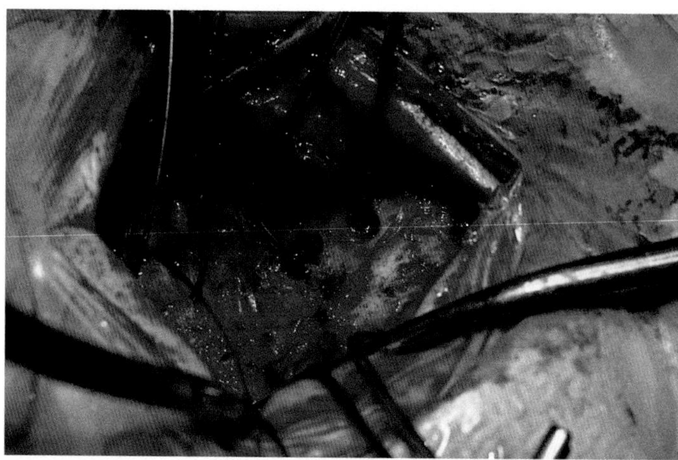

Figure 6. The occipitocervical area is exposed. The head is to the right, the occipital wires are in paired full-thickness bur holes, the C1 wire is passed, and the C2 wires are on the left.

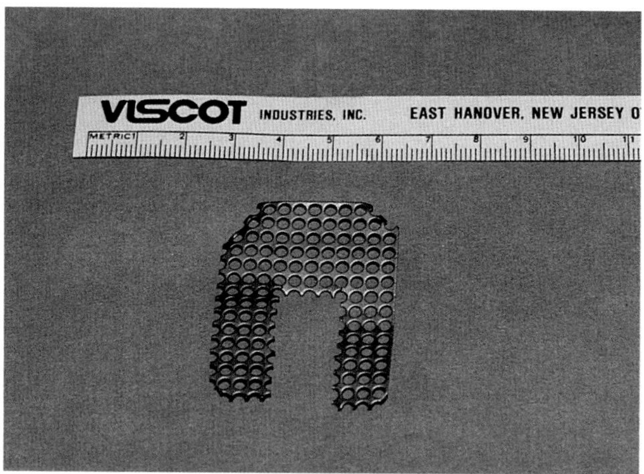

Figure 7. A 0.025-inch Howmedica mandibular mesh cut into a "hot-pants" configuration.

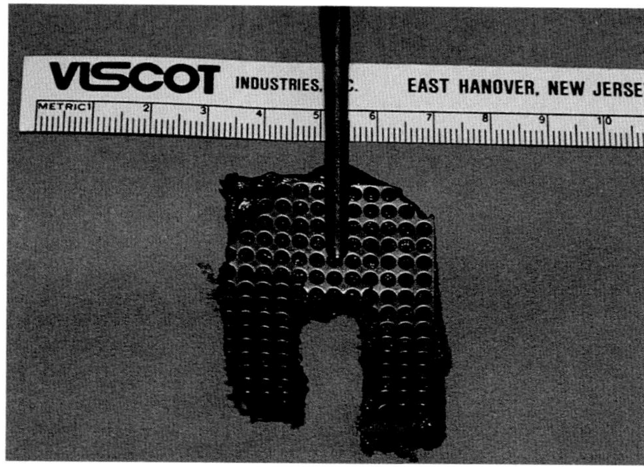

Figure 8. Corticocancellous bone graft is shaped to conform to the mesh and clamped to it. The cancellous surface will lie against the host surface.

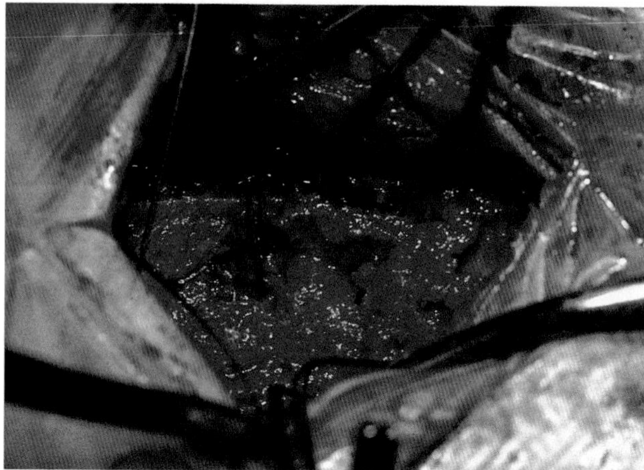

Figure 9. The host surface has been decorticated and packed throughout with cancellous bone.

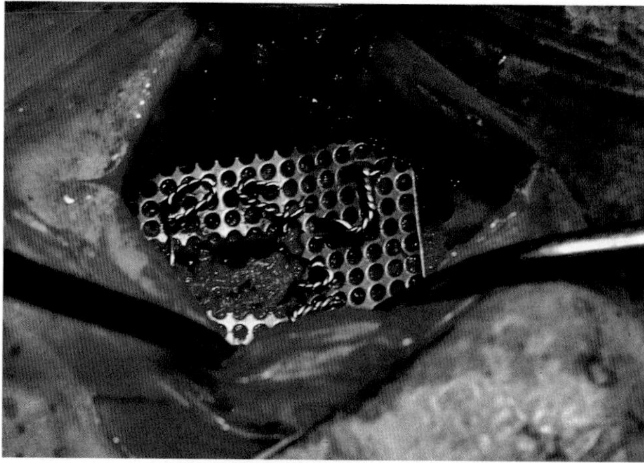

Figure 10. The metal mesh-backed bone graft is wired down and impacted against the host surface. The wires have been cut and twisted down.

At this stage, the bone graft is taken from the iliac crest. A large piece of corticocancellous bone is taken with osteotomes and further cancellous strips taken with Capener gouges. The wound is packed and the cervical spine approached again. Because the bone is fragile, metal mesh backing is used. This technique allows the construct to become a satisfactory biomaterial for successful arthrodesis. The metal mesh provides a backing against which wires can be tightened without cutting through the soft bone graft, fills the entire host surface with bone instead of an implant, compresses the bone onto the host surface, and provides immediate stabilization so as to avoid a halo vest for external immobilization. Howmedica 0.025-inch mandibular mesh is used and cut into a ''hot-pants'' configuration so as to cover the occiput and straddle the spinous processes of C2 and below (Fig. 7). The bone graft is clamped to the metal mesh and trimmed so as to conform to it (Fig. 8).

The graft is positioned so its cancellous surface will lie against the host surface. If the graft is fragmented, as much as possible is applied to the mesh. Small holes are cut through the bone via the holes in the mesh so as to allow passage of wires through the metal-backed graft. All the areas of the occiput, except the bridges between the bur holes, the posterior arch of C1, and the laminae of C2 are decorticated with an air-powered bur. Cancellous bone is placed to cover the surfaces (Fig. 9). The wires are then passed through the metal-backed graft. The double-occiput wires are kept double and the C1 double wire is cut so as to allow one wire on each side. A #14 gauge Angiocath needle is useful as an aid to wire passage since the wires will slip inside the needle when it is passed through the holes in the mesh-backed bone graft. Once the wires are passed and it is certain that no cancellous bone will be pushed into the canal, the clamp attaching the mesh and bone is released, and the metal-backed bone graft is gently pushed down onto the host surface. The wires are then tightened down, compressing the cancellous bone onto the host surface. When they are fully tightened, the wires are cut off and turned down. The final assembly is shown in Fig. 10. The wound is then closed, with care to do the muscle layers and then the fascia. In the past, methylmethacrylate was placed over the mesh to intercalate the wires. This was found to be unnecessary and led to difficulty in wound closure (Fig. 11).

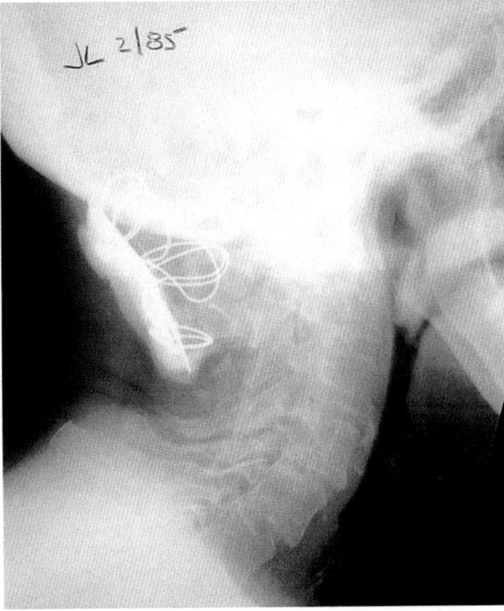

Figure 11. A lateral radiograph of an occiput-C2 arthrodesis in which methylmethacrylate was used over the mesh.

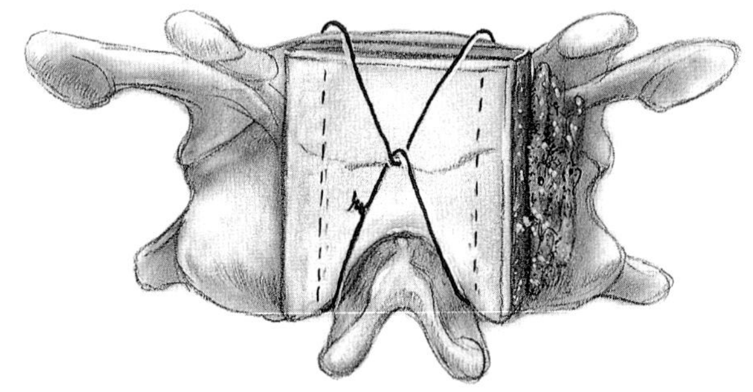

A

Figure 12. Four wire configurations **(A–D)** for atlantoaxial arthrodesis.

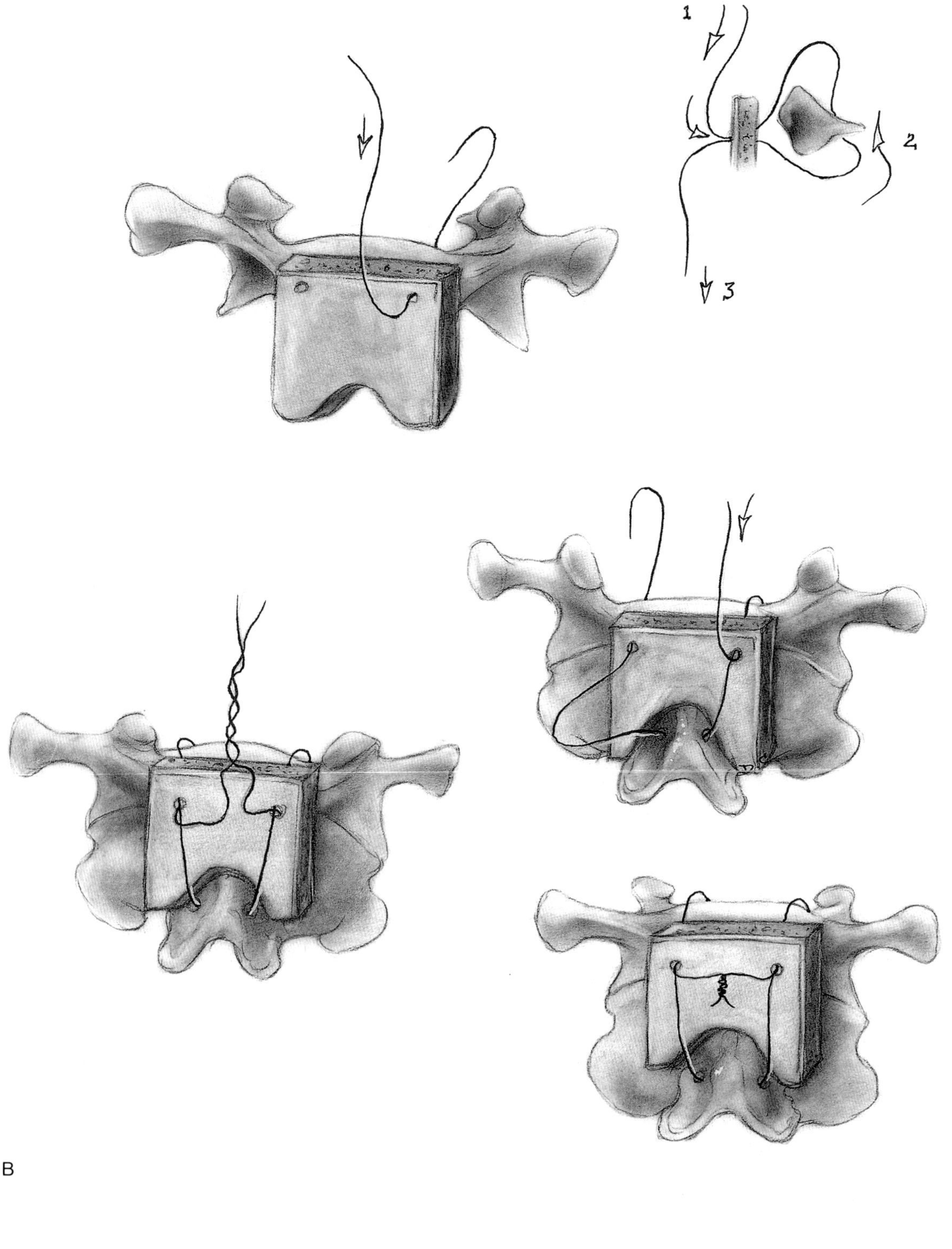

B

Atlantoaxial Arthrodesis

Atlantoaxial arthrodesis can be accomplished with a variety of wire techniques. No technique is best, and a variety of configurations are shown in Fig. 12. They all depend on the same wire passage technique under C1. A Brooks fusion can be done with passage of the wire under the laminae of C2 and grafts placed between C1 and C2 (Fig. 13) or a "hot-pants" graft.

Subaxial Arthrodesis

Subaxial arthrodesis has been used with the metal mesh backing and wires placed into the subaxial spinous processes (Fig. 14). Laminectomy can be accomplished with the construct bridging the laminectomy defect. Rheumatoid arthritics typically have eroded cervical facet joints, requiring gentle dissection on initial exposure so as to not to enter the spinal canal. This pathology also mitigates against the successful use of Southwick lateral facet wiring of grafts. After closure, the traction device is removed and the patient returned to bed in a soft collar and

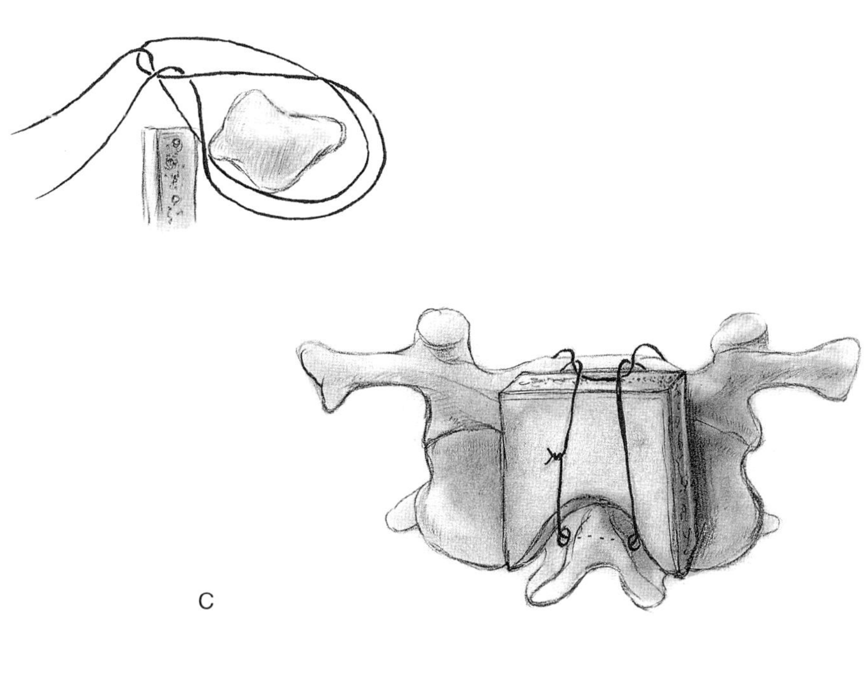

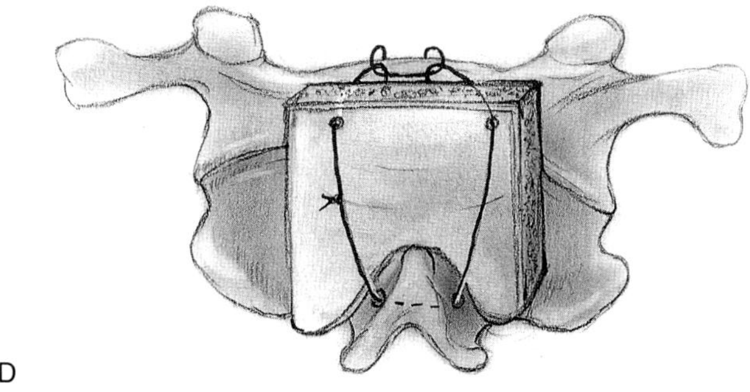

Figure 12. *(Continued.)*

left intubated overnight to be extubated the next morning once fully awake and once swelling in the face and airways has decreased. This protocol (particularly the fiberoptic intubation) has avoided the problem of postoperative airway obstruction particular to rheumatoid arthritic patients who have undergone posterior spine surgery.

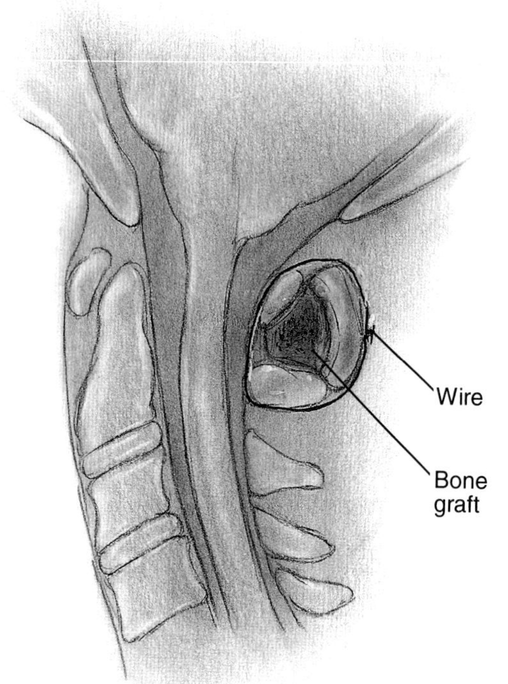

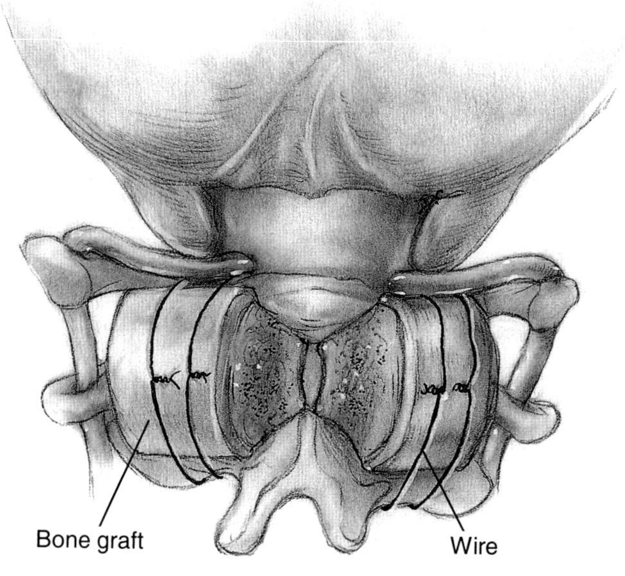

Figure 13. A Brooks fusion construct utilizing bone grafts interposed between C1 and C2.

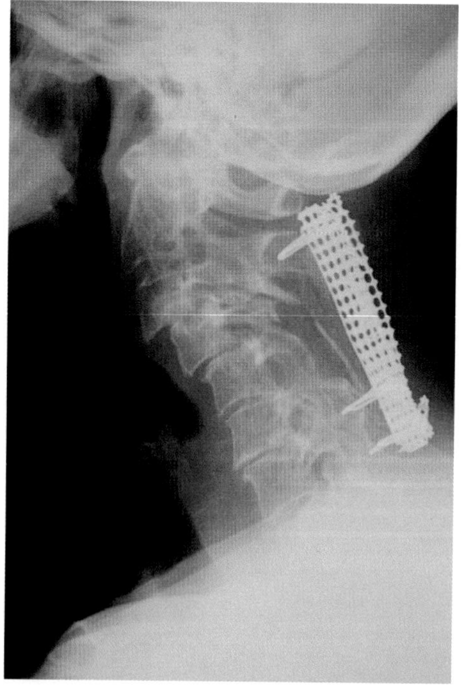

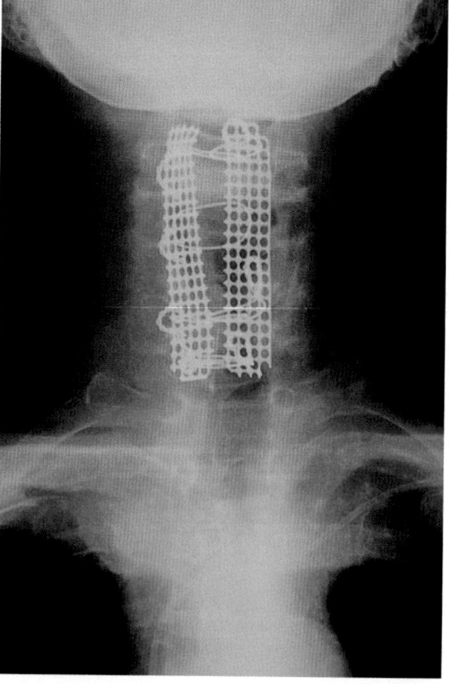

Figure 14. A metal mesh-backed subaxial arthrodesis of C2–C6 with a laminectomy at C3–C4 for subaxial subluxation is shown. **A:** The arthrodesed graft can be seen on the lateral view. **B:** The wires attached to spinous processes are seen on the antero-posterior view with one wire in the middle to connect the two pieces of mesh.

POSTOPERATIVE MANAGEMENT

The patient is left intubated overnight on a ventilator to avoid airway problems from obstruction and hypoventilation following extubation. These patients have orofacial swelling from the prone position, fragile oropharyngeal tissues, and airway trauma (which is reduced by fiberoptic intubation). They typically have difficult airways, making urgent reintubation hazardous. Fiberoptic intubation and prolonged postoperative ventilation have avoided disastrous problems (7). The head of the bed is elevated for 2 days to help reduce edema. Once extubated,

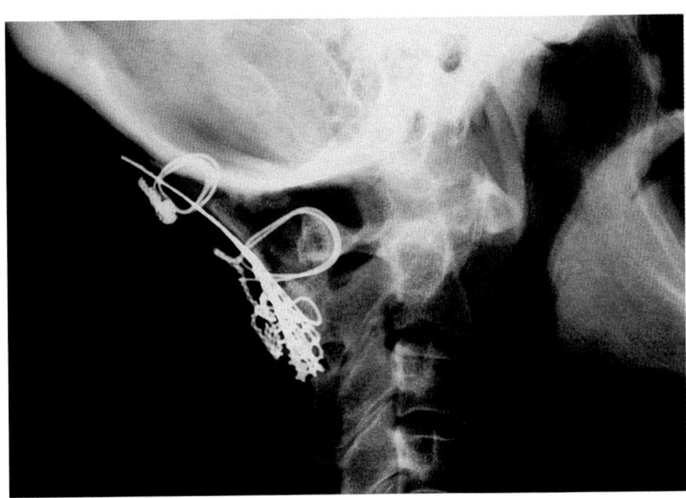

Figure 15. An occiput-C2 arthrodesis with residual atlantoaxial subluxation.

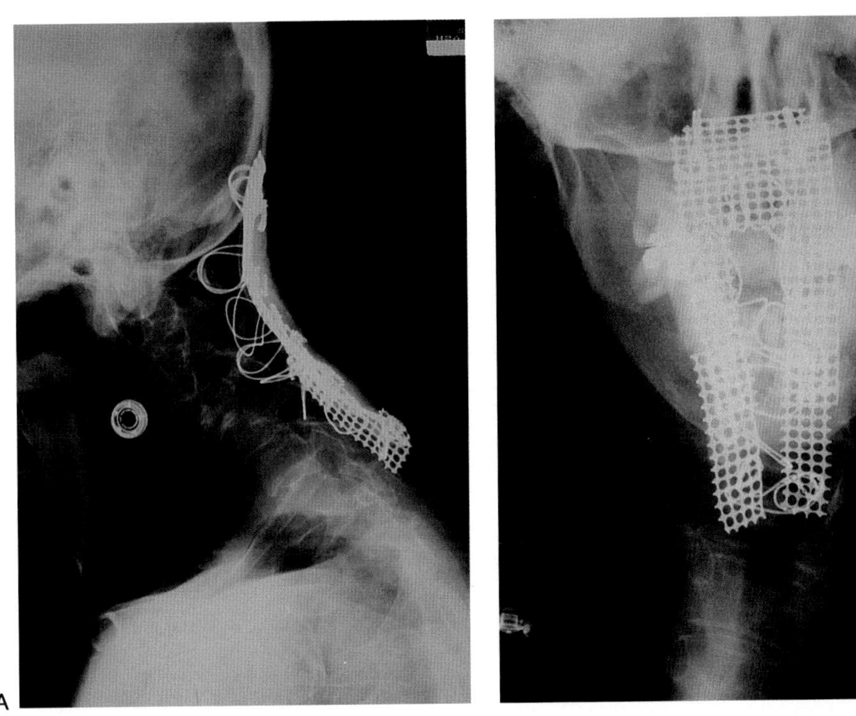

Figure 16. An occipitocervical arthrodesis involving the entire cervical spine for occipitocervical and multilevel subaxial subluxations as seen on lateral **(A)** and anteroposterior **(B)** views.

these patients are fitted with plastizote collars and mobilized by physical therapists to the highest ambulatory status possible. Soft cervical collars are initially used and replaced by front- or side-opening customized plastizote collars. These patients typically do not fit into off-the-shelf collars. No special rehabilitation is required. The avoidance of halo vest immobilization permits rapid rehabilitation. Rubbing alcohol applied to the chin skin twice daily toughens the skin to avoid irritation from the plastizote collar.

The patient is seen at 4 to 6 weeks with radiographs and checked for progress and functional problems and again at 12 weeks with radiographs. The collar is used for up to 12 weeks and then removed. Patients are followed long term at 6 months, 1 year, and 2 years with radiographs including flexion-extension lateral views.

Metal mesh backing for occipitocervical fusions has been very successful. A study of 70 patients demonstrated that 47 improved more than one Ranawat grade. Marked pain relief occurred in 63 (6). In the subaxial spine, a study of 42 posterior arthrodeses demonstrated that 82% had neurologic improvement and 92% significant reduction in pain or neurologic improvement (4). Duration of neurologic symptoms was the most significant predictor of neurologic outcome. Metal mesh backing is used most often in occiput-to-C2 constructs (Fig. 15) but can be extended through the subaxial spine if needed for adjacent instabilities (Fig. 16).

COMPLICATIONS

The airway is a major concern and is addressed by the fiberoptic intubation technique and postoperative ventilation (7). A study of 124 posterior procedures in rheumatoids identified 7 of 55 (13%) who had postoperative airway obstruction versus 1 of 69 in those treated with fiberoptic intubation and overnight ventilation (7).

Infection is a concern in the neck and donor site. Six deep infections (three donor site, three neck) occurred in the 70 occipitocervical patients (7). If an infection occurs, open debridement, antibiotics, and delayed primary closure are used. Long-term antibiotic suppression is used to maintain suppression of the infection.

Nonunion has not been a significant clinical problem. Four asymptomatic nonunions were seen in the 70 occipitocervical arthrodeses (6). In the subaxial series, 15% of patients had fibrous union and 7% nonunion (4). Nonunion requires rearthrodesis if it is clinically problematic. If fibrodesis results in a satisfactory clinical outcome, it may not require further surgery.

Mesh breakage with nonunion has not been a significant problem in this series. A noncompliant patient may benefit from the use of a halo vest and may be able to tolerate it well. Additionally, to avoid mesh breakage, it is probably best to leave the width of each limb of the mesh with three or more holes to avoid a weak construct (Fig. 7). I do not recommend this construct in the nonrheumatoid patient who has good bone and who can tolerate a halo vest. The construct has been used for pathologic fractures and offers the same benefits to this category of patients as it does in rheumatoid arthritics.

ILLUSTRATIVE CASE FOR TECHNIQUE

A 65-year-old woman with a 35-year history of polyarticular rheumatoid arthritis complained of a few years of neck pain with headache in the occipitocervical area accompanied by crepitance. She also reported a Lhermitte's phenomenon radiating into all four extremities, right-hand numbness, and bilateral hand paresthesias. Physical examination revealed tenderness in the occipitocervical junction, limited extension and rotation of the neck, a positive Sharpe-Purser test, mild hyper-reflexia throughout the four extremities, positive finger jerk reflexes, and extensor toe responses, but no weakness or loss of pin sensation in the four extremities. Radiologic evaluation demonstrated anterior atlantoaxial subluxation of 5 mm in extension, 8 mm in flexion, atlantoaxial impaction with a Ranawat measure of 11 mm, and subaxial spondylodiscitis at C2–C3, C3–C4, and C4–C5 (Fig. 17). Examination by MRI demonstrated the dens above the foramen magnum and a cervicomedullary angle of 139 degrees (Fig. 18). An occiput-C2 arthrodesis with metal mesh backing was undertaken in Trippe-Wells tong traction. At 1 year post-

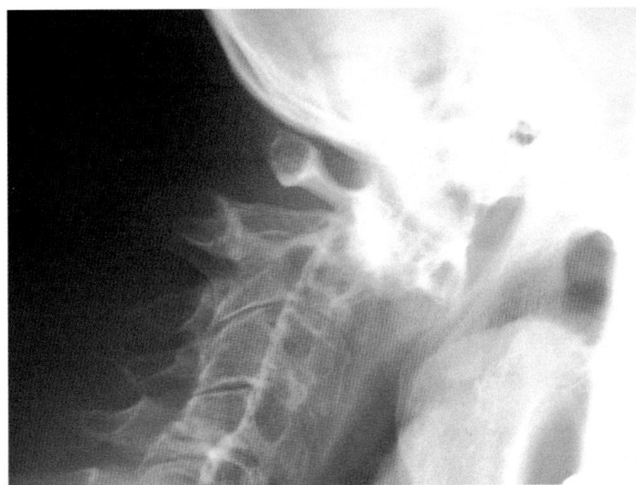

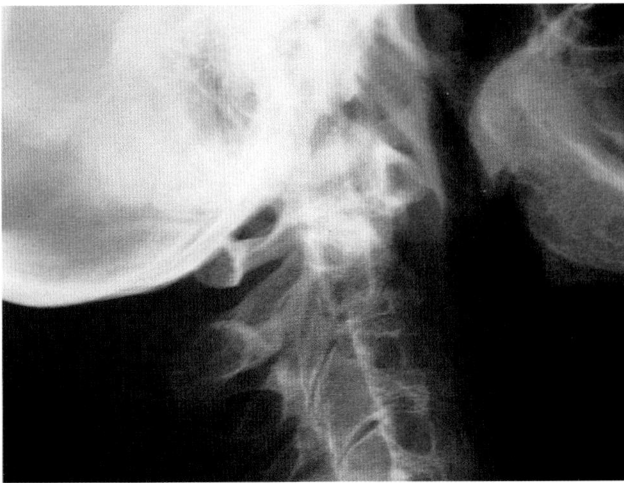

Figure 17. Flexion **(A)** and extension **(B)** radiographs of the illustrative case with atlantoaxial subluxation, atlantoaxial impaction, and subaxial spondylodiscitis.

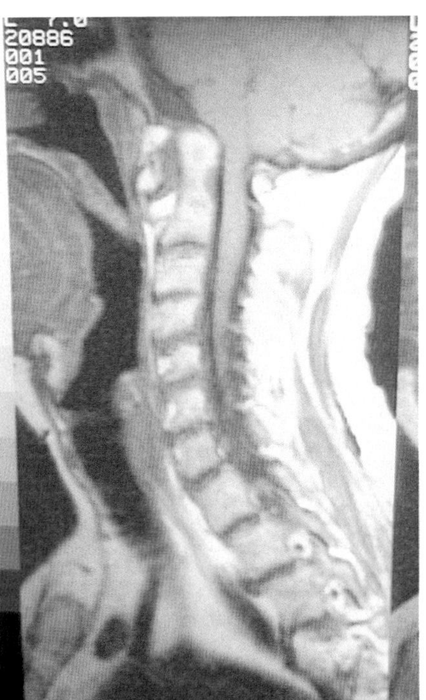

Figure 18. An MRI of the illustrative case with atlantoaxial impaction. The dens lies just above the level of the clivus with a cervicomedullary angle of 139 degrees.

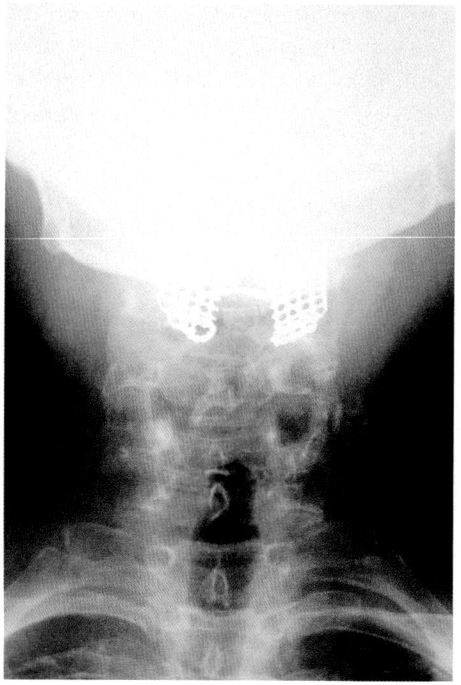

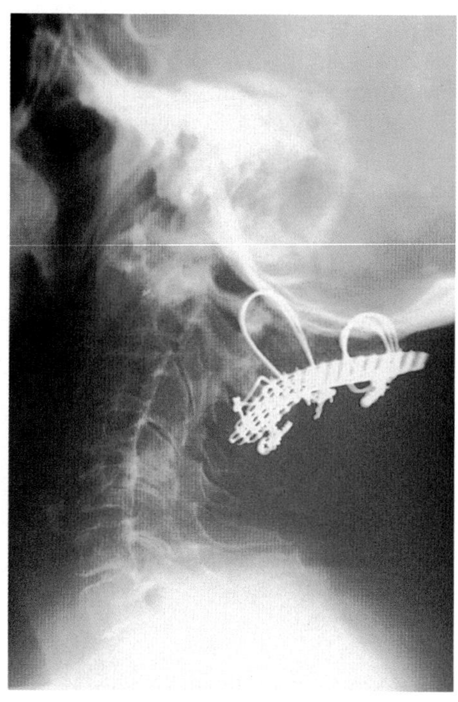

Figure 19. A 1-year follow-up of the illustrative case demonstrates the arthrodesis of occiput to C2 on the anteroposterior **(A)** and lateral **(B)** radiographs.

operatively, she complained of no pain or neurologic symptoms and had minimal residual upper motor neuron findings. A successful arthrodesis was found on radiologic follow-up (Fig. 19).

RECOMMENDED READING

1. Boden, S. D., Dodge, L. D., Bohlman, H. H., and Rechtine, G. R.: Rheumatoid arthritis of the cervical spine. A long term analysis with predictors of paralysis and recovery. *J. Bone Joint Surg.*, 75A: 1282–1297, 1993.
2. Clark, C. R., Goetz, D. D., and Menezes, A. H.: Arthrodesis of the cervical spine in rheumatoid arthritis. *J. Bone Joint Surg.*, 71A: 381–392, 1989.
3. Klein, J. D., Hey, L. A., and Lipson, S. J.: Predictors of preoperative neurologic deficit and postoperative outcome in patients with rheumatoid arthritis of the subaxial cervical spine. In: *Proceedings of the Cervical Spine Research Society*, 23–24, 1993.
4. Klein, J. D., Hey, L. A., and Lipson, S. J.: Arthrodesis of the subaxial cervical spine in rheumatoid arthritis. *Orthop Trans*, 18:716, 1994.
5. Lipson, S. J.: Rheumatoid arthritis in the cervical spine. *Clin. Orthop.*, 239: 121–127, 1989.
6. Tsahakis, P., and Lipson, S. J.: Occipito-cervical fusion with metal mesh backing in rheumatoid cervical spine disease. *Orthop Trans*, 16: 789, 1992–1993.
7. Wattenmaker, I., Concepcion, M., Hibberd, P., and Lipson, S. J.: Upper-airway obstruction and perioperative management of the airway in patients managed with posterior operations on the cervical spine for rheumatoid arthritis. *J. Bone Joint Surg.*, 76A: 360–365, 1994.

Master Techniques in Orthopaedic Surgery,
THE SPINE, edited by D. S. Bradford,
Lippincott-Raven Publishers, Philadelphia, © 1997.

8

Cervical Spine Plate Fixation

Max Aebi

INDICATIONS/CONTRAINDICATIONS

The choice between anterior and posterior surgery depends not only on the biomechanical conditions of an implant construct for a specific cervical spine lesion, but also on factors like surgical trauma, the need for decompression, conditions for graft healing, availability of a trained surgeon, rate of infection, and rehabilitation potential. In these areas anterior surgery is clearly superior to posterior surgery (2, 3, 8–11).

Anterior Fixation

The AO/ASIF cervical spine plate fixation is either an anterior or posterior procedure. With anterior plate fixation two options are possible. The Orozco-plate fixation is the original anterior cervical plate fixation of the AO/ASIF group (10, 11) (Fig. 1). The connection between the screw and the plate is not angle stable, and a solid bone graft is necessary against which the plate must be loaded under a tension banding stress. The second option from the AO/ASIF group is the cervical spine locking plate (CSLP), which is made out of titanium (Fig. 2). This plate is characterized by a stable angle between screw and plate because of a firm anchorage of the screw head within the screw hole of the plate. This plate, therefore, has a strong buttressing effect. Because the screws have better anchorage to bone as well as the plate, it is not necessary that they penetrate the posterior cortex of the vertebral body.

M. Aebi, M.D.: Division of Orthopaedic Surgery, McGill University; and Department of Orthopaedic Surgery, Montreal General Hospital and Royal Victoria Hospital, Montreal, Quebec, Canada H3A 1A1.

I feel an anterior plate is indicated for anterior surgery, following a decompression and/or grafting, in which the cervical spine is left with a certain degree of instability. This is usually the case in trauma, tumors, and (not as frequently) degenerative cervical spine disease as well as other cervical spine disorders. Anterior surgery may be problematic in fractures of the cervical spine, when disruption of the facet capsule ligamentous complex or dislocation of the facet joints is present. Anterior surgery has many advantages over posterior surgery, such as decreased blood loss, soft-tissue trauma, infection, and incidence of neurologic sequelae. Bone graft healing is hastened since the graft is put under a compressive load (2,4,8,11). When both the vertebral body and posterior elements are destroyed, a combined procedure may be chosen.

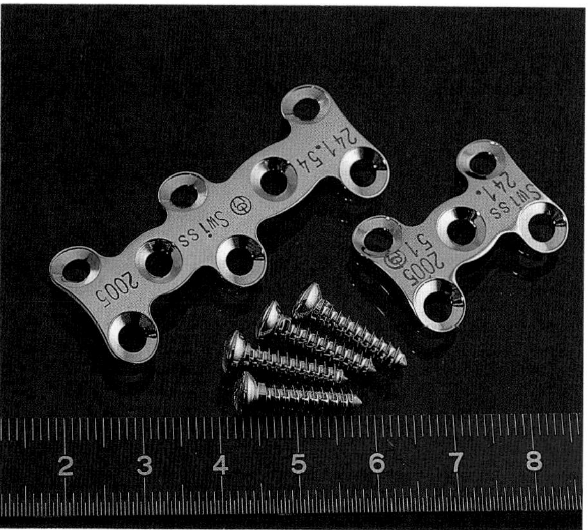

Figure 1. The Orozco plate. Different sizes are available.

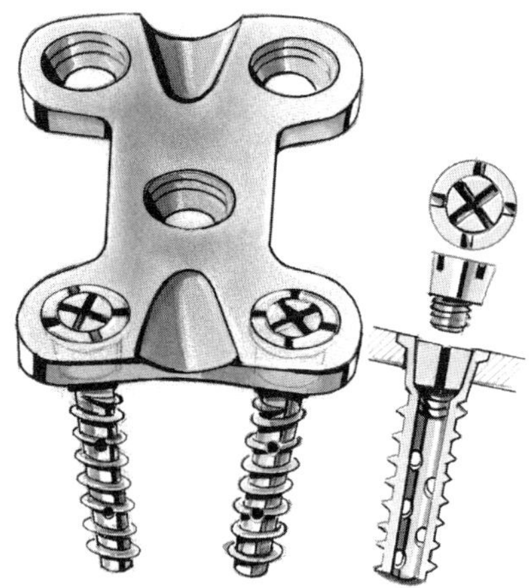

Figure 2. The cervical spine locking plate (CSLP), made of titanium. Different sizes are available.

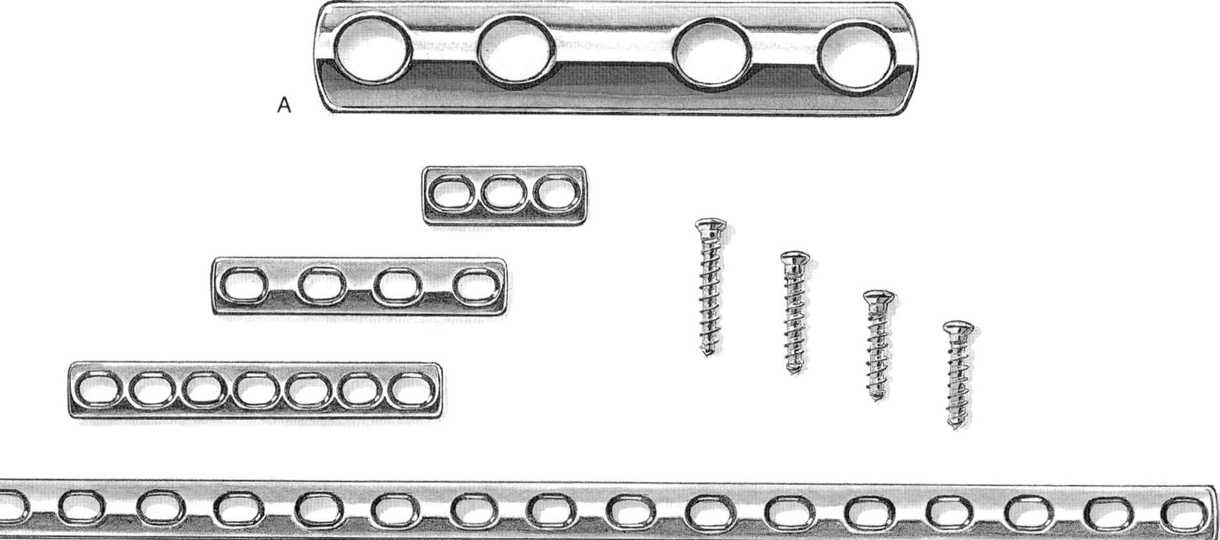

Figure 3. **A:** One-third tubular plate. **B:** The posterior cervical spine titanium plate with a hole distance of 8 to 12 mm.

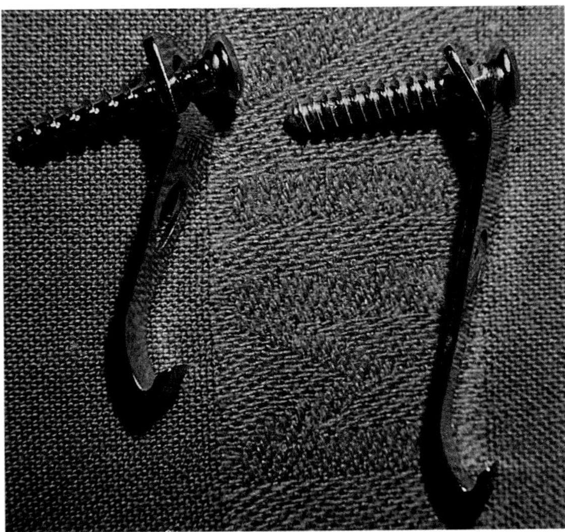

Figure 4. Magerl's cervical spine hook plate, available for one- or two-segment fixation.

Posterior Fixation

The original posterior plate fixation of the AO/ASIF group was carried out with the one-third tubular plate, which is hammered flat and contoured to the lordosis of the cervical spine either uni- or multisegmentally (1). For the same reason, the 3.5-mm steel or titanium reconstruction plate was used until very recently, when posterior titanium plates were introduced with a hole distance of 8 or 12 mm (Fig. 3) to fit individually to intervertebral distances of the lateral mass for the screw fixation (3).

A different concept of posterior plate fixation has been introduced by Magerl with the posterior hook plate (6,7). This plate has a cranial hole, which fits to the massa lateralis, and a caudal hook, which fits to the lamina. The plate clearly acts as a tension-banding system against an interspinous graft (Fig. 4).

Posterior plate fixation is indicated when the posterior ligament/capsular complex is ruptured in trauma with dislocation and cannot be reduced by closed reduction. Irreducible facet-joint dislocation sometimes may only be reduced by a posterior open reduction or even joint resection. However, care must be taken not to displace disc material into the spinal canal. The disc cannot be controlled from a posterior approach. This can only be done by an appropriate anterior approach. Posterior plating may also be indicated after wide posterior decompression to avoid late deformity and instability. The posterior plate fixation is biomechanically more stable and rigid than the anterior plate fixation (5,13). However, for practical use, sufficient stability can also be reached most of the time with an anterior plate fixation, when indicated (2).

PREOPERATIVE PLANNING

In the process of establishing the correct pathologic diagnosis, imaging procedures and electrophysiologic evaluations are necessary. In most pathologies of the cervical spine, specifically in traumatic and degenerative instability, the conventional anteroposterior (AP), lateral, and oblique radiographs provide the appropriate diagnosis in more than 90% of cases. However, when a neurologic deficit is present, more precise diagnostic workup is necessary. Computed tomography

(CT) scans are indicated when the lesion is mostly located in the bone, in combination with a myelogram when a root or foraminal involvement is assumed. Magnetic resonance imaging (MRI) is called for when a cord or root compression by soft or tumor tissue, a direct root or cord involvement, or a disc pathology is suspected. The MRI is extremely helpful in defining lesions, mainly at the craniocervical junction in rheumatoid arthritis and in tumor and infection involvement of the cervical spine. The combination of imaging techniques with electrophysiologic evaluations, such as sensory or motor evoked potentials, is increasingly important and helpful, as it may give more or less significance to structural pathologic findings in terms of true or pending neurologic deficit and the necessity of treatment.

Cervical spine stabilizing surgery is not stressful to the patient's general homeostasis. This is especially true for atraumatic anterior surgery. Therefore, basically no age limit exists for this surgery as long as the patient is in a stable general condition. Blood loss is minimal, except in the case of posterior surgery, during which the patient's morbidity may be increased through the unfavorable prone position. To establish the extent of a necessary fixation and the location for the screw fixation, conventional radiographs (AP and lateral views) are usually sufficient. The length of the plate and screws can be measured on the radiographs by respecting the magnification factor. Instability, deformities, and destruction of bony and ligamentous elements can be detected in most instances and addressed accordingly with an appropriate plate-screw and bone graft or bone substitute construction. The amount of correction of a kyphotic or scoliotic deformity can be measured and planned on the radiographs.

SURGERY

Anterior Surgery

The patient is positioned supine with the head located in a head rest or fixed by the Mayfield clamp, in slight hyperextension maintaining cervical lordosis. The neck is free and above the table to ensure free access for the image intensifier for the AP and lateral projection. The image intensifier for the lateral projection is integrated in the patient's sterile draping (Fig. 5). Usually, when the patient's head is positioned in a head rest, traction is applied by the Gardner-Wells tong (Fig.

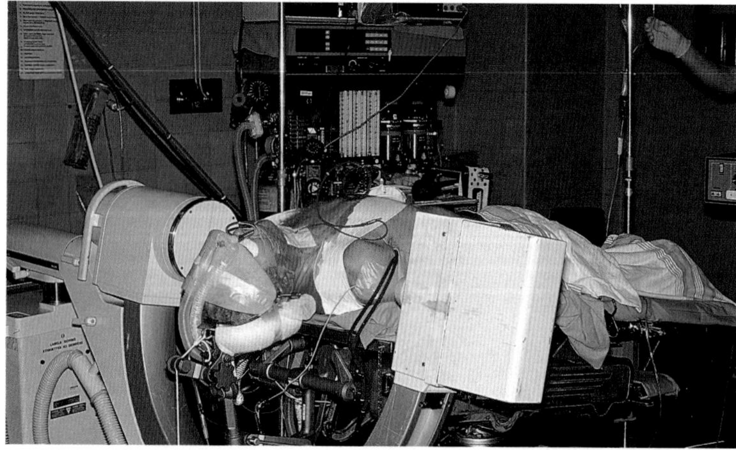

Figure 5. Image intensifier integrated in the patient's sterile draping. The position of the image intensifier is demonstrated without covering by drapes.

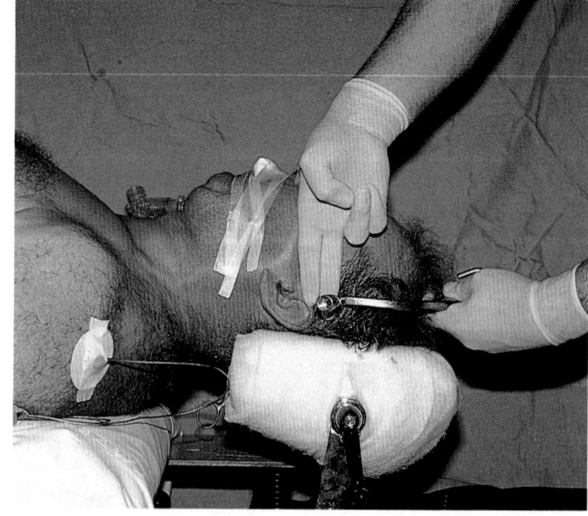

Figure 6. Gardner-Wells tong for longitudinal traction. The shoulders are pulled distally with strips and the arms are positioned adducted toward the body.

6). The starting traction weight is about 3 to 4 kg and can be increased or lowered according to the intraoperative needs. The arms of the patient are adducted to the body and fixed with strips (Fig. 7). The shoulders are pulled caudally with large self-fixing straps attached to the contralateral side at the pelvis. Care must be taken to leave the iliac crest on the right side of the patient free for the incision in order to harvest the necessary corticocancellous bone for the anterior fusion.

The anesthesiologist should use long tubes for the airway connection, in order to stay away from the head, preferably situated at the left caudal end of the patient (Fig. 8). This allows completely free access to the neck from both sides as well as from the top of the head. The surgeon is positioned on the right side looking toward the head of the patient. The assistants are positioned at the top and on the left side of the head. The scrub nurse is located at the left side of the surgeon (Fig. 9). The whole head and body are covered by sterile towels, except the anterolateral aspect of the neck and the right iliac crest, which are only covered by an adhesive plastic drape (Fig. 10). The pedal to operate the image intensifier is within the surgeon's reach. The image intensifier in the lateral projection is used to identify the level of the surgery as well as the penetration of the drill bit and the inserted screws within the vertebral body.

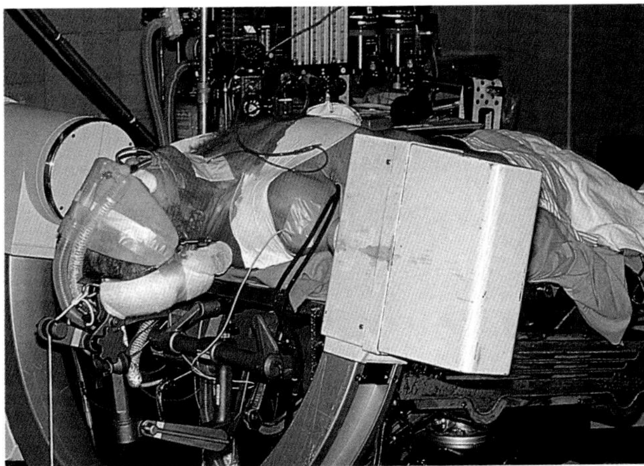

Figure 7. The arms of the patient are adducted to the body and fixed with strips.

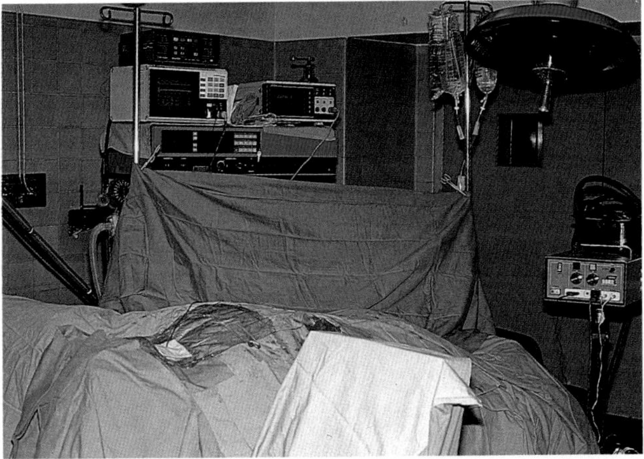

Figure 8. Patient draped. The left lower end and the left side of the patient show the drape that separates the anesthetist. The image intensifier is integrated under the draping.

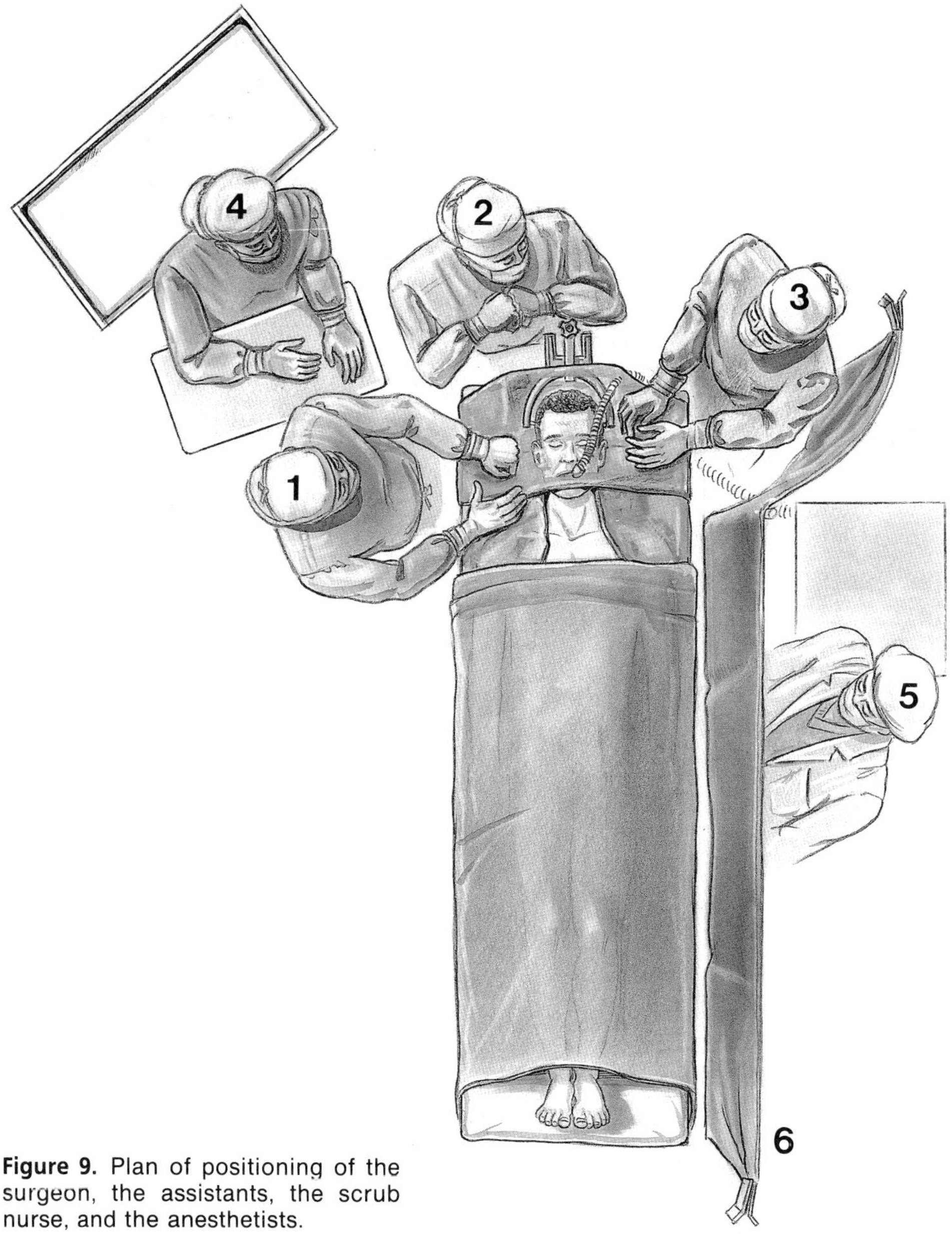

Figure 9. Plan of positioning of the surgeon, the assistants, the scrub nurse, and the anesthetists.

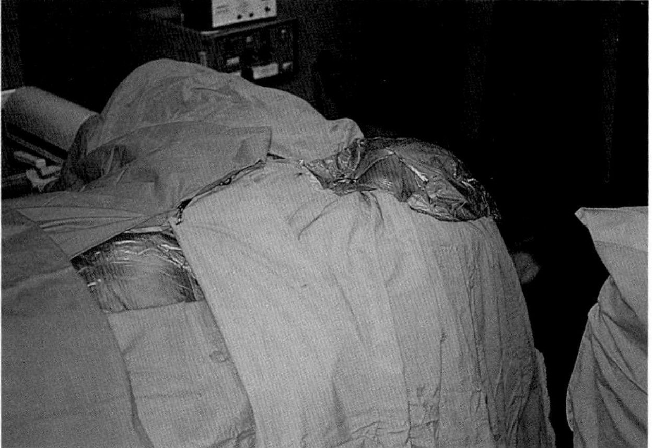

Figure 10. The operation sites at the neck and at the right iliac crest are covered by an adhesive plastic drape.

For the anterior plate fixation, which is only possible from C2 to T1, a classic anterolateral approach is used. The access between the sternocleidomastoid muscle and the neuromuscular bundle on the lateral side and the short straight colli muscles, the trachea and thyroid, and the esophagus on the medial side is extremely atraumatic and the approach to the vertebral C2 to T1 is quite easy (Fig. 11). Depending on the number of levels that should be included in the fixation, a horizontal (for one level) or an oblique skin incision (for two or more levels) is chosen. Once the anterior aspect of the cervical spine is exposed, the wound is held open with Hohmann hooks, which are inserted at the anterolateral aspect of the vertebral body or the disc. With three or four Hohmann hooks, the exposure is usually sufficient and acts as dynamic tension on the soft-tissue structures, in contrast to the cervical self-retractor, which acts statically (Fig. 12).

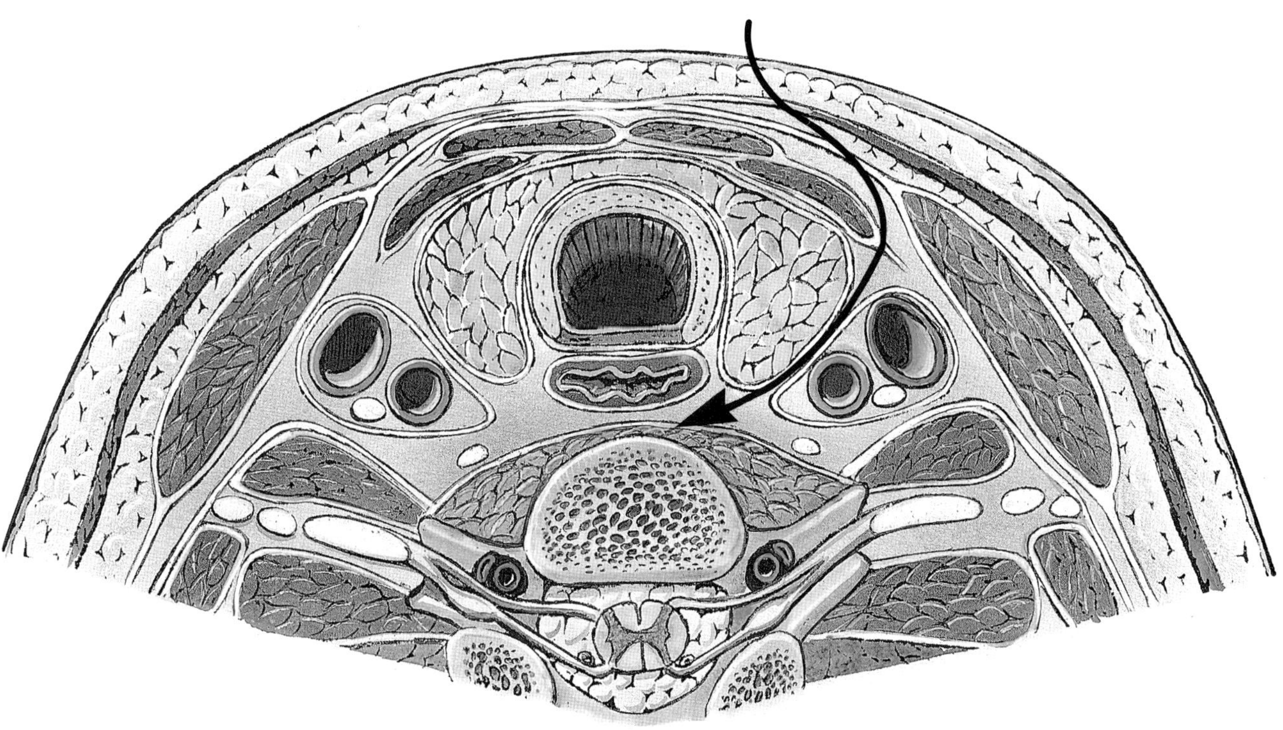

Figure 11. Access from C2 to T1 between the sternocleidomastoid muscle and the neuromuscular bundle on the lateral side and the short straight colli muscles, the trachea, thyroid gland, and esophagus on the medial side.

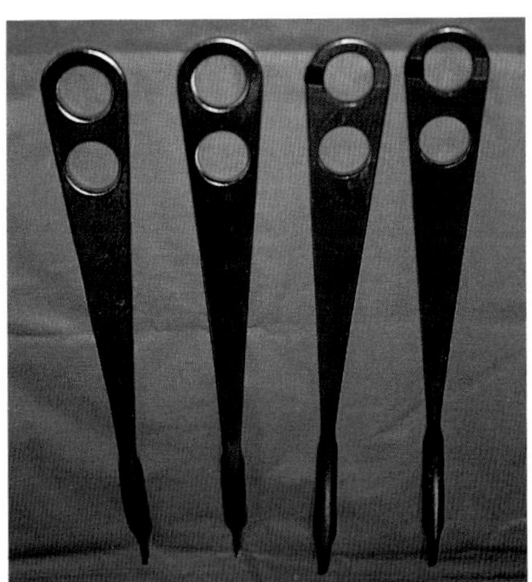

Figure 12. Hohmann hooks for the exposure of the operating field. The Hohmann hooks are introduced subperiosteally and anchored at the anterolateral aspect of the vertebral bodies.

Anterior Plate Fixation with the Standard Orozco Plate. It is essential to know the sagittal diameter of the vertebral body to prevent penetration of the posterior cortex with the drill. In most cases, the disc at the site of injury is removed prior to fusion and at this stage the depth of the vertebral body is measured with the depth gauge (Fig. 13A). A special drill guide with an inside diameter of 2.7 mm is set to the appropriate length and the length of the protruding 2.5-mm drill measured with a ruler (Fig. 13B). Make sure that the nut on the drill guide is tightly locked. Before drilling, an Orozco plate is applied to the anterior aspect of the vertebral bodies and held in place with a clamp or with pins located in each hole. Using the AO special drill guide, the hole is drilled through the plate hole and the length measured with the depth gauge (Fig. 14). If the posterior cortex has not been penetrated, then the special drill guide is adjusted to allow a further 1 mm of drilling. This is repeated if necessary and must be done with great care to prevent injury to the contents of the spinal canal. The use of special titanium-covered screws avoids the need for penetration of the posterior wall.

The anterior cortex of the vertebral body is tapped with 3.5-mm tapping. The appropriate length 3.5-mm cortex screw is inserted. A similar procedure is performed with the other screw holes. The Orozco plate is only a valid construct when used in combination with a strong corticocancellous bone graft. This bone graft is shaped to a trapezoid form to adapt the fused segment to the cervical lordosis and to lock the facet joints (Fig. 15). The bone graft is then brought under compression by applying the plate as a tension-banding device. This can be achieved by drilling the screw holes eccentrically within the round plate holes. When tightening the screws, a dynamic compression of the vertebral bodies against the bone graft is then achieved, like using a DC-plate on a long bone (1,2). This is a very subtle trick; however, it increases the stability of the construct significantly and enhances the healing at the graft-host bone interface.

The temporary fixation of the plate at the anterior aspect of the cervical spine is sometimes difficult when drilling the screw holes. During this procedure the plate may be displaced and the screw hole may get lost. We therefore use simple sterile pins, like those used to pin paper to a bulletin board, to temporarily fix the

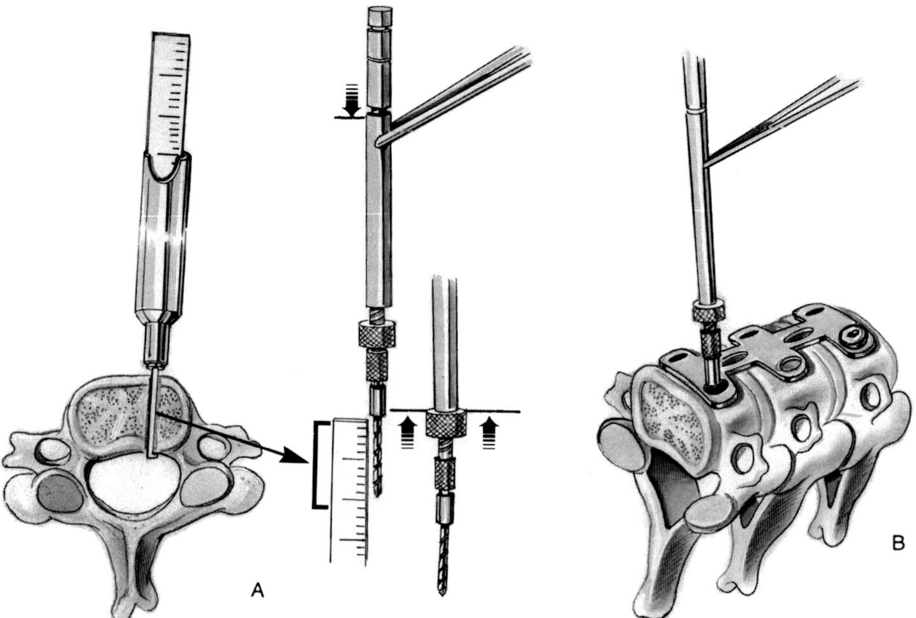

Figure 13. **A:** Measuring the sagittal diameter of the vertebral body through the adjacent disc space with a depth gauge. **B:** A special drill guide to set the length of the drill.

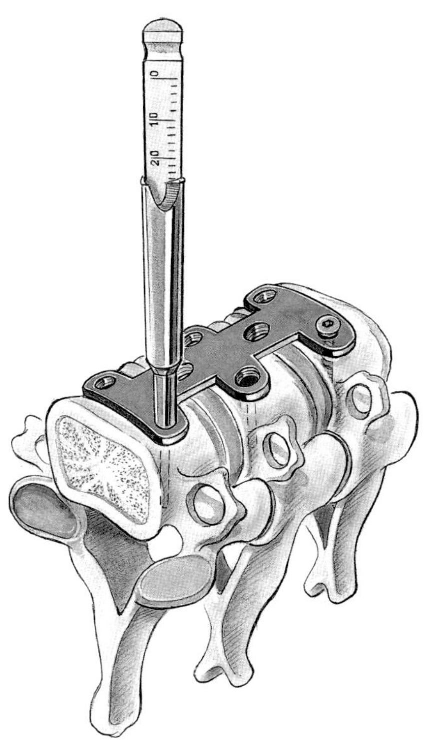

Figure 14. Measuring the screw hole with the depth gauge.

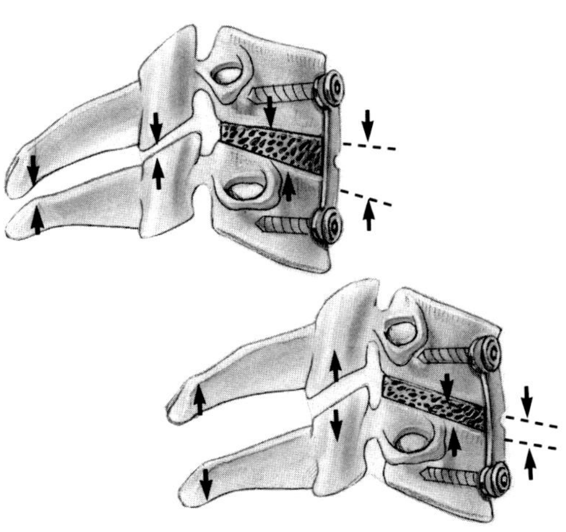

Figure 15. The shape of the graft is trapezoid (*above*) in order to adjust the lordotic form of the cervical spine. A rectangular graft (*below*) would open the interspinous space posteriorly.

A

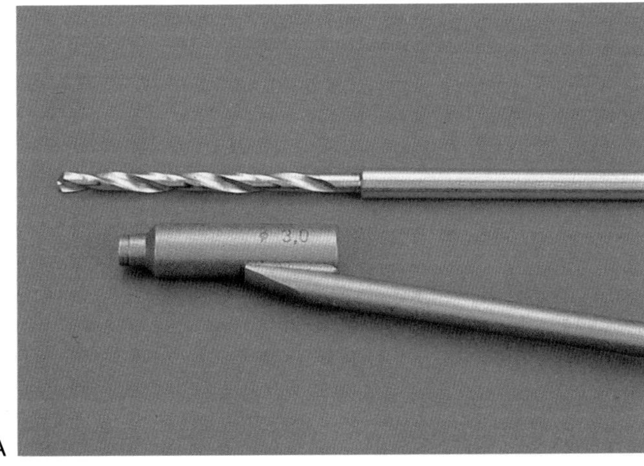

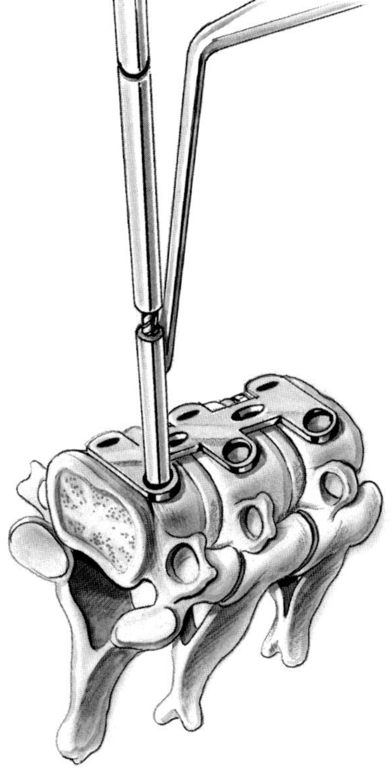

B

Figure 16. A,B: Special drill guide of the CSLP instrumentation, which stops the drill at a 16-mm length.

plate against the bone. They have the advantage of not interfering with the other instruments used, and they can be easily inserted and removed.

Anterior Plate Fixation with Cervical Spine Locking Plate. The spine is approached anteriorly through an anterolateral approach at the appropriate level. Since the discs are angled in the horizontal plane such that their direction changes from caudal to cranial as they extend from anterior to posterior, the plate size is selected to ensure that the screws penetrate the upper region of the lateral bodies. This prevents the screws from entering into the intervertebral disc above and below the level that requires fusion. Anterior overlapping of a normal disc by the plate must be avoided. The plate is positioned and the first screw hole drilled with the aid of a special drill guide. The drill stops automatically, allowing only 16 mm of penetration into the vertebral body (Fig. 16). The soft-tissue protector is used when tapping the thread, and the tap also stops automatically to prevent overpenetration (Fig. 17).

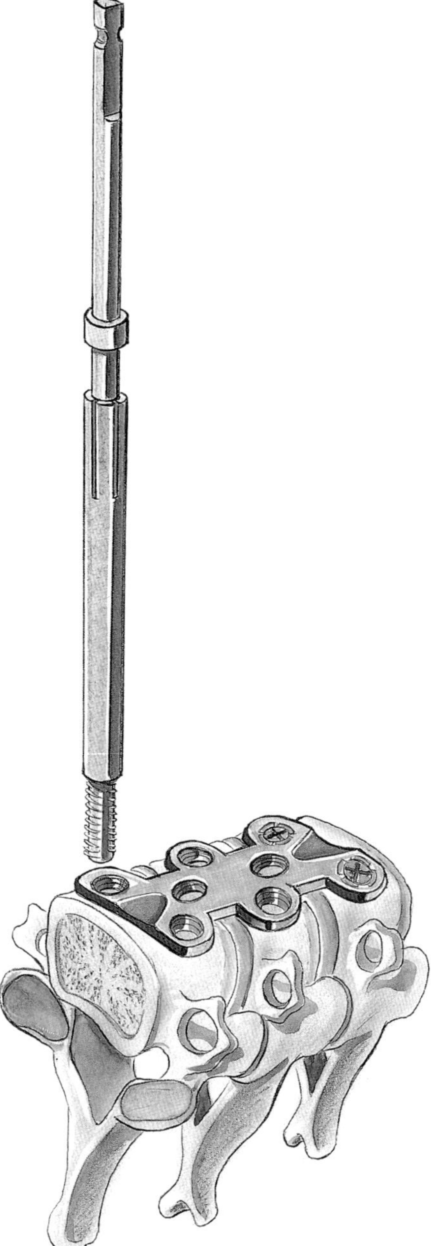

Figure 17. Special tapping instrument, with the sleeve to make sure that the exact tapping direction and depth are maintained.

The screws are applied using the crosshead screwdriver. The crosshead screwdriver is first inserted into the screw head and then the split sleeve is pushed over the screw head to hold it in position. The second split sleeve is necessary to prevent the cross split screw head from expanding on insertion. The perforated hollow cylindrical screw is screwed down until the rim of the screw head is flush with the plate surface. The two split sleeves automatically disengage when tightened but remain on the screwdriver for easy removal (Fig. 18).

The plate is finally locked in place by the insertion of a small screw with a cortical head. The small screw is held on the screwdriver by a split sleeve in the same way as the screw used previously. When the small screw is driven home, it expands the head of the larger screw and locks it into the plate (Fig. 19).

Posterior Surgery

The patient is placed in prone position, with the head fixed either in a Mayfield clamp or in a head rest. In the latter case the patient is put under traction with the installation of a Gardner-Wells tong. The traction weight is about 3 to 4 kg and can be increased or lowered according to the intraoperative needs. The neck is free and above the table to ensure free access for the image intensifier for the AP and lateral projection. The image intensifier for the lateral projection is integrated in the patient's sterile draping. The patient's arms are adducted to the body and fixed with strips. The shoulders are pulled caudally with large self-fixing straps

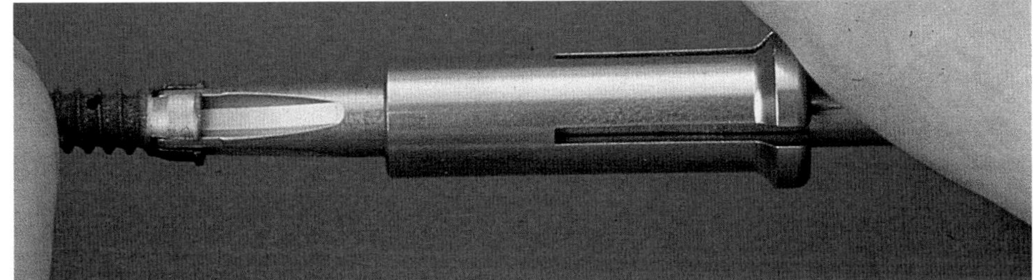

Figure 18. Screwdriver for the locking screw.

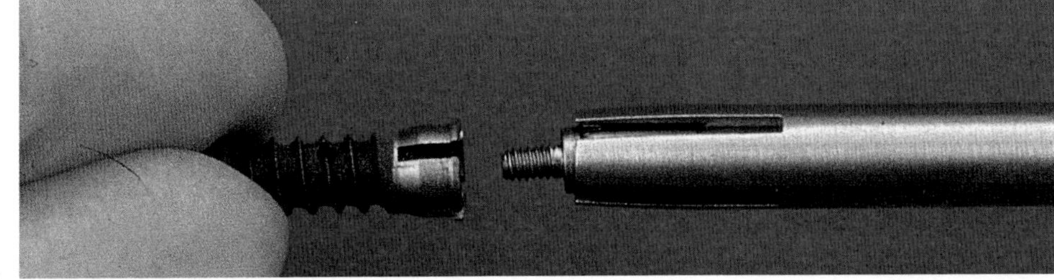

A

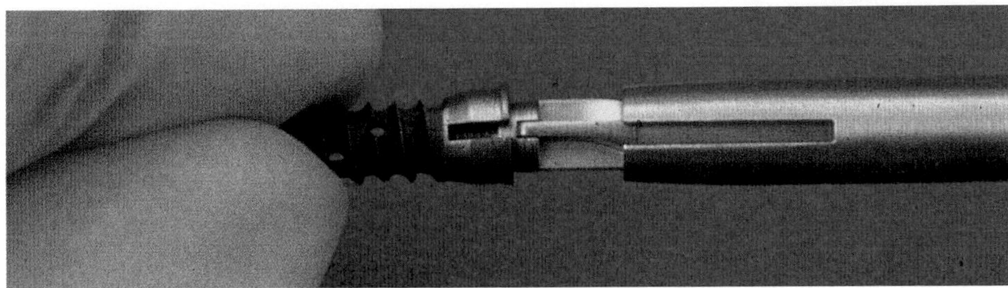

B

Figure 19. A: Screwdriver with a split sleeve holding the small screw. **B:** The small screw expands the big screw head when driven home and locks the head in the plate hole.

attached to the contralateral side at the pelvis. Care must be taken to leave the iliac crest on the right side of the patient free for the incision in order to harvest the necessary corticocancellous bone for the posterior fusion. The anesthetists are located away from the head and to the right side of the patient's leg. The surgeon is positioned on the left side of the patient's body (patient prone) and the left posterior iliac crest is exposed in order to harvest bone. The scrub nurse and the assisting surgeons are positioned as they would be for anterior surgery, always in relationship to the leading surgeon. Depending on the pathology that needs surgery, the neck is either extended or held in forced flexion to allow easier access to the facet joints or the occipitocervical junction.

The posterior approach is a median incision over the spinous processes and/or the protuberance occipitalis, again depending on how many segments are to be included in the fixation. It is recommended that the length of the incision extend one spinous process above and below the planned fixation area, in order to have easy access when performing the osteosynthesis. The muscles need to be dissected and stripped subperiosteally as far lateral as the massa articularis of the vertebral joints. The wound is held open by self-retractors, which statically retain mainly muscles (Fig. 20), unlike the anterior approach in which vessels, nerves, esophagus, trachea, and thyroid need a dynamic, careful retraction.

Posterior Plate Fixation with a 3.5-mm Reconstruction Plate or One-Third Tubular Plate. After performing a midline posterior approach, it is essential to identify radiographically the levels to be fused. Kirschner wires are then inserted in the lateral masses of the end vertebrae (Fig. 21). The entry points and directions are the same as for the hook plates (see also Figs. 26 and 27). A one-third tubular plate (hammered flat) (Fig. 22), or 3.5-mm reconstruction plate of appropriate length is chosen, contoured (Fig. 23), and positioned over the protruding Kirschner wires (Fig. 24), to check whether the end holes of the plate correspond to the entry points of the Kirschner wires. If they do not, the entry points have to be altered accordingly. The Kirschner wires are then individually removed and replaced by 3.5-mm cortex screws in the usual way (Fig. 25). Care must be taken not to perforate the lateral mass. If more than one motion segment is to be included, the end screws are not fully tightened, so that the plate can be adjusted and the remaining screws inserted. Since anatomic landmarks are hidden by the plate, check the entry point and direction of the drill in these holes with the image

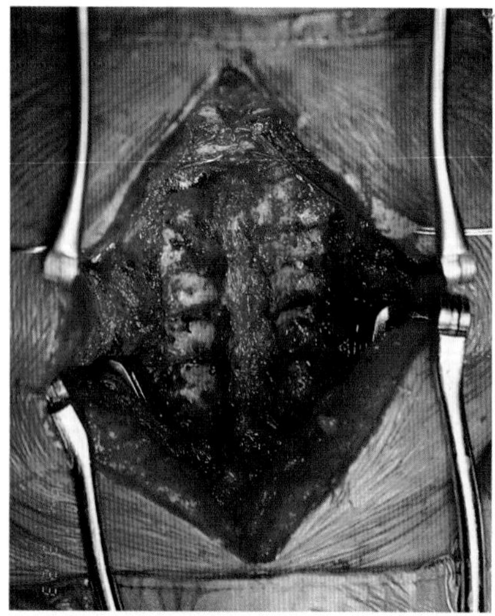

Figure 20. Posterior cervical spine exposures with two self-retainers. The massae laterales are exposed and anatomically identified.

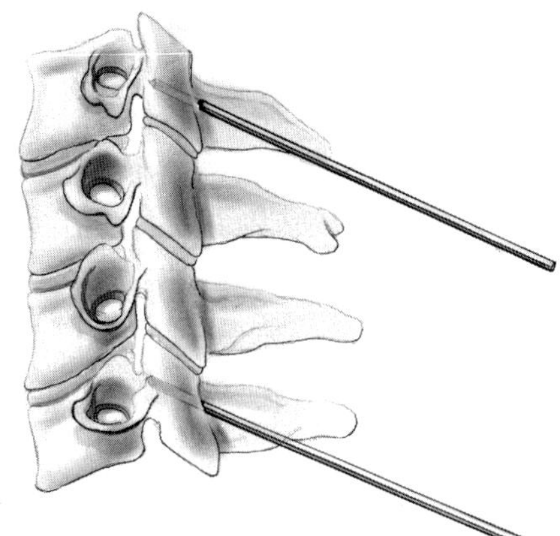

Figure 21. K-wires are positioned in the lateral mass.

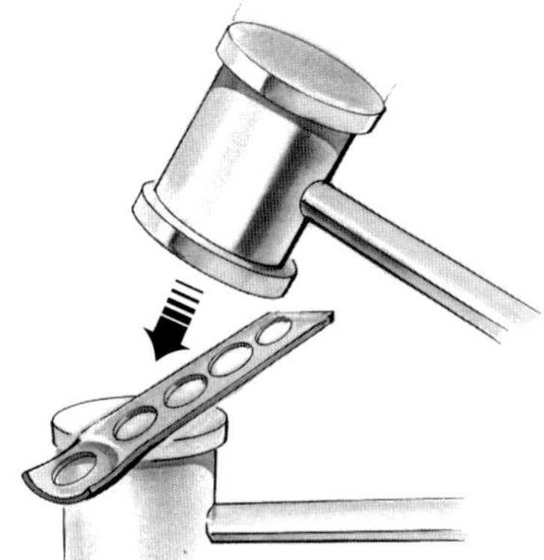

Figure 22. The one-third tubular plate, when used instead of the titanium posterior cervical plate, is hammered flat.

intensifier. The remaining screws are then introduced and all are tightened. The laminae are decorticated and the cancellous bone graft applied for the fusion. The recently developed reconstruction plates with an 8- or 12-mm distance between the screw holes allow for easier adjustment to the massa lateralis than the one-third tubular or the ordinary 3.5-mm reconstruction plate.

In performing an occipitocervical fusion with plates from the occiput to the C3 or C4, sometimes the incision does not allow for drilling and inserting the screw in C2, which is used as a transarticular screw C1–C2. This is because the drill or screwdriver cannot be held inclined obliquely enough due to the height of the wound edges. In this case, the drill bit or the screw can be driven through a percutaneous stab wound outside the wound, allowing the exact inclination necessary. Furthermore, it is advisable to work with instruments that are both long and flexible at the occipitocervical junction because the angle between the occiput and the cervical spine may be very acute and therefore not allow for appropriate inclination of the drill and screwdriver.

Posterior Plate Fixation with the Hook Plate According to Magerl. After a midline incision and subperiosteal dissection of the posterior spinal elements, the entry points of the screws in the anterior masses are identified. The entry point lies 2 to 3 mm medially and cranially to the middle of the articular mass (Fig. 26). Each screw diverges by 15 to 25 degrees anterolaterally (Fig. 27) and runs parallel

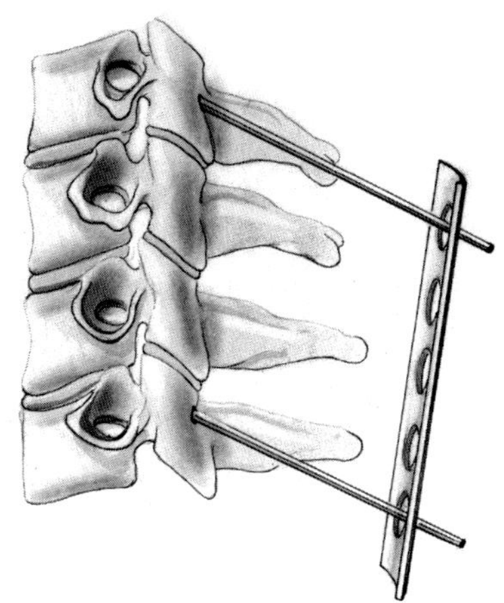

Figure 23. The plate is contoured.

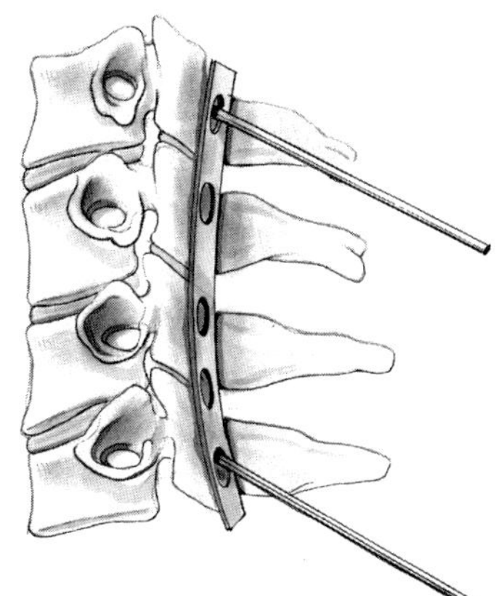

Figure 24. The plate is positioned over the K-wires.

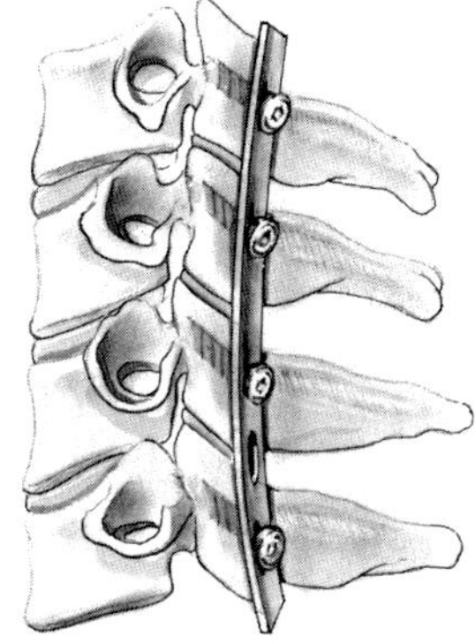

Figure 25. K-wires replaced by 3.5-mm cortical screws.

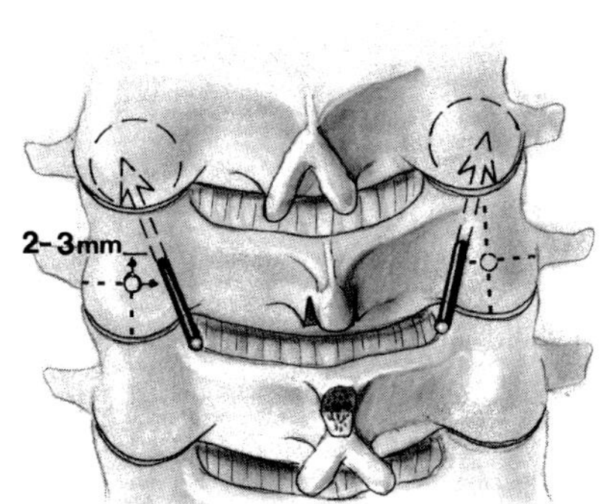

Figure 26. Entry point for the lateral mass screws according to Magerl.

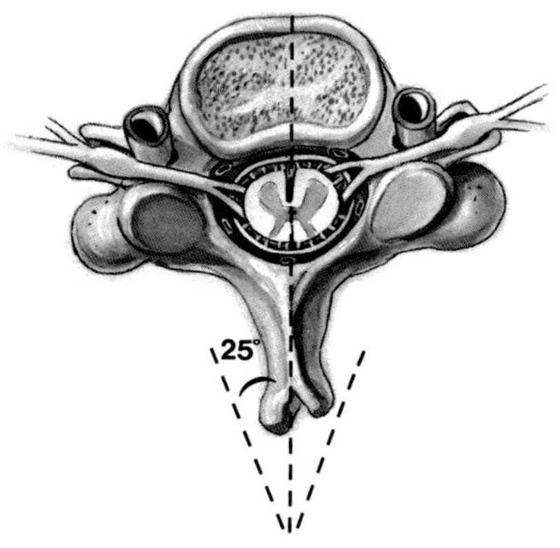

Figure 27. Position of the lateral mass screw in the horizontal projection.

to the surface of the intervertebral joints (Fig. 28). The inclination of the surfaces may be determined by inserting a fine dissector into the joints. The screw canals are prepared using long 2.5-mm drills. The cortex of the articular processes on the far side is carefully perforated. The length of the drill hole is measured by a 3.5-mm depth gauge and the canal is tapped only two-thirds of the distance. If a long spinous process hinders the preparation of the screw canal, it may be shortened.

Screws inserted into C2 must be directed 25 degrees toward midline (Fig. 29) and 25 degrees cranially to avoid the vertebral artery passing through the isthmus of the C2 vertebral into the body of C2, leaving the C1–C2 joints intact (Fig. 30). Perforation of the articular surface must be avoided. In order to prevent the hooks from sliding into the intervertebral joints, corresponding notches are made into the lamina medial to the joints where the hook side of the hook plate is prepared (Fig. 31). The site of the H-graft is prepared using an oscillating saw (Fig. 32). The lower notch must not be too deep in order to avoid a fracture of the spinous process.

To stabilize one motion segment, the plates are contoured by torque and bent to match the posterior aspect of the lamina as well as the articular mass (Fig. 33). A corticocancellous H-graft is inserted between the spinous processes with a neutral vertebral position. The contoured hook plates are placed into the prepared

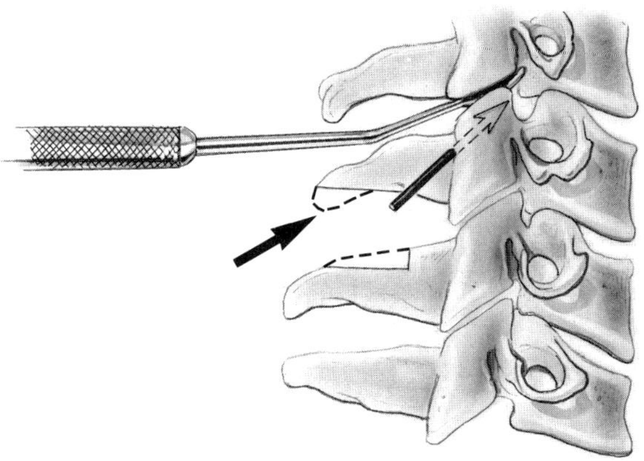

Figure 28. Position of the screw in the lateral projection, parallel to the joint surfaces, which can be identified by dissector introduced in the joint.

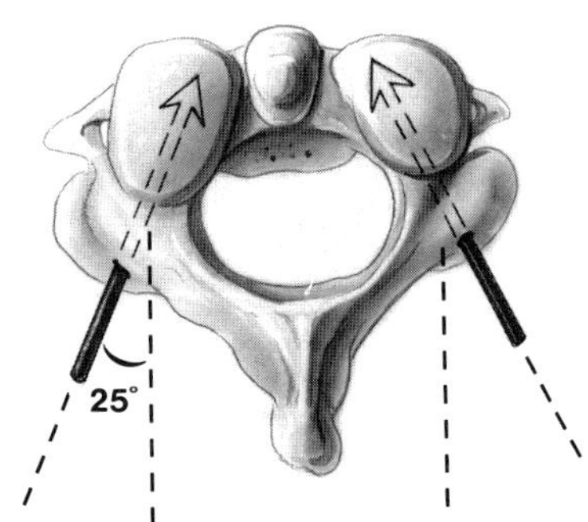

Figure 29. Position of the screws in the C2-mass in the horizontal projection.

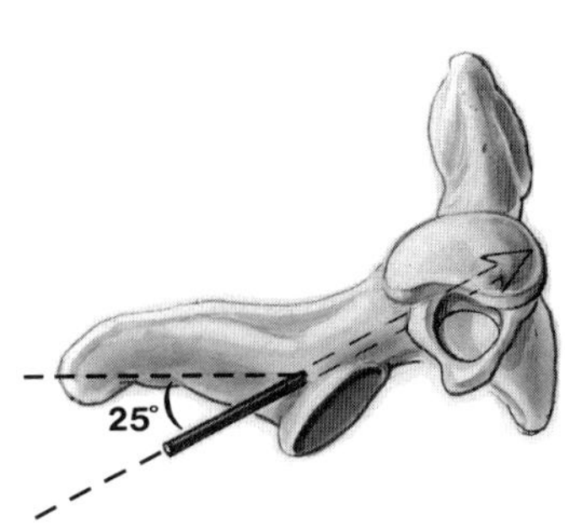

Figure 30. Position of the screws in the C2-mass in the lateral projection.

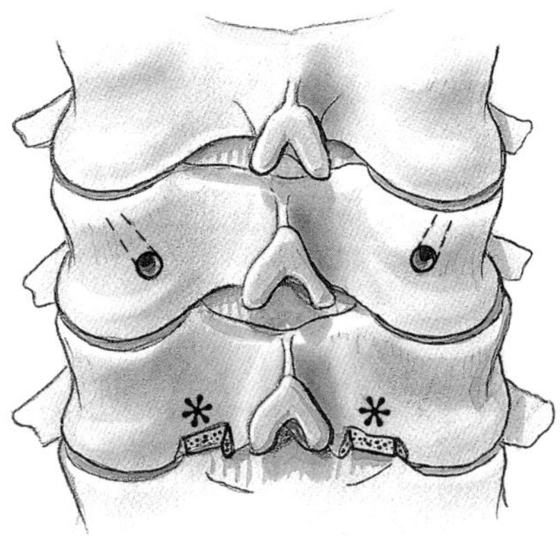

Figure 31. Preparing the hook site by cutting notches out (*).

notches, and 3.5-mm cortex screws are inserted in a very small articular mass, using 2.7-mm cortex screws.

Tightening the screws sandwiches the H-graft (Fig. 34). If a hook begins to lift out, the curvature of the hook should be increased. With two hole plates, it is possible to secure the hook by inserting a short screw into the lower lamina, but this is rarely necessary. Finally, a cancellous bone graft is applied between the lamina and the facet joints (Fig. 35).

To stabilize two motion segments (Fig. 36) with the long hook plates, two motion segments must be fused. The middle spinous process is removed and the upper two screw canals, hook notches, and graft bed are prepared. Plates of appropriate length are chosen and centered. They should be about 2 mm shorter to allow for compression. The H-graft is inserted, the plates applied, and the upper screws inserted. They are tightened until some compression results. This is followed by drilling the lower screw holes, parallel to the screws above. The drill is placed

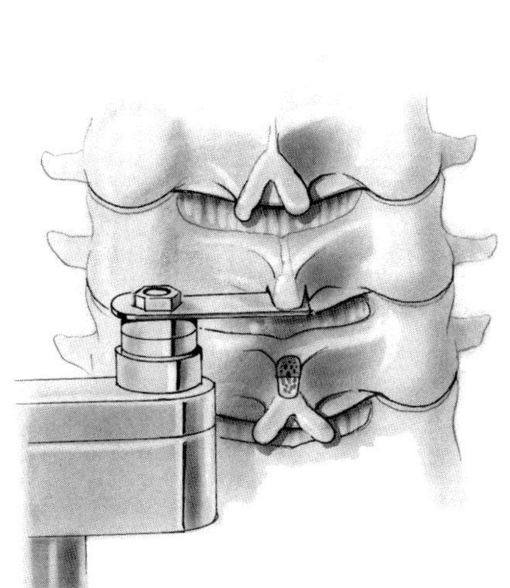

Figure 32. Preparing the graft side with the oscillating saw.

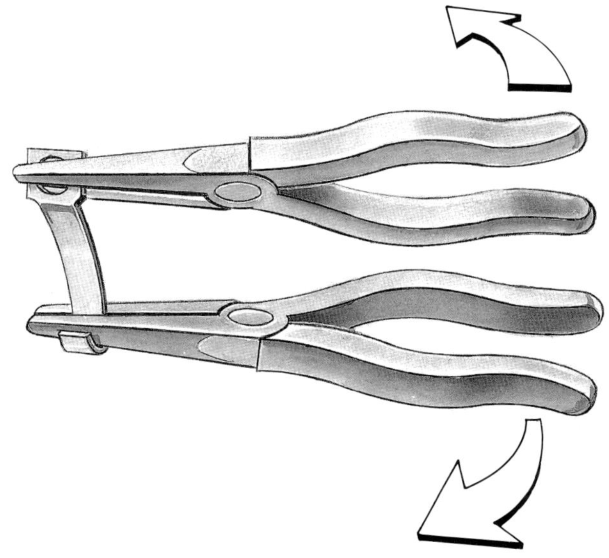

Figure 33. Contouring of the hook plate by torsion. Usually the plate has to be bent more sharply in the area of the hook.

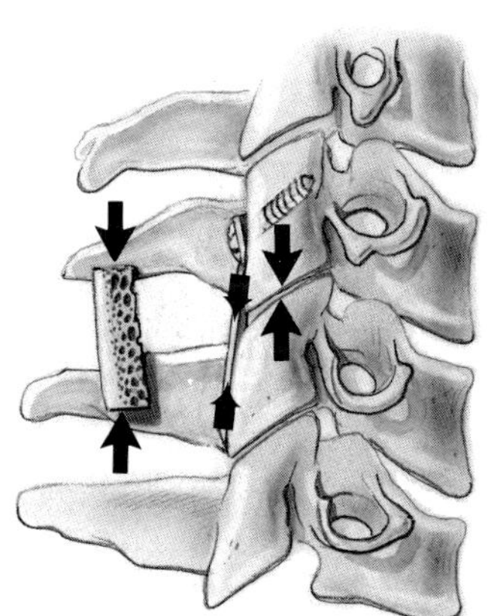

Figure 34. Tightening the screws sandwiches the H-graft.

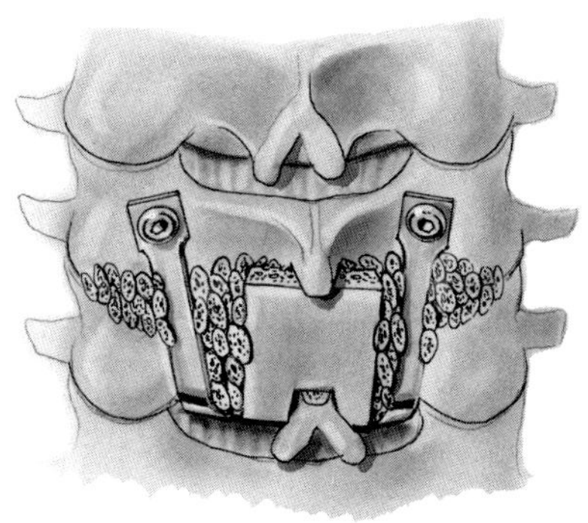

Figure 35. Applying cancellous bone graft between the laminae and the facet joints.

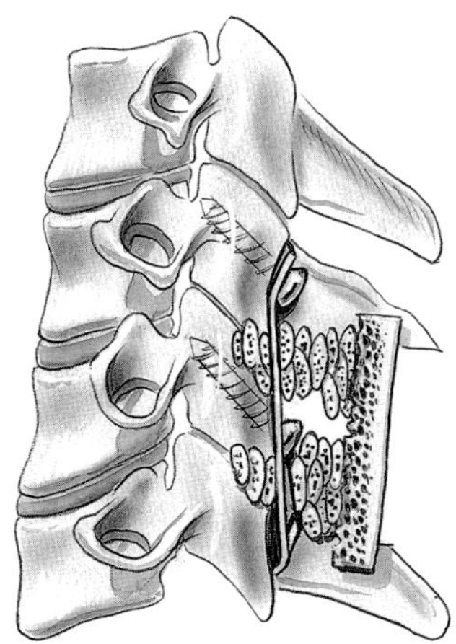

Figure 36. Application of the hook plate when bridged to motion segments.

through the upper part of the plate holes. First the lower screws are tightened and then the upper screws. This technique provides for compression in both motion segments.

POSTOPERATIVE MANAGEMENT

Postoperative management for both anterior and posterior plate fixation is simple and well standardized because of the high degree of stability achieved by an appropriate internal fixation and bone graft placement. Postoperatively the patient is partially immobilized by a Plastozot collar (see Fig. 38) for at least 6 weeks, to a maximum of 10 weeks. Six weeks postoperatively, a radiograph is taken and if the healing process is significant, a soft Schanz collar may be applied instead of the Plastozot collar. If functional stability can be confirmed during surgery, a soft collar may be used immediately after surgery. Instructions are given to the patient about isometric exercises for the long collis and the neck muscles. The patient should perform these exercises twice daily for 10 minutes. Three months after the operation, motion is usually unrestricted and the patient's life and work are back to normal, but heavy physical stress like contact sports is prohibited for at least another 3 months.

A solid fusion can be expected in both anterior and posterior instrumented fusions in more than 95% of cases. After a learning curve for the surgeon who begins to perform this kind of surgery, the complications or failure due to the instrumentation are almost none, at least in our personal experience. However, neither anterior nor posterior plating replace a critical indication for surgery and a firm judgment of the surgeon's capabilities and possibilities in performing this kind of surgery.

COMPLICATIONS

The possible pitfalls are twofold: from the approach and from the instrumentation and/or graft positioning. Complications are certain when the screw placement is incorrect and the graft plate combination is not well balanced. Screw loosening has repeatedly been reported. In our experience, this only happens when a screw is located in either the disc or the construct graft plate and vertebral bodies are not stable. It is important that the bone graft be well shaped and sized to fit in the bone bed and able to transfer load from above to below. The simple Orozco

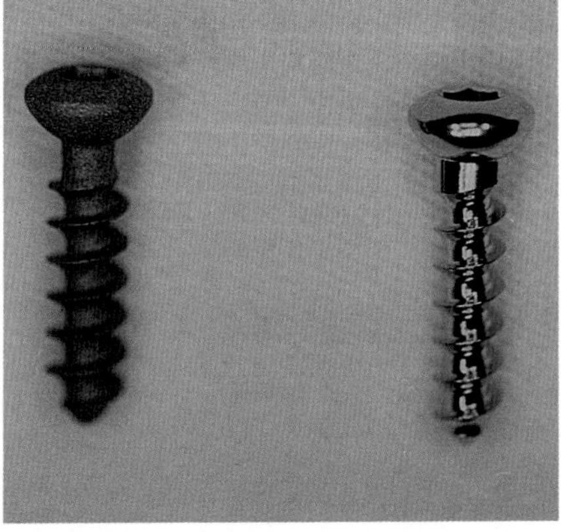

Figure 37. Cortical screws covered with a titanium plasma layer for use with the simple Orozco plate.

plate should not be used as a buttressing plate, but as a tension-banding plate only, in combination with solid bone graft. We have also addressed the problem of screw loosening by using screws covered with a titanium plasma layer (Fig. 37), which contributes to a firm bone implant interlocking. A few centers used these screws long before the titanium CSLP system appeared on the market. With these screws it is not necessary to use the posterior vertebral bony wall for screw fixation. These titanium plasma-covered screws can also be used for the posterior plate fixation.

A posterior wall perforation with the drill or the screw can be avoided with the proper technique, including preoperative and intraoperative measurement of the sagittal diameter of the vertebral bodies. The sagittal diameter of the vertebral body is best measured through the adjacent disc space, once the disc has been removed. The variable drill guide is then adjusted to the measured length or 1 mm less, and the drill hole is made. By adjusting the drill guide 1 mm at a time, a progressive slow approximation to the real screw hole length is done. Consequentially, no abrupt perforation of the cortex of the dorsal wall is possible, and a cord lesion is highly improbable. This has never been a problem in our experience.

A postoperative drain needs to be inserted in anterior surgery, because even relatively little blood accumulation may create an external constraint for the trachea, causing secondary respiratory problems.

It is extremely important that all maneuvers performed with drills, tappers, and screwdrivers be done with meticulous precision and under systematic protection of the adjacent vital soft-tissue structures by guides and retractors in order to avoid any lesion of the vessels, nerves, esophagus, trachea, or thyroid.

In traumatology of the cervical spine we must be extremely careful when dealing with dislocations in which disc material is ruptured in fragments, which may be dislocated into the spinal canal when a reduction is done. The disc can be held under control quite well by an anterior approach; however, when using a posterior approach, an MRI may be indicated to evaluate the condition of the disc before the reduction maneuver is started.

The main technical complication that may occur in posterior plating is injury of the vertebral artery and root caused by an inappropriate screw position outside the massa lateralis. A compromise of the spinal canal, or medial screw misplacement, is almost never the problem. In the posterior approach, the likelihood of infection is at least double that of anterior surgery, probably because of the more significant soft-tissue damage in posterior surgery (4).

ILLUSTRATIVE CASE FOR TECHNIQUE

A 32-year-old man fell from the back of a horse and sustained a C5–C6 cervical spine injury with an immediately present incomplete quadriplegia (Frankel grade C) at the level of the injury. The injury consisted of a complete disruption of the posterior ligament/joint-capsule complex of C5–C6 segment and consecutive 80% displacement of C5 over C6 (flexion distraction injury).

The only intact ligament structure was the anterior longitudinal ligament; therefore we were faced with a highly unstable lesion (Fig. 38A,B). Because of this high degree of instability and because the patient needed to be optimally rehabilitated as soon as possible, we decided on a combined anterior-posterior procedure. This technique gives optimal stability to the C5–C6 segment and allows postoperative mobilization without external fixation (just a soft collar). It was decided to begin anteriorly to gain control over the disrupted and partially dislocated C5–C6 disc. Under traction of 6 kg with a Gardner-Wells tong, it was possible to reduce the dislocation intraoperatively, which confirmed the high degree of disruption. A slightly oversized tricortical bone graft was placed in the intervertebral C5–C6

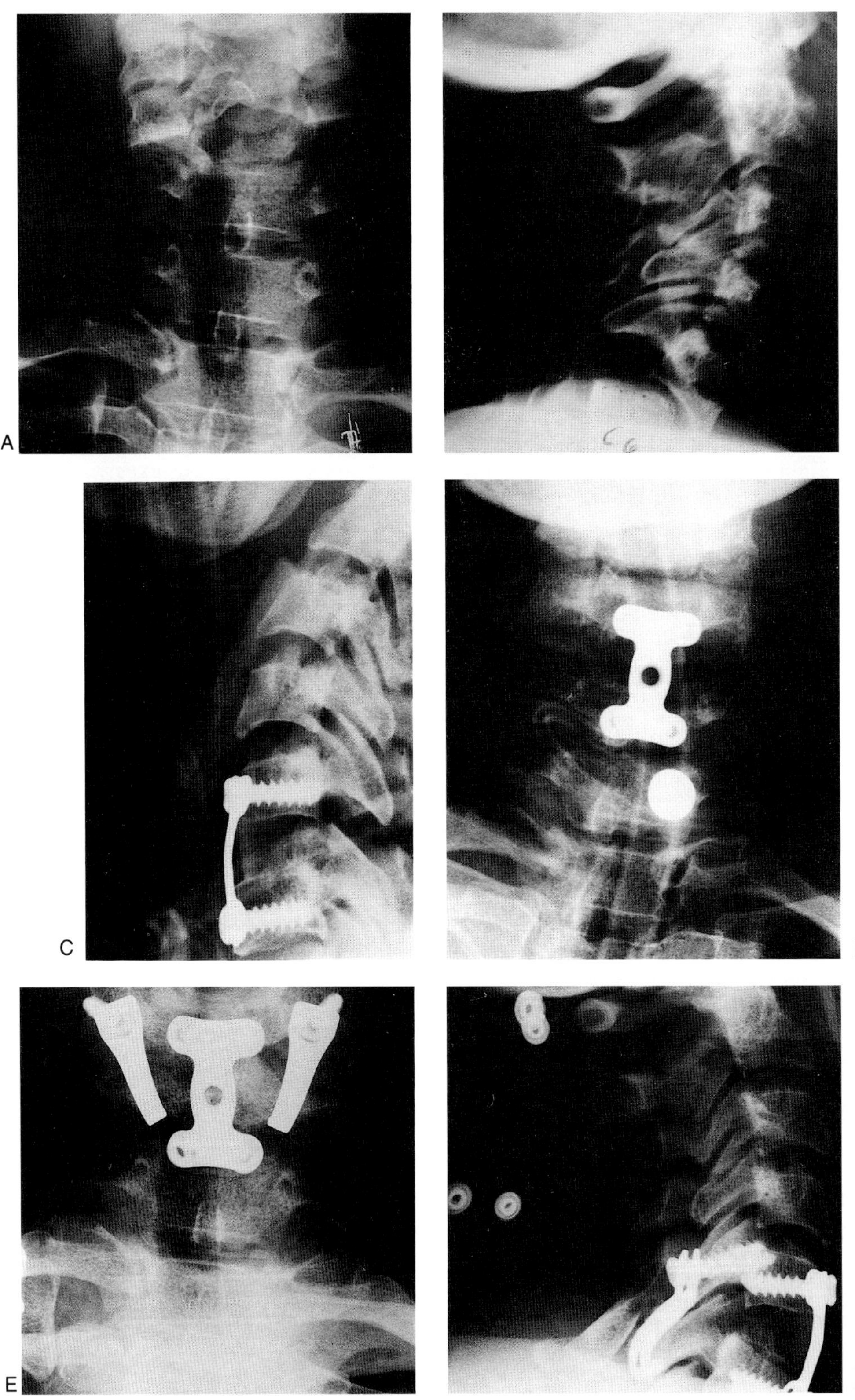

Figure 38. A,B: The anterior longitudinal ligament is the only intact ligament structure. **C,D:** Tricortical bone graft placed in the intervertebral C5–C6 space. The graft is trapezoid-shaped. **E,F:** Magerl's hook plate used to achieve a major tension-banding effect.

space after the destroyed disc was removed. The graft was shaped in a trapezoid form in order to support the cervical lordosis (Fig. 38C,D).

It may be noted that separation of the C5–C6 facet joints was significant after anterior plating and thus posterior tension banding by plates was required to close the joint space and to enhance the stability of the C5–C6 motion segment. Under the same anesthesia, the patient was flipped over into a prone position and a posterior approach was used, exposing the massa lateralis of C5 and C6. Magerl's hook plates were used, and a major tension-banding effect was achieved: the joint space of the C5–C6 facet was closed and the lordosis well established (Fig. 38E,F). Note the direction of the massa lateralis screws: slightly upward, parallel to the facet joint bone, and 15 to 20 degrees toward the outside, thus avoiding the nerve root and the vertebral artery. A posterior fusion was added.

The patient did extremely well postoperatively and became an independent walker with minimal residual signs of incomplete quadriplegia.

RECOMMENDED READING

1. Aebi, M., and Webb, J. K.: The Spine In: *Manual of Internal Fixation*, edited by M. E. Müller, M. Allgöwer, R. Schneider, and H. Willenegger. 3rd ed. Springer Verlag, Berlin, Heidelberg, New York, Tokyo, 1991.
2. Aebi, M., Zuber, K., and Marchesi D.: Treatment of cervical spine injuries with anterior plating. *Spine* 16: 538–545, 1991.
3. Anderson, P. A., Henley, M. B., Grady, M. S., Montesano, P. X., and Winn, H. R.: Posterior cervical arthrodesis with AO-reconstruction plates and bone graft. *Spine* 16: S72–S79, 1991.
4. Bombart, M., Canevet, D., and Deckard, J.: Comparaison sur l'ensenble de la série des résultats de la chirurgie par voie antériure et par voie postérieure. *Rev. Chir. Orthop.* 70: 533–536, 1984.
5. Coe, J. D., Warden, K. E., Sutterlin, C. E., and McAfee, P. C.: Biomechanical evaluation of cervical spinal stabilization methods in a human cadaveric model. *Spine* 14: 1122–1131, 1989.
6. Grob, D., and Magerl, F.: Dorsale Spondylodese der Halswirbelsäule mit der Hakenplatte. *Orthopäde* 16: 55–61, 1987.
7. Jeanneret, B., Magerl, F., Ward, E. H., and Ward, J-CH.: Posterior stabilization of the cervical spine with hook plates. *Spine* 16: S56–S63, 1991.
8. Mestadgh, H.: Resultate der ventralen Spondylodese der Halswirbelsäule (C2–C7): *Orthopäde* 16: 70–80, 1987.
9. Morscher, E., Jenny, H., and Suter, H.: Die vordere Verplattung der Halswirbelsäule mit dem Hohlschrauben—Plattensystem. *Der Chirurg.* 57: 702–707, 1986.
10. Orozco Delclos, R., and Liovet Topes, J.: Osteosintesis en las fracturas de raquis cervical: nota de technica. *Revista Orthop. Traumatol.* 14: 285–288, 1970.
11. Senegas, J., and Gauzère, J. M.: Plaidoyer de la voie antérieure dans les traumatismes sévères des cinq dernières vertèbres cervicales. *Rev. Chir. Orthop.* (Suppl. 2) 62: 123–128, 1976.
12. Stauffer, E. S., and Kelly, E. G.: Fracture-dislocations of the cervical spine. *J. Bone Joint Surg.* 59A: 45–48, 1977.
13. Ulrich, C., Wörsdörfer, O., Claes, L., and Magerl, F.: Comparative study of the stability of anterior and posterior cervical spine fixation procedures. *Arch. Orthop. Trauma Surg.* 106: 226–231, 1987.

Master Techniques in Orthopaedic Surgery,
THE SPINE, edited by D. S. Bradford,
Lippincott-Raven Publishers, Philadelphia, © 1997.

9

Cervical Laminoplasty

Hiromi Matsuzaki

INDICATIONS AND CONTRAINDICATIONS

Cervical laminoplasty, using the posterior approach, is indicated for spinal lesions that affect more than two cervical vertebrae and require multivertebral decompression. On the other hand, the anterior approach is indicated for spinal lesions contained within a region of two intervertebral spaces or when an anterior bone spur is the source of a lesion, even if the lesion involves more than one intervertebral space. Such an operation must include anterior fusion, which is inevitably accompanied by a restriction of cervical vertebral mobility.

Posterior laminoplasty has the major advantage of providing multivertebral decompression without sacrificing vertebral mobility. Furthermore, in contrast to laminectomy, it can preserve the posterior tissues, including the vertebral arch, thus reducing structural disruption of the spine. This has particular anatomic significance for the cervical vertebra (C2), which serves as the pivot connecting the occipital bone to the third and succeeding vertebrae. Preservation of the posterior structures of C2, including the spinous process, is therefore very important.

Various surgical methods have been devised in Japan to decompress C3 and the succeeding vertebrae. I use a modified method based on Hirabayashi's open-door laminoplasty. However, when intraoperative ultrasonography reveals compression of the spinal cord by an anterior element, I employ expansion of the cervical spinal canal accompanied by hemifusion (Matsuzaki's method), in which the expanded vertebral arches are fused. In order to decompress C2, I use this method with a domelike laminoplasty. The major indications for this procedure include cervical myelopathy, ossification of the posterior longitudinal ligament (OPLL), developmental stenosis of the spinal canal, and spinal cord tumors. The method is not indicated for kyphotically aligned cervical vertebrae or unstable cervical vertebrae. The principle of the laminoplasty in my method is to decom-

H. Matsuzaki, M.D.: Department of Orthopaedic Surgery, Nihon University School of Medicine, 1-8, Kandasurugadai, Chiyoda-ku, Tokyo 101, Japan.

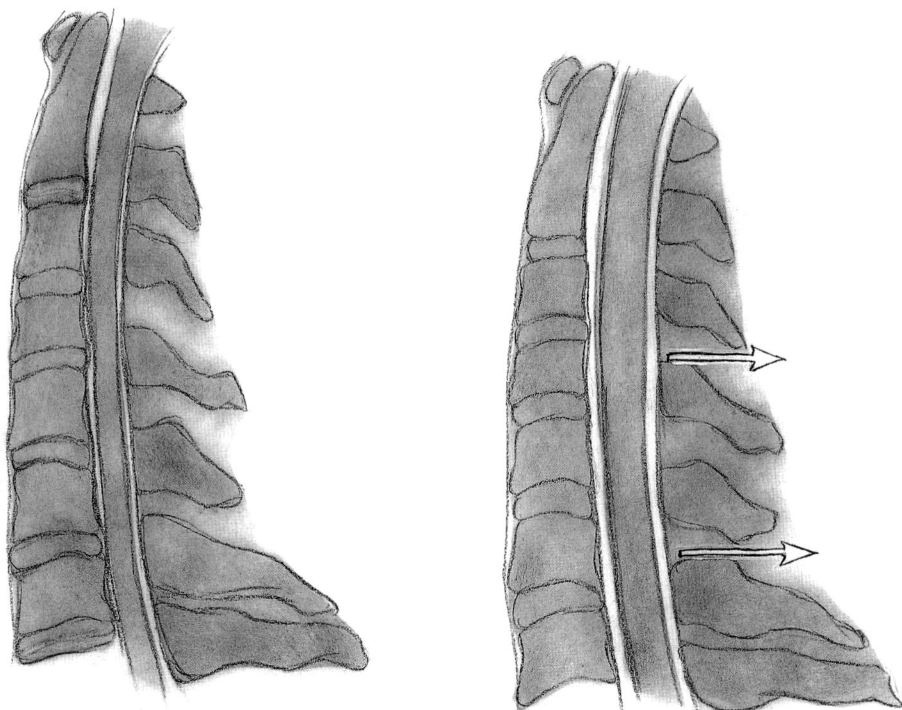

Figure 1. Posteriorly achieved expansion induces the posterior displacement of the spinal cord, which in turn brings about decompression.

press the spinal cord by displacing it posteriorly (Fig. 1). If the vertebrae are kyphotic, however, the decompression tends to be insufficient. If they are unstable due to rheumatoid arthritis, for example, the slippage of the vertebral bodies may be intensified, or kyphosis may result. In short, Matsuzaki's method is indicated when: (a) the lesion involves two or more intervertebral areas, (b) the cervical vertebrae are aligned lordotically, and (c) no severe instability exists in the region.

PREOPERATIVE PLANNING

The range of decompression is determined by the clinical symptoms and findings on myelography and magnetic resonance imaging (MRI). The procedure should include the lesion, as demonstrated on the MRI scan, plus at least one normal vertebral arch above and one below the lesion. Before the range of expansion is ultimately determined, the posterior displacement of the spinal cord to be brought about by the decompression should be estimated, particularly on the basis of a sagittal MRI scan. Careful preoperative assessment of the need for surgical decompression, using MRI, is important because posterior displacement of the spinal cord may result in new compression of C2, leading to yet another spinal disorder.

SURGERY

Positioning the Patient

In order to minimize bleeding from the extradural veins with the patient in the prone position, it is essential to reduce abdominal pressure and prevent venous congestion. The patient's trunk is supported at four points in a Hall frame. The head, encased in a three-point holder (Mayfield's tongs), is raised by approximately 20 degrees, with the neck slightly flexed. Utmost care should be taken not to increase abdominal pressure during the procedure. Slight traction on the head will help stabilize the vertebral arches and increase the safety of surgical maneuvers (Fig. 2). When additional hemifusion is required, the posterior superior iliac spine should be prepared for the possible excision of a bone graft.

Surgical Technique (Modified Open-Door Laminoplasty)

The incision made to expose the surgical field in the modified open-door laminoplasty should extend from the vertebral arch immediately above the lesion to the immediately adjoining arch below. The nuchal, supraspinous, and interspinous ligaments are carefully spared from invasion. The nuchal ligament attaching to C7 and T1 should particularly be spared by severing it from the upper end of the spinous processes of these vertebrae. The arches are exposed as far as the middle of the facet joint, leaving the rest of the joint intact (see Figs. 4 and 29). This is done because the soft tissue surrounding the lateral half of the joint is later needed to suture the expanded arches with nylon thread in order to secure them in place (see Fig. 11).

The expansion of the spinal canal from C3 through C6 is done as described here. When the vertebrae are affected by myelopathy but not radiculopathy, facetectomy is not needed. In this case a right-handed surgeon should attempt the expansion on the left side of the vertebrae. The large spinous processes of C5 and C6 are truncated so that they will be level with the processes of C3 and C4. Diagonal resection of the right sides of the spinous processes will prevent serious deviation of the processes from the median line when the expansion is achieved (Fig. 3). With the nuchal ligament severed at the expansion borders between C2 and C3 and between C6 and C7, two bony gutters are drilled, one for expansion and the other as a hinge. Both gutters should be positioned at the midpoint where

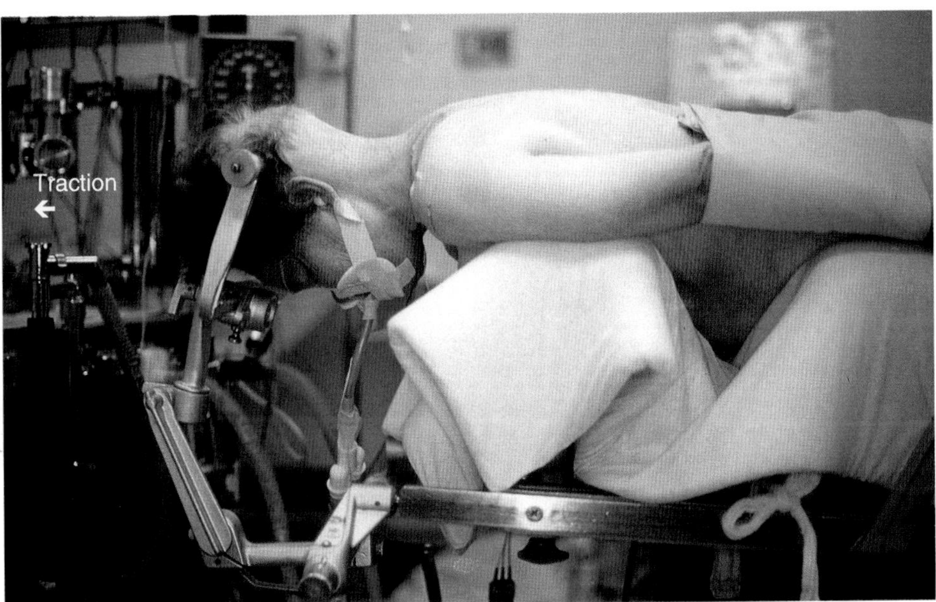

Figure 2. The patient's trunk is supported at four points by a Hall frame; the head is secured by a three-point holder (Mayfield's tongs), with the neck slightly flexed.

the vertebral arch curves to form the facet joint. If the gutters are located more laterally than this point, the facet joint tends to be destroyed and cause cervical pain and other complaints after the operation (Fig. 4). Marking with ink will help locate the right positions for drilling of the gutters (Fig. 5). With a high-speed drill (cutting bur) of 4-mm diameter, the expansion gutter is drilled on the left side of the vertebral arch until the inferior lamina of the arch is exposed. The lamina is safely removed by inserting the thin tip of a small punch between the lamina and

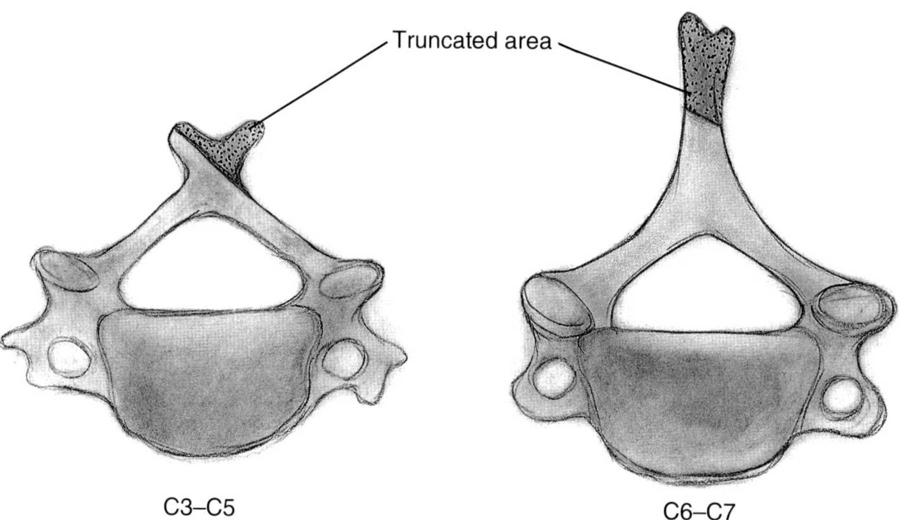

Figure 3. The spinous processes on the hinge side are diagonally truncated, while those on the expansion side are left intact to offer support for the suture with nylon thread to the soft tissue in the hinge area.

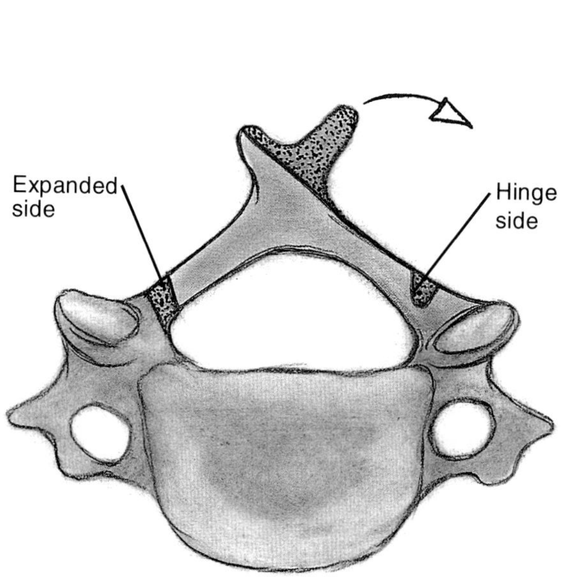

Figure 4. The location of the bony gutter: the point where the arch curves into the facet joint.

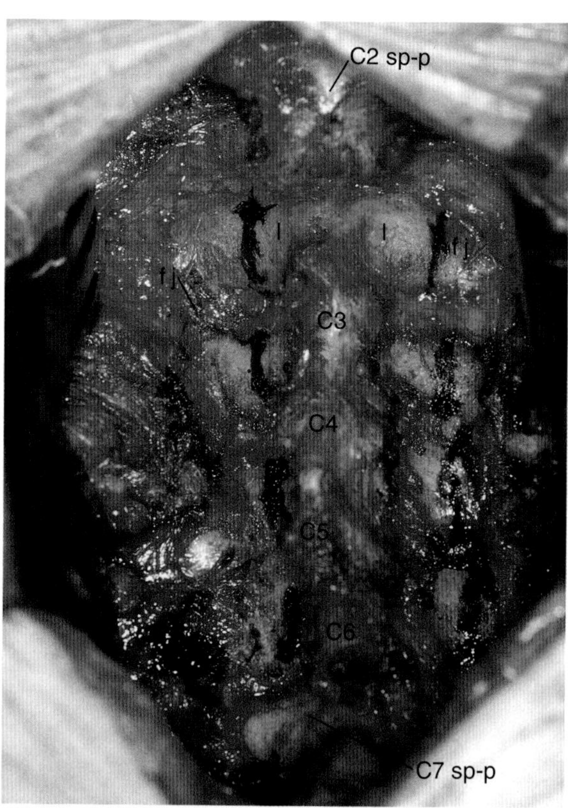

Figure 5. The gutter position is marked with ink. *fj*, facet joint; *l*, lamina; *sp-p*, spinous process.

the ligamentum flavum and snipping it away. This procedure enables the surgeon to avoid injuries to and bleeding from the extradural veins.

When the expansion gutter is completed, the ligamentum flavum is cut over a distance of three-quarters of the exposed semicircumference of the vertebral arch at the levels of C2–C3 and C6–C7, in preparation for the expansion (Fig. 6). The portion of the ligament trapped in the expansion gutter is then resected. This completes the pretreatment of the area to be expanded.

Next, the hinge gutter is drilled along the mark on the right side of the vertebral arches from C3 to C6, also with a high-speed drill. The surgeon must be very careful not to overdrill, or the function of the gutter as a hinge will be impaired. This can be done by attempting exploratory expansion of the arch from the left (expansion) side with a punch or a finger, while the bony gutter is still being drilled, in order to determine the appropriate depth of the hinge (Fig. 7). The

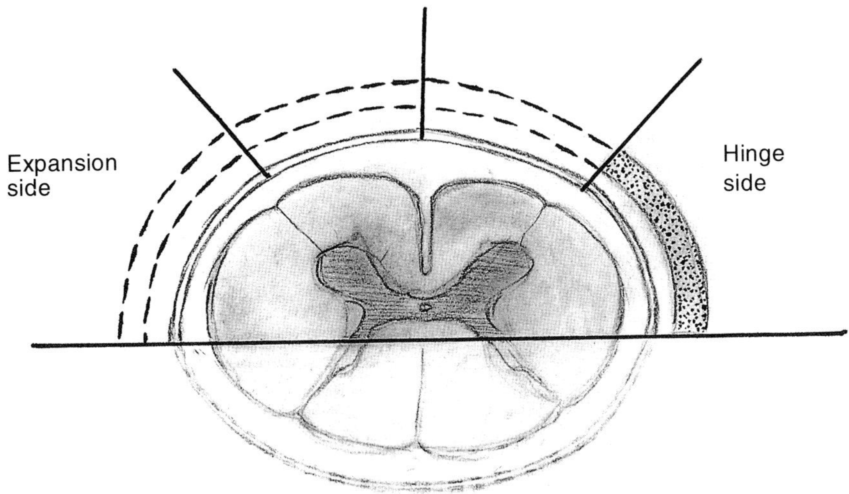

Figure 6. The ligamentum flavum is cut for three-fourths of the exposed semicircumference at the borders of the expansion, and one-fourth remains on the hinge side.

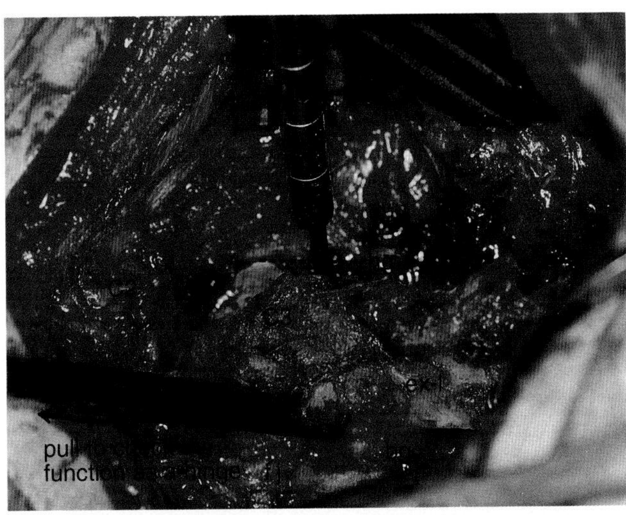

Figure 7. The procedure shown in Fig. 6 can be accomplished attempting exploratory expansion of the arch from the left (expansion) side with a punch and thus determining the appropriate depth of the hinges, while the bony gutter is still being drilled. *bg*, bony gutter; *ex-l*, expanded laminae; *fj*, facet joint; *hg*, hinge gutter.

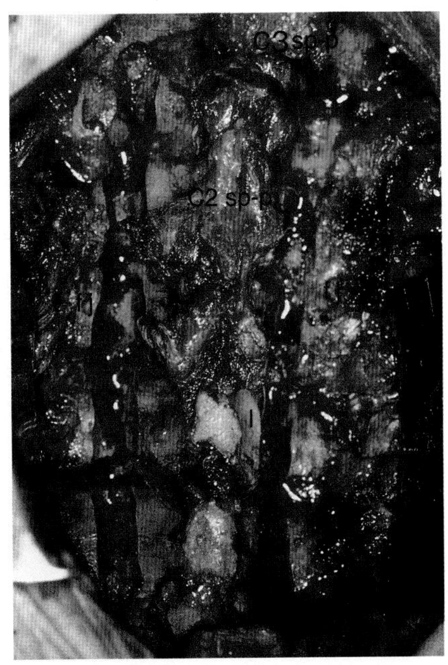

Figure 8. The bony gutter at completion. *bg*, bony gutter; *fj*, facet joint; *l*, laminae; *sp-p*, spinous process.

procedure should be applied to one vertebral arch at a time, in a craniad-to-caudad direction. If the arches of C6 and C7 are too hard to yield a flexible hinge, which is sometimes the case, the gutter should be deepened for greater flexibility. The construction of a suitable hinge is the crucial feature of the operative procedure; a broken hinge can cause neurologic impairment, as discussed later in this chapter (Fig. 8).

In order to expand the spinal canal, the spinous processes are slowly pushed up with both thumbs, left to right in the dorsal direction (Fig. 9). In many cases the ligamentum flavum and dura mater will have adhered to the vertebral arches. In such cases sudden expansion of the arches results in simultaneous elevation of the dura mater, leading to a traction injury of the nerve roots. Sufficient expansion can be expected if the expansion gutter is 15 mm wide (Fig. 10).

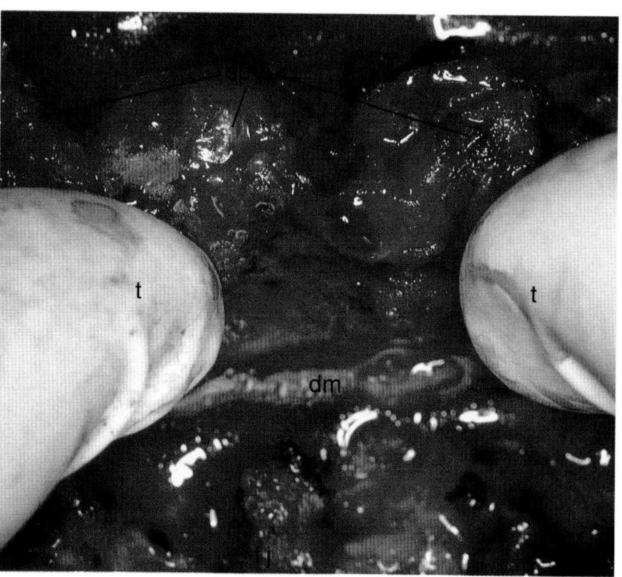

Figure 9. To achieve expansion, the vertebral arches are slowly pushed up with both thumbs. *dm*, dura mater; *fj*, facet joint; *t*, surgeon's thumb; *sp-p*, spinous process.

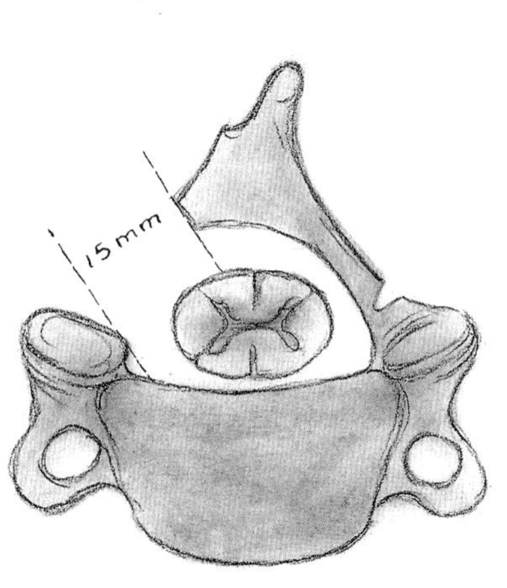

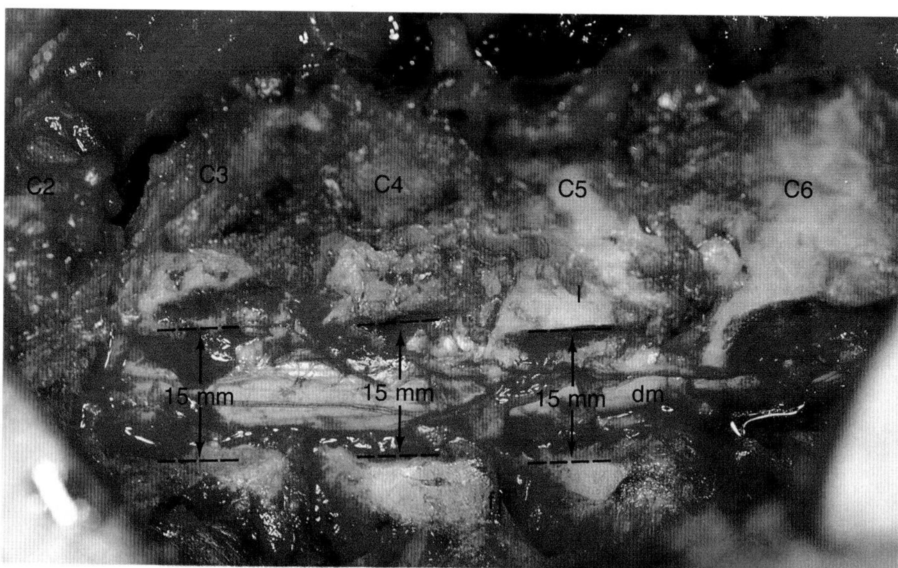

Figure 10. The arches are expanded until the aperture between the arches reaches 15 mm. *dm*, dura mater; *fj*, facet joint; *l*, laminae.

When, after the expansion maneuver, decompression of the spinal cord is confirmed ultrasonography, each expanded spinous process is sutured to the soft tissue as close to the facet joint as possible with nylon thread, in order to maintain the expanded contour (Fig. 11). Each muscle and the nuchal ligament are sutured back into their original positions so that the nuchal ligament will support the expanded spinous processes (Fig. 12). Drainage is established to prevent the formation of hematomas before the surgical wound is closed. Spinal cord tumors can be removed after the vertebral arches are expanded by laminoplasty.

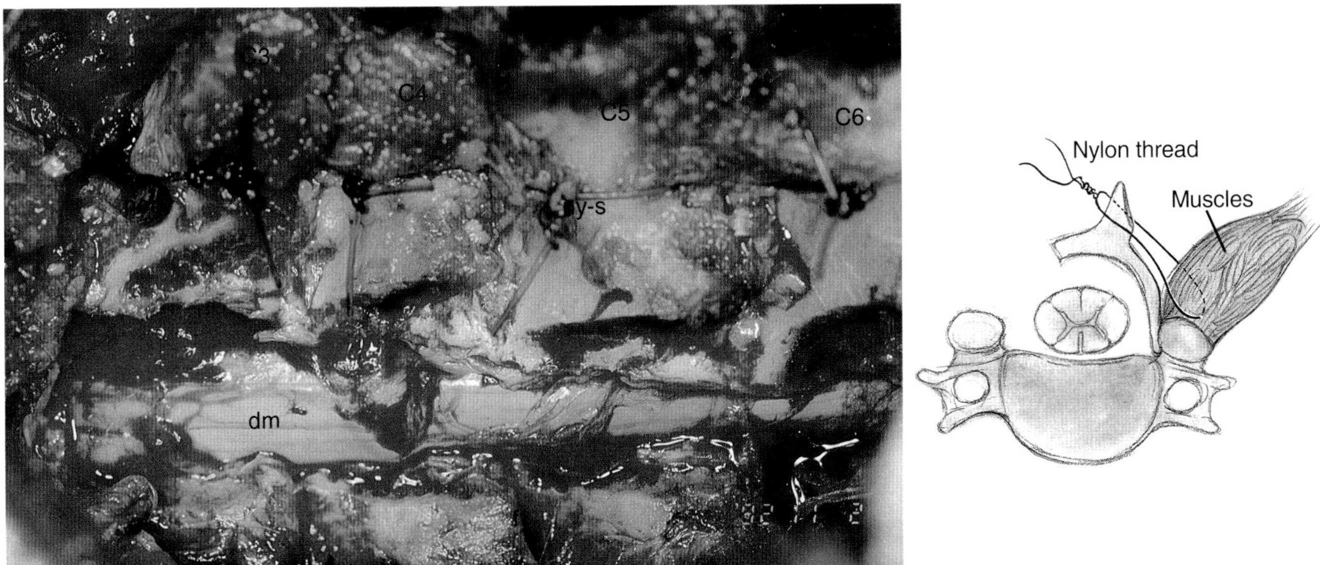

Figure 11. To maintain the expanded contour, the arches are sutured with nylon thread to the soft tissue in the bottom of the hinge area. *dm*, dura mater; *fj*, facet joint; *not*, notch for suture; *ny-s*, sutured with nylon thread.

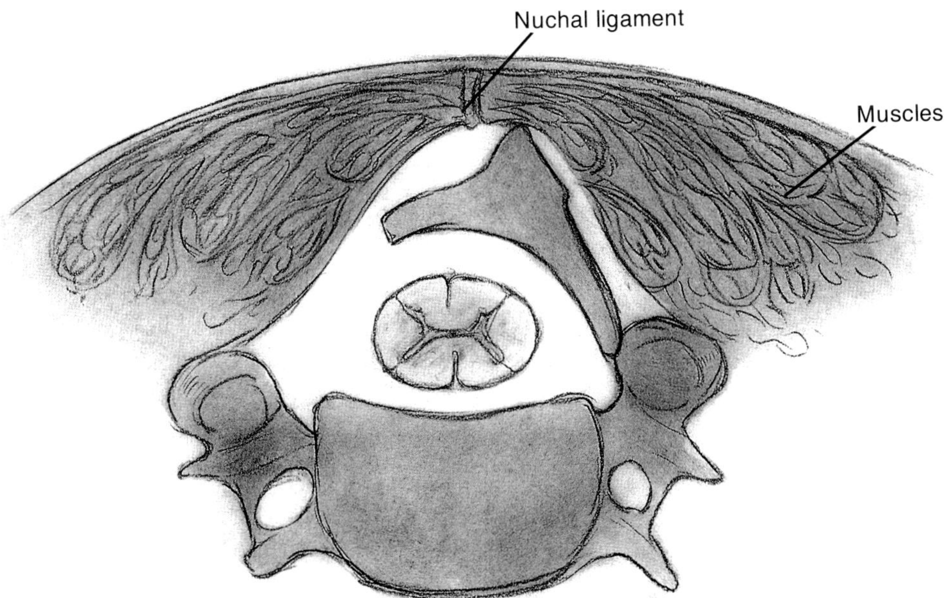

Figure 12. The expanded processes will be supported by the nuchal ligament.

Cervical Canal Expansion with Hemifusion (Matsuzaki's Method)

Matsuzaki's (5) method for expanding the cervical canal is the same as the modified open-door laminoplasty until the conclusion of vertebral arch expansion.

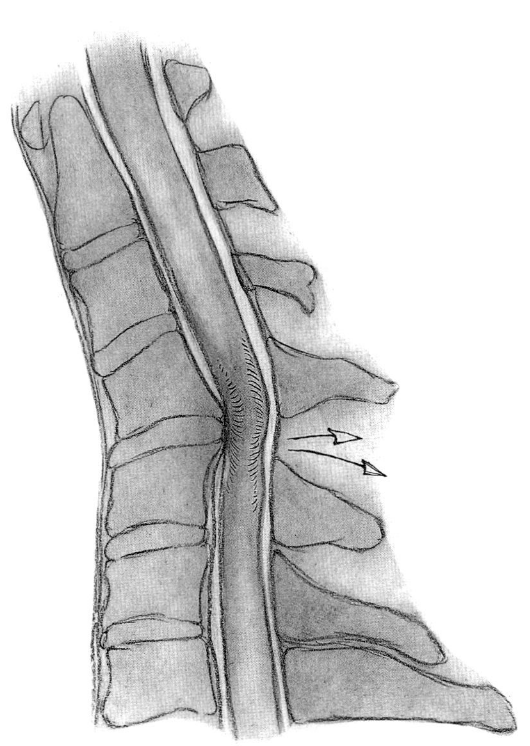

Figure 13. If the neck is flexed, the compression on the spinal cord exerted by the anterior bony spur or OPLL lesion increases.

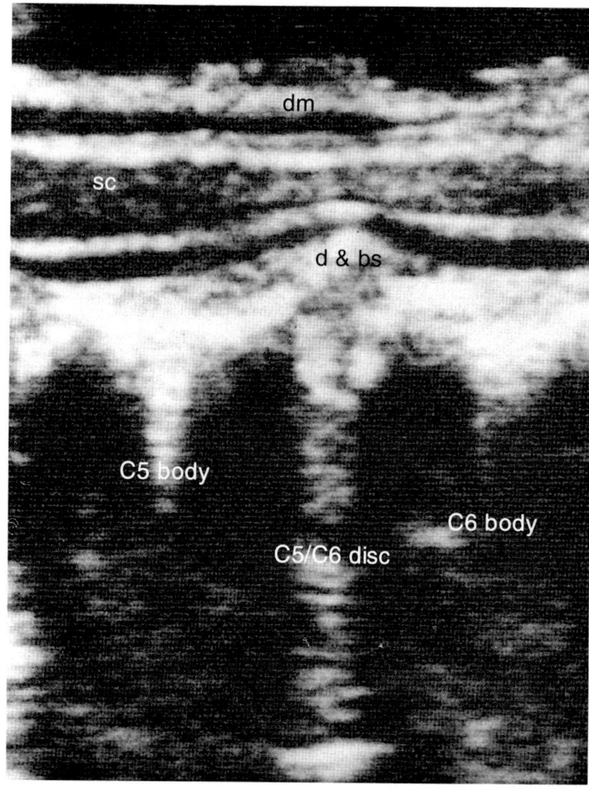

Figure 14. The expansion has not fully relieved the compression exerted by the bony spur; hemifusion on the expanded arches is indicated (intraoperative ultrasonogram). *sc,* spinal cord; *dm,* dura matter, *d&bs,* disc, bony spur.

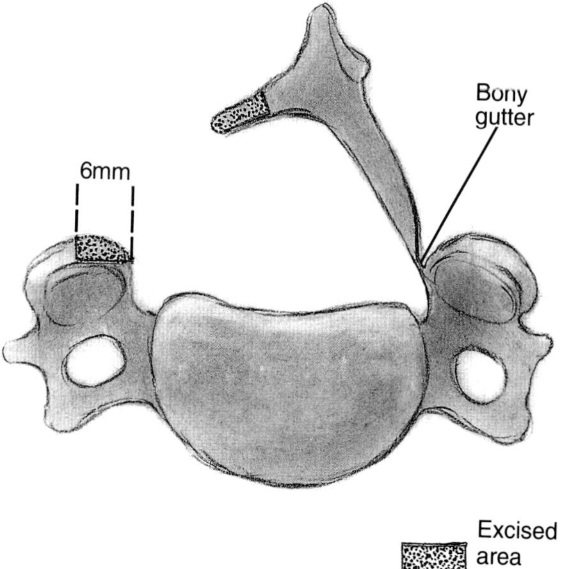

Figure 15. The preparation of the grafting bed for hemifusion.

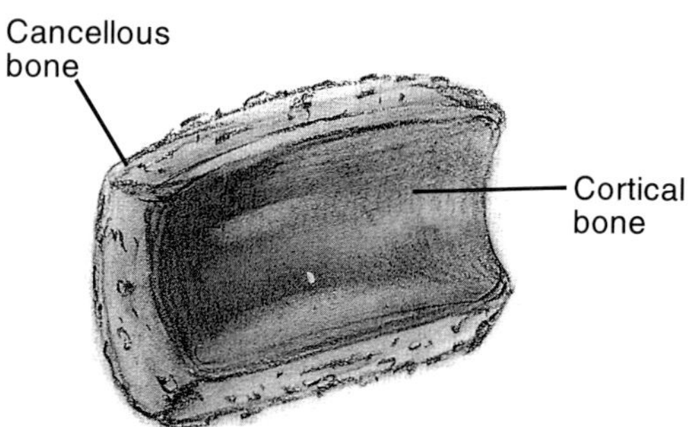

Figure 16. The bone graft obtained from the ilium; the curving cortex is to face the dura mater.

If at this point the spinal cord has not been fully displaced dorsally, but remains under compression from an anterior bone spur or lesion of the OPLL, movements of the cervical spine will enhance the spinal compression in the area, resulting in so-called dynamic mechanical compression (Fig. 13). This problem can be mitigated by fusing the expanded arches and the facet joint with a bone graft. Hemifusion should cover the area at risk for dynamic mechanical compression, which usually involves two, and occasionally three, arches. Ultrasonography is indispensable in laminoplasty as a means of detecting a compressed portion of the spinal cord during the operation (Fig. 14).

Preparation of the Grafting Bed

In preparing the bed for a bone graft to prevent dynamic mechanical compression of the spine, the edges of the expanded vertebral arches and the facet of the intervertebral joint are appropriately shaped with a high-speed drill. The lateral portion of the facet is drilled off at a width of some 6 mm until the spongiosa is barely visible (Fig. 15).

Procurement and Shaping of the Bone Graft

To procure the graft, a piece of bone 6-mm-thick is cut from the area extending from the posterior superior iliac spine to the iliac spine. The length and width of the graft are determined as the case requires, with the cortex to be used as one surface of the graft. Fat is also obtained for transplantation onto the exposed dura mater. The cortical surface of the graft is positioned to face the dura mater, with which it fits well owing to its natural curvature (Fig. 16). The areas of the cortex

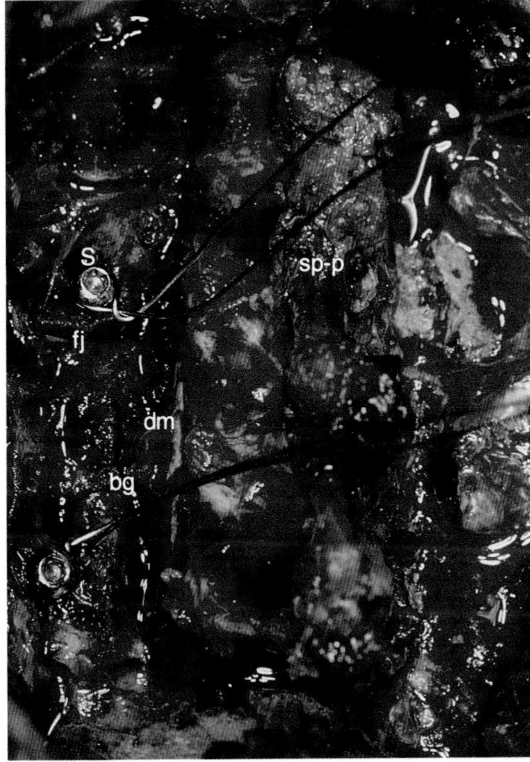

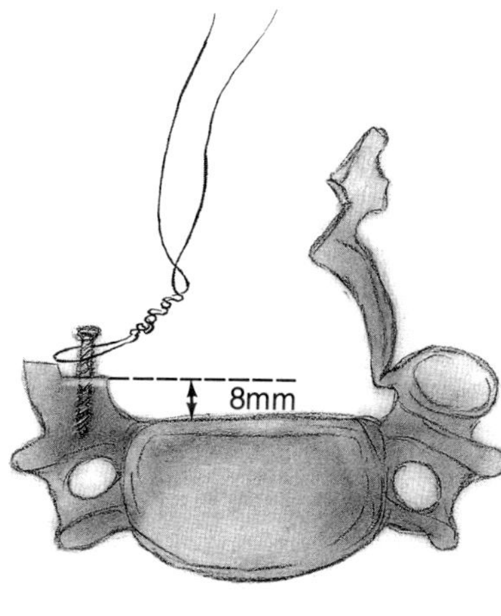

Figure 17. An 8-mm-deep screw hole is drilled at the center of the facet joint. *bg*, bony gutter; *dm*, dura mater; *fj*, facet joint; *S*, screw with wire; *sp-p*, spinous process.

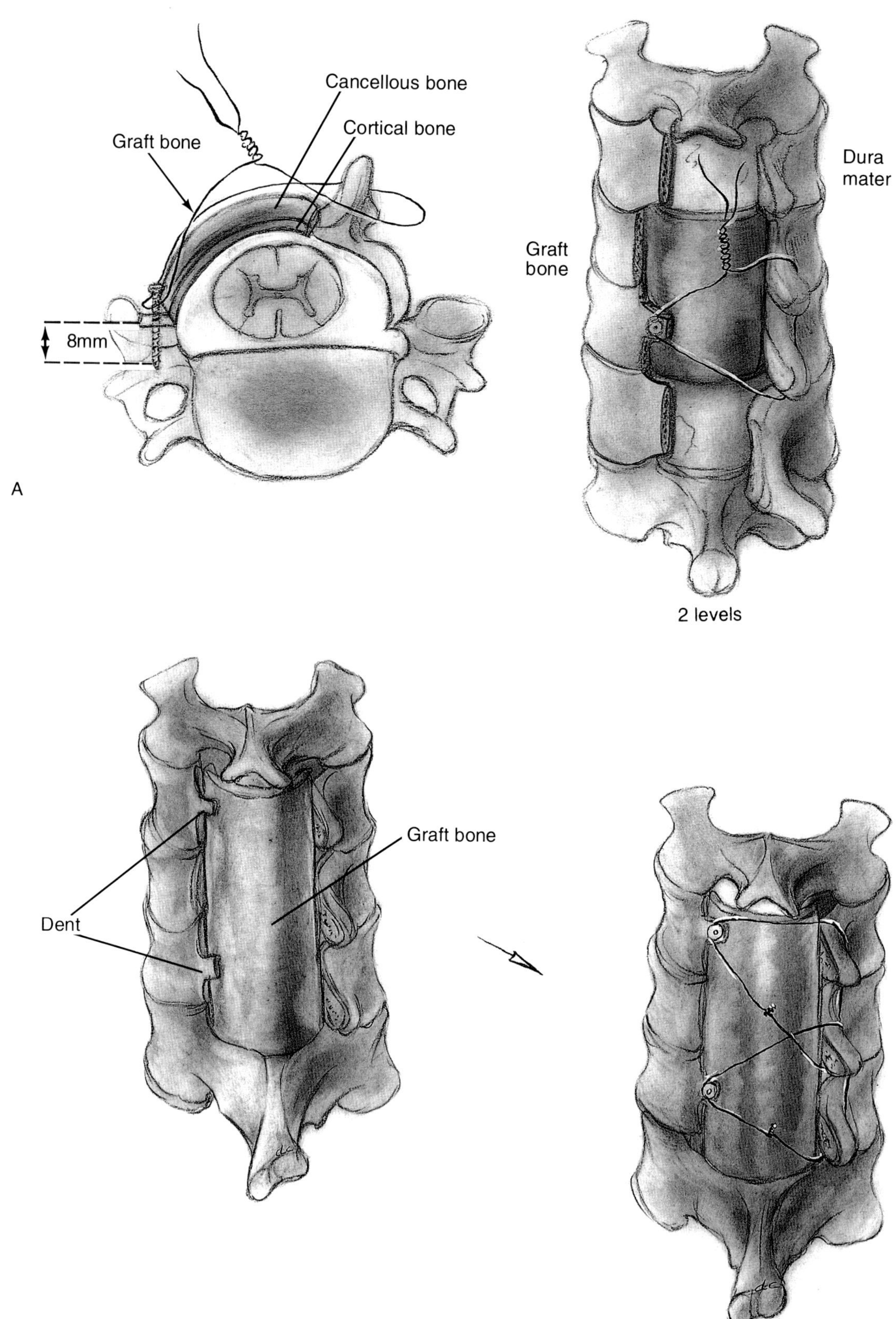

Figure 18. The screw is secured into the facet joint. A dent is drilled at the point where the screw is to be inserted.

that will meet the grafting bed are scraped to facilitate bone union. As mentioned above, the 15-mm aperture in the expansion gutter should permit sufficient expansion and, consequently, decompression.

Fixation of the Bone Graft

The bone graft is secured with an AO-OR-202-12 screw or a sapphire screw entwined with a strand of 0.6-mm wire or nylon thread. A hole approximately 8 mm deep is drilled for the screw in the center of the grafting bed on the facet. The procedure must be done very carefully without excessive drilling; a screw that penetrates too deeply may damage the blood vessels and nerve roots (Fig. 17).

A single screw is used to secure the graft to two vertebral arches; two screws are necessary to fuse three or more arches. A dent is drilled into the bone graft at the point at which the screw is to be inserted. When the screw is in place, the wire attached to it is passed through the interspinous space and wound around the base of the spinous process of one arch. After the wire is tightened and secured, the procedure is repeated for the other arch, thus securing both vertebral arches (Figs. 18 and 19). A notch in the base of the spinous process will prevent the wire from slipping off. The gap between the graft and the bed is filled with bone chips.

Treatment of Unfused Arches

A free fat graft is placed onto the exposed dura mater. If the expanded vertebral arches are unfused and appear unstable, a supportive suture should be added to

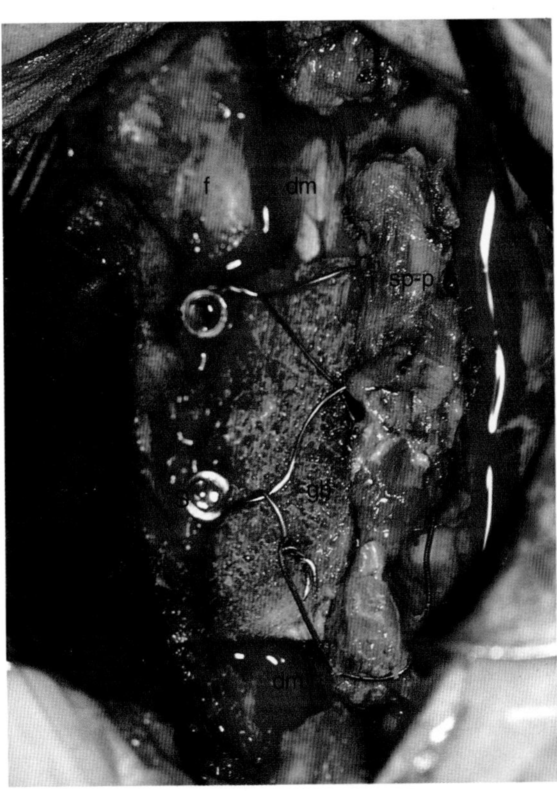

Figure 19. The bone graft is fixed to the expanded arches. *dm*, dura mater; *f*, facet; *gb*, graft bone; *S*, screws with wire; *sp-p*, spinous process.

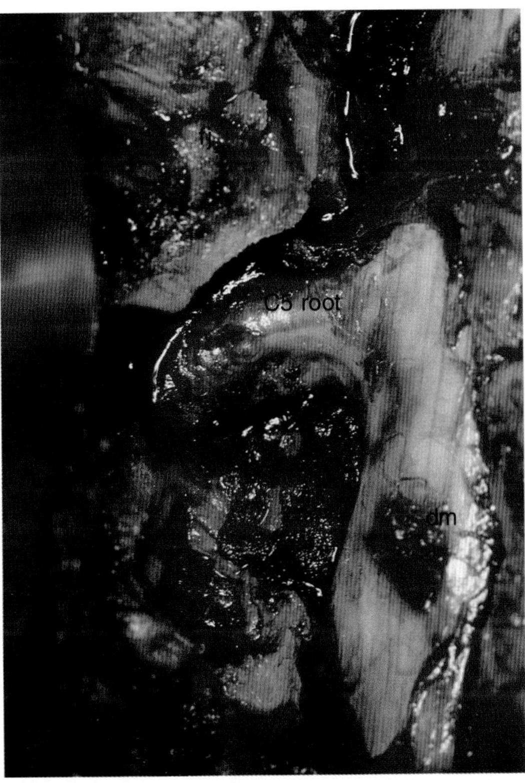

Figure 20. After a facetectomy, the C5 root is decompressed but still remains flattened from the anterior compression. *dm*, dura matter; *fj*, facet joint.

maintain the expansion. The subsequent steps in the procedure are the same as in the modified open-door laminoplasty. In patients with a compressed nerve root, facetectomy is first done with a high-speed drill to remove the causative anterior bone spur. The area is then subjected to hemifusion. Figure 20 shows the decompressed C5 nerve root immediately after the procedure. The root is flattened from the sustained anterior pressure.

Matsuzaki's Method Applied to C2 (C2 Domelike Laminoplasty)

Decompression of the C2 vertebra is indicated when the spinal cord is directly compressed by a lesion of the OPLL and also when, after the posterior decompression of C3 and succeeding vertebrae, the dorsally displaced spinal cord is in turn compressed by the arch of C2. In the operation it is essential to preserve the posterior structures of C2, in view of the anatomic specificity of this vertebra, which, as the connecting pivot between the occipital bone and the cervical vertebrae below C2, has a convergence of muscles extending to both areas (Fig. 21).

The domelike laminoplasty on C2 should be done before the expansion of C3 and the subtopical vertebrae. First, the muscles attached to the caudal side of the

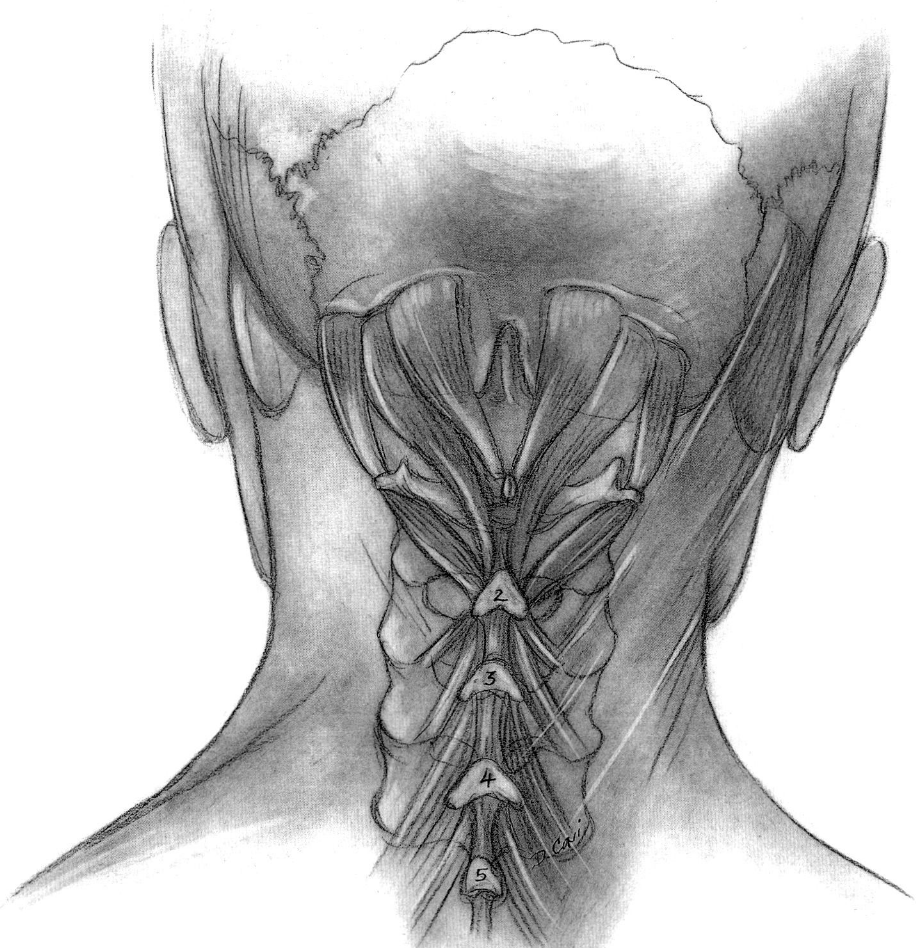

Figure 21. Posterior muscles around the C2.

spinous process of C2, including the multifidus, are detached after marking the point of attachment, in order to facilitate the restoring suture that is inserted later. Because the spinal canal widens toward the cranial end of C2, the extent of the domelike expansion needs to reach only two-thirds of the way up the vertebra from its caudal end (Fig. 22). With a high-speed drill (diamond bur), the inside of the vertebral arch is drilled away, from its caudal end toward the center of the spinal canal and anterior cranial end of the arch, leaving from 5 to 6 mm of the exterior layer of the arch (Fig. 23). If the spinous process of C3 interferes with this procedure, its tip is truncated. When the ligamentum flavum becomes barely visible, it is nipped away, along with the thinned arch, with a punch. As the punch approaches the cranial end of the arch, the procedure becomes quite difficult;

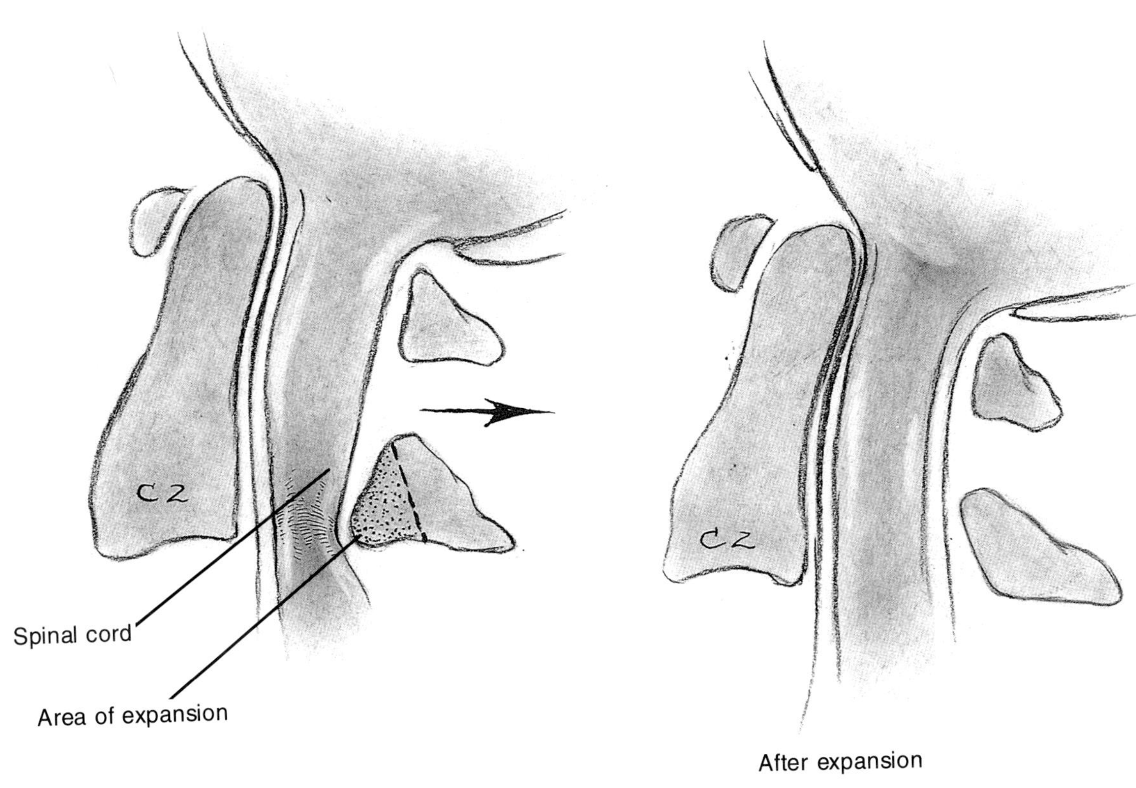

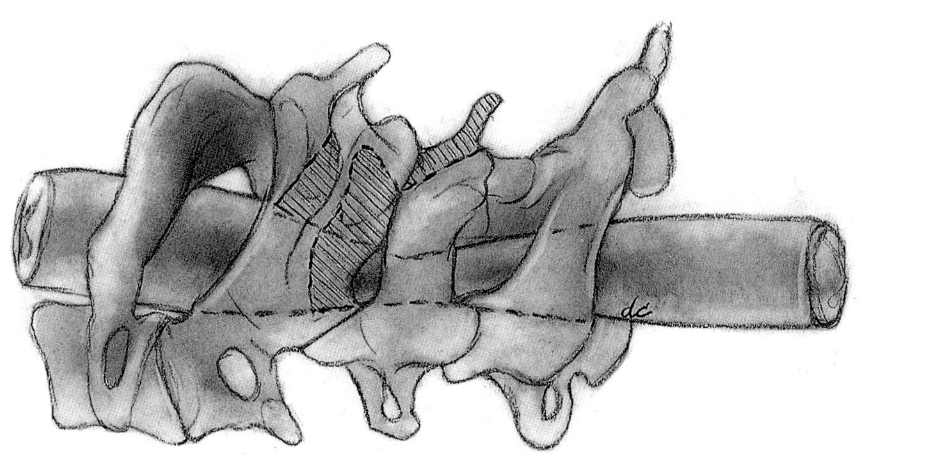

Figure 22. A,B: The spinal canal in the C2 tapers down toward its caudal end.

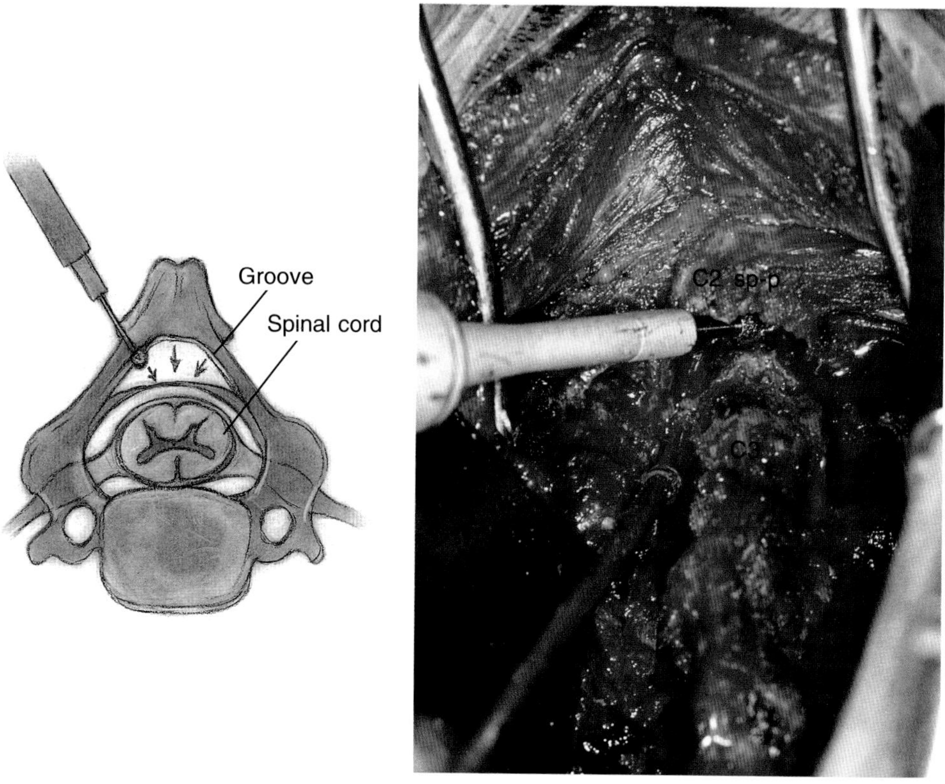

Figure 23. With 5 mm to 6 mm of the external layer left, the C2 arch is drilled with a diamond bur, anteriocranially from the caudal end.

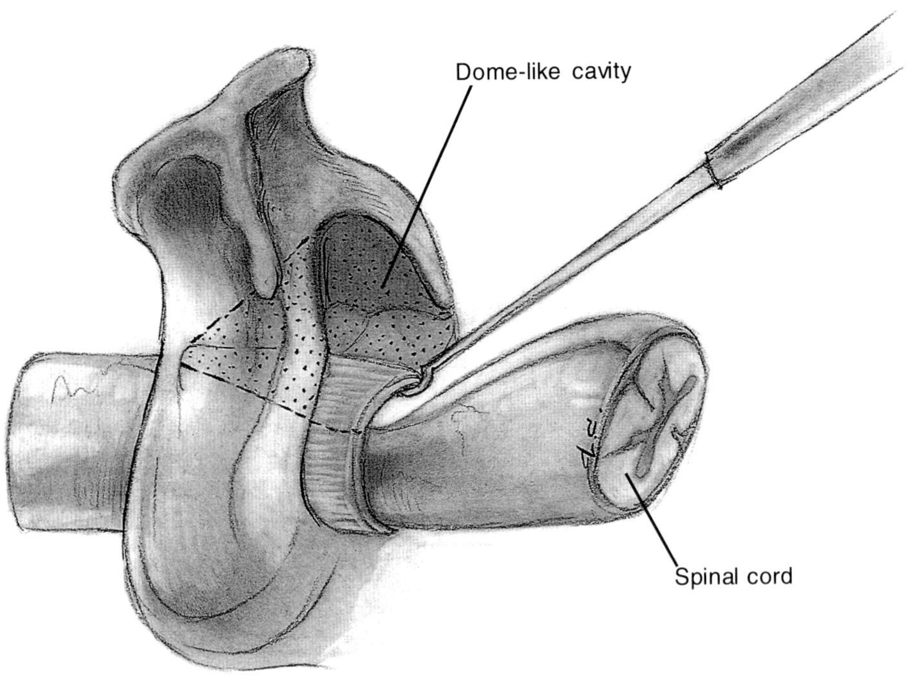

Figure 24. Osteotomy is safely performed with the bone curette directed dorsally.

consequently, the rest of the procedure is done with a bone curette, taking care not to compress the spinal cord. This can be done with the tip of the curette pointed dorsally (Fig. 24).

Figure 25 shows a C2 vertebra before and after the domelike expansion. The dura mater now lies within the dome. A free fat graft is placed onto the decompressed area. The detached musculus multifidus is sutured into its original location and secured with thread passed through the holes drilled in the spinous processes (Fig. 26). When complete hemostasis is confirmed, the incision is closed with a drain placed in the vertebral arch. Figure 27 shows a myelographic computed tomography scan of a C2 vertebra following a domelike laminoplasty. The contrast medium filling the subarachnoid space attests to adequate decompression.

POSTOPERATIVE MANAGEMENT

In order to move the patient immediately after cervical laminoplasty, a Philadelphia brace is applied for stability. For 1 or 2 weeks thereafter the patient is kept at rest, with the head on a low pillow raised at an angle of 20 to 30 degrees. Rotation of the head is prevented by sand bags placed on both sides of the face. The drain in the vertebral arch is removed after 48 hours. Seven or fifteen days after the operation the patient can generally begin to walk in a step-by-step manner while wearing a Philadelphia brace. Patients who have undergone a modified open-door laminoplasty must wear the brace for 6 weeks, whereas those who have had a cervical canal expansion and hemifusion must wear the brace for 8 weeks. The degree of postoperative improvement rate should be 60.5% according to the Cervical Myelopathy Score established by the Japanese Orthopaedic Association. This means the restoration of walking ability and marked improvement in the kinetic function of the fingers.

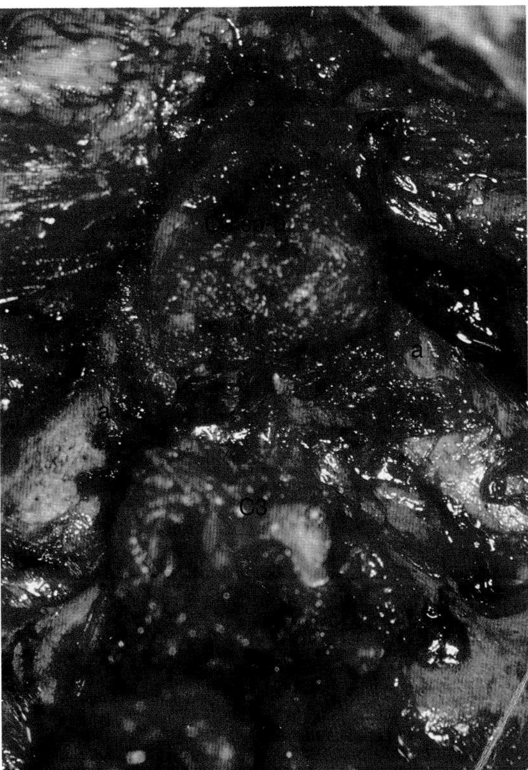

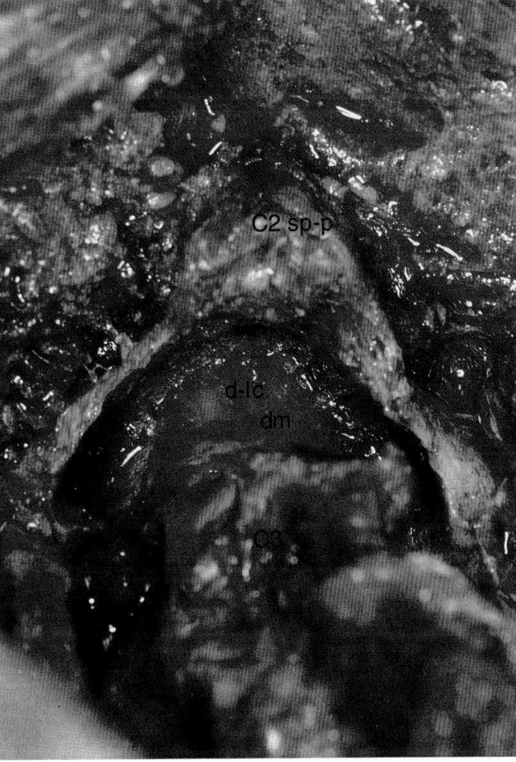

Figure 25. The dura mater (*dm*) is seen within the spinal canal expanded like a dome. *a*, arch; *dc*, dome-like cavity; *sp-p*, spinous process.

The range of motion (ROM) of the neck after cervical laminoplasty appears to decrease by 30% to 40%. When the spinal cord is prone to anterior compression, however, this restriction in the ROM is therapeutically desirable in that it reduces the risk of dynamic injury to the cord.

COMPLICATIONS

Sagging of the Expanded Arch into the Hinge Gutter

When the hinge gutter is being drilled, its flexibility or resilience should be constantly tested by exploratory opening of the treated arches from the left side.

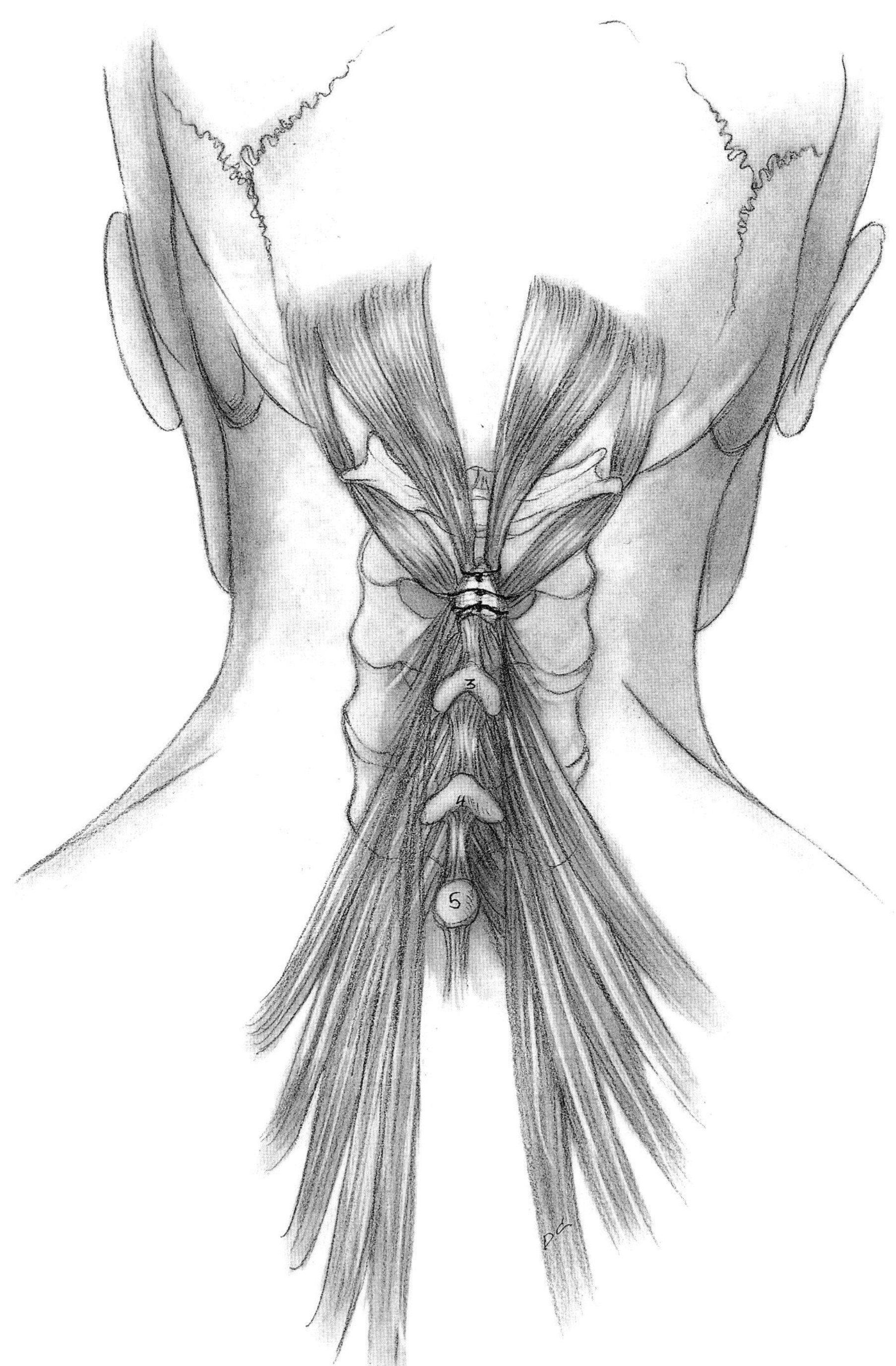

Figure 26. The muscles are firmly sutured to their original positions.

If the gutter is made too thin, it loses the function of a hinge, and the expanded arch may sag into the gutter, resulting in spinal pathology. As noted earlier, the construction of the bony gutters is therefore the crucial point in the laminoplasty (Fig. 28).

Development of Kyphosis

The laminoplasty procedure is contraindicated for patients with kyphosis because of the inevitable exacerbation of this condition after the operation. Yet kyphosis can develop even in patients with straight alignment of cervical verte-

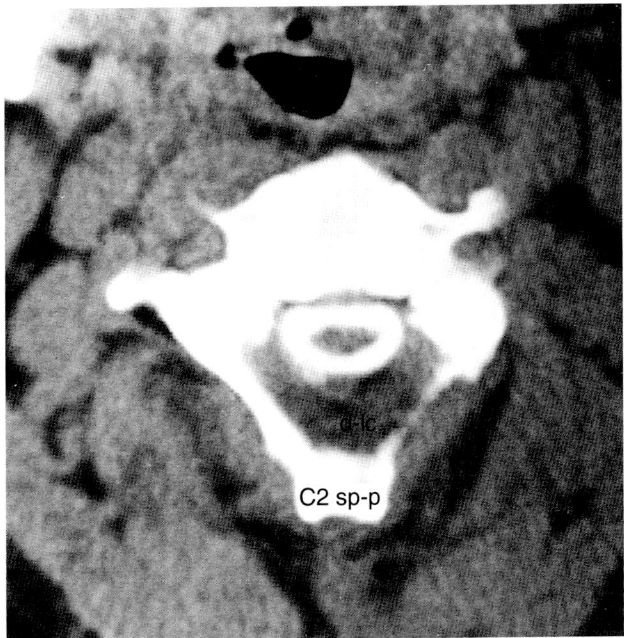

Figure 27. Myelographic computed tomography after the domelike laminoplasty; decompression achieved sufficiently. *dc*, dome-like cavity; *sp-p*, spinous process.

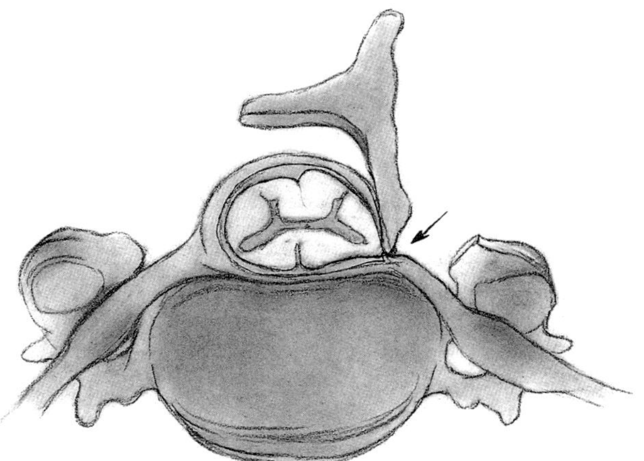

Figure 28. When the hinge gutter breaks down or is made too thin, the vertebral arch may sag, inducing spinal disorders.

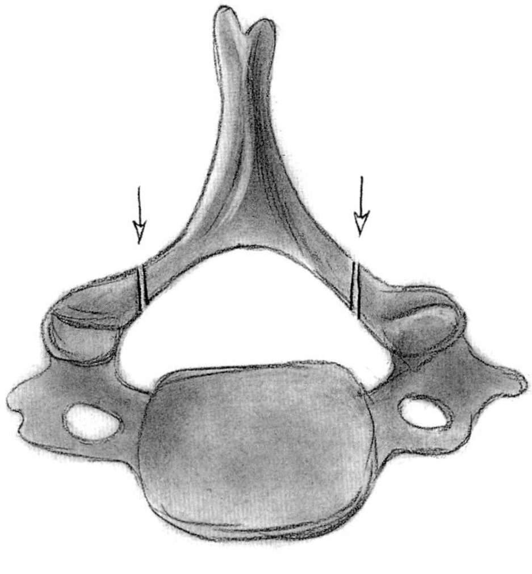

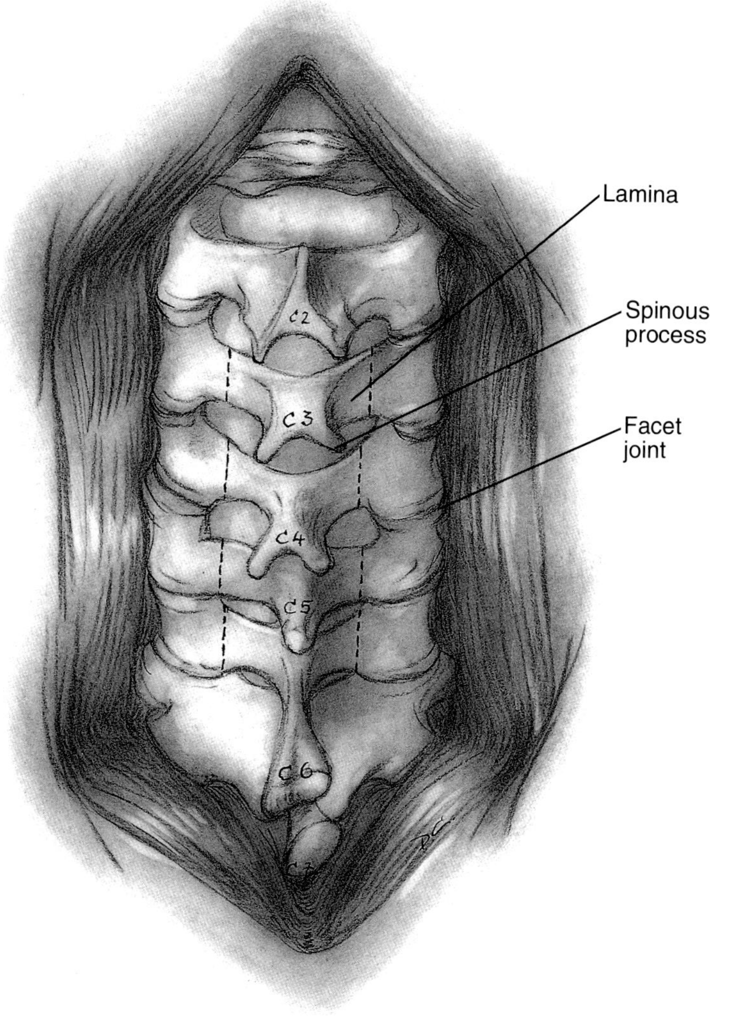

Lamina
Spinous process
Facet joint
C2
C3
C4
C5
C6

Figure 29. If the bony gutter is constructed too laterally, it destroys the facet joint and leads to complications.

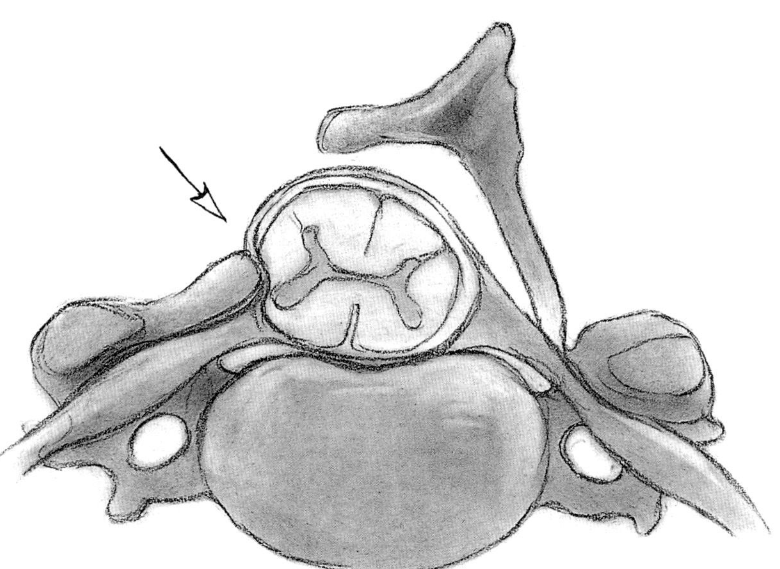

Figure 30. The intrusion of the gutter edge into the spinal canal can also cause neurologic impairment.

brae, and has occurred in 20 of my own cases among 200 (10%). Kyphosis especially tends to develop if the bony gutter is made in the periphery of the facet joint, and neck pain or stiff shoulders can also result from this. The gutter should therefore be created in such a way that both of its ends lie tangent to the spinal canal (Fig. 29). It must be also kept in mind that intrusion of the edge of the vertebral arch into the spinal canal may impair the posterior nerve roots (Fig. 30).

Enhanced Slippage of the Vertebral Body

In patients with slippage of a vertebral body, the laminoplasty may later enhance this slippage. It is therefore all the more important not to injure the facet joint and posterior ramus of the treated vertebra, which govern the neck muscles.

Tethering Effects on the Nerve Roots

The laminoplasty may be followed by complications suggesting the impairment of nerve roots in the region of the operation. These become manifest, in most cases from immediately after the procedure to 2 or 3 days later. Six of 200 (3%) patients of my own developed such symptoms as difficulty in abducting the shoulder and reduced grasping power. Because the ligamentum flavum and dura mater are often adherent to the vertebral arch, they are raised along with the elevated arch when the spinal canal is expanded abruptly, applying a strong traction to the nerve roots (tethering effect; Fig. 31). A period of at least several minutes should be allowed to elapse during the expansion, with the spinous processes pushed slowly dorsally with both thumbs.

Bone Regeneration in the Area Decompressed by C2 Domelike Laminoplasty

In the early phase of development of the domelike laminoplasty, I was concerned about possible bone regeneration in the spinal canal affected by the proce-

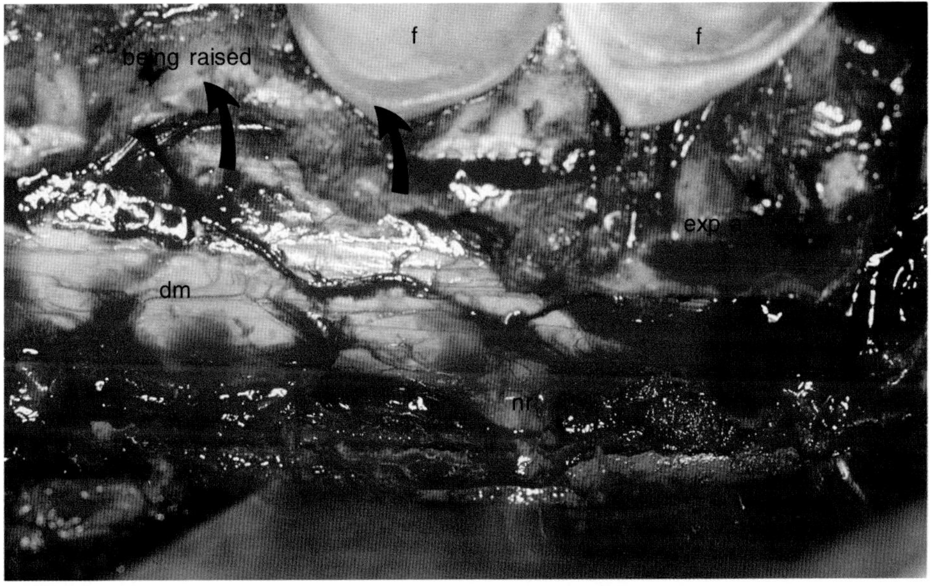

Figure 31. The nerve roots were raised (*arrows*) as the arches (*a*) were expanded; the nerve roots (*nr*) are seen strained. *dm*, dura mater; *f*, finger.

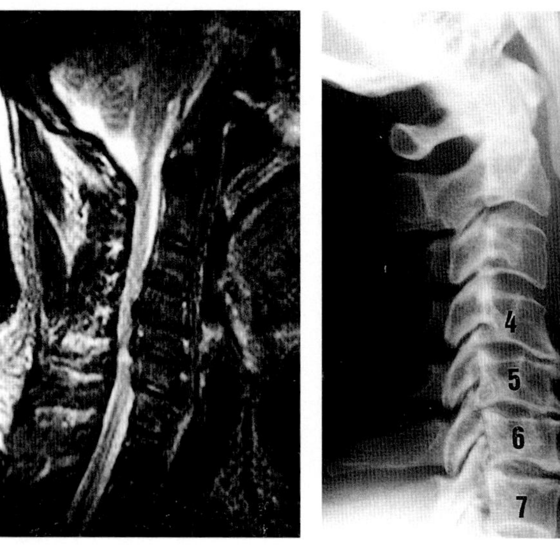

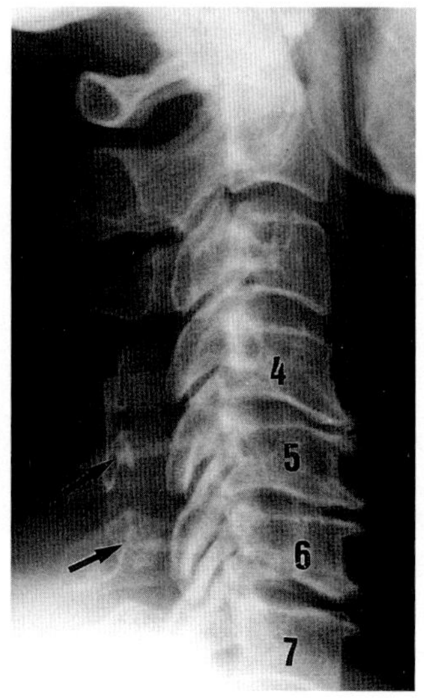

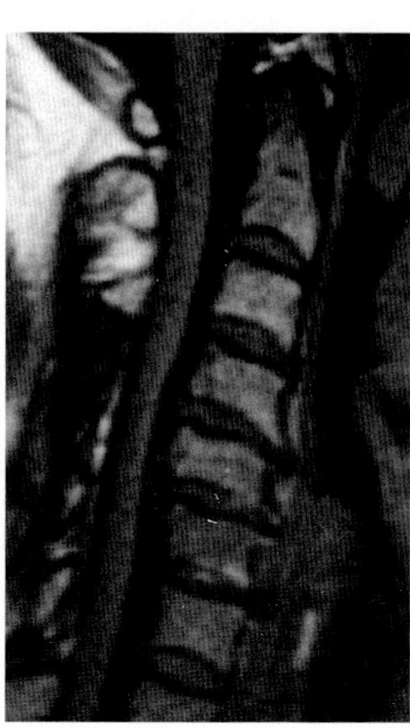

A, B

C, D

Figure 32. Preoperative MRI scan (**A**) and radiograph (B) showing remarkable stenosis due to OPLL at each disc level. C: Postoperative expansion laminoplasty with hemifusion using two sapphire screws (*arrows*) with nylon thread. Expansion area: C4–C7; hemifusion area: C4–C6. D: The postoperative MRI scan taken a year later showed a morphological improvement in the spinal cord.

dure, which might have led to a recurrence of spinal compression. After a lapse of 10 years, however, the only reported effect is mild osteogenesis in some patients, which does not appear to present serious problems. Both the risk of compression and the other complications mentioned above are preventable if the precautions described in this chapter are taken.

ILLUSTRATIVE CASE FOR TECHNIQUE

A 59-year-old man had paresis in all of his limbs caused by OPLL. He was unable to walk and had a neurologic deficit in the cervical vertebrae below C5. Preoperative lateral radiograms revealed OPLL of the continuous type in the C4–C7 region. Because the cervical alignment was straight, a hemifusion of the C4–C6 vertebrae was done as a supplementary procedure. After the operation, the patient's spinal canal was found to have been enlarged by 60%. An MRI scan done a year after the operation showed morphologic improvement in the spinal cord compared with a preoperative MRI scan. The patient exhibited a 75% clinical recovery, with remarkable improvement in his activities of daily living (Fig. 32).

RECOMMENDED READING

1. Hirabayashi, K., Watanabe, K., Wakano, K., et al.: Expansive open-door laminoplasty for cervical spine stenotic myelopathy. *Spine*, 8: 693–699, 1983.
2. Itoh, T., and Tsuji, H.: Technical improvements and results of laminoplasty for compressive myelopathy in the cervical spine. *Spine*, 10: 729–736, 1985.
3. Kawai, S., Sunago, K., Doi, K., et al.: Cervical laminoplasty (Hattori's method): procedure and follow-up results. *Spine*, ad: 1245–1250, 1988.
4. Kurokawa, T., Tsuyama, N., Tanaka, H., et al.: Enlargement of the spinal canal by the sagittal splitting of spinal processes. *Bessatu Seikeigeka*, 2: 234–240, 1982 (in Japanese).
5. Matsuzaki, H., Toriyama, S., Koyama, I., et al.: Cervical expansive laminoplasty with posterolateral hemifusion. *Shujutu*, 41: 529–536, 1987 (in Japanese).

6. Matsuzaki, H., Hoshino, M., Toriyama, S., et al.: Dome-like expansive laminoplasty for the second cervical vertebra. *Spine*, 14: 1198–1203, 1989.
7. Miyazaki, K., and Kirita, Y.: Extensive simultaneous multisegment laminectomy for myelopathy due to the ossification of the posterior longitudinal ligament in the cervical region. *Spine*, 11: 531–542, 1986.
8. Tsuji, H.: Laminoplasty for patients with compressive myelopathy due to so-called spinal canal stenosis in cervical and thoracic regions. *Spine*, 7: 28–34, 1982.
9. Tsuzuki, N., Hotta, Y., Imai, T., et al.: Tsuzuki's laminoplasty. *Bessatsu Seikeigeka*, 2: 255–262, 1982 (in Japanese).

PART III

Techniques—Thoracic/Lumbar Spine

Master Techniques in Orthopaedic Surgery,
THE SPINE, edited by D. S. Bradford,
Lippincott-Raven Publishers, Philadelphia, © 1997.

10

Anterior Thoracic Fusion

James W. Ogilvie

Anterior Thoracic Fusion

INDICATIONS/CONTRAINDICATIONS

Anterior thoracic fusion is performed for one or a combination of the following indications:

Decompression of the spinal canal: When an intervertebral herniation is decompressed through the anterior approach, anterior interbody fusion is often performed. The absolute indications for fusion in this situation have not been clearly defined, but the morbidity of fusion is small and the rationale for arthrodesis of a degenerated motion segment is intuitively attractive.

Stabilization of vertebral motion segments after partial or complete vertebrectomy: Following decompression of the spinal canal by removal of all or a portion of the vertebral body whether it be for tumor, trauma, infection, or congenital or degenerative conditions, the spinal column may be rendered mechanically unstable. Anterior fusion, sometimes in conjunction with posterior instrumentation and fusion, is indicated to restore stability.

To mobilize the spine in conjunction with staged kyphosis or scoliosis surgery: Stiff spinal deformities may require anterior release and intervertebral bone grafting in conjunction with staged anterior-posterior reconstruction. When correcting kyphosis deformity in the adult, release of the anterior longitudinal ligament and interbody bone graft increases the amount of correction possible when the posterior instrumented fusion is performed and decreases the incidence of pseudarthrosis.

J. W. Ogilvie, M.D.: Department of Orthopaedic Surgery, University of Minnesota, Minneapolis, Minnesota 55455

PREOPERATIVE PLANNING

Upright 2 m lateral and anteroposterior (AP) radiographs are obtained for examination of the spine and to document the sagittal contour. Some idea of the exact rib through which the exposure is to be obtained will be evident from the lateral views. If the ribs are sloping, the incision should be two levels above the vertebra in question. Otherwise, the exposure is best achieved through the rib one level above (6). Spot radiographs may demonstrate greater bony detail. Appropriate imaging studies are also obtained depending on the diagnosis to ascertain canal compromise, adjacent disc pathology, and the integrity of the vertebral bodies. Magnetic resonance imaging (MRI) of the thoracic spine is often the study of choice.

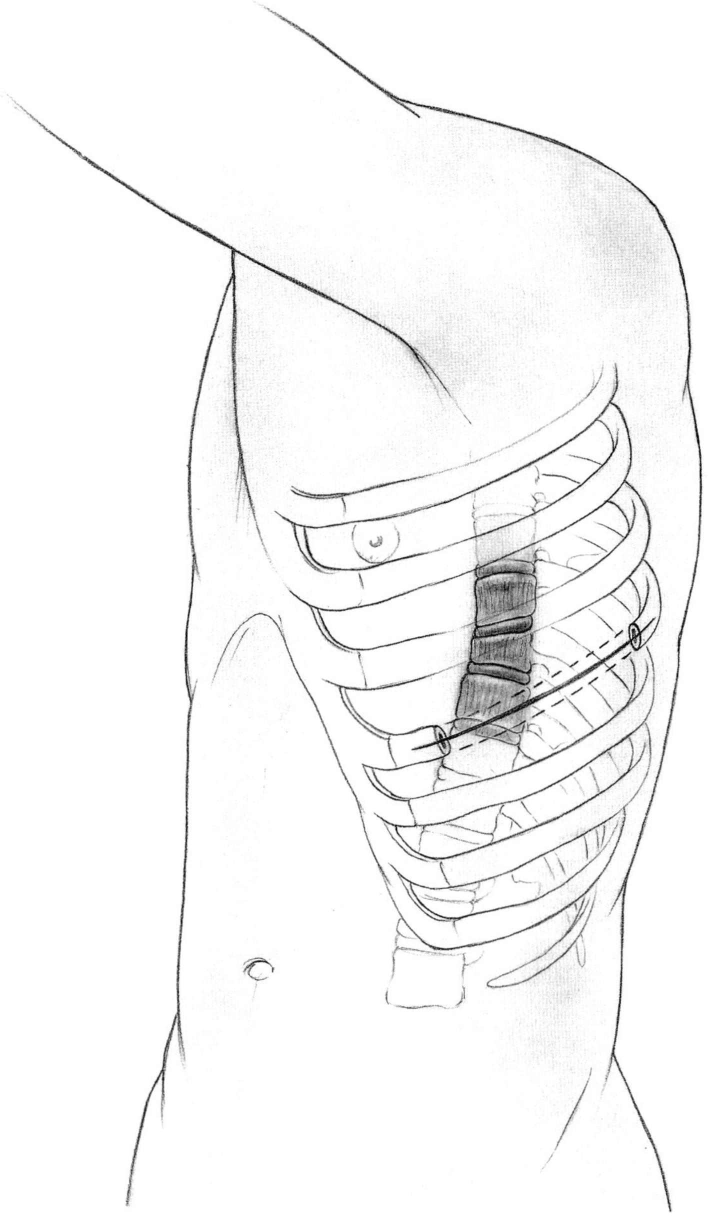

Figure 1. With the patient in the right lateral decubitus position, an incision is made over the rib one or two levels proximal to the disc space to be exposed.

Following physical examination for diagnosis of the patient's disorder, attention should be turned to the chest wall through which transthoracic exposure is made. Cutaneous infection, extensive scarring, or previous adjacent parallel incisions may contraindicate surgery through this area. In severe scoliosis, the spinal column may be lying adjacent to the chest cage, and entrance through a rib bed may provide only limited exposure of one or two vertebral bodies. In general, an incision is planned through the rib one level cephalad to the vertebra desired (Fig. 1). If the ribs are more obliquely oriented it may be necessary to make the incision two levels above the desired vertebral level. If a complete discectomy to the posterior longitudinal ligament is desired, the surgeon must have direct line of vision into the disc space in order to minimize inadvertent trauma to the canal contents. It is imperative that the thoracic incision be placed with this in mind. Entrance to the chest through the left side allows one to deal with the aorta rather than the vena cava. The aorta is more resistant to incidental trauma and easier to repair than the vena cava in case of such an event.

The sixth rib usually passes under the tip of the scapula; if exposure above that level is required, an angled incision is needed so that medial scapular musculature can be taken down, the scapula retracted, and entrance into the chest accomplished through the third, fourth, or fifth rib bed. Access to the T3 vertebral body is possible through this incision.

If thoracolumbar exposure is needed, usually for a thoracolumbar fracture or scoliosis, an incision is made through the tenth rib. The diaphragm inserts over the bed of the 11th rib and an approach one level above allows a less complicated closure since the diaphragm and the rib bed can be closed separately.

SURGERY

If pulmonary function is not a contraindication, it is often advisable to ask the anesthesiologist to insert a double-lumen endotracheal tube so that the lung can be more completely collapsed in the operative field. This is more important above the level of the sixth rib since the lung can be easily compressed with a moist laparotomy pad when operating below that level.

The patient is placed in the lateral decubitus position, with an axillary roll to prevent traction on the brachial plexus. The pelvis and upper thorax are taped to the table so that the table can be flexed to enhance exposure by opening the intercostal spaces. The thorax should be sterilely prepared and draped from midline anteriorly to midline posteriorly and from the nipple to the groin. Palpation is used to count up from the 12th rib, and an incision is made over the appropriate rib. Since the latissimus dorsi and serratus anterior are innervated proximally, they are divided in layers along the inferior border of the incision in order to denervate the minimum amount of muscle mass.

Subperiosteal exposure of the rib allows the rib to be cut posteriorly just beyond the angle (Fig. 2). Because of the obliquity of the intercostal insertion, subperiosteal dissection of the rib is carried out posterior to anterior along the superior border of the rib and anterior to posterior along the rib's inferior border. Anteriorly the rib is divided medial to the anterior axillary line. Care should be taken to avoid cutting the subcostal neurovascular bundle. After incising the parietal pleura, moist sponges are placed on the wound edges, and a chest retractor is placed to maintain exposure while the lung is gently compressed with moist laparotomy pads. Confirmation of the correct levels of dissection is obtained with an intraoperative radiograph or by palpating the ribs from inside the thorax. Although it requires experience, the first rib can usually be palpated. When performing a thoracolumbar exposure, the diaphragm is bluntly dissected free and divided at the periphery, leaving a 5- to 10-mm cuff. The dendritic pattern of vagus innervation of the diaphragm is thereby preserved.

The parietal pleura is incised with a Metzenbaum scissors, and the segmental vertebral vessels are visualized (Fig. 3). If a single-level anterior fusion is the objective, it may not be necessary to ligate these vessels. If the exposure requires multiple vertebral levels, the segmental vessels are ligated with silk sutures or metallic clips (Fig. 4). This ligation should be at the level of the midvertebral body. Nutrient vessels to the spinal cord have their collateralization at the level of the foramen, and if ligation is accomplished there, the cord's blood supply may be compromised (3). Gentle blunt dissection allows the great vessels and mediastinal contents to be isolated with a moist gauze sponge. For safety reasons, a broad smooth retractor should always be placed between the great vessels and the disc space undergoing excision during the dissection.

The intervertebral disc is excised in a stepwise fashion: (a) the disc margin is outlined with electrocautery both for hemostasis and to identify precisely the

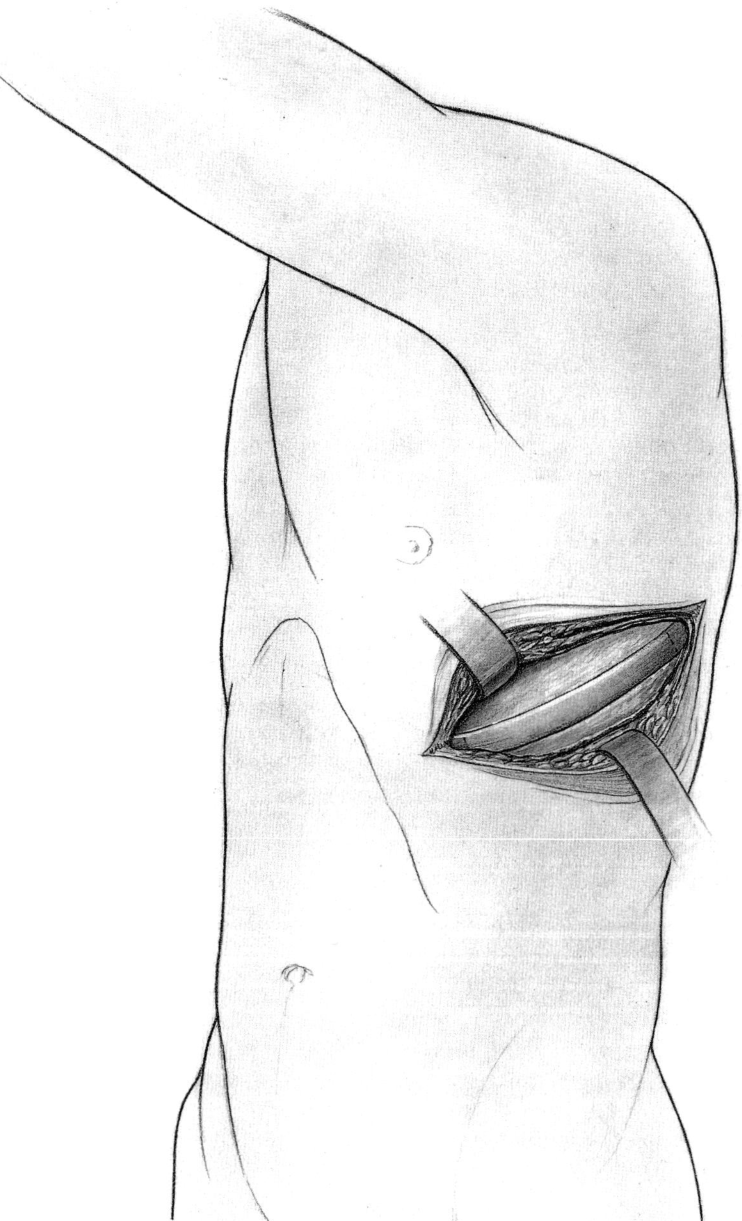

Figure 2. Subperiosteal exposure of the rib is made through the latissimus dorsi anteriorly to beyond the anterior axillary line and posteriorly to the angle of the rib.

margins of the disc (Fig. 5), (b) a #15 blade is used to dissect the anulus from the end plate, (c) further dissection of the end plate is done with a medium Cobb elevator, (d) a narrow rongeur is used to remove anular and nuclear fragments, and (e) sharp curettes are used to "melon-ball" remaining disc material until the posterior longitudinal ligament is reached. It is mandatory that the curettes be sharp so that excessive force need not be applied to cut into the disc. Knowing that an inadvertent slip may occur, it is also important that the forces used in curetting the disc be directed away from the great vessels or the spinal cord, preferably toward the vertebral end plate.

Throughout this part of the procedure, the vertebral end plate is preserved to avoid excessive bleeding and to provide a counter cutting surface during the use of the curette. After the disc space is prepared, the bony end plates are excised with a curette or osteotome and the disc space is packed with bone graft. Autoge-

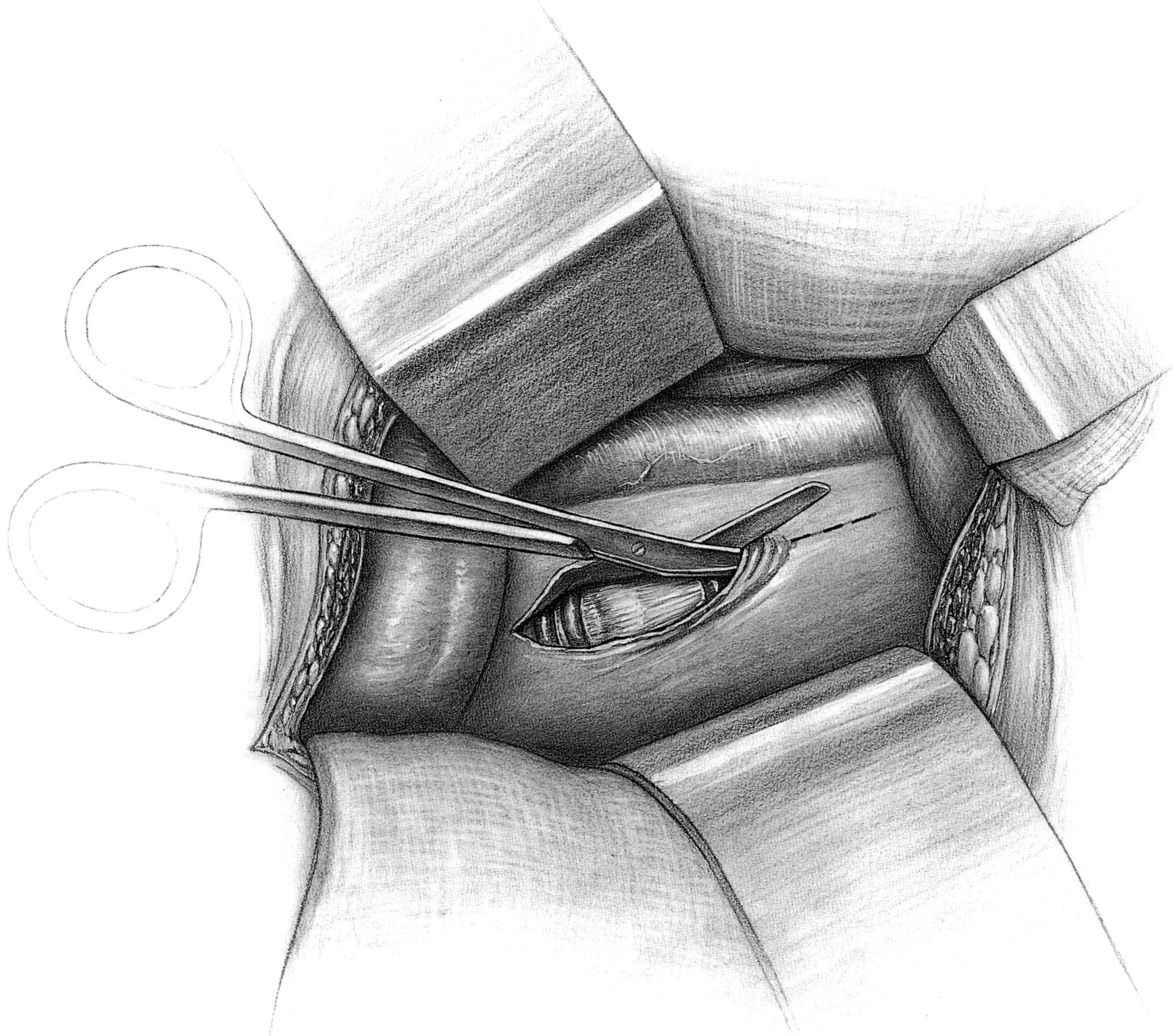

Figure 3. After the rib is removed, the lung is packed off with moist sponges and the parietal pleura is incised overlying the vertebra to be exposed.

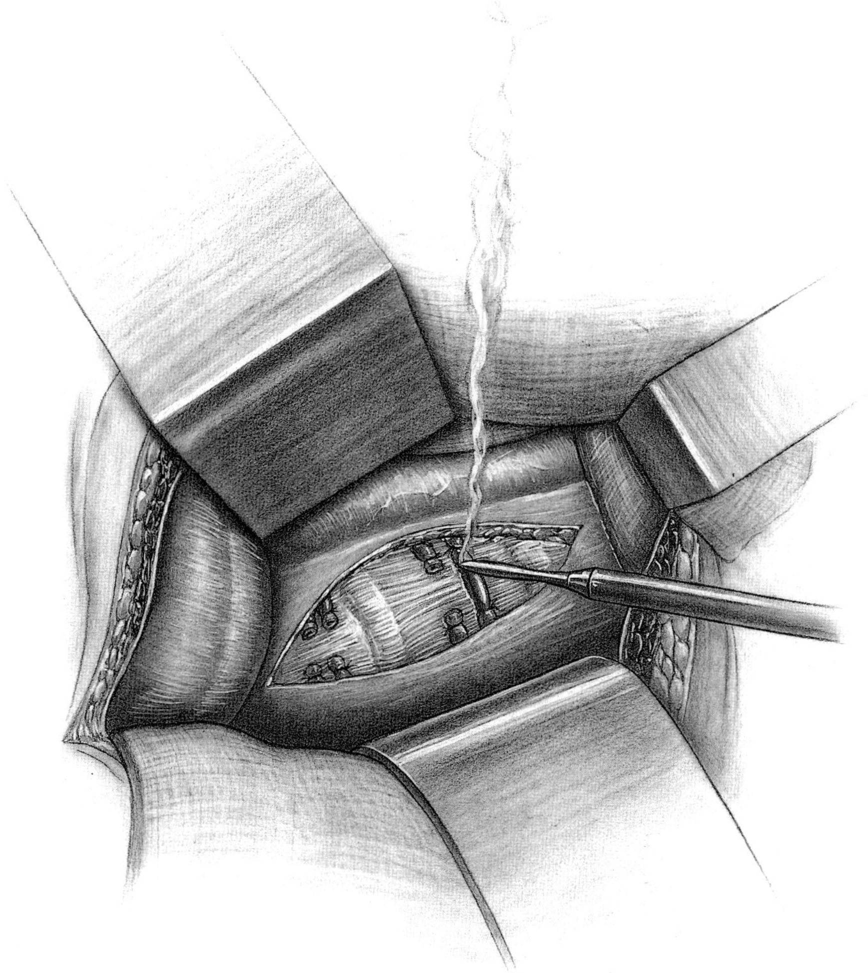

A

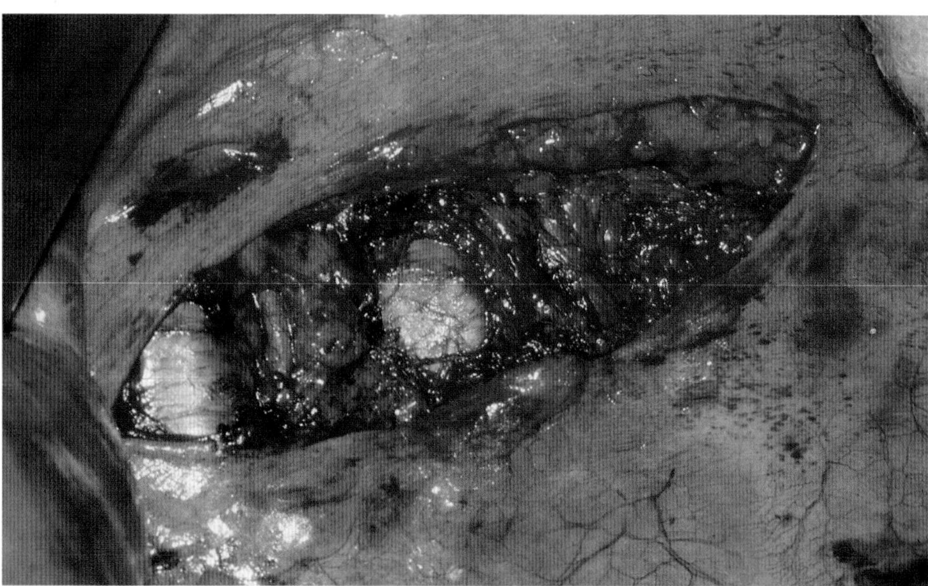

B

Figure 4. A,B: Ligation of the segmental artery and vein is done at the midvertebral body to avoid disturbance of the collateralization of the cord's blood supply at the foramen posteriorly.

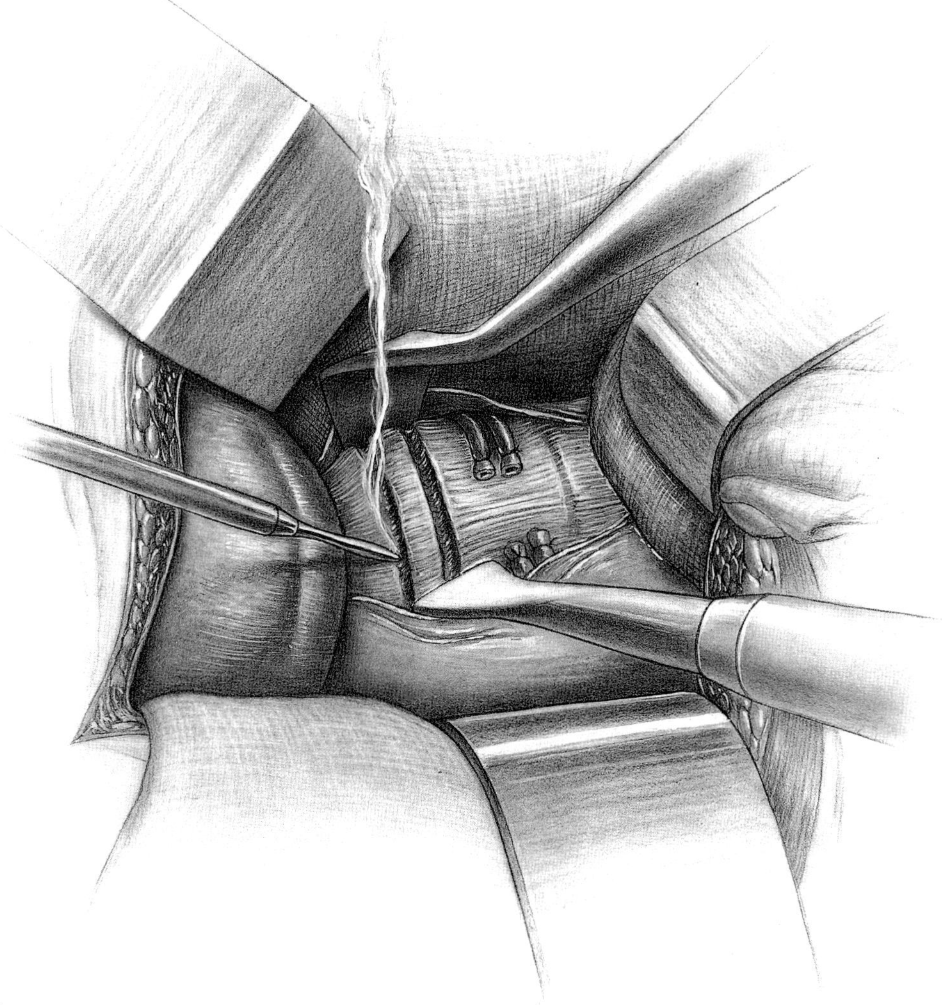

A

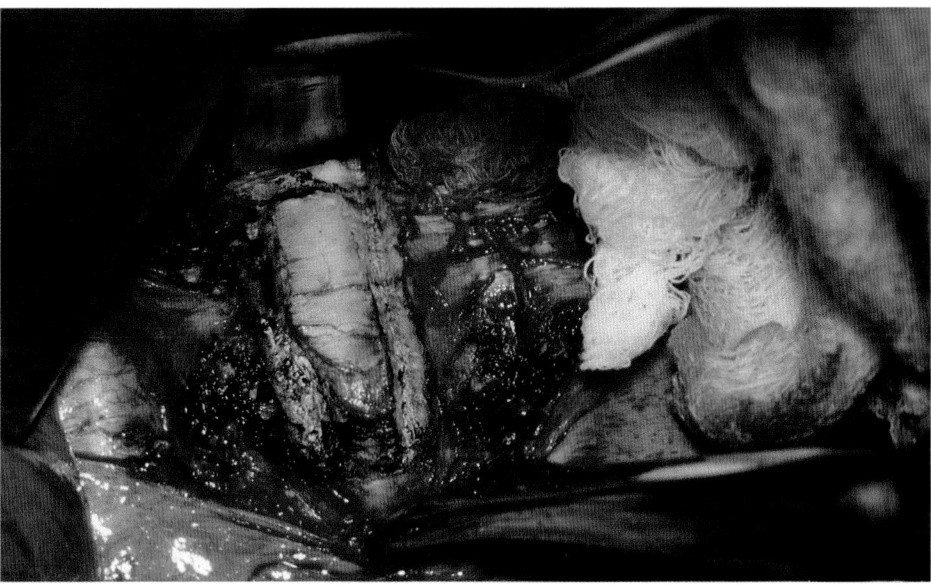

B

Figure 5. A,B: Excision of the intervertebral disc is done using curettes and rongeurs after outlining the disc with electrocautery. The bony vertebral end plate is preserved during removal of the disc.

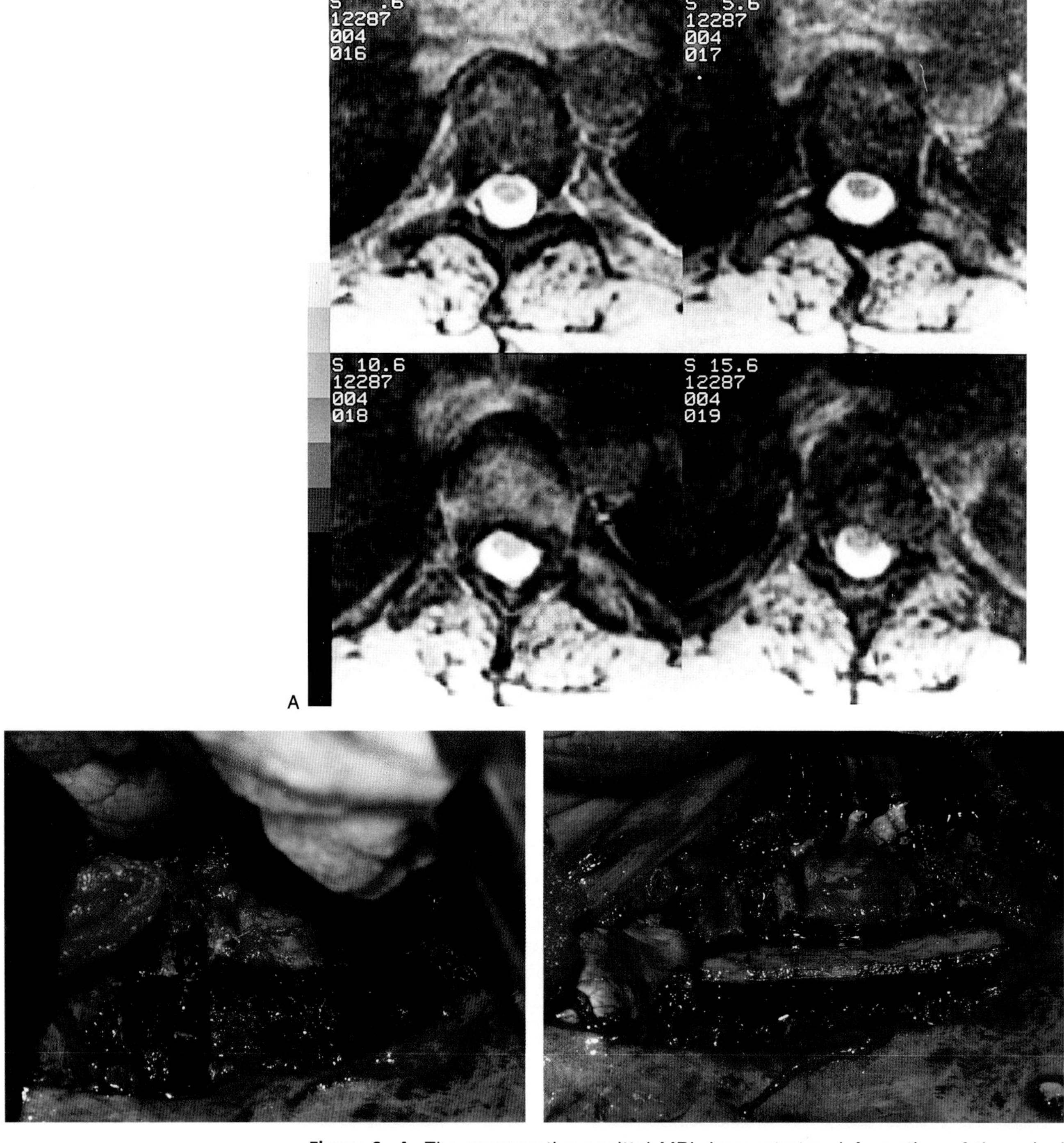

Figure 6. **A:** The preoperative sagittal MRI demonstrates deformation of the spinal cord at the T10 level corresponding to the area of thoracic back pain and the patient's T10 sensory deficit. Decompression of the canal is done by removal of the disc back to the posterior longitudinal ligament. If an extruded fragment is present, the canal is entered and explored after excising the ligament. **B:** After decompression, a trough is created across the motion segments to be fused. **C:** Two rib struts can usually be press-fit into the slot. The disc space anterior to the rib struts is filled with autogenous cancellous bone taken from the trough.

nous rib is usually preferred, but other sources including fresh-frozen femoral head and freeze-dried femoral rings or cancellous cubes may be used. If more than one contiguous disc space is to be fused, a trough may be fashioned with a rongeur and osteotomes (Fig. 6). The length of the trough is measured with a paper template constructed from a suture package or other malleable material. Two rib struts are then cut to the proper length and placed in the trough. The cancellous bone from the trough is packed into the disc space anterior to the struts. Two years after surgery the rib strut is well incorporated (Fig. 7); this patient returned to his employment 7 months after surgery with a lifting restriction of 25 pounds.

Following the fusion, closure of the parietal pleura is done with a running absorbable 3–0 suture (Fig. 8) and a #28 chest tube is placed in the posterior axillary line, at least one interspace away from the thoracotomy. If the thoracolumbar approach has been used, the diaphragm is closed with either interrupted or continuous sutures placed at 7-mm intervals. Two retention sutures are placed in the rib bed at equal intervals. These are of doubled absorbable #1 suture on a large tapered needle and are placed subperiosteal to avoid trauma to the intercostal nerve. It is not uncommon for the patient to notice these retention sutures spontaneously breaking 4 weeks after surgery. Absorbable material is used to minimize long-term irritation of the retention sutures. A rib approximator is used to draw the ribs together and layered closure of the intercostal (and serratus anterior if at that level) and latissimus dorsi muscles is done with continuous 2–0 absorbable suture. Prior to closure of the rib bed, the lung is re-expanded under direct vision.

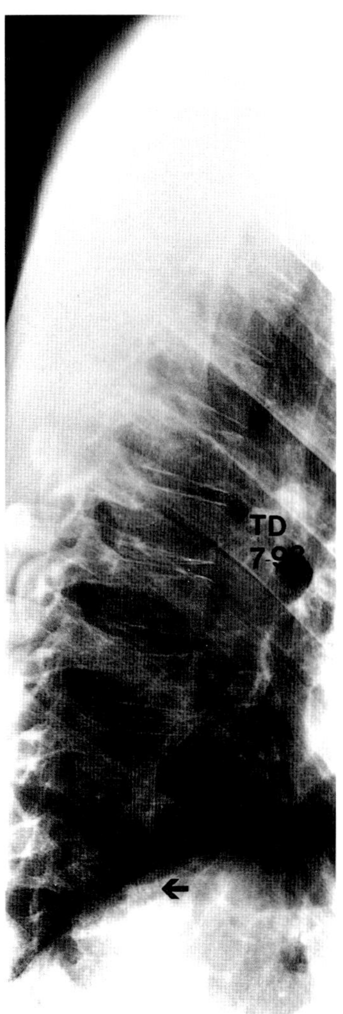

Figure 7. Two years following surgery, the rib strut, (*arrow*) is well incorporated.

POSTOPERATIVE MANAGEMENT

The chest tube is placed on continuous suction at 15 cm of water. When the drainage has decreased to 100 to 150 ml/24 hr or when the drainage is no longer bloody but mostly serous, the tube is removed. A reactive pleuritis from the presence of a chest tube can produce several hundred milliliters of serous drainage. This usually occurs at the 2nd to 4th postoperative day. A postextubation chest radiograph is obtained to exclude a significant pneumothorax. The chest tube wound should be reapproximated with tape 24 hours after removal of the chest tube to avoid an unsightly scar.

Initially the patient may require nasogastric suction since the occurrence of a significant ileus is common. In the absence of nasogastric suction, acute gastric dilatation may occur with the serious consequences of decreased ventilation and aspiration. Pain management is provided with intravenous patient-controlled analgesia; some surgeons use intrapleural local anesthetic or epidural catheters to deliver analgesics. Infiltration of the intercostal nerves with long-acting local anesthetic prior to closure of the chest provides only limited benefits. Vigorous pulmonary toilet diminishes the incidence of atelectasis and pneumonia. The patient may be more comfortable and have better respiratory excursion with a rib binder on the thorax.

A follow-up visit is made at 3 or 4 weeks after surgery. The patient is encouraged to make contact earlier if temperature elevation above 100 degrees, drainage from the wound, dyspnea, increasing pain, or any neurologic abnormality are present. As incisional pain diminishes, progressive passive and then active range of motion of the ipsilateral shoulder is encouraged to prevent adhesive capsulitis. A physical therapist may be needed for selected patients. Thereafter, visits are made at 2- to 3-month intervals depending on the clinical situation. It is common for the patient to feel the rib retention sutures spontaneously break at 4 to 6 weeks after surgery. By this time the incision has structurally healed and the patient needs only reassurance.

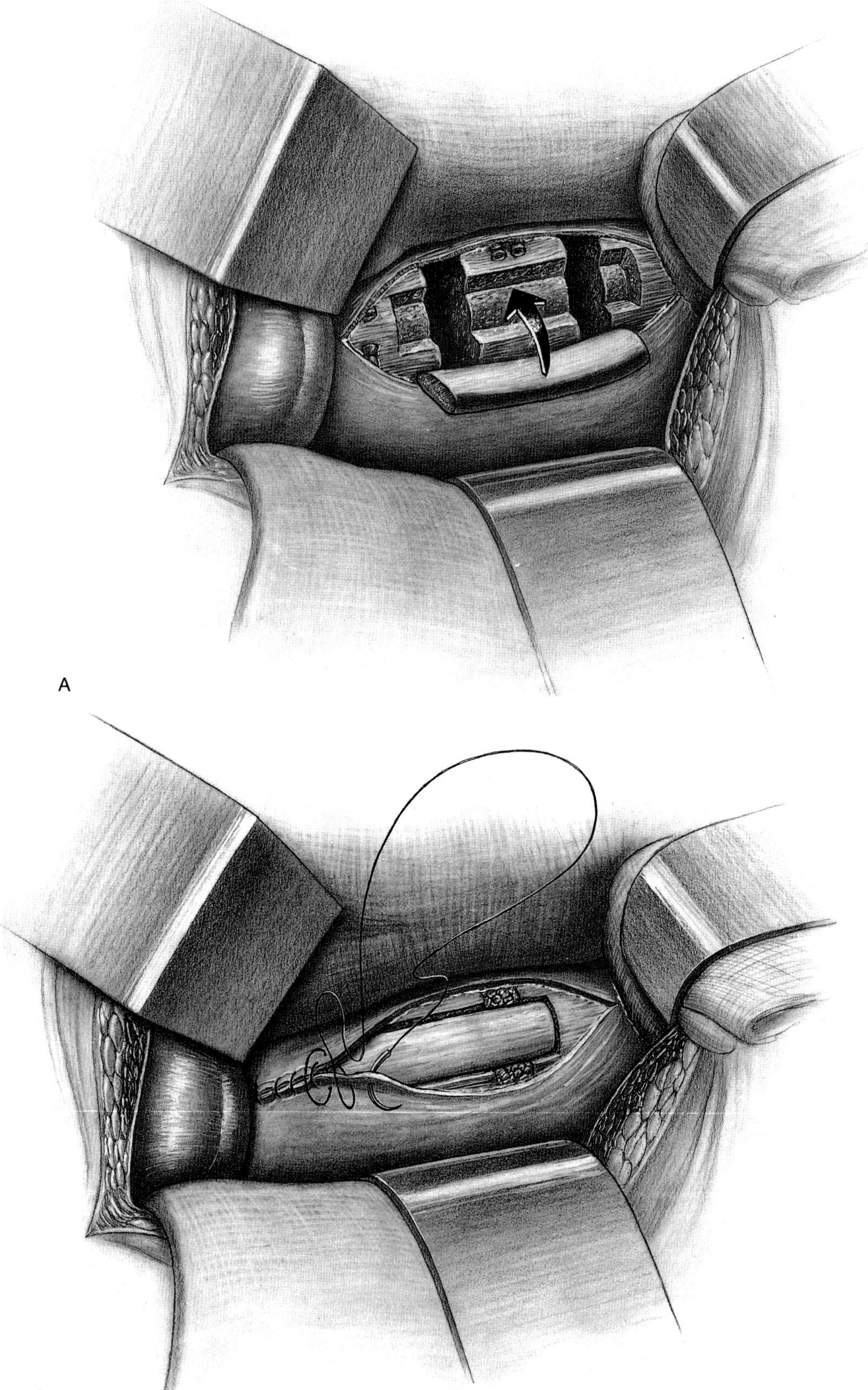

Figure 8. After the bone graft is placed **(A)**, the parietal pleura is closed in a watertight fashion **(B)**, a 24 or 28 Fr chest tube is placed in the posterior axillary line, the lung is re-expanded, and the chest is closed in an anatomic manner.

Anterior fusions may take more than 6 months to heal, and lateral tomograms are necessary if routine radiographs do not adequately visualize the area. Maximum medical improvement is not achieved until the fusion has healed and the patient has accomplished the requisite physical reconditioning. Depending on the extent of fusion, intrinsic stability of the spine, and concomitant posterior instrumentation, a brace may be worn until fusion has occurred. Walking and stationary cycling are usually allowed; but bending, twisting, and lifting are restricted. Rehabilitation may require the services of an exercise therapist to guide the tentative patient. Many patients experience severe deconditioning during a prolonged preoperative course and the postoperative convalescence. Optimal results cannot be expected until endorphin levels are restored through large-muscle exercise and cardiovascular conditioning.

COMPLICATIONS

Intraoperative complications can be life-threatening. These include direct trauma to the great vessels, spleen, liver, or pericardium. The immediate assistance of a vascular or general surgeon should be available during surgery. Chylothorax is a rare complication that may result from disruption of the mediastinal lymphatics (4). In most cases it is initially diagnosed by the presence of chylous fluid in the chest tube drainage. Spontaneous resolution is usual. When pleural adhesions are present from previous surgery or infection, small air leaks may be created while mobilizing the lung. These should be oversewn or stapled after clamping with a Duval clamp. At the periphery of the lung such leaks rarely create a bronchopleural fistula.

Postoperative problems such as infection or empyema require a multidisciplinary approach with consultations from infectious disease and a thoracic surgeon. Dehiscence of the thoracotomy wound is a rare but serious complication. Postthoracotomy pain and intercostal neuralgia usually resolve but may necessitate injection of the intercostal nerve with steroid.

Anterior Lumbar Fusion

INDICATIONS/CONTRAINDICATIONS

Anterior interbody fusion in the lumbar spine is performed for the following indications:

Mobilization of a scoliotic or kyphotic deformity: Anterior instrumentation and/or vertebrectomy of the lumbar spine for deformity, fracture, and tumor are discussed elsewhere and will not be covered here. Uninstrumented discectomy and fusion are utilized when subsequent posterior instrumentation is planned and the coronal deformity cannot be corrected to less than 50 degrees on side-bending radiographs.

A sagittal deformity requires anterior mobilization in the skeletally immature patient if the thoracic kyphosis cannot be corrected to 65 degrees or less on hyperextension and in most kyphotic deformities in the adult patient whether they are in the thoracic or lumbar spine. Hyperlordotic deformity in the lumbar spine, as seen in spinal muscular atrophy and some muscular dystrophies, cannot be corrected without multiple-level anterior discectomy and fusion.

Circumferential arthrodesis: When long fusions of the thoracolumbar spine are extended to the pelvis, the incidence of failed fusion is reduced by performing anterior and posterior fusion initially. In those with a posterior lumbar pseudarthrosis with or without infection, anterior fusion may be indicated as the primary treatment.

Discogenic pain is a controversial indication for anterior fusion in the lumbar spine. Anterior abdominal wall skin lesions, previous colostomy, ileostomy, or vesicostomy may contraindicate an anterior incision. Anterior fusion is difficult, if not contraindicated, when previous infection, previous surgery, or tumor has scarred the vena cava or aorta, preventing mobilization for exposure. Incidental trauma to the great vessels in this circumstance may precipitate bleeding that cannot be controlled. Previous therapeutic radiation to the abdomen or pelvic area may produce a friable and avascular abdominal wall, bowel, or great vessels. The threat of spontaneous visceral rupture, wound dehiscence, or abdominal wall slough may obviate the anterior approach.

PREOPERATIVE PLANNING

When anterior lumbar surgery is performed for spinal deformity, preoperative lateral and AP radiographs are needed to evaluate the lumbar spine. Supine side-bending radiographs can help to determine whether a rigid lumbosacral take-off is present. When the lumbar spine is being fused from cephalad, stopping in the

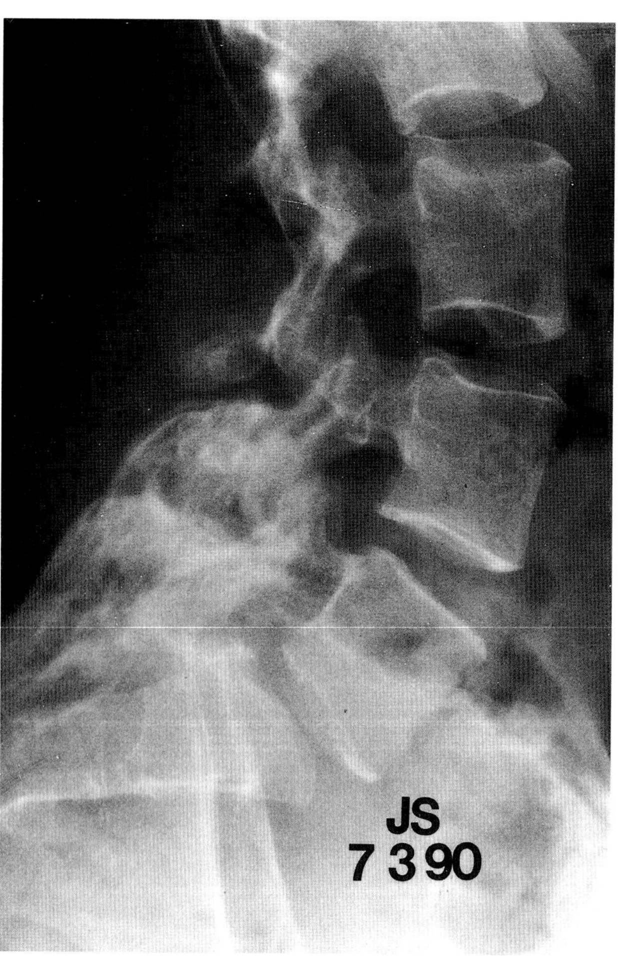

Figure 9. Lateral radiograph of a 30-year-old woman who had undergone an uninstrumented L5–S1 bilateral lateral fusion for a painful spondylolisthesis secondary to a pars interarticularis defect.

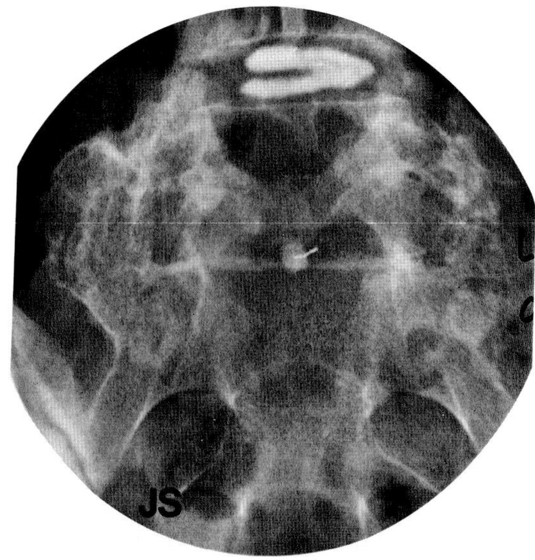

Figure 10. The patient's low back pain was unchanged following surgery, and lumbar discography was performed. Discography at the L4–L5 disc was minimally painful, whereas attempted discography at L5–S1 reproduced her characteristic pain.

lumbar spine, the caudal end vertebra should come to the midline on side-bending radiographs. The cephalad-most vertebra should also have less than a 15-degree tilt from the intercrestal line to lessen the likelihood of premature degeneration. Standing full-spine radiographs are necessary if the coronal or sagittal spinal contour must be evaluated. If decompression is the objective of the surgery, imaging studies of the canal are also necessary. Unless there are metallic implants in the lumbar spine, MRI is usually preferred Myelography with computed tomography is necessary if an MRI is not possible in the assessment of the lumbar nerve roots and dura.

If anterior surgery is done as part of lumbar pseudarthrosis repair, AP tomography is the author's preferred method of documenting the condition if routine radiographs are not definitive. The medical history is an important part of the preoperative evaluation for pseudarthrosis. Pain attributed to a failed fusion is mechanical in nature (e.g., better when the patient is in the horizontal position and worse with superincumbent weight on the spine).

When anterior surgery is performed for discogenic pain, an evocative test should be performed to add a measure of validity for the procedure. Discography can exclude discs from a proposed fusion when they are found not to be a pain focus, and it can also confirm that other discs are the source of pain. Properly performed discography is done with the double-needle technique, by which a larger bore needle penetrates the superficial structures and only the #25 gauge needle penetrates the anulus. If the contrast medium is injected into the anulus or end plate, a factitious finding may result. The pain produced from a pain-provocation discogram should be significant (e.g., greater than 7 on a digital analog scale of 10 as the worst pain). It should also reproduce the patient's chief symptoms qualitatively, but not necessarily quantitatively. When positive, discography-reproduced pain is usually more intense than the patient's normal pain pattern (see Figs. 9–12).

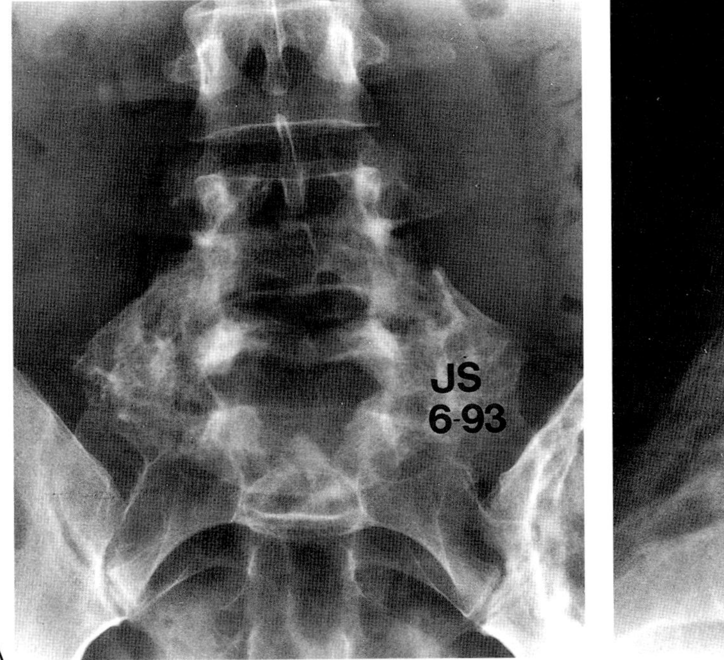

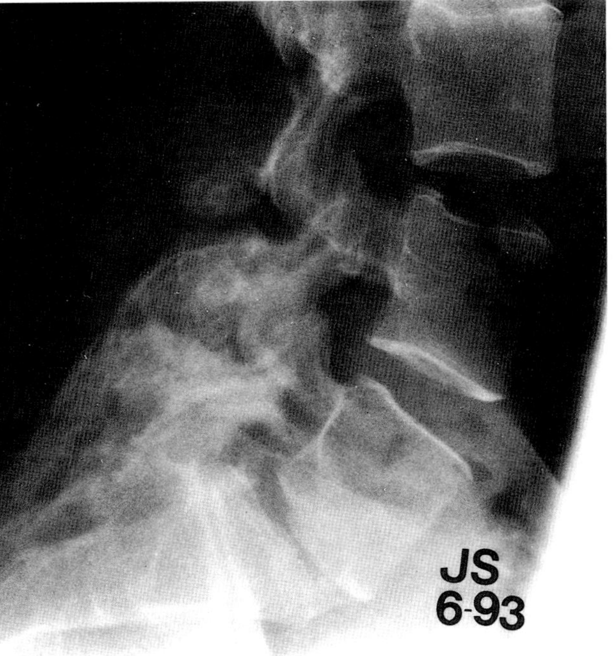

Figure 11. A,B: Following anterior L5–S1 fusion with autogenous cancellous bone, her pain was relieved. Anteroposterior and lateral radiographs 3 years later demonstrate the previous bilateral lateral fusion and the anterior L5–S1 anterior fusion.

SURGERY

It is the author's preference to approach the lumbar spine (L2 and below) with a left sided, subdiaphragmatic, retroperitoneal exposure. Avoiding the peritoneal cavity decreases the incidence of small bowel obstructions from peritoneal adhesions. The left-sided approach allows one to deal with the aorta rather than the vena cava. The aorta is more resistant to incidental trauma and is more easily repaired should that unfortunate complication occur. Flank incisions also allow ready exposure to the iliac crest for harvesting autogenous bone graft material. Alternately, an oblique or longitudinal incision in the anterior abdominal skin permits exposure of the properitoneal fat by incising the abdominal fascia along the lateral border of the abdominis rectus muscle. The incision is then developed in a method similar to the oblique muscle-splitting incision described.

Several exceptions to this preference are worth mentioning, most notably to scoliotic deformities, which are approached from the convexity. When performing an L5 vertebrectomy for spondyloptosis, the low transperitoneal approach is preferred since it allows easier access to both sides of the vertebral body. Local skin conditions may contraindicate a flank incision. When performing a combined AP short-segment fusion (one or two levels), the posterior approach is done first in order to harvest abundant iliac bone graft for both the posterior and anterior fusions.

Correct placement of the patient on the operating table is critical. The patient is placed in the lateral decubitus position tilted back 20 degrees. Flexion of the operating table further opens the interval between the thorax and pelvis, enhancing exposure. Following sterile preparation and draping from midthorax to pubis and anterior midline to posterior midline, an incision is made from the tip of the 12th rib anteriorly and inferiorly to a point 3 cm medial to the anterior superior iliac crest (2) (Fig. 12).

A further 3- to 4-cm distal extension of the incision allows exposure to the level of S1. At the tip of the 12th rib, which may be electively removed, although it provides very little bone graft material, blunt dissection exposes the properitoneal fat (Fig. 13). The plane between properitoneal fat and the transversalis fascia is

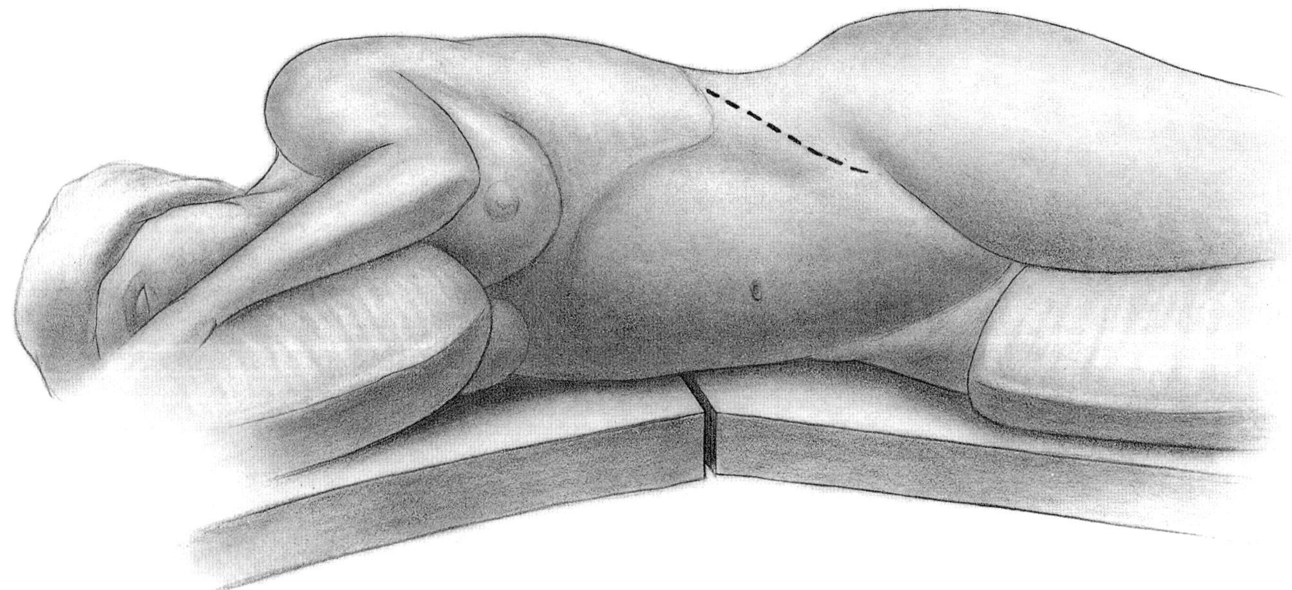

Figure 12. The patient is positioned in the right lateral decubitus position for an incision through the left flank. Immobilization of the torso is done with 3-inch tape across the table at the level of the greater trochanter. For exposure of the lumbosacral disc space, the incision usually extends 4 to 5 cm distal to the iliac crest.

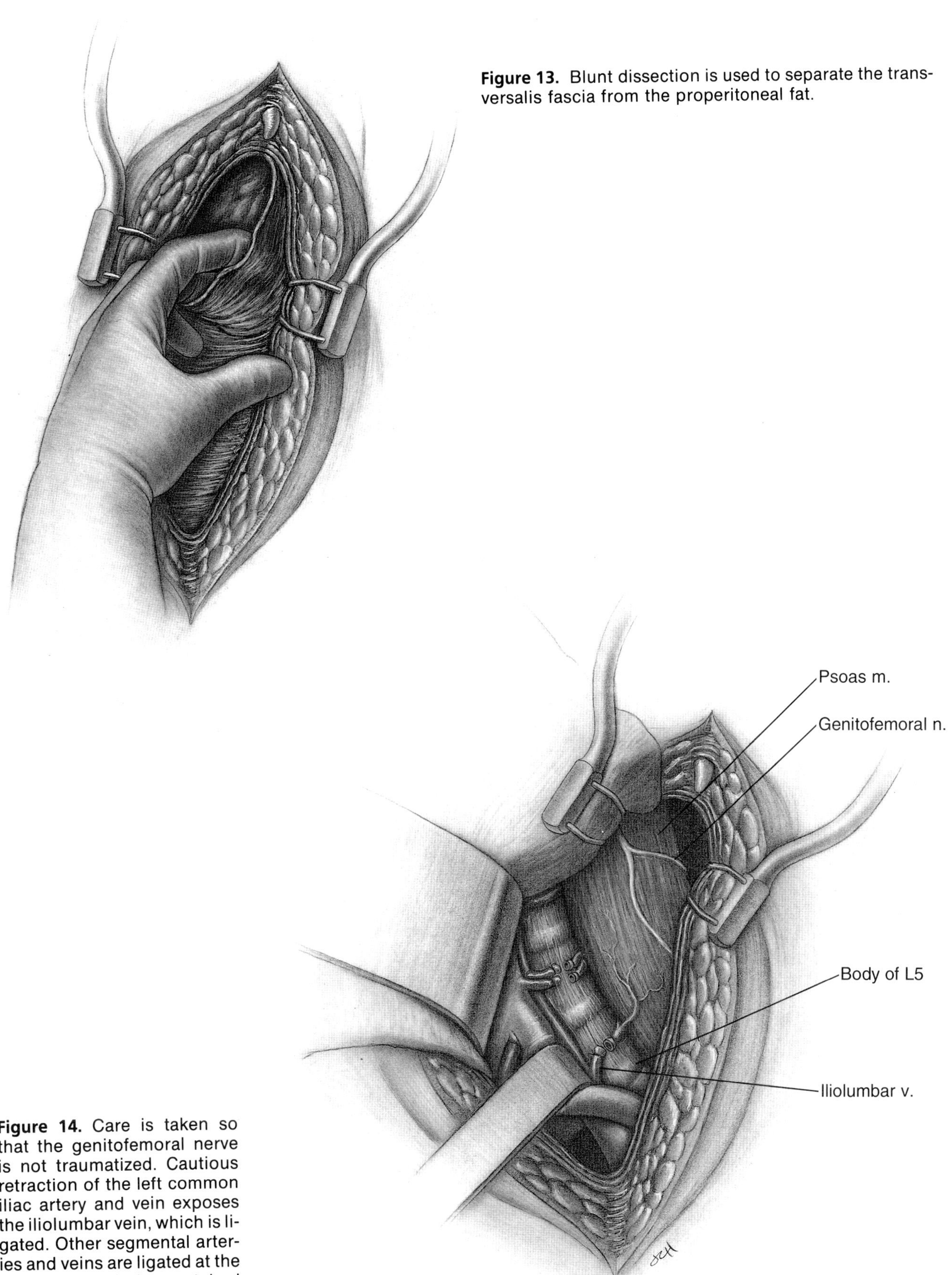

Figure 13. Blunt dissection is used to separate the transversalis fascia from the properitoneal fat.

Figure 14. Care is taken so that the genitofemoral nerve is not traumatized. Cautious retraction of the left common iliac artery and vein exposes the iliolumbar vein, which is ligated. Other segmental arteries and veins are ligated at the midportion of the vertebral body.

developed with blunt dissection. Dissection is continued behind the investing fascia of the kidney (Gerota's fascia) if the dissection is carried to the level of the renal vessels (2). As the peritoneal sack is reflected medially, the ureter is left with the peritoneum. There may be a tendency to initiate the dissection directly on the psoas fascia in order to avoid the ureter; however, this may traumatize the ilioinguinal or genitofemoral nerves, which lie on the muscular fascia (Fig. 14). This can result in an uncomfortable dysthesia of the groin that may not resolve spontaneously. It is best to leave some of the fat on the psoas fascia and thus avoid these sensory nerves.

After the peritoneum has been reflected, a moist laparotomy pad is used to protect fragile viscera such as the kidney, spleen, or liver from the retractor. The periaortic lymphatic system is often richly vascularized; pre-emptive ligation will enhance exposure and minimize blood loss. Palpation of the concave midportion of the vertebral body will identify the area where the segmental artery and vein are located. They are under the muscular origins of the psoas and crux of the diaphragm. After they have been exposed with a combination of sharp and blunt dissection, the vessels are ligated with silk sutures or metallic clips in the midbody to preserve the collateralization that occurs at the neural foramen. The plane between the anterior longitudinal ligament and the great vessels is bluntly developed, and a medium-sized malleable or Chandler retractor is placed at the level of the disc to protect the vessels during discectomy and fusion.

If the common iliac vessels are to be mobilized for discectomy and fusion at L4–L5 or L5–S1, the iliolumbar vein should be identified and ligated if possible. Traumatic avulsion of this vein is difficult to control (Fig. 15). Unless an unusually

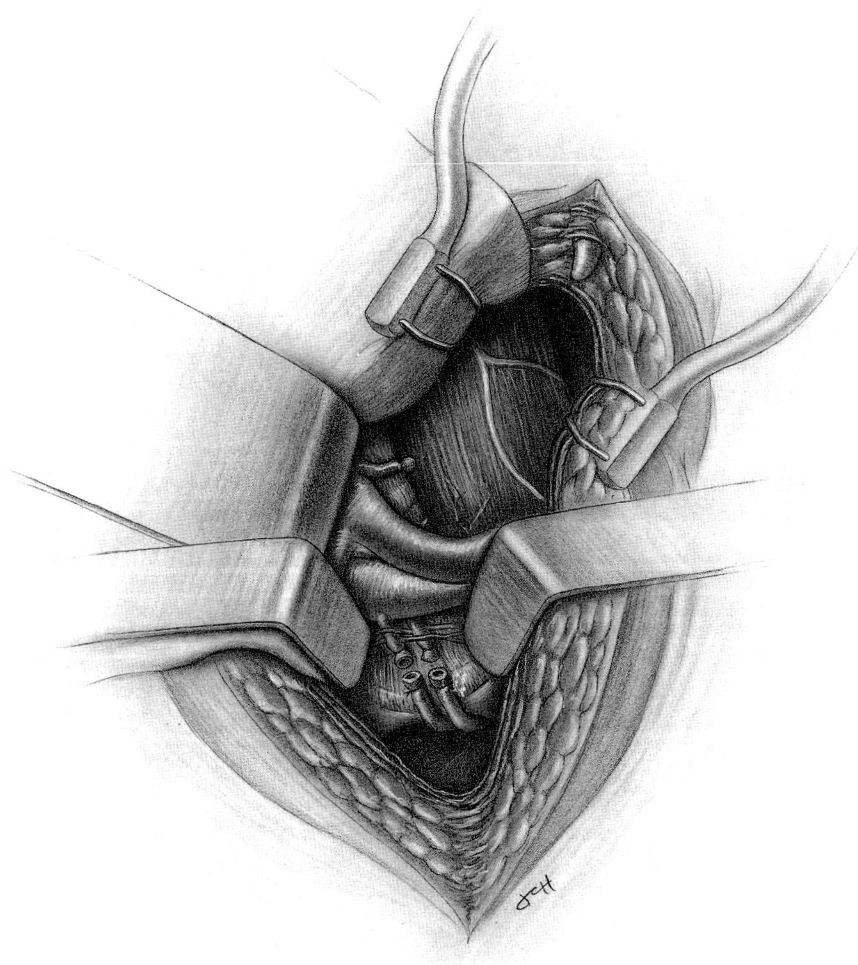

Figure 15. If exposure of the lumbosacral disc is needed, the middle sacral artery and vein are ligated as they cross the disc space in the iliac vessel bifurcation.

low bifurcation of the great vessels exists, the approach to the L5–S1 disc space is done between the bifurcated vessels. The middle sacral artery should be identified and ligated as it crosses the disc space.

After retractors have been placed to protect the adjacent vessels, discectomy is performed in a stepwise fashion: (a) the disc space is outlined with electrocautery to define the limits of the disc space and to enhance hemostasis; (b) a #15 blade is used to divide the anulus as far anterior and posterior as safely possible, and (c) the Cobb elevator is then used to develop the plane between the bony end plate and the cartilage disc. Rongeurs and curettes are used to remove additional disc material. The curettes are used to "melon ball" the disc material, always cutting against the intact bony end plate and not applying force in the direction of the great vessels anteriorly or the spinal canal posteriorly. Sharp curettes are mandatory.

Bone grafting the disc space should be done in accordance with the objective of the operation (i.e., simple decortication of the end plate and cancellous bone grafting if it is not important to add stability to the motion segment). If the disc space graft must also impart resistance to axial load, the space can be filled with tri- or bicortical iliac struts, allogenic femoral ring grafts filled with autogenous cancellous bone, allogenic femoral calcar, or rib struts in a slot (Fig. 16). Any bony end plate that is not in contact with such grafts should be decorticated and grafted with autogenous bone if available.

After the operating table has been straightened out, the abdominal wound is closed without drains in two layers. It is not uncommon to visualize chylous fluid

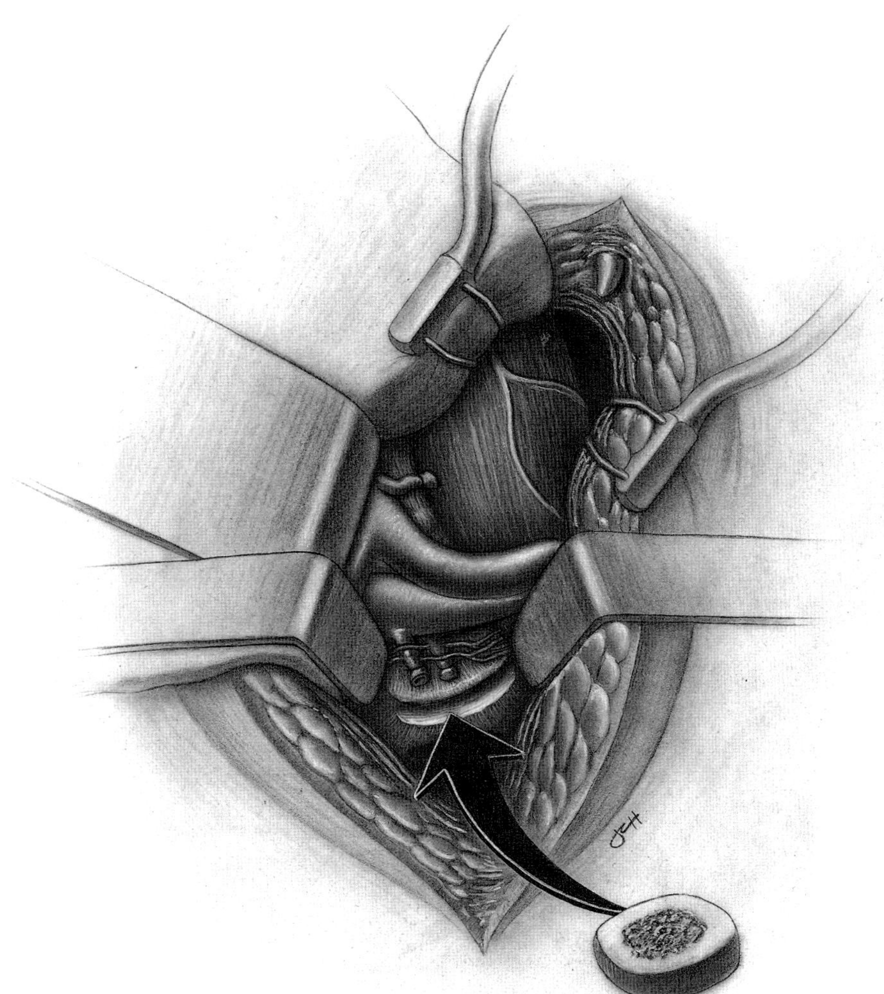

Figure 16. Instruments are placed to retract and protect the iliac vessels as the intervertebral disc is excised. An allograft femoral ring filled with autogenous cancellous bone is then inserted in the disc space.

from the periaortic lymphatic. This resolves spontaneously and it is not necessary to attempt ligation of the source. The transversalis and internal oblique muscles are closed together, and the external oblique is closed separately. Monofilament absorbable #1 or #0 sutures are used to minimize "sawing" through the muscles as they are closed.

POSTOPERATIVE MANAGEMENT

Postoperative ileus is the rule rather than the exception and should routinely be addressed with nasogastric tube suction initiated intraoperatively. An abdominal binder may reduce incisional pain and allow better respiratory effort. Early ambulation is encouraged. Sequential compression hose and frequent in-bed isometric isotonic exercise of the lower limbs may reduce venous stasis and lessen the incidence of deep vein thrombosis.

If the lumbar spine is stable as the result of posterior instrumentation or if posterior fusion is already present, bracing is not necessary for reasons other than comfort. Radiographs are obtained at 2-month intervals until healing is evident, usually at 4 to 6 months. Complete maturation of the interbody graft may require 1 year or more. Maximum medical improvement may take 8 to 12 months following surgery if preoperative deconditioning was prolonged.

As spinal stability and comfort increases, more vigorous supervised low-impact aerobic conditioning exercises are prescribed. Reconditioning exercises depend on the stability of the spine. If mechanical stability is present, low-impact aerobic exercises such as walking or stationary cycling may be initiated when incisional pain permits. The patient is advised not to do lifting, bending, or twisting until fusion healing is well under way.

COMPLICATIONS

After the abdominal musculature is divided and the peritoneal sack bluntly reflected medially, care should be taken not to traumatize the ilioinguinal or genitofemoral nerves, which may cause a bothersome dysthesia that does not always resolve. During surgery blunt or sharp trauma to the great vessels, spleen, ureter, liver, or bowel may occur. Inadvertent tears of the iliolumbar vein are particularly troublesome. Repair is difficult and at times impossible. Bypass of the common iliac vein with a vascular allograft may be needed. It is my practice to isolate and ligate the iliolumbar vein whenever possible to avoid inadvertent avulsion.

In lower lumbar spine surgical approaches, chylous fluid may leak from the periaortic lymphatics. If simple ligation does not stop the flow, the fluid is *not* treated with a retroperitoneal drain. Such fluid is reabsorbed, and no ill effects have been encountered. Incisional hernia may occur and requires subsequent repair, usually with the assistance of a general surgeon. It is common to experience a sympathectomy effect due to division of the lumbar sympathetic chain. The patient may even complain that the contralateral limb has been cold since surgery. In reality it is the ipsilateral limb that is warm and dry. This usually resolves spontaneously within 12 to 18 months and seldom has long-term consequences.

Incidental trauma to the spleen, liver, or kidney can occur during the course of the surgery (7). Careful technique will minimize the incidence, but unexplained acute hypovolemia, hematuria, or signs of hemoperitoneum should alert the surgeon. Late retroperitoneal fibrosis is uncommon but may occur (1, 8). Male sexual dysfunction in the form of functional impotence or retrograde ejaculation occurs in approximately 1% of patients (5). Because the anterior dissection is carried out above the sacral nerve roots, postoperative impotence should not be anatomic. Causes other than sacral nerve root injury should also be investigated in the evaluation of such impotence. Retrograde ejaculation may spontaneously resolve and thus should not be considered as a reliable contraceptive alternative. Failure of anterior fusion (2% to 35%) is the most common complication.

ILLUSTRATIVE CASE FOR TECHNIQUE

T.N., a 28-year-old woman, injured her midback 11 months before evaluation while lifting a box weighing 25 pounds. She heard a snapping sound and felt a burning sensation under her left scapula. Extensive nonoperative treatment including nonsteroidal antiinflammatory drugs, physical therapy, bed rest, and pain medication failed to relieve her symptoms. At that point she sought an orthopaedic consultation. Physical examination demonstrated decreased trunk mobility secondary to midthoracic pain. Decreased sensation to pinprick was found on her left anterior chest from below her breast to below the umbilicus. Deep tendon reflexes were normal and no Babinski reflexes or clonus were seen. The superficial abdominal reflex on the left was diminished. Routine radiographs of the spine were normal and the thoracic MRI revealed a left-sided disc herniation at T7–T8 with cord deformation (Fig. 17). Through a left T6 thoracotomy, the T7–T8 disc was removed and an interbody fusion was performed with an autologous rib graft (Figs. 18 and 19). At 6 months following surgery she returned to work. She also had two full-term pregnancies at 3 and 5 years following surgery giving birth to normal infants. Eight years after surgery she returned for evaluation of chronic lumbar back pain. Her neurologic examination was normal and she had minimal thoracic back pain.

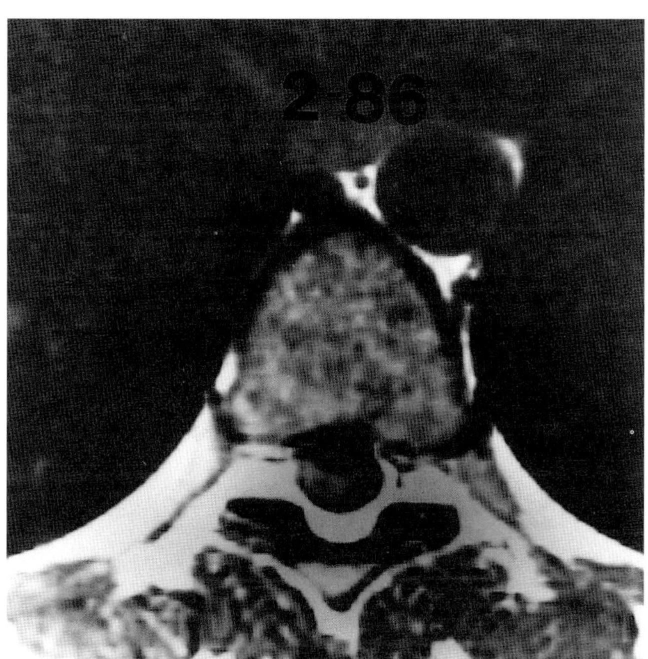

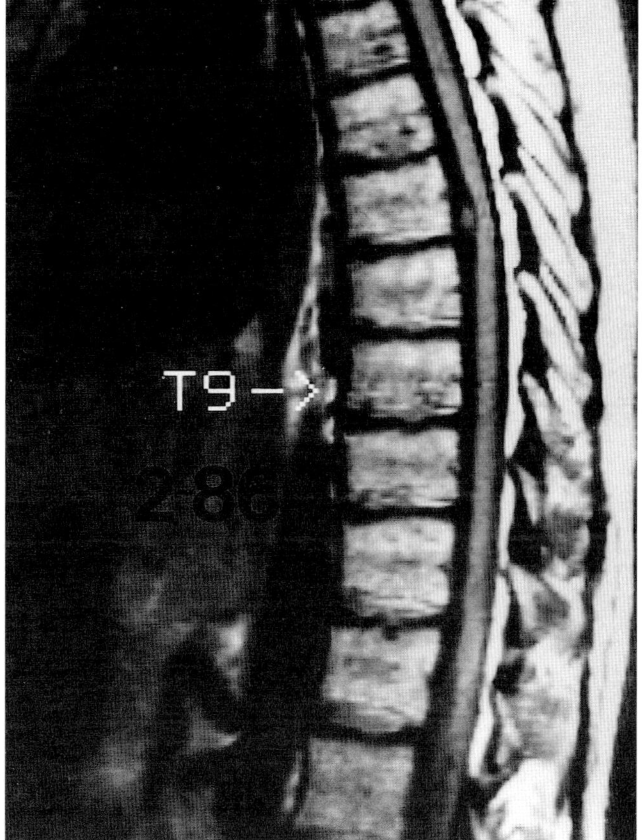

Figure 17. A,B: Thoracic MRI revealed a left-sided disc herniation at T7–T8 with cord deformation.

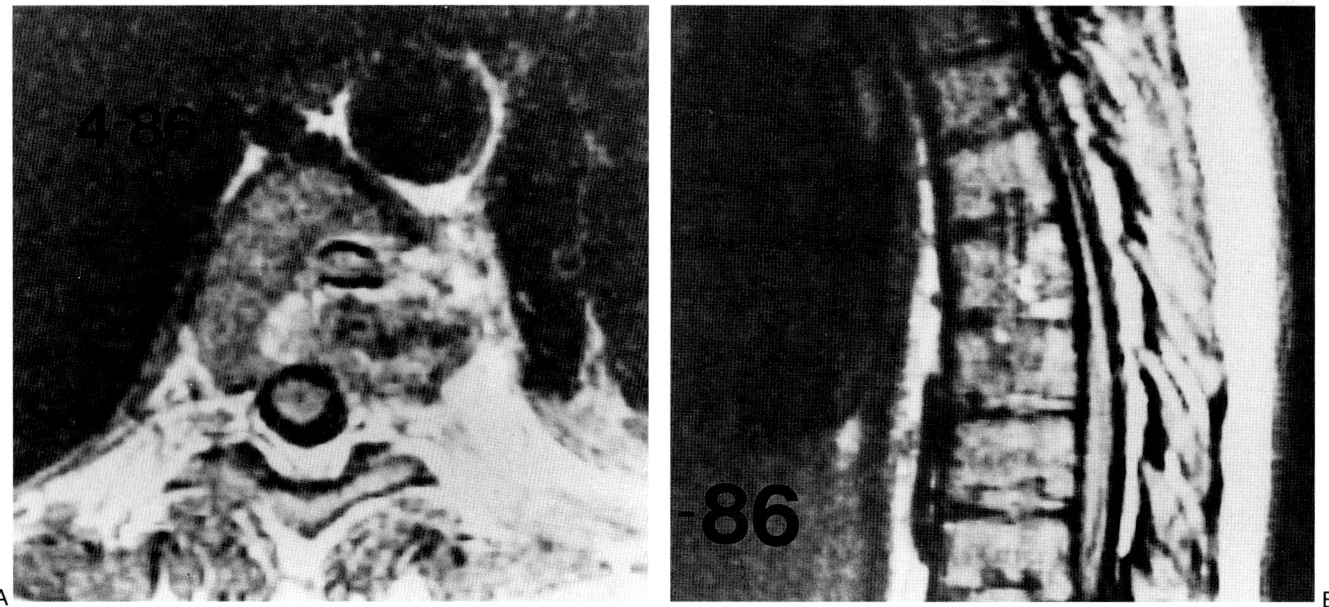

Figure 18. A,B: A postoperative MRI confirmed decompression of the cord at the T7–T8 level.

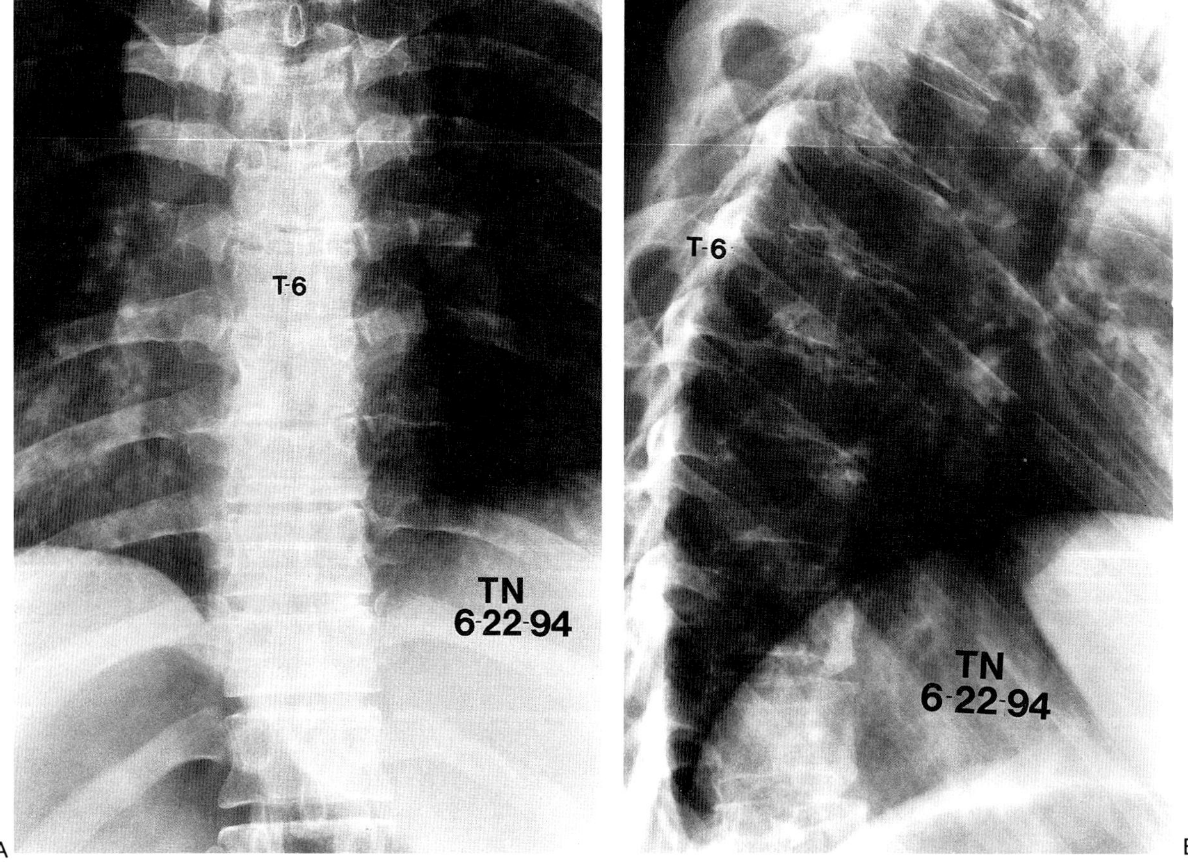

Figure 19. A,B: Radiographs of the thoracic spine showed consolidation of the rib graft fusion at T8–T9.

RECOMMENDED READING

1. Chan, F. L., and Chow, S. P.: Retroperitoneal fibrosis after spinal fusion. *Clin. Radiol.*, 34: 331–335, 1983.
2. Digby, K. H.: Twelfth rib incision as approach to kidney. *Surg. Gynecol. Obstet.*, 73: 84–85, 1941.
3. Dommisse, G. G.: The blood supply of the spinal cord. *J. Bone Joint Surg.*, 56B: 225–235, 1974.
4. Eisenstein, S., and O'Brien, J. P.: Chylothorax: a complication of Dwyer's anterior instrumentation *Br. J. Surg.*, 64: 339–341, 1977.
5. Flynn, J. C., and Price, C. T.: Sexual complications of anterior fusion of the lumbar spine. *Spine*, 9: 489–492, 1984.
6. Hodgson, A. R., and Stock, F. E.: Anterior spinal fusion. *Br. J. Surg.*, 44: 266, 1956.
7. Johnson, R. M., and McGuire, E. J.: Urogenital complications of anterior approaches to the lumbar spine. *Clin. Orthop.*, 154: 114–118, 1981.
8. Silber, I., and McMaster, W.: Retroperitoneal fibrosis with hydronephrosis as a complication of the Dwyer procedure. *J. Pediatr. Surg.*, 12: 255–257, 1977.

Master Techniques in Orthopaedic Surgery,
THE SPINE, edited by D. S. Bradford,
Lippincott-Raven Publishers, Philadelphia, © 1997.

11

Excision of Hemivertebrae

David S. Bradford and Serena S. Hu

INDICATIONS AND CONTRAINDICATIONS

Congenital scoliosis can be divided into those deformities that are: (a) secondary to failure of formation, (b) secondary to failure of segmentation, and (c) mixed lesions. Hemivertebrae are examples of failure of formation, whereas congenital bars and blocked vertebrae are examples of failure of segmentation. A unilateral unsegmented bar, especially one associated with a contralateral hemivertebra, has the worst prognosis for progression. Isolated hemivertebrae are less predictable in their growth potential, and consequently the magnitude of the deformity that may result from continued spinal growth is uncertain. Hemivertebrae in the cervicothoracic and lumbosacral junctions are more likely to result in more noticeable deformity because of the inability of the spine above or below to compensate adequately (7). Surgery is indicated in those children presenting with a significant deformity greater than 40 degrees with coronal imbalance secondary to a hemivertebra, in patients presenting with a deformity that on sequential radiographs has shown progression, or patients presenting with a lumbar sacral hemivertebra associated with pelvic obliquity and/or lumbar scoliosis. There are several surgical options: (a) posterior spinal fusion, (b) combined anterior and posterior fusion, (c) hemiepiphysiodesis, and (d) hemivertebra excision.

Posterior spinal fusion has been reported as a gold standard in managing spinal deformity. It is a relatively straightforward procedure with minimal risks. However, in young patients with a hemivertebra, an isolated posterior fusion carries a high probability of continued bending and rotation of the fusion mass with anterior vertebral growth. A combined anterior and posterior fusion improves the fusion rate, may facilitate some correction if instrumentation is used and/or a postoperative cast is added, and decreases the likelihood of bending and rotation of the fusion mass with further growth. Hemiepiphysiodesis is a useful procedure if done

D. S. Bradford, M.D. and S. S. Hu, M.D.: Department of Orthopaedic Surgery, University of California San Francisco School of Medicine, San Francisco, California 94143–0728.

in a young patient, preferably under 6 years of age, with mild-to-moderate curvatures (under 30 to 40 degrees). However, even when convex fusion includes the involved segments of the curvature and not just the apical segments, correction of the deformity with growth is unpredictable. The early improvement may deteriorate with the adolescent growth spurt.

Excision of the hemivertebra can achieve a more reliable and greater degree of correction as well as improvement in coronal balance. The optimal age for hemivertebra excision is 3 to 10 years of age, after the growth potential of the hemivertebra has been demonstrated and before compensatory curves become structural. In older patients, a resection is still feasible even after the compensatory curves become less flexible, but the corrective surgery will require addressing these compensatory deformities by a more extensive fusion with instrumentation.

Hemivertebra excision would be contraindicated in the cervical spine, is less likely to achieve maximum correction in the thoracic spine, and is most optimally carried out at the thoracolumbar, lumbar, and lumbosacral area. Patients with hemivertebrae associated with minor curvatures (20 to 30 degrees) above the lumbosacral joint, without documentation of progression, should not be considered candidates for this procedure.

PREOPERATIVE PLANNING

A routine history and physical examination should be carried out as one would normally do for any patient with spinal deformity. A careful examination of the spine for evidence of a hairy patch, skin discoloration, or a sacral dimple or sinus is important. Evidence of pelvic obliquity, leg-length inequality, trunk decompensation, or neurologic dysfunction should be noted. Routine standing anteroposterior (AP) and lateral radiographs of the spine from occiput to sacrum are necessary on all patients. Bending films are helpful to determine flexibility of the curvature proximally and distally to the congenital abnormality. Widening of the interpedicular distance suggests intrinsic spinal cord abnormalities such as diastematomyelia. Routine myelography or computed tomography (CT) scanning is not carried out. However, magnetic resonance imaging (MRI) evaluation of the cervical, thoracic, and lumbar spine should be done in patients who have abnormal neurologic findings, in patients being prepared for operative intervention, or in patients with demonstrated widening of the interpedicular distance on routine radiographs. The MRI is important in order to rule out intracanal abnormalities such as a tethered cord, which may occur in from 10% to 50% of patients with congenital scoliosis (3). It is also useful in the MRI study to obtain a coronal view in the region of interest to delineate exactly where the segmentation has occurred and whether an unsuspected bar exists on the contralateral side. Finally, as with any patient who has a congenital spine deformity, genital-urinary abnormalities are not uncommon. Patients should be evaluated with ultrasound or an intravenous pyelogram to rule out pathology.

SURGERY

The patient is brought to the operating room and prepared in a routine fashion. Following the induction of anesthesia and intubation, the patient is positioned in the lateral decubitus position with the convex side up, and a Foley catheter is inserted. A roll may be placed under the patient at the level of the deformity to facilitate the approach (Fig. 1). The table is flexed to open up the level and to facilitate exposure. For lumbosacral excision, the patient should be prepped and draped down to the pubis. It is advisable to prep and drape anterior midline to posterior midline. A standard retroperitoneal thoracoabdominal or thoracic approach is used depending on the level of the hemivertebra. Lumbosacral lesions may be approached through a retroperitoneal incision (Fig. 2), whereas hemivertebra lying at the thoracolumbar junction down to L2–L3 should be approached through a thoracoabdominal approach, removing the 10th or 11th rib. In the thoracic spine, the rib removed is the one lying one or two levels above the hemivertebra to be excised. It may be possible to stay extrapleural with the approach after removing the rib by carefully and bluntly dissecting off the pleura from the chest wall and vertebral bodies. Once the vertebral bodies are identified (Fig. 3), the segmental vessels above and below the level of the excision are carefully identified and then clipped with vascular clips or tied and divided. Exposure is facilitated with appropriate pediatric-size chest retractors. It is useful at this stage to take a radiograph with metal markers in both the proximal and distal disc spaces to delineate better the level and outline of the hemivertebra (Fig. 4).

The dissection of the pleura off the spine is then carried out extraperiosteally to avoid excessive bleeding. Dissection must proceed around to the opposite side to allow adequate exposure and prevent damage to the arterial or venous circulation.

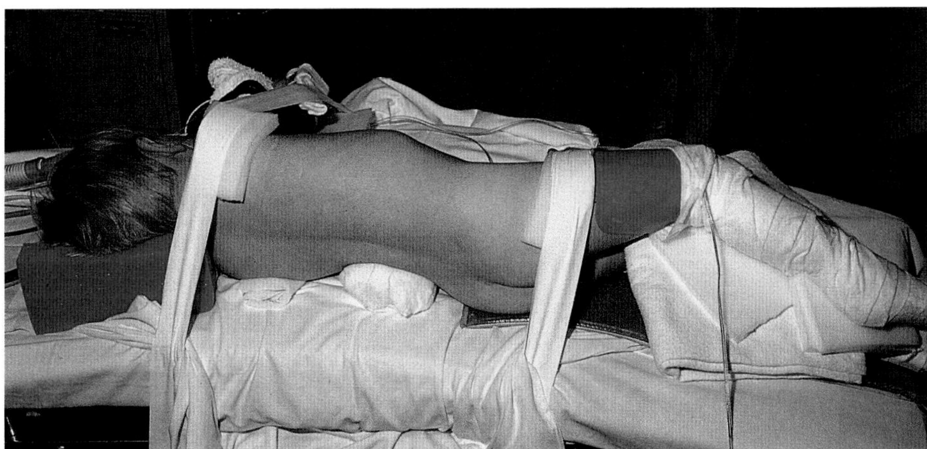

Figure 1. A patient positioned in the lateral decubitus position with a roll under his waist at the level of his lumbosacral hemivertebra.

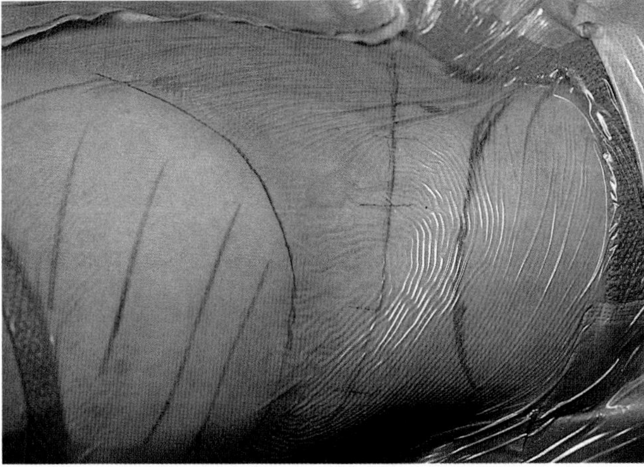

Figure 2. Retroperitoneal flank incision on the patient's right side.

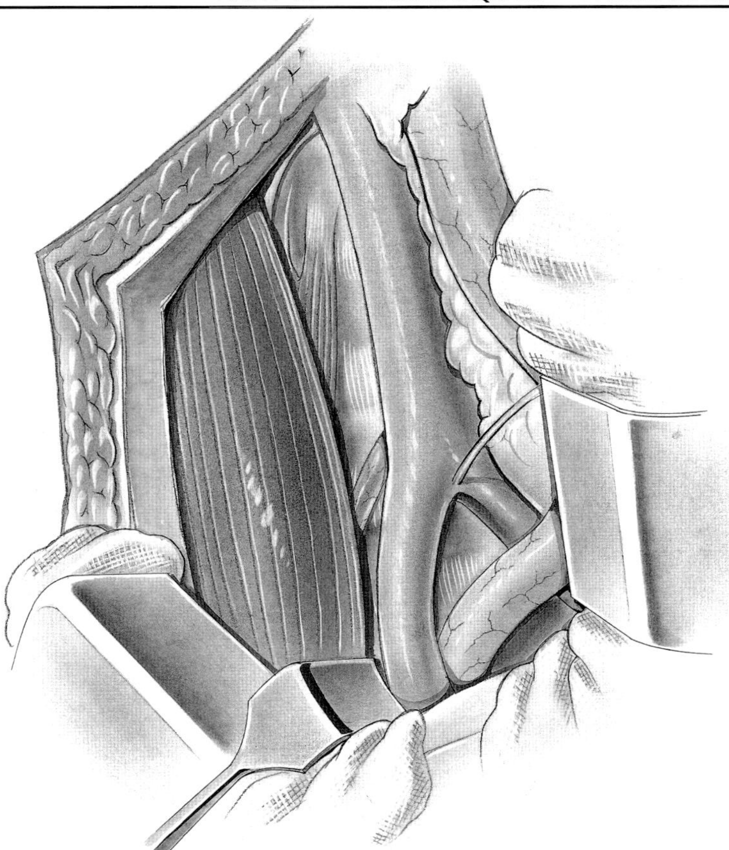

Figure 3. The segmental vessels prior to ligation. The inferior vena cava and common iliac veins are seen with the intervertebral discs and vertebral bodies palpable.

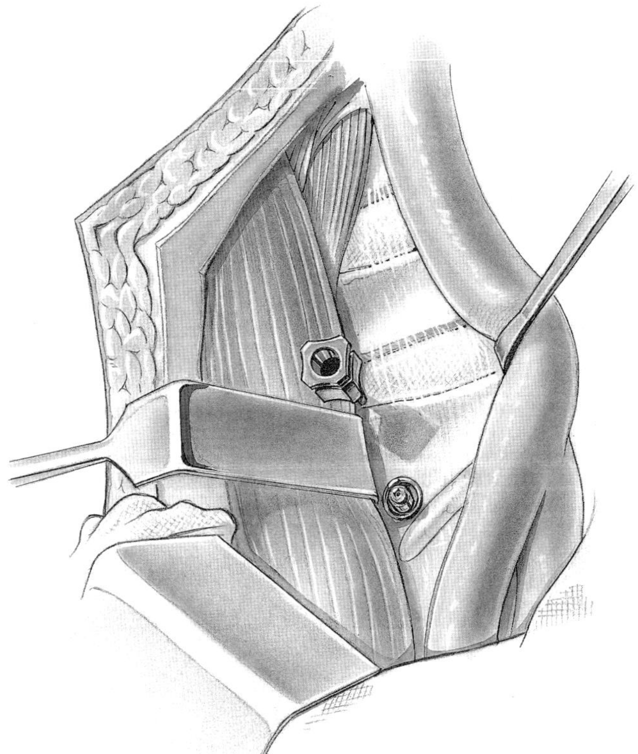

Figure 4. After segmental vessels have been ligated and divided, the great vessels are swept to the contralateral side of the disc space and vertebral body. Metallic markers are placed in the superior and inferior disc spaces for radiographic confirmation of the level.

Excision of the hemivertebra begins with excision of the disc on each side of the hemivertebral body. The disc is first incised (Fig. 5) with a scalpel along with the anterior longitudinal ligament and then removed with a combination of curettes and rongeurs. The disc should be excised carefully across the vertebral interspace to the opposite concave side, removing the anulus and nucleus back to the posterior longitudinal ligament. It is desirable to leave a small portion of the anular fibers on the concave side approximately 6.5 to 1.0 cm in width to act as a tether, preventing translation during the second-stage corrective procedure. After the disc has been totally removed back to the posterior longitudinal ligament, the vertebral body is excised with rongeurs and curettes (Fig. 6). This bone is saved to use for later bone grafting.

If one is in the thoracic spine, the head of the rib that is articulating with the hemivertebra and interspace is removed to facilitate exposure as well as eventual closure of the space once the vertebra has been excised. It must be stressed that the disc should be removed all the way back to the posterior longitudinal ligament. The outer disc fibers are quite fibrotic and cartilaginous, particularly posteriolaterally, and during the process of deformity correction they may retropulse, causing neurologic pressure if the cartilaginous rim is not completely removed. It is desirable also to smooth down or shave the ends of the vertebra above and below the hemivertebra once the hemivertebra is excised in order to allow better closure with contact following the posterior procedure (Fig. 7). If excessive bleeding is encountered through tears in the posterior longitudinal ligament from epidural veins, hemostasis is adequately secured with Gelfoam soaked in thrombin solu-

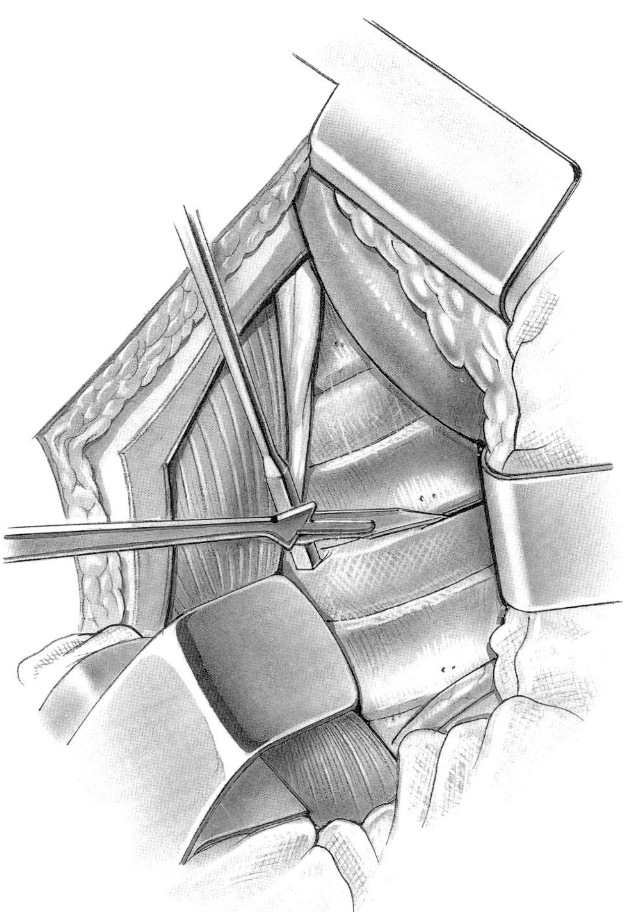

Figure 5. A sharp scalpel blade is used to incise the superiormost disc.

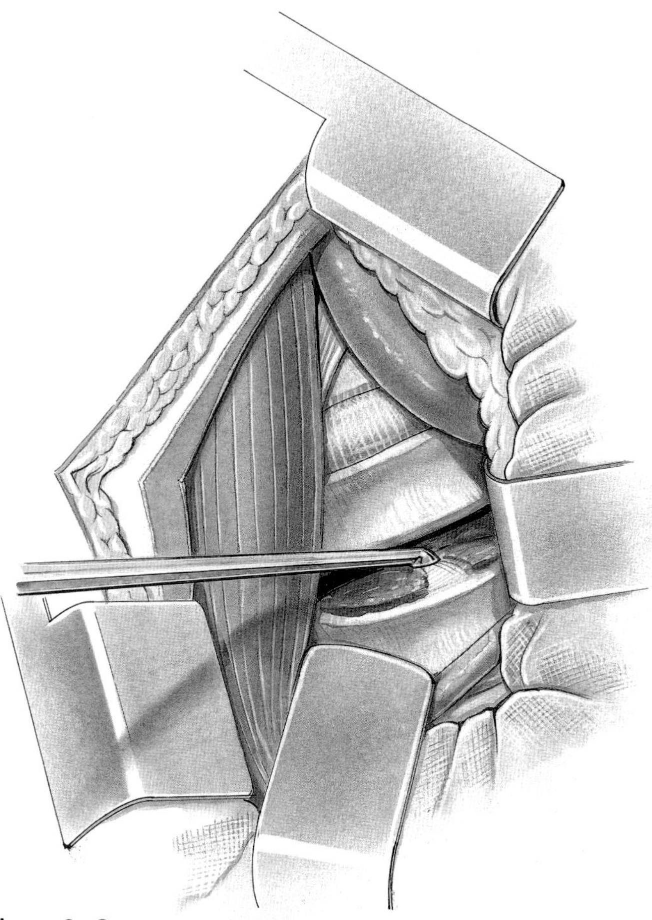

Figure 6. Curettes and rongeurs are used to remove the superiormost disc. Note visualization of the inferior disc space as it intersects with the superior disc.

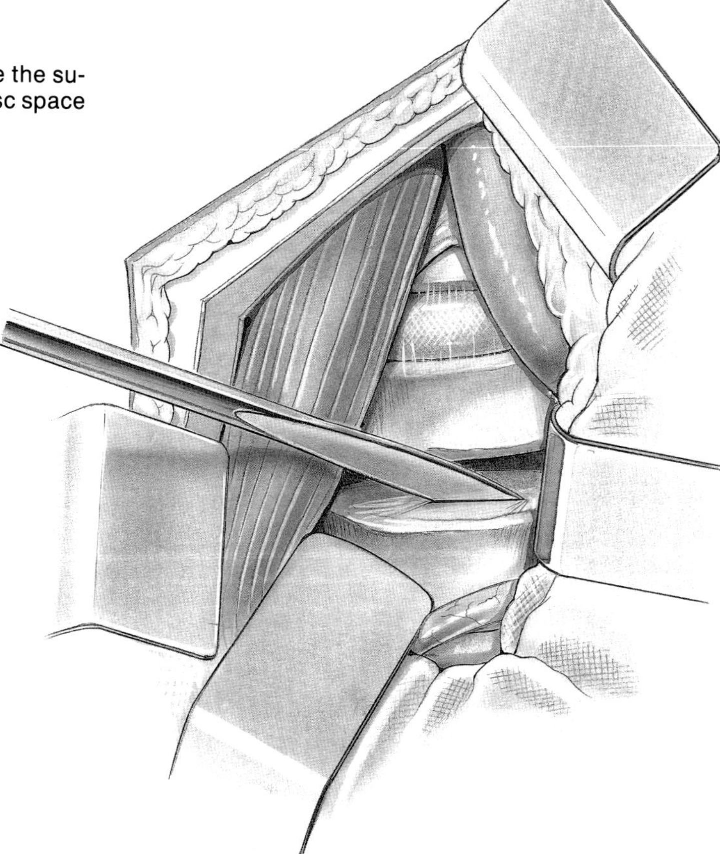

Figure 7. Because the hemivertebra is partially incarcerated, a curved osteotome is used to even the resection so as to leave a triangular defect that can be smoothly closed down.

tion. Topical collagen (Avitene) is also helpful. It is also very important to remove all the cartilage from the vertebral body above as well as below to ensure arthrodesis. Partial removal of the pedicle is performed with a high-speed bur (Fig. 8). Gelfoam is placed loosely over the posterior longitudinal ligament, and then the space between the two vertebral bodies created by the excision may be filled partially with very finely cut up pieces of the excised vertebral body. The space obviously must not be packed too tightly with bone as it may jeopardize correction, but bone may be placed in the space loosely to facilitate arthrodesis (Fig. 9).

If the deformity is substantial, and it is unlikely that anatomic correction will be achieved from the excision, it is often desirable to do a hemiepiphysiodesis at the segments above and below the site of hemivertebral excision. In this case, the convex half of the disc of the motion segment above is excised with a scalpel and rongeurs back to the bony end plate from the anterior ligament back to the posterior ligament, and the space is packed loosely with residual bone from the hemivertebra that was removed. By doing an epiphysiodesis in this fashion above and below the site of vertebral excision, with eventual arthrodesis, a tethering effect is created, allowing improvement of the deformity with continued growth.

The pleura overlying the vertebral bodies is then closed with a running 2–0 absorbable suture, and the chest tube is placed in position through a stab incision and put to underwater seal suction. The chest is closed in a routine fashion. If a retroperitoneal approach only has been used, no drain is necessary. The skin is closed cosmetically with a subcuticular 3–0 Vicryl stitch.

The patient is then positioned for the posterior approach. This may be facilitated by bringing in an additional operating table on which a four-poster frame has already been applied and transferring the patient to the new operating table. If

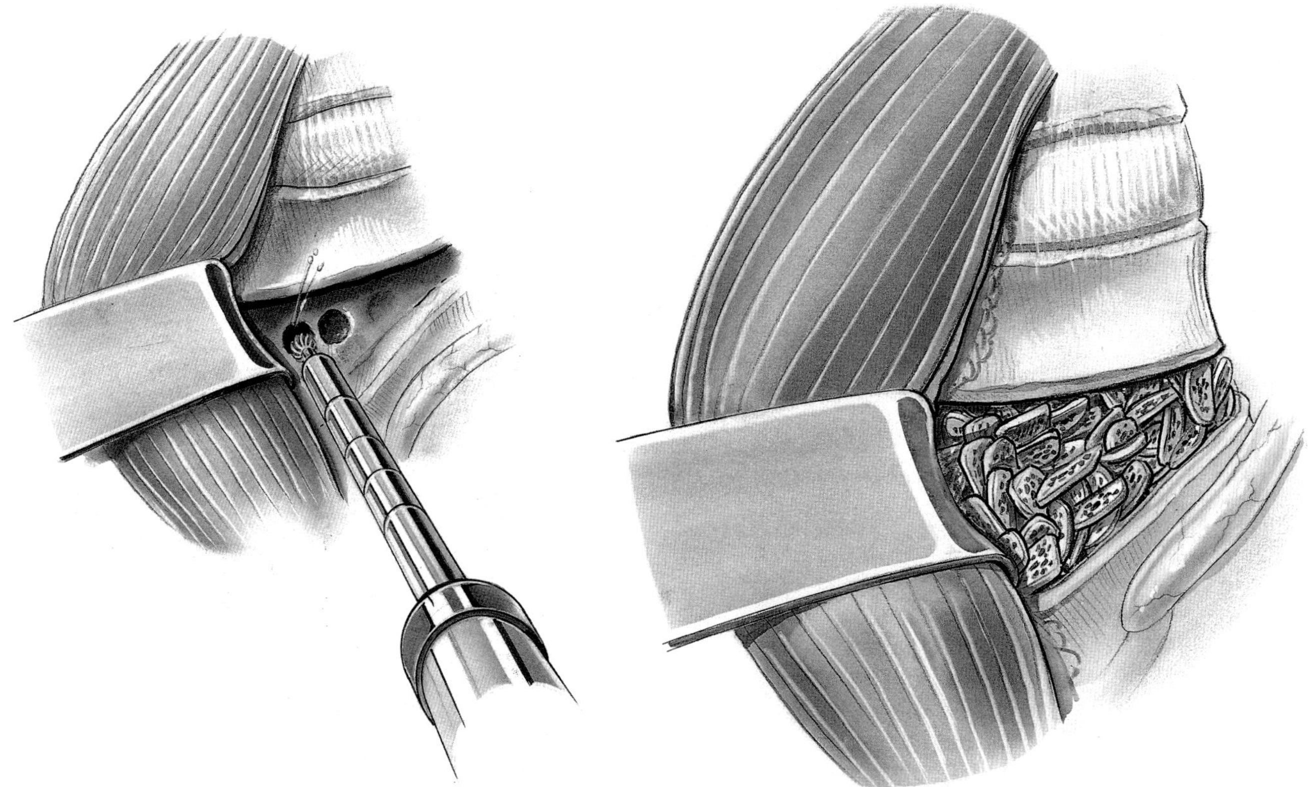

Figure 8. The resected area that has been smoothed out to form an isosceles triangle. After adequate resection of the contralateral anulus has been performed, partial removal of the pedicle is performed with the high-speed bur.

Figure 9. The area of the resection is loosely filled with fragments of resected bone.

the patient is small, however, it is very easy to turn the patient in the prone position and slide a four-poster frame or rolls under the patient (Fig. 10). It is important to pad the chest and the iliac crest bilaterally adequately, allowing ample space over the abdomen to prevent increased venous pressure. We prefer to do the surgery (second-stage posterior procedure) all under one anesthetic. We have seen no complications from this, and, in fact, the morbidity is decreased. Hospitali-

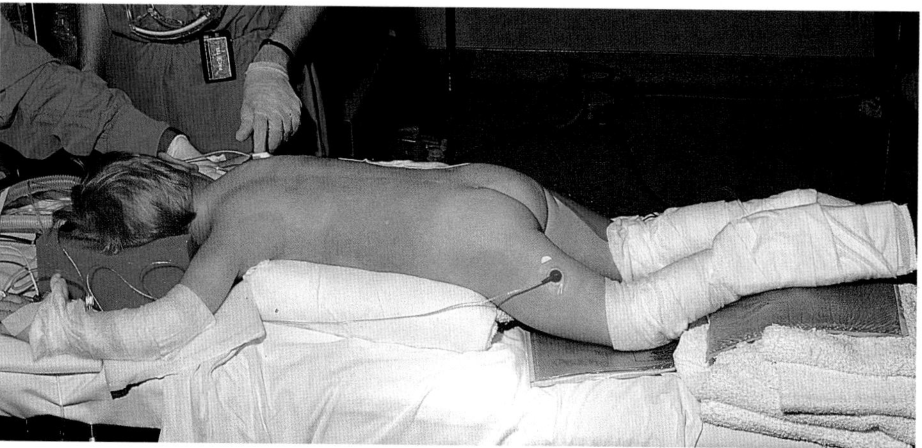

Figure 10. The patient is prone on a roll with the abdomen free.

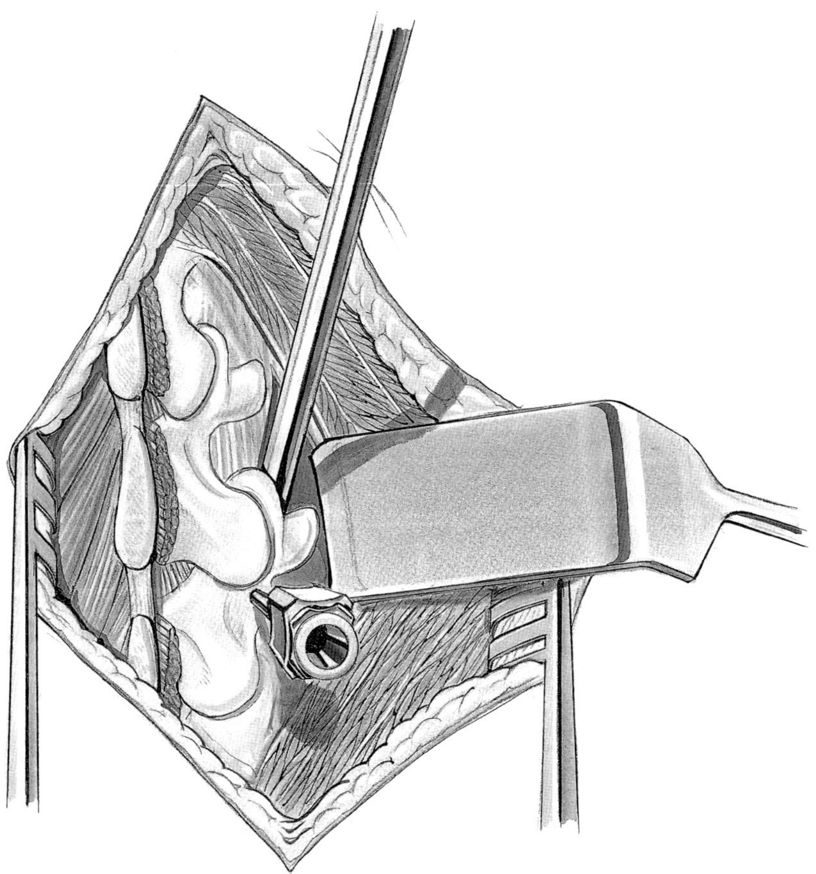

Figure 11. Exposure of the hemivertebra posteriorly. A retractor is placed around the transverse process and a metallic marker placed at the level of the pedicle for radiographic confirmation.

zation time is shortened, and the overall cost is substantially less. The instrument trays are kept sterile during the repositioning process, and the patient is reprepped and draped in a routine fashion. A routine midline exposure is then carried out overlying the hemivertebra, and, after subperiosteal exposure, a radiograph is taken to determine the proper level (Fig. 11).

Once the level has been adequately identified and complete exposure posteriorly obtained, the hemivertebra (laminae) is excised with a variety of rongeurs and curettes. Removal of the posterior arch is greatly enhanced by removing most of the pedicle during the anterior procedure. If during the anterior procedure the pedicle has not been drilled down flush to the nerve root, the removal is a bit more difficult from the posterior approach. Once the lamina, facets, and transverse process have been completely removed, the lamina above and below is decorticated carefully with a high-speed Surgairtome and local bone graft is laid over the posterior elements one level above and one level below the excised lamina (Fig. 12). If a hemiepiphysiodesis anteriorly has been done, more than one additional level above and below the excised segment, then the posterior fusion should be added to the convex side over these additional segments. If a thoracotomy has been done, usually sufficient bone exists for the fusion from the rib. If the procedure has been done in the retroperitoneum only, as in the case of a lumbar hemivertebra, it may be necessary to expose the iliac crest and to obtain iliac crest bone or to use bone bank bone. We prefer to use autologous bone for this procedure.

If the patient has sufficient bone stock and is approaching skeletal maturity, it may be quite possible to use a short compression rod on the convex side to correct the deformity and provide adequate fixation. Furthermore, this compression im-

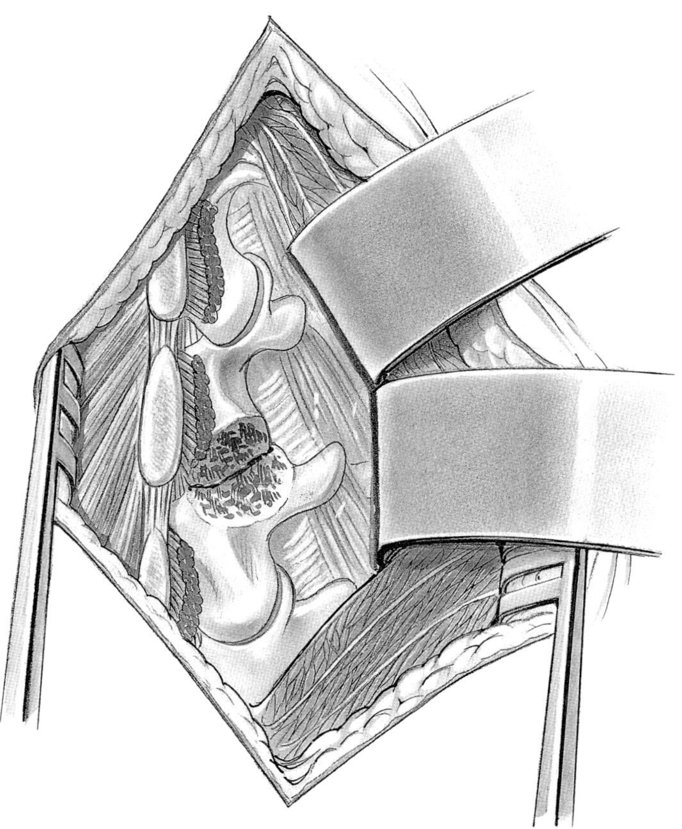

Figure 12. After resection of the lamina and residual pedicle of the hemivertebra, bone graft is laid loosely prior to closure.

plant on the convex side will prevent the slight tendency toward kyphosis that often occurs with hemivertebra excision. In these cases we have found that the pediatric CD lumbar hooks with the rod are quite adequate to compress the two vertebrae together. A wake-up test is then done to be assured that neurologic function remains intact. The procedure may also be done with spinal somatic sensory evoked potentials as a spinal cord monitor. We feel that a wake-up test, however, is sufficient.

If the patient is skeletally immature with bone stock not sufficient in size to secure with an implant, the wound is closed, and after a dressing is applied, the patient is placed on a pediatric spica table. Anesthesia is maintained and a plaster body spica including both legs from the ankles to the upper chest is applied. The patient is bent into the convexity to maximize correction. Slight overcorrection is desired. A radiograph is taken with the patient still under anesthesia to ensure closure of the wedge and adequate correction of coronal deformity. It is very important during the application of the plaster to be certain that the patient's spine does not drift into kyphosis, since this is a normal tendency following hemivertebra excision. This can be avoided by maintaining posterior pressure over the apex of the deformity while the plaster is drying. A wake-up test is again performed prior to extubation once the radiograph appears satisfactory.

If correction is not felt to be sufficient, the cast can be wedged, and additional correction can be obtained. It is very important to pad the cast adequately, particularly over the iliac crest and the area of the deformity to prevent skin ulceration from excessive pressure.

POSTOPERATIVE MANAGEMENT

The patient is maintained in a double spica cast with the abdomen and chest, as well as perineal area, adequately cut out, allowing for proper nutrition and hygiene. The chest tube can generally be pulled in 48 hours and the patient discharged in approximately 7 days. If internal fixation has not been used, the patient is kept at bed rest for 3 to 4 months, being allowed only to semirecline in a wheelchair or chaise lounge during this period. A local patient is seen in 6 to 8 weeks for repeat radiographs and inspection of the cast for any pressure sores. If a return visit at this time is not possible, radiographs are sent in for evaluation to be certain loss of correction has not occurred. At the 4-month visit, the patient's cast is removed, radiographs are obtained to ascertain the status of the fusion, and a brace is fabricated, a body jacket without leg extension, to be worn for an additional 2 to 4 months. If the fusion appears solid at that time, progressive activities can be undertaken. The patient should avoid competitive sports for at least 8 months after surgery.

If internal fixation has been used, then it is possible to place the patient in a brace immediately after operation. The postoperative degree of mobility would be directly related to the security of fixation. As a general rule, even with internal fixation we prefer to keep the patient sedentary for 2 to 4 months after surgery in order to ensure solid fusion.

The magnitude of correction is directly related to the level of the deformity and the age of the patient. As a general rule, deformity secondary to a lumbar hemivertebra can be corrected up to 70 to 80%. Certainly 100% is possible. In the thoracic spine, however, we have not found the correction to be as good, although substantial improvement is nonetheless possible. The advantages of the procedure lie in the fact that correction is obtained over a short segment. Hence a greater degree of spine flexibility is possible following this procedure than is possible with standard spinal fusions over multiple segments. It is important to stress to the patient, however, and particularly to the parents, that although correction is substantial, it is nonetheless essential to continue to follow the patient through skeletal maturity, since progression above or below the area of hemivertebra excision is still possible during the stage of active growth. Additional surgery may therefore be necessary in select patients who demonstrate the progression of compensatory curves following hemivertebra excision.

COMPLICATIONS

Complications inherent in hemivertebra excision are similar to those expected with any spinal procedure. Theoretically, one would assume there may be a greater risk of neurologic injury as a result of excision. That has not been our experience. In fact, in the series reported by Slabaugh et al. (6), only one case of transient quadriceps weakness occurred early on in their series of eight hemivertebra excisions. No patients were noted to have neurologic deficits in the other series reported (1,4,5).

Incomplete correction secondary to inadequate excision or loss of correction may occur and hence is more likely to lead to progressive deformity with growth. Compulsory follow-up with repeat radiographs is therefore essential to identify this condition. Should it occur, further surgery with extension of the fusion and instrumentation may be the treatment of choice.

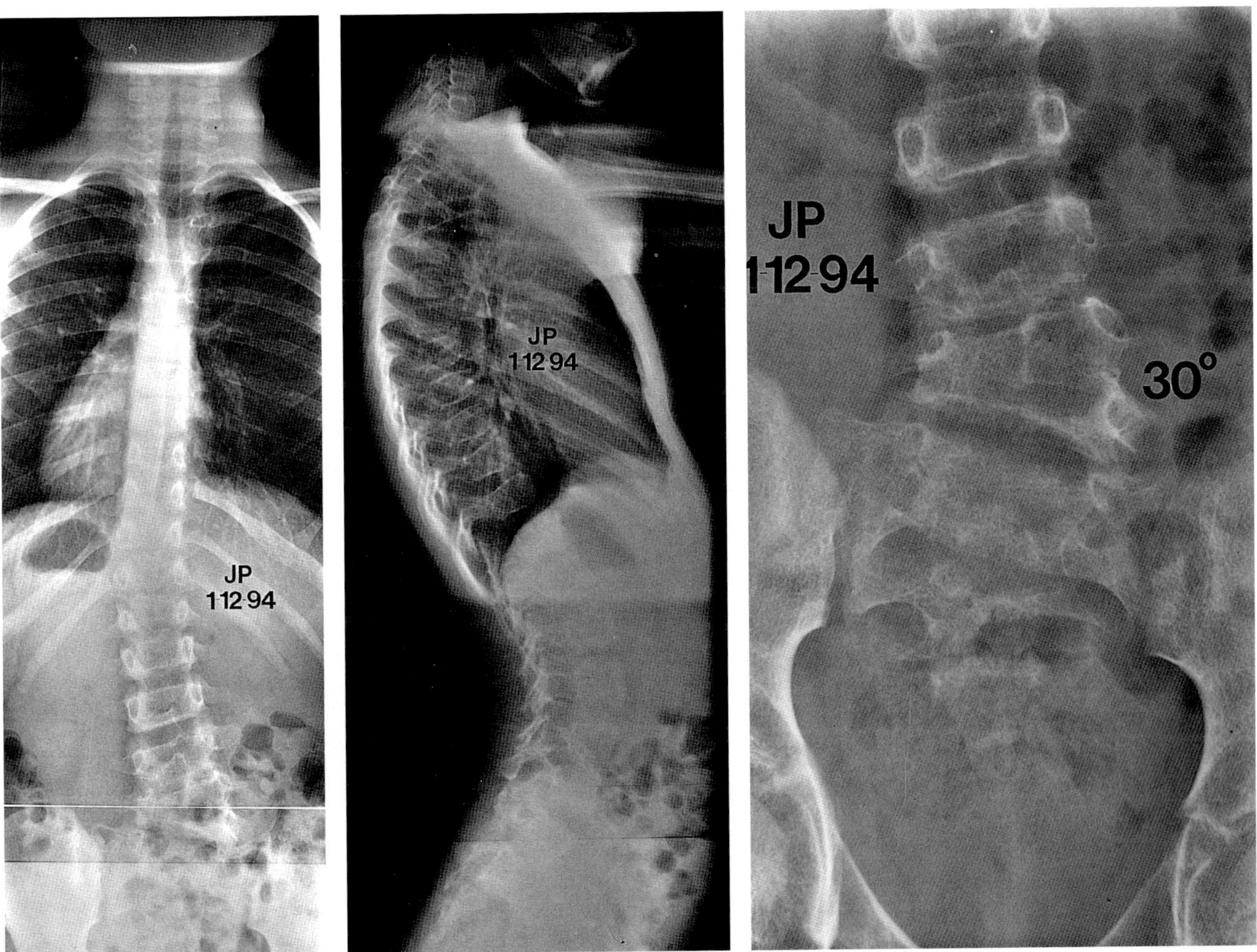

Figure 13. Anteroposterior **(A)**, lateral **(B)**, and AP lumbar **(C)** preoperative radiographs of 8-year-old girl with an L6 hemivertebra on the right causing truncal imbalance.

Pseudarthrosis may occur following this procedure and is more likely to occur in those patients who are not instrumented. However, adequate cast correction, restricted activities, and continued immobilization until the fusion is solid should prevent this complication.

Junctional kyphosis at the site of hemivertebra excision may occur as the spine drifts into slight sagittal deformity. This may be prevented by internal fixation or postoperative casting in an extension mode counteracting the kyphotic tendency. It is also less likely when the fusion extends posteriorly on the convex side two segments above and two segments below the hemivertebra excision. Finally, it is important to remember that these patients often have multiple congenital anomalies, particularly intrinsic spinal cord pathology. Adequate evaluation with MRI studies of the spine will rule out intrinsic cord pathology, which if present should be addressed and treated prior to hemivertebra excision.

ILLUSTRATIVE CASE FOR TECHNIQUE

Several weeks before this 8-year-old girl was examined, her parents noticed that she had truncal imbalance. Radiographs showed an L6 hemivertebra on the right (Fig. 13). Her physical examination revealed pelvic obliquity. She plumbed 2 to 2.5 cm to the left of the midline. Her neurologic exam was normal. It was felt that surgery was necessary because of the truncal imbalance and the high probability of progression.

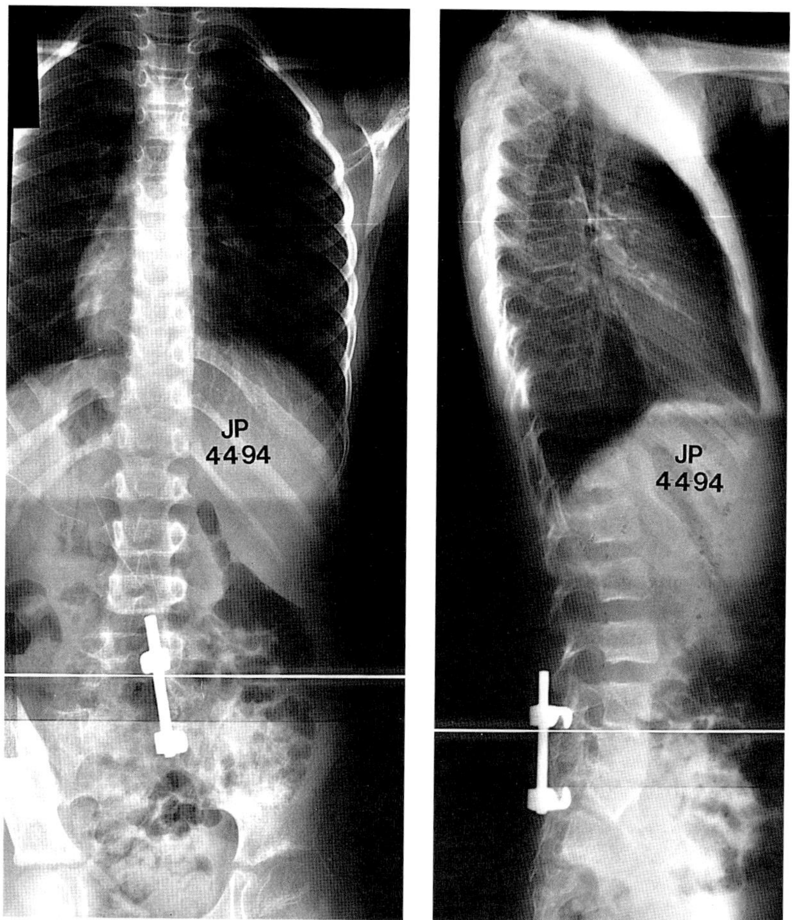

Figure 14. Postoperative AP **(A)** and lateral **(B)** radiographs reveal excellent truncal balance. Her hardware is in excellent position and evidence of early fusion is present.

The patient underwent combined anterior and posterior surgery under one anesthetic. Through a retroperitoneal approach to the lumbosacral spine, an L6 vertebrectomy, L4–L5, L5–S1 discectomy, L4–L5, L5–S1 interbody fusion was performed with local bone graft. The patient was turned and through a posterior approach had an L5 laminectomy with removal of the hemivertebra and removal of the residual portion of the pedicle along with the transverse process. Laminotomies were also done at L4 and S1 along with nerve root exploration, and spinal fusion using iliac crest bone autograft of L4–S1 with internal fixation using a small pediatric CD set. She was given a wake-up test and showed no evidence of neurologic deficit.

After the surgeries she was placed in a long-leg spica cast. She was noted to have decreased extensor hallucis longus and tibialis anterior function (4/5) postoperatively. At 3 months after surgery she had improved function. Her postoperative radiographs (11 weeks) showed that her hardware was in excellent position with evidence of early fusion (Fig. 14).

RECOMMENDED READING

1. Bergoin, M., Bollini, G., Taibi, L., and Cohen, G.: Excision of hemivertebrae in children with congenital scoliosis. *Ital. J. Orthop. Traumatol.*, 12: 179–184, 1986.
2. Bradford, D. S., and Boachie-Adjei, O.: One-stage anterior and posterior hemivertebral resection and arthrodesis for congenital scoliosis. *J. Bone Joint Surg.*, 72A: 536–540, 1990.
3. Bradford, D. S., Heithoff, K. B., and Cohen, M.: Intraspinal abnormalities and congenital spine deformities: A radiographic and MRI study. *J. Pediatr. Orthop.*, 11: 36–41, 1991.
4. Carcassonne, M., Gregoire, A., and Hornung, H.: L'ablation de l'hémi-vertèbre (libre): Traitement préventif de la scoliose congénitale. *Chirurgie*, 103: 110–115, 1977.
5. Leatherman, K. D., and Dickson, R. A.: Two-stage corrective surgery for congenital deformities of the spine. *J. Bone Joint Surg.*, 61B: 324–328, 1979.
6. Slabaugh, P. B., Winter, R. B., Lonstein, J. E., and Moe, J. H.: Lumbosacral hemivertebrae: A review of twenty-four patients, with excision in eight. *Spine*, 5: 234–244, 1980.
7. Winter, R. B., Moe, J. H., and Eilers, V. E.: Congenital scoliosis: A study of 234 patients treated and untreated. *J. Bone Joint Surg.*, 50A: 1–15, 1968.

Master Techniques in Orthopaedic Surgery,
THE SPINE, edited by D. S. Bradford,
Lippincott-Raven Publishers, Philadelphia, © 1997.

12

Eggshell Procedure

Samuel J. Chewning, Jr. and Charles F. Heinig

INDICATIONS/CONTRAINDICATIONS

The eggshell procedure is an operative technique that allows the experienced spine surgeon to operate on the anterior column of the spine through a posterior approach. This is accomplished by using the pedicle as a conduit to the anterior column. The term *eggshell* is a descriptive one for the appearance of the vertebral body once the cancellous part of the vertebral body has been removed, leaving only a very thin cortical shell similar to an empty eggshell. This procedure is not usually used as an isolated operation but rather as a component of an operative procedure (i.e., as the osteotomy portion for the correction of a rigid kyphotic deformity).

The eggshell procedure or transpedicular vertebrectomy may be used for a variety of indications. It was first described by Michelle and Krudger (1) in 1949 for biopsy and drainage of a vertebral body. Currently it is used in its simplest form for the same indication, transpedicular biopsy of a vertebral body lesion, or as a means for draining a disc space or bony abscess. The transpedicular approach and partial removal of cancellous bone allow the spine surgeon to create a potential space within the vertebral body that permits decompression of the anterior portion of the spinal canal in either tumor or fracture cases. As one becomes more comfortable with the operation, it can be expanded into a complete vertebrectomy and/or osteotomy for correction of a fixed deformity. The primary contraindication to this procedure is the lack of proper training. It is not usually done on normal spinal anatomy. With the exception of a routine biopsy, most eggshell procedures are done for chronic or acute deformity. It is necessary, therefore, that the spinal surgeon understand the normal anatomy of the level involved as well as have a thorough understanding preoperatively of the pathologic anatomy.

S. J. Chewning, Jr., M.D., and C. F. Heinig, M.D.: Miller Orthopaedic Clinic, Charlotte, North Carolina 28203.

PREOPERATIVE PLANNING

Before any eggshell procedure is performed, it is strongly recommended that a thorough radiographic evaluation be done. This may include myelography, computed tomography (CT), magnetic resonance imaging (MRI), tomography, or three-dimensional CT reconstructions of the involved spinal segment. A thorough neurologic examination is required. Subtle changes in gate pattern or bowel and bladder function may necessitate more extensive neurologic evaluation, such as electromyelograms or cystometrograms. Since there is no one indication for the eggshell procedure, no single preoperative protocol is best for the evaluation of these patients. At a minimum, standing radiographs [anteroposterior (AP) and lateral] and a tomographic study (CT or MRI) are recommended.

SURGERY

Anesthesia and Positioning

Anesthetic considerations must be based on the patient's overall condition and the magnitude of the procedure to be performed. Most of these cases will be carried out under general, endotracheal anesthesia. The anesthesiologist's ability to provide moderate hypotension (mean arterial pressure, 70 to 80 mm Hg) will help control bleeding. The surgeon's need for interoperative spinal cord monitoring will also affect the choice of anesthetic agents. For procedures such as vertebral body biopsy, the patient is placed in the prone position. When an osteotomy is to be performed, the positioning becomes more critical. If an extension osteotomy is carried out, the patient must be positioned and secured to the intraoperative table in a manner that allows an extension moment to be applied to the spine as the osteotomy is reduced or closed. An operating table that permits interoperative biplanar radiographs is also necessary.

The surgical approach is posterior, and the magnitude of the exposure is dictated by the overall surgical goal. For a simple biopsy, the exposure is unilateral and is centered directly over the desired vertebral pedicle.

Simple Application

Decompression of a vertebral body abscess or a vertebral body biopsy is the most basic application of the eggshell procedure. The location of the pedicle is identified (confirmed by intraoperative AP and lateral radiographs). As a general rule, the pedicle lies at the point of intersection between a midline drawn through the transverse process, the lower-most aspect of the superior articular facet, and a line drawn along the lateral margin of the pars interarticularis. Pedicles are usually larger and more cylindrical in the lumbar spine and become smaller and more elliptical in the thoracic spine.

Once the approximate area of the pedicle has been identified, the posterior cortical bone is removed with a rongeur, curette, osteotome, or high-speed bur. Removal of the cortical bone reveals the well-vascularized cancellous bone of the pedicle. A probe is then placed down through the pedicle much like an intramedullary nail. Several different diameters of probes should be available. A very small #000 curette makes an excellent initial instrument to place into the pedicle. A modified ganglion knife (developed by Arthur Steffee) is also an excellent instrument to make the initial pass through the pedicle into the body. The opening within the pedicle is enlarged using progressively larger curettes until the cancellous bone within the pedicle has been removed. The operator now has a cortical tube leading into the vertebral body. If biopsy or drainage is to be carried out, curettes may be introduced through the conduit of the pedicle and into the body where tissue may be obtained. Biopsy needles may also be used through the hollow pedicle to obtain direct biopsy of the vertebral body. Until the surgeon is familiar with this procedure, it is strongly recommended that either fluoroscopic control or biplane radiographs be obtained frequently. Biopsy of vascular lesions or decompression of acute fractures may be complicated by significant bleeding. The surgeon may simply plug the opening in the pedicle to obtain hemostasis by tamponade. This may be done with bone, Gelfoam, bone wax, or a cottonoid.

Complex Application

A more complex application of the eggshell procedure is a complete vertebrectomy and/or osteotomy. A fixed short-segment kyphotic deformity secondary to a pathologic fracture is a good example of this application. In this model, the anterior body height is less than one-third of its normal height, with the posterior height being fairly well maintained. This creates an acute short-segment kyphotic deformity. The overall operative goal is to perform a debulking of the tumor and an extension osteotomy to correct the kyphotic deformity. The center or rotation for this operation will be the anterior longitudinal ligament. Balance will be obtained by removing the posterior elements and the middle column. The spine will be shortened to the height of the remaining height of the anterior body wall. Therefore, it is necessary to remove most of the bone within the body, the posterior margin of the body, the pedicles, lamina, spinous process, and facets.

In the example given, the surgeon would identify the pedicles from both the left and right sides of the spine, as described previously for the biopsy (Figs. 1 and 2). The cancellous bone is then removed from within both pedicles and curettes are introduced into the cancellous bone of the vertebral body (Figs. 3–7). The cancellous bone has a definite feel compared with the cortical margins of the vertebral body. By curetting bone from within the body and removing it out of the pedicle, the surgeon begins to enlarge the opening at the junction of the pedicle with the vertebral body (Fig. 8). The surgeon will be able to operate at an angle of roughly 45-degrees from lateral to medial and to decancellate an area directly anterior to the spinal canal (Fig. 9). The same procedure is done through the opposite pedicle (Figs. 10 and 11). It is now possible for an operator and assistant to carry out a "mining operation." One surgeon uses a curette to loosen the

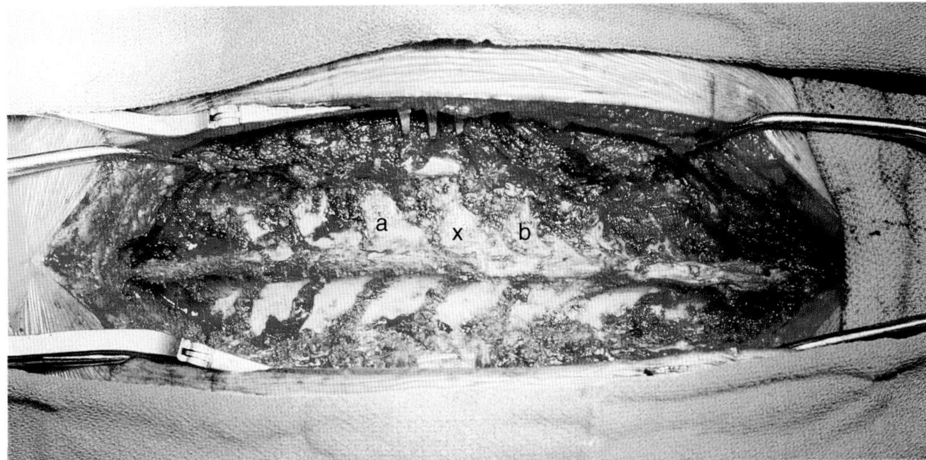

Figure 1. Subperiosteal exposure of the spine that is to be instrumented and fused. *x* indicates the level that is to be removed, in this case T7. With the correction of the kyphosis *a* will be approximate to *b* or T6 (*a*) will be closed to T8 (*b*).

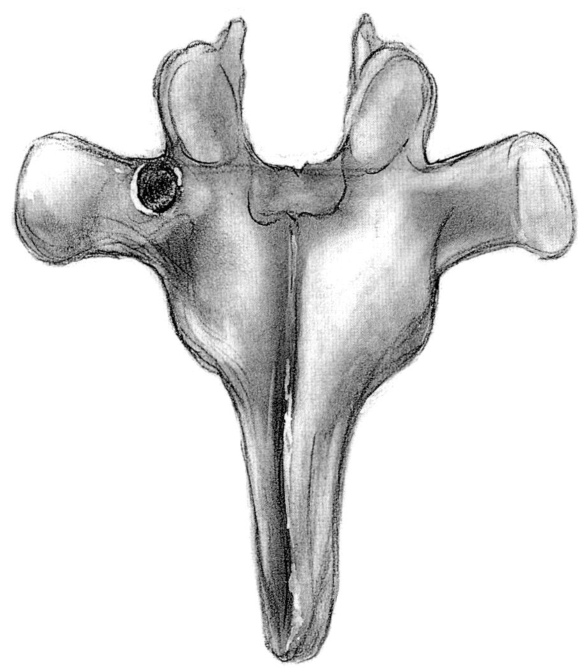

Figure 2. Location of the opening to the pedicle relative to the transverse process superior and inferior facets.

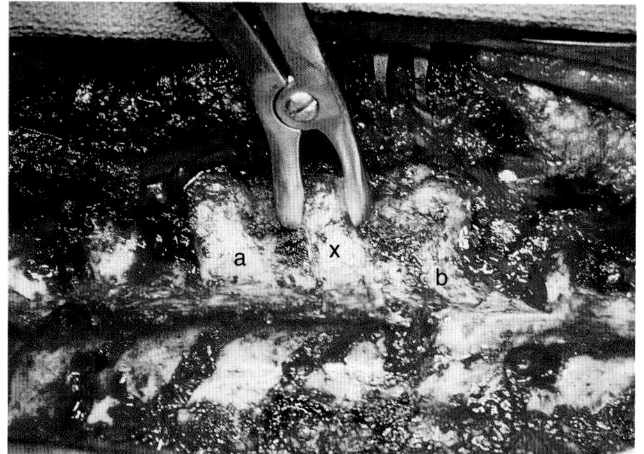

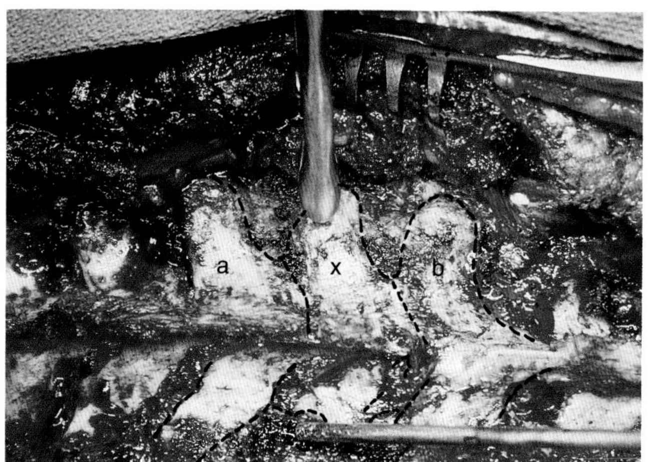

Figure 3. A,B: Removing the cortical bone from the base of the transverse process as it joins the lamina to expose the opening of the desired pedicle.

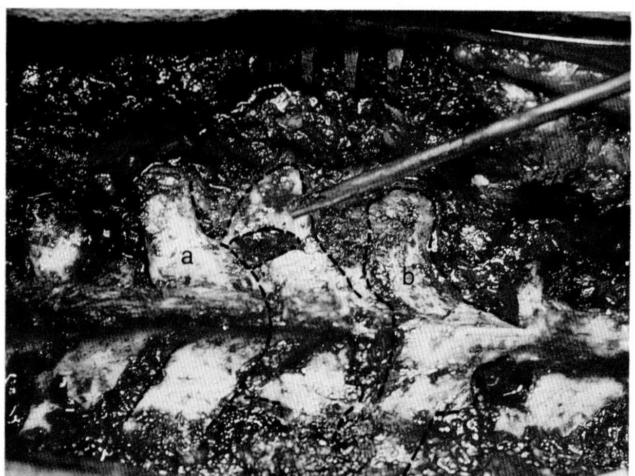

Figure 4. *X* marks the spot where the cancellous bone is exposed directly over the pedicle of (in this case) T7.

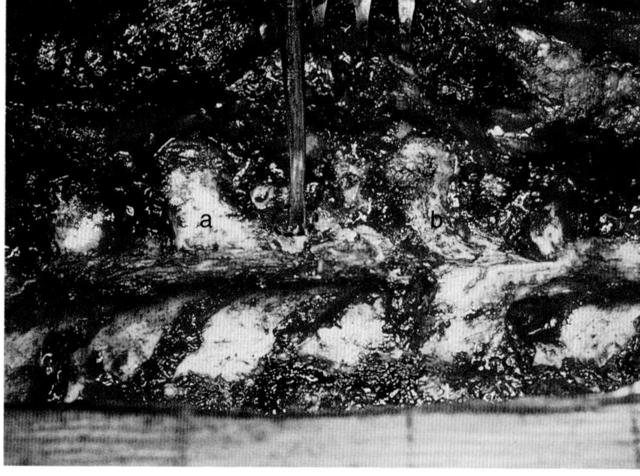

Figure 5. Probe is introduced into the pedicle of T8.

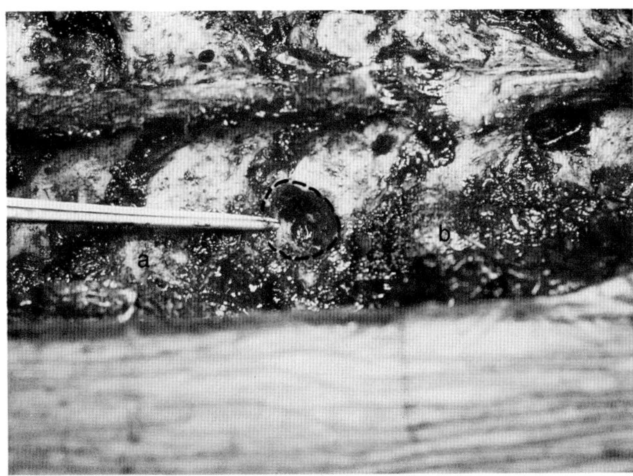

Figure 6. Cortical bone has been removed on the opposite side to allow exposure for the opposite pedicle.

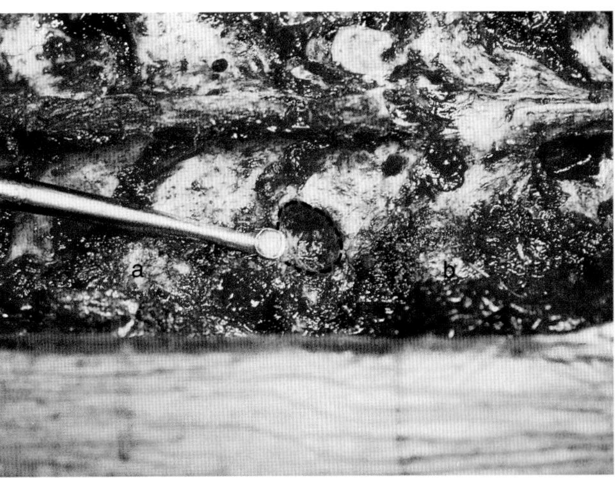

Figure 7. Curette is used to enlarge the opening and place the pedicle into the vertebral body.

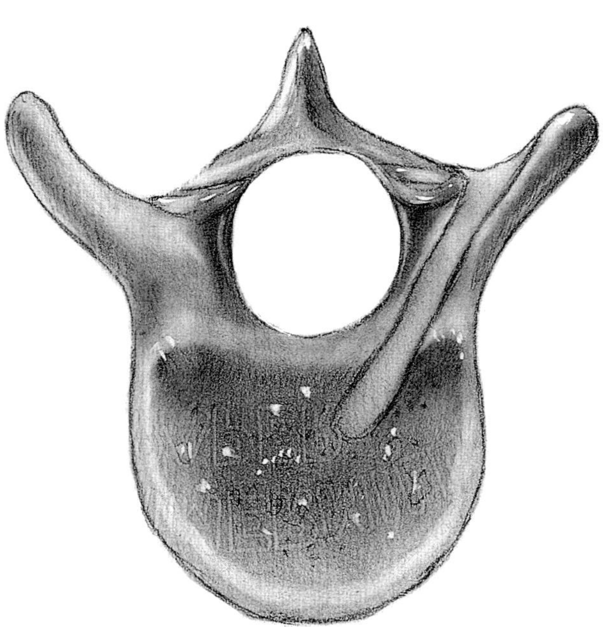

Figure 8. The path of the curette and bone removal into the vertebral body.

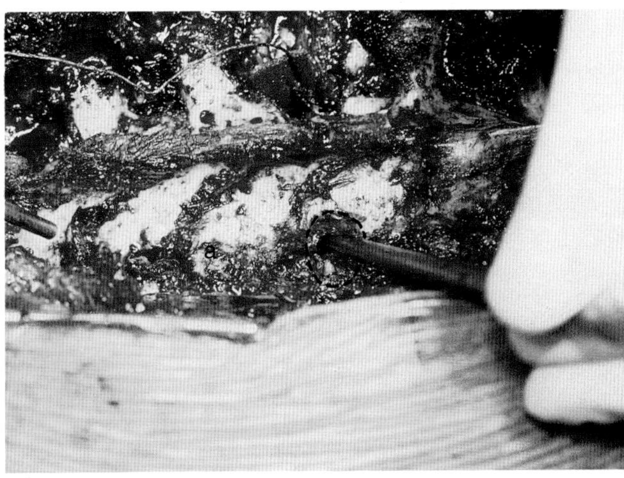

Figure 9. Curette is used to remove more bone from within the vertebral body.

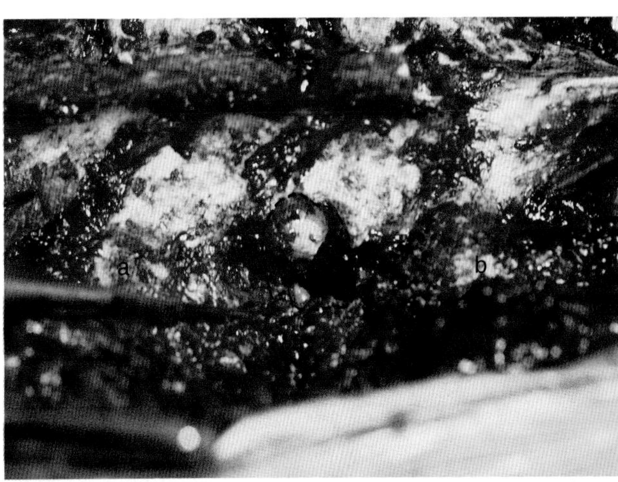

Figure 10. Lateral wall of the pedicle and transverse process had been broken down and a large opening has been created into the vertebral body.

cancellous bone, and the other surgeon uses suction and a pituitary rongeur to bring the cancellous bone out the opposite pedicle (Figs. 12 and 13). This provides a very rapid and efficient means for removing cancellous bone or tumor from within the body. This process is continued until the desired amount of tumor or bone has been removed.

In the thoracic region, the most difficult area from which to remove the cancellous bone is the central area of bone directly anterior to the spinal canal. Since the pedicle lies in the upper one-third to one-half of the vertebral body, it is very easy to break through the superior end plate and enter into the superior disc space. The disc is removed and bone graft packed in its place to obtain an interbody fusion. To remove additional bone from anterior to the spinal canal, it may be necessary to break down the lateral wall of the pedicle carefully. This allows the instruments to come in at a more oblique angle. A large curette is used to remove

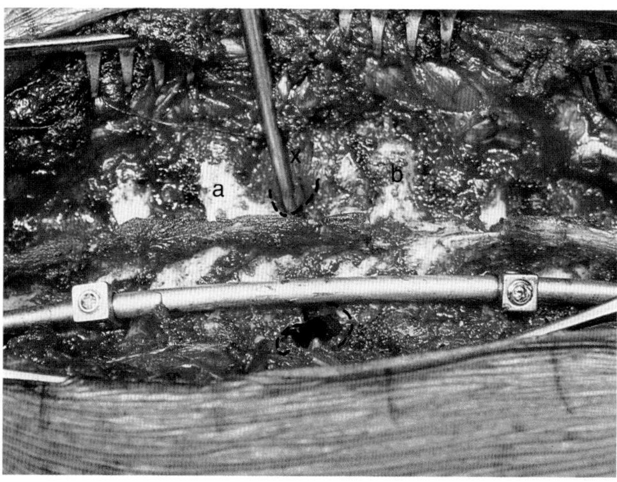

Figure 11. A provisional rod is in place to stabilize the spine. The opposite side pedicle is now entered to remove bone from the opposite pedicle.

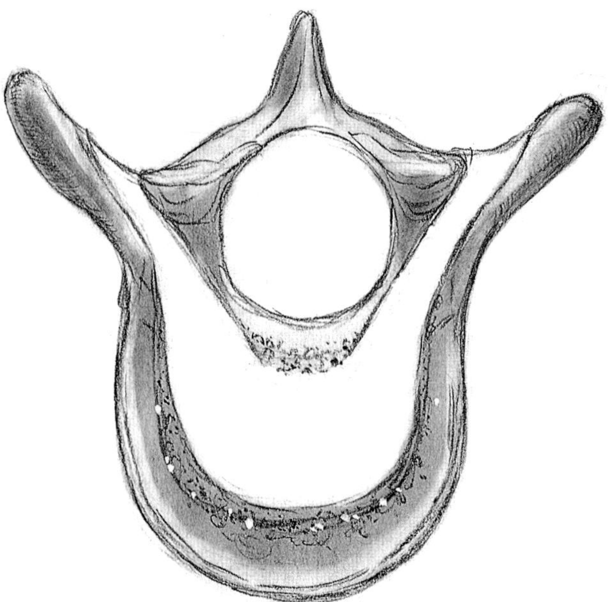

Figure 12. Bone being removed from within the body from both sides, creating a thin cortical or eggshell rim.

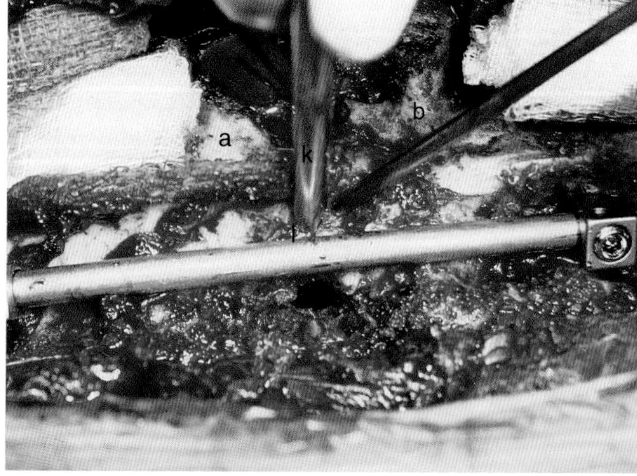

Figure 13. Kerrison rongeur (*k*) is used to finish the removal of the superior facet, inferior facet, and lamina (*l*) of T7.

the cancellous bone from directly anterior to the canal. The operator has now created an eggshell. The cancellous bone is missing, and a cortical shell of bone remains. With a surgical suction in the body a radiograph may be obtained. This will give an "air-vertebrogram" delineating the amount of bone removed. The surgeon now plugs the openings in the pedicles to control the bleeding and proceeds with preparation for instrumentation.

Some general considerations should be apparent to the surgeon at this time. The posterior elements have been left totally intact and the medial wall of the pedicle has not been violated. The medial wall and the posterior elements provide protection for the neural elements within the spinal canal. As long as their integrity has been maintained, the spinal contents are protected from the effects of temperature change, the drying effects and heat from the operative lights, and mechanical trauma from suction, instrumentation, and pressure. The beginning surgeon seems to have an almost irresistible urge to want to visualize the neural elements so as "not to damage them." This desire may have the opposite effect in that it allows the neural elements to be exposed to mechanical trauma. Again, a thorough understanding of the anatomy is mandatory.

In this model the purpose of the operation is to create an extension moment. Note at this time that the posterior elements as well as the medial wall of the pedicle are still intact. The surgeon should not succumb to the urge to have the neural elements exposed throughout the entire case. Once the medial pedicle wall is removed, the dura expands laterally, which cuts off the access to the vertebral body. The next step is to fracture the lateral pedicle wall and allow this fracture to extend into the vertebral body wall. This creates a fracture line similar to scoring a piece of glass prior to breaking it.

Attention is next directed to the posterior elements. The spinous process is removed. The lamina and facets are removed. The surgeon now has exposure of the posterior dura with a very wide decompressive laminectomy and foraminotomy. The only bony structures that are visible posteriorly are the medial walls of the pedicles. Using pituitary rongeurs, long-handled elevators, curettes, and Kerrison rongeurs, the operator carefully peels down and removes the medial walls of the pedicles. Next, a long-handled elevator is passed ventral to the dural sac to collapse the posterior wall of the vertebral body into the space created by the decancellation. The entire neural tube is now exposed, and a 360-degree decompression has been carried out (Fig. 14). In addition, a wedge osteotomy has

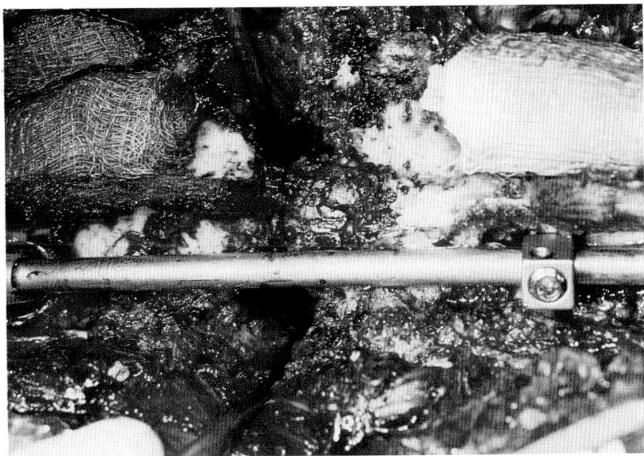

Figure 14. Both pedicles have been removed. The superior and inferior end plates of T7 have been removed through the pedicles. All the posterior elements have been removed. The posterior bone of the body has been removed to free the anterior canal completely, and the 360-degree decompression of the spinal cord has been carried out. The area between the arrows indicates the fully exposed spinal cord.

been created. Posteriorly, this wedge is the height of the superior-to-inferior facet distance. Anteriorly, it is the height of the remaining anterior cortical wall. The angular correction that may be obtained can be judged from the preoperative radiographs by measuring the facet-to-facet height posteriorly and the remaining vertebral body height anteriorly. Fixation points have already been prepared above and below the osteotomy level. The kyphotic deformity is carefully corrected by contraction or compression to close the osteotomy (Figs. 15–17). This has shortened the spinal canal and protected the neural elements from elongation. For tumor patients this technique allows a complete one-level vertebrectomy and shortening of the spine.

In the thoracic spine it is often necessary to remove the proximal ribs and rib heads at this level. If necessary, prior to closure of the osteotomy, cancellous bone graft may be placed anteriorly to create an interbody fusion. The neural elements are observed as the osteotomy is closed to make sure any remaining bone that has been placed anteriorly does not retropulse into the canal. The inferior edge of the remaining superior lamina and the superior edge of the remaining inferior lamina may be undercut to keep them from impinging on the neural tube.

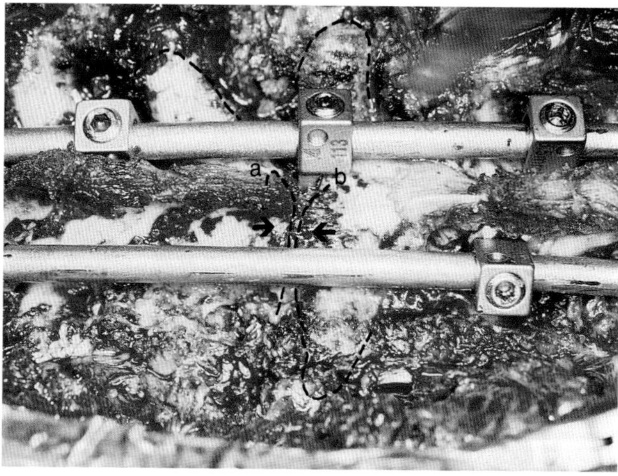

Figure 15. Compression has been carried out along the instrumentation and has approximated the facets of *a* down onto *b*, closing T7 to T8 lamina to lamina.

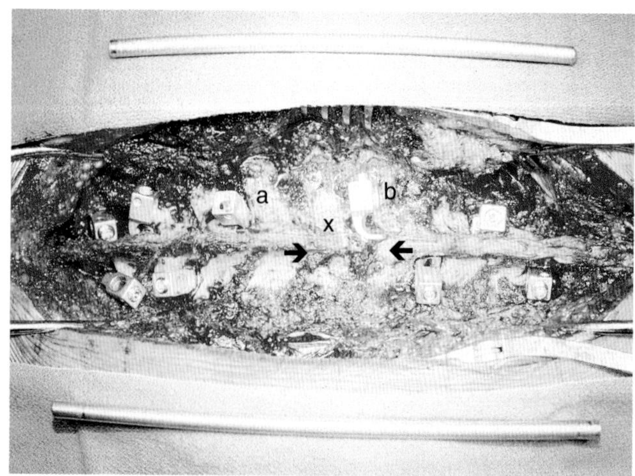

Figure 16. Intraoperative photograph showing hook placement, rod contour, and T6 (*a*) relative to T8 (*b*) with T7 (*X*) prior to removal.

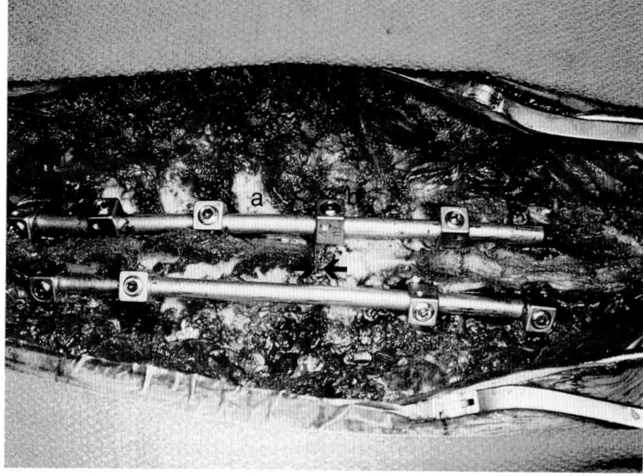

Figure 17. T7 has been completely removed and T6 has been approximated to T8 lamina to lamina, or as labeled here, *a* has been brought to *b*.

The ultimate stability of the spinal construct depends on whether or not facet-to-facet or bone-to-bone apposition is obtained. A posterior/posterior lateral fusion is now completed. Autologous bone graft is placed after decortication of the posterior elements. Care is taken during decortication not to weaken the force-bearing posterior elements (i.e., the lamina, where a hook has been placed). Make sure that all hardware has been inserted and secured in the fashion specific for the system used. The fascia should be closed over suction drains. The subcutaneous layer is approximated with absorbable suture, and the skin is closed.

POSTOPERATIVE MANAGEMENT

The postoperative routine will vary depending on the complexity of the pathology. Patients undergoing vertebrectomy or osteotomy are kept at bed rest until they have been fitted with a custom-molded thoracolumbosacral orthosis (TLSO). They may then ambulate in the brace. Drains are removed when the drainage is less than 20 to 30 mls in an 8-hour period. Bracing is continued full time (when out of bed) for 3 months. The patient is then weaned from the brace over a 6- to 12-week period.

The timing of office visits is tailored to the specific needs of a particular patient. As a general rule the patient is seen at postoperative months 1, 3, 6, 9, 12, 18, and 24. Radiographs (AP and lateral) are obtained at each of these office visits. These patients should have obtained maximal medical improvement by 12 to 18 months.

COMPLICATIONS

The eggshell procedure is usually not used as an isolated procedure (other than for vertebral biopsy). Complications are related to the overall operative procedure.

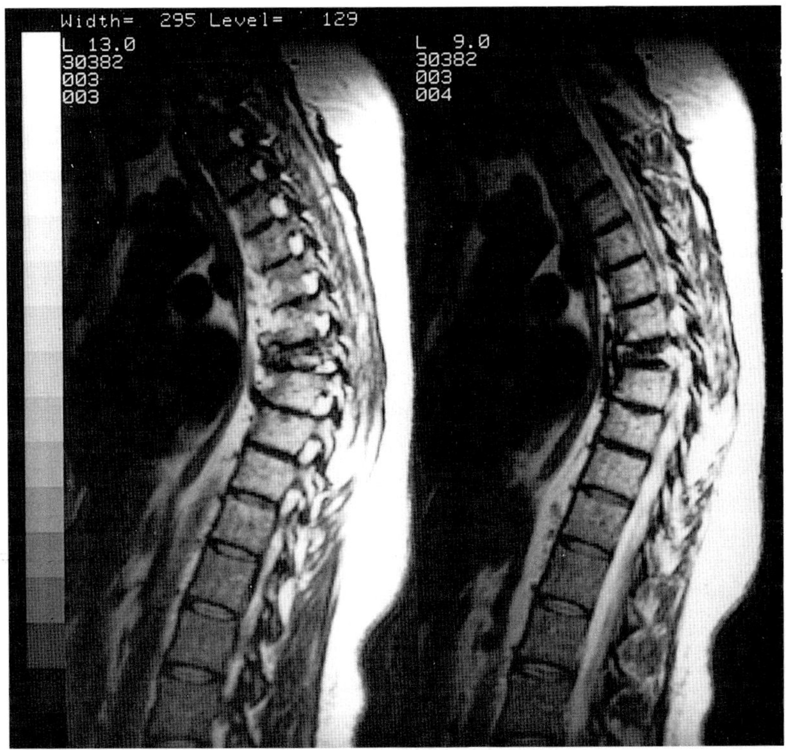

Figure 18. MRIs of a patient with plasma cytoma of T7 causing cord compression and short-segment kyphotic deformity.

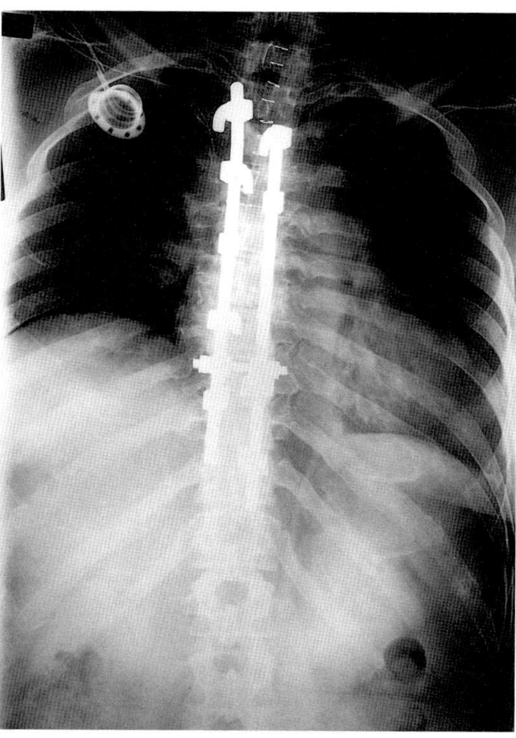

Figure 19. Postoperative radiograph showing removal of T7.

Deep wound infections are managed with irrigation, surgical debridement, closure over drains (when the wound is ready), and appropriate antibiotics. Prominent hardware may require removal. Hardware failure and pseudarthrosis may lead to a repair of the failed fusion and possibly reinstrumentation. A nondiagnostic biopsy may be addressed with a larger open procedure.

ILLUSTRATIVE CASE FOR TECHNIQUE

A 49-year-old woman was referred for the surgical treatment of multiple myeloma. Her spine lesion was in T7 (Fig. 18). Over the preceding 4 months she had experienced progressive collapse of the T7 lesion with increasing back pain and pain radiating down her legs. She had been treated with maximum radiation and chemotherapy. Surgical treatment consisted of an eggshell or transpedicular vertebrectomy and decompression at the T7 level. All the posterior elements of T7 including the spinous processes, laminae, facets, and transverse processes were also removed. The rib heads were resected. Instrumentation loaded in compression was utilized to pull her spine into extension and approximate the osteotomy. The osteotomy posteriorly was closed by placing the lamina and facets of T6 down onto the facets of T8. The interbody space was filled with bone graft prior to closure of the osteotomy (Fig. 19). A formal posterior fusion was carried out as well.

RECOMMENDED READING

1. Michelle, A., and Krudger, F. J.: A surgical approach to the vertebral body. *J. Bone Joint Surg.*, 31A: 873–878, 1949.
2. Heinig, C. F.: Eggshell procedure. In: *Segmental Spinal Instrumentation*. pp. 221–234, 1984.
3. Kostuik, J. P.: Laminoplasty of the thoracic and lumbar spine: eggshell procedure. In: *The Adult Spine: Principles and Practice*, edited by J. W. Frymoyer. pp. 1838–1840. Raven Press, New York, 1991.
4. Chewning, S. J., and Heinig, C. F.: Osteotomy. In: *The Pediatric Spine: Principles and Practice*, Vol. II, pp. 70–71, 1994.

Master Techniques in Orthopaedic Surgery,
THE SPINE, edited by D. S. Bradford,
Lippincott-Raven Publishers, Philadelphia, © 1997.

13

Thoracoplasty for Rib Deformity

Randal R. Betz, and Howard H. Steel

INDICATIONS/CONTRAINDICATIONS

The posterior rib prominence is the major cosmetic concern of patients presenting with scoliosis. The surgeon should remember this when discussing surgery with the patient. Our philosophy is that if the patient needs to undergo surgery for stabilization of a progressing curve, maximal safe cosmetic correction of a rib prominence should be obtained at that time. With rigid curves, the trunk does not always derotate despite current advanced spinal instrumentation systems, and a thoracoplasty is an excellent adjunctive procedure to posterior spinal fusion.

Although subjectively increased flexibility appears to occur following rib resection, Barnes (1) did not find it a help in treating infantile idiopathic scoliosis. Halsall et al. (4) found increased flexibility in a cadaver study when rib osteotomies were performed on the concave side only. We feel that rib resection is indicated primarily for cosmesis and psychological reasons, as do others (6); we also feel it is useful when rib prominence adversely affects the ability to sit in a chair. Secondary considerations would include increasing flexibility during surgical correction, but a concave rib osteotomy would probably be required as well.

Adolescent Scoliosis

Thoracoplasty is primarily indicated in patients with thoracic and double major curves. Although it is less commonly indicated, a patient with a thoracolumbar

R. R. Betz, M.D. and H. H. Steel, M.D.: Shriners Hospitals for Crippled Children, Philadelphia Unit, Philadelphia, Pennsylvania 19152–1299.

curve undergoing a posterior approach may need to have the distal ribs resected. From a review of 98 patients with adolescent idiopathic scoliosis who underwent posterior spinal fusion with Cotrel-Dubousset instrumentation, it appears that a rib resection is indicated in 25% of patients (5). A strong indication for rib resection is a preoperative rib angle on radiograph or clinical examination of 15 degrees or more (Fig. 1) (5). Relative indications include rib angle on radiograph greater than 10 degrees, curve severity greater than 60 degrees, curve flexibility less than 20% on bending films, and/or postoperative correction of the Cobb angle of less than 50 percent based on a intraoperative radiograph (5).

Adult Scoliosis

Generally most adult patients (older than 21 years of age) have rigid curves that will not derotate following posterior instrumentation. In these patients, a convex thoracoplasty is almost always beneficial. Rarely, a patient has a stable curve but experiences discomfort when sitting; in this situation, a thoracoplasty without a spinal fusion may be indicated.

Following Successful Posterior Spinal Fusion with Residual Rib Prominence

Patients with residual rib prominence who complain of discomfort when they sit in a chair or lean against a wall or who have psychological disruption from the cosmesis (psychological consults recommended) are candidates for a rib resection as a secondary procedure. Careful reassessment of the posterior trunk deformity with a rib prominence radiograph and computed tomography (CT) scan are essential because a rib deformity in a severely rotated spine may actually be caused by the most posterior bony elements of the spine, not the ribs.

Thoracoplasty is not appropriate in patients with a severely rotated spine when the ribs do not protrude beyond the posterior margin of the spine. This can be assessed by a preoperative radiograph and CT scan. Be aware that some patients with existing fusions complaining about the cosmesis are upset with trunk asymmetry, which won't be corrected by thoracoplasty. Careful assessment may indicate that an osteotomy of the previous fusion to bring the apex of the curve closer to the midline should be combined with thoracoplasty.

A

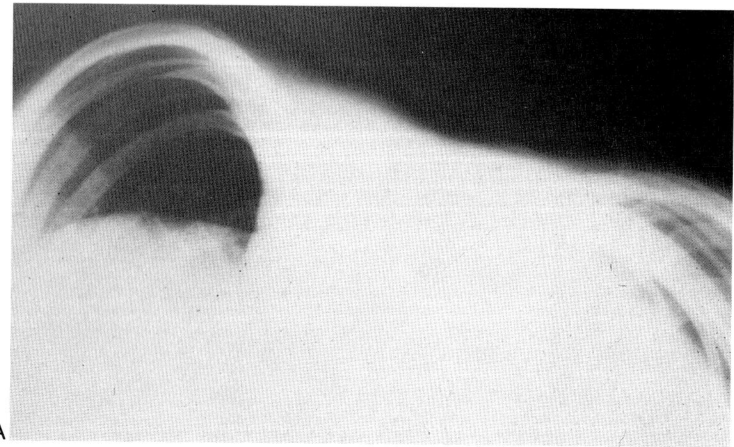

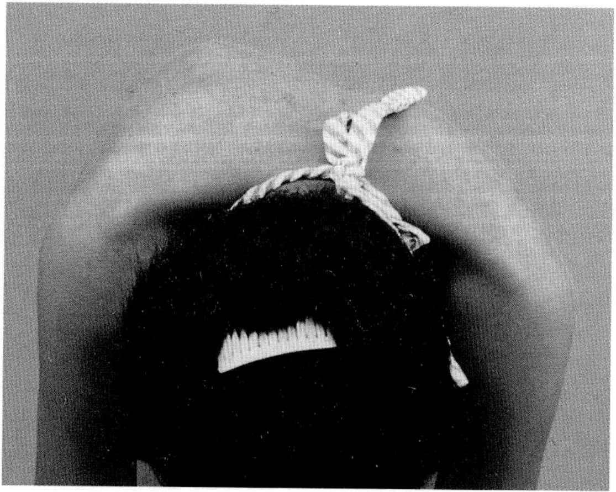

B

Figure 1. Radiograph **(A)** and clinical photograph **(B)** of preoperative rib prominence.

PREOPERATIVE PLANNING

Routine scoliosis films are obtained, including anteroposterior (AP), lateral, both bends, and a rib prominence view (Fig. 2). These films are used to assess curve flexibility and preoperative rib angle to determine if the indications are present. However, the final decision is made on the operating room table. Once the patient is under general anesthesia and positioned on the table, the rib prominence is pushed. If it does not reduce completely and very easily, a rib resection is indicated. If doubt exists, the thoracoplasty procedure can be performed following spinal instrumentation, although we prefer to do it prior to insertion of the instrumentation to minimize blood loss. It is important to drape the patient so that the rib prominence can be visualized and to bear in mind that it will always look worse postoperatively than prone on the operating table.

SURGERY

The patient is positioned in the manner standard in a posterior spinal fusion for idiopathic scoliosis (Fig. 3) and is washed and prepped in standard fashion. The patient is draped from C7 to the midgluteal crease with wide margins posteriorly

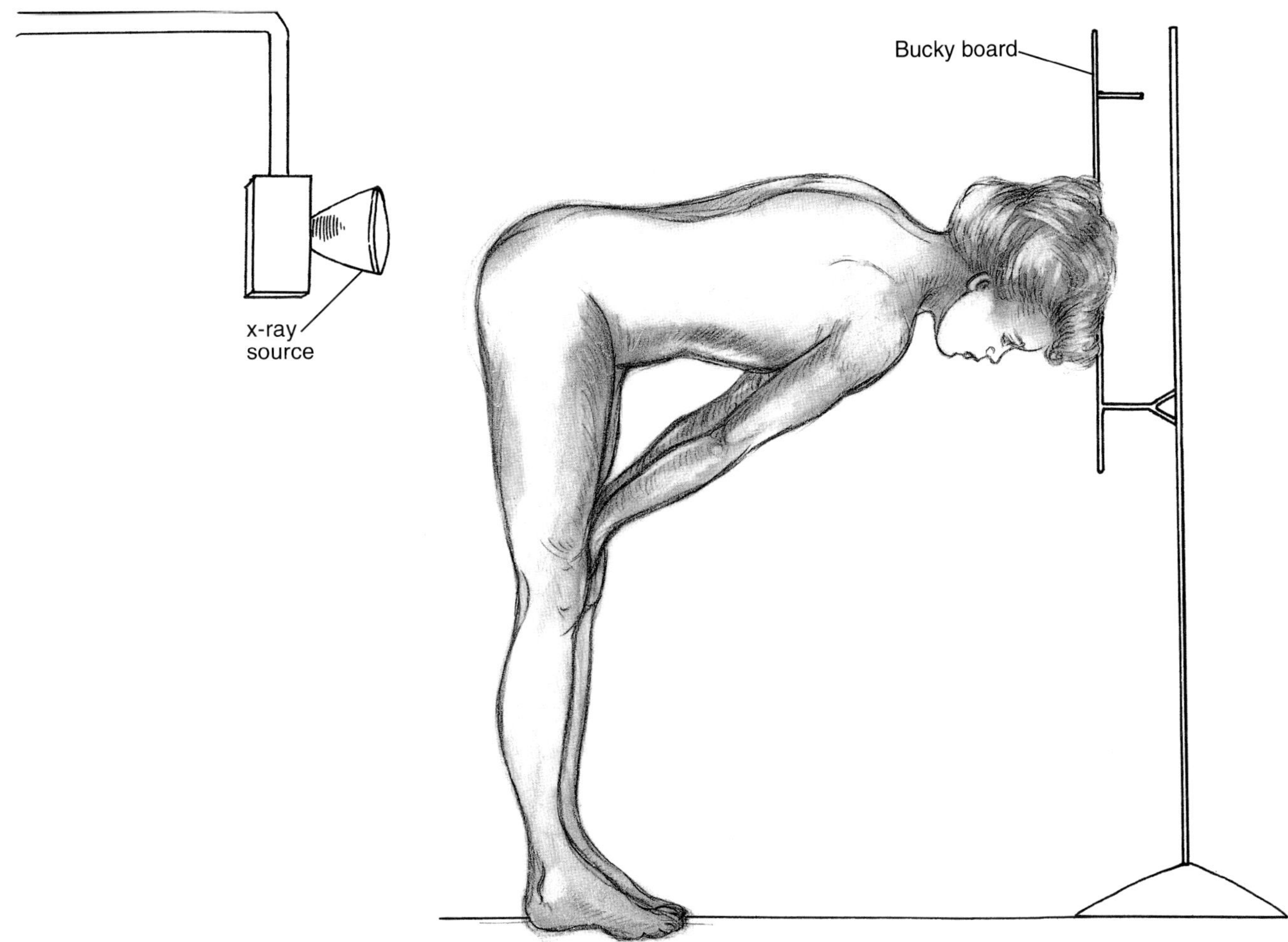

Figure 2. Schematic drawing of positioning for rib prominence radiograph.

for adequate visualization of the rib prominence (the lateral drapes should lie at the posterolateral axillary line and wider if possible). Following draping, an incision is drawn with a marking pen using the electrocautery cord (Fig. 4). The top of the cord is placed at C7 and the bottom at the midgluteal crease, and a straight line is drawn down the spine. For a selected right thoracic fusion with thoracoplasty, it is necessary to extend the skin incision distally to approximately L2 or L3 in order to retract the thoracolumbar fascia adequately from the midline. Stopping the skin incision at T12 does not provide adequate lateral exposure for this single-incision technique. Likewise, proximally the skin incision needs to be carried approximately ½ to 1 inch further. Despite the slight increase in length in the incision, it is still much more cosmetically appealing than two incisions. Besides cosmesis, the other reason we now use the midline incision instead of a two-incision technique is because with better translation of the apex of the curve to the midline, less rib needs to be resected laterally than was necessary with a Harrington rod fusion. With Harrington rod distraction for severe curves needing a rib resection, the apex was minimally translated, and therefore most of the rib resection occurred laterally. Most of the rib resection now takes place at the medial-most attachment.

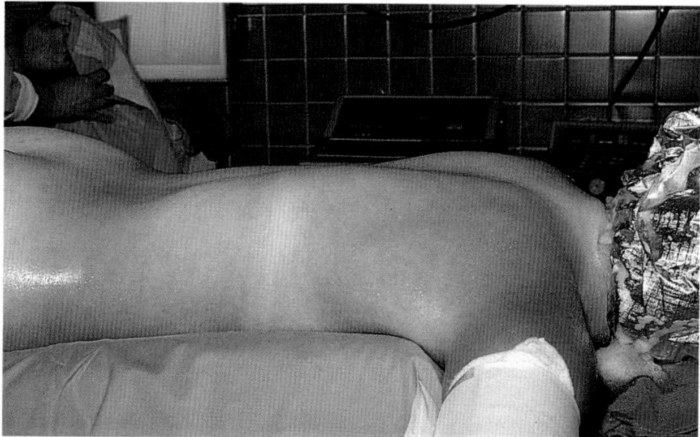

Figure 3. The patient is placed in a prone position, standard for any posterior spinal fusion for scoliosis.

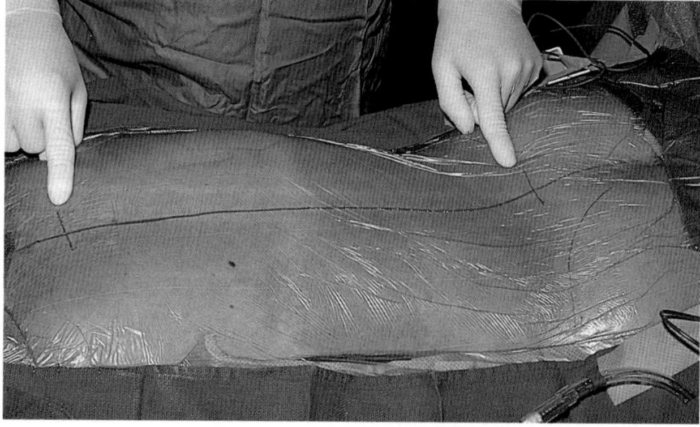

Figure 4. A single incision is drawn with a marking pen centered over the spinous processes at the top and bottom of the spine. It is necessary to extend the skin incision distally to about L2 or L3 in order to use a single incision to resect the ribs. This is different from the two-incision technique published by Dr. Steel (8).

After skin incision, the spinous processes are outlined and the thoracolumbar fascia incised off the spinous process (Fig. 5). In the L2–L3 region, the surgeon must be careful to pick up the very thin layer of thoracolumbar fascia with forceps. Then, using sharp and blunt dissection, this fascia is elevated off the paravertebral muscle fascia, developing a plane by working laterally and proximally at the same time. The thoracolumbar fascia needs to be incised sequentially off the spinous processes as one proceeds proximally (Fig. 6). This is a very easy and identifiable plane in a patient who has not previously had a spinal fusion. It can be tedious and more complex in revision spine surgery, but it can be done. Once the fascia

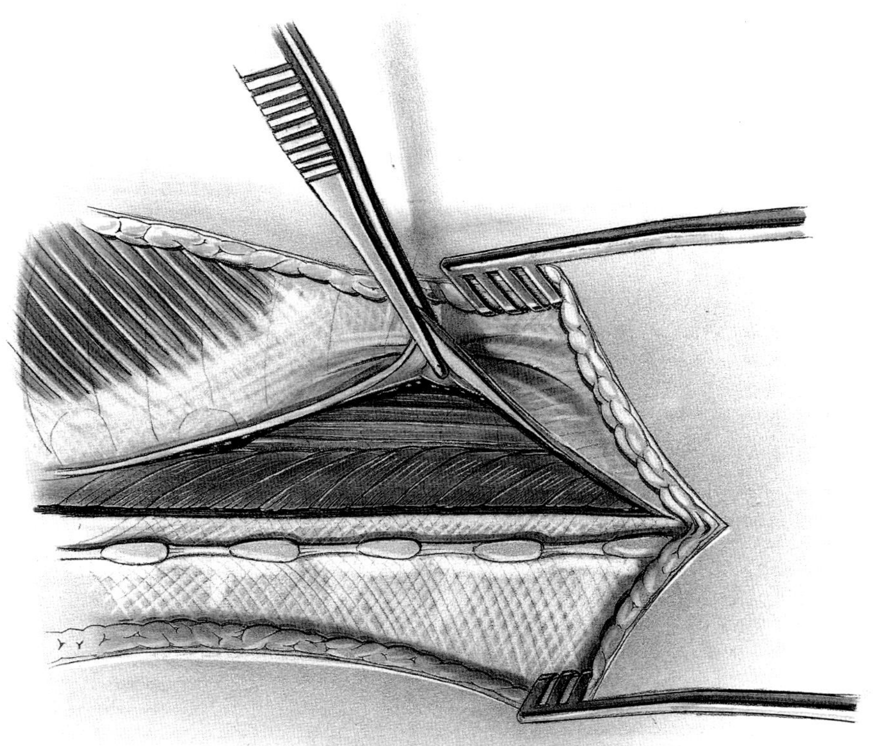

A

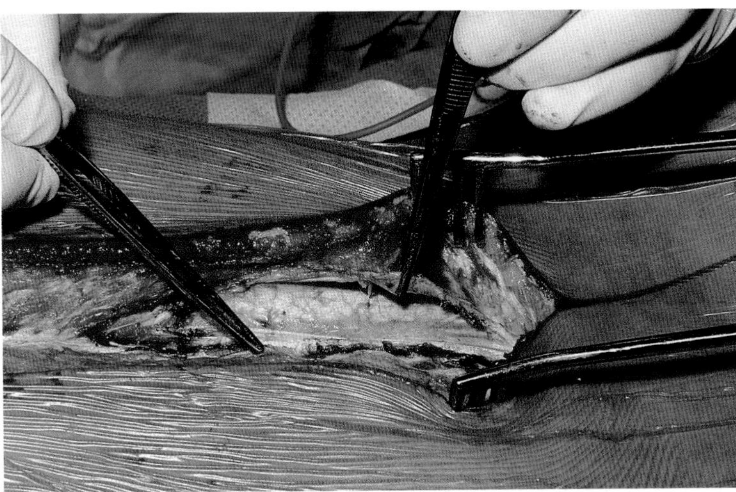

B

Figure 5. A,B: At the distal end of the wound, the thoracolumbar fascia is incised off the spinous process, illustrated here by the fascia held in the forceps of the left hand with the other forceps pointing to the spinous process.

is retracted laterally, two Weitlaner self–retaining spring retractors are used at top and bottom to hold it (Fig. 7). The patient should be told before surgery that some of the sensory nerves to the skin do transfer across this area and will need to be incised during the retraction. The ribs are then palpated, starting at the apex of the deformity (Fig. 8). The most prominent are palpated first, and then, working symmetrically (one distal, one proximal, two distal, two proximal), a symmetrical resection is made (Fig. 9).

The most important part of the procedure is deciding how much rib deformity to resect. The philosophy to keep in mind is that you can always take more rib out, but you can't put it back. Taking too much rib and creating a concavity is worse than leaving residual rib deformity. If the rib deformity is long and six or seven ribs need to be resected, the patient should be told prior to surgery that a second surgery may be necessary. Many factors are out of the surgeon's control, such as the degree to which the rib compresses in when it is cut. Some ribs are very rigid and continue to stick out, but upon resection others immediately lie down flat.

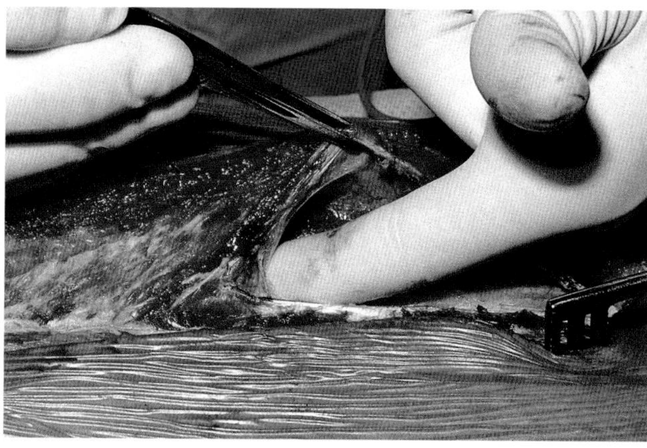

Figure 6. Holding the thoracolumbar fascia elevated, a finger is slipped between the fascia and the paravertebral muscle fascia and used to develop a plane. Using electrocautery, the thoracolumbar fascia is then excised off the spinous processes proximally.

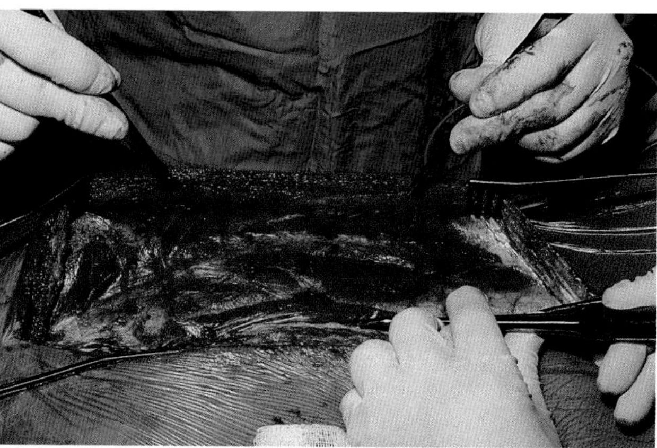

Figure 7. The entire thoracolumbar fascia is then retracted toward the convexity of the curve over the rib deformity.

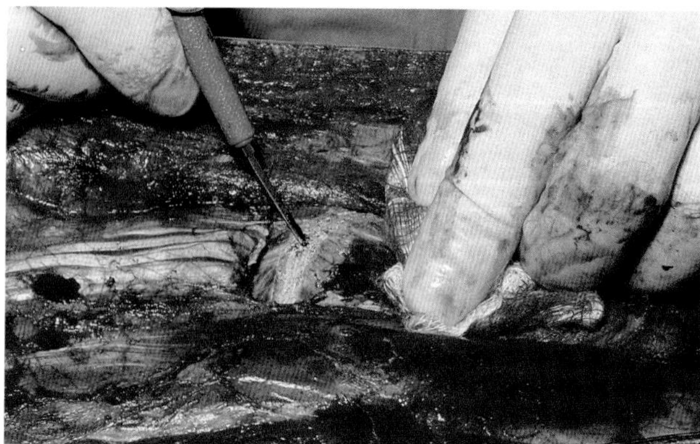

Figure 8. Using electrocautery, the ribs are then palpated and the muscle covering the rib is incised parallel to the rib and through to the periosteum.

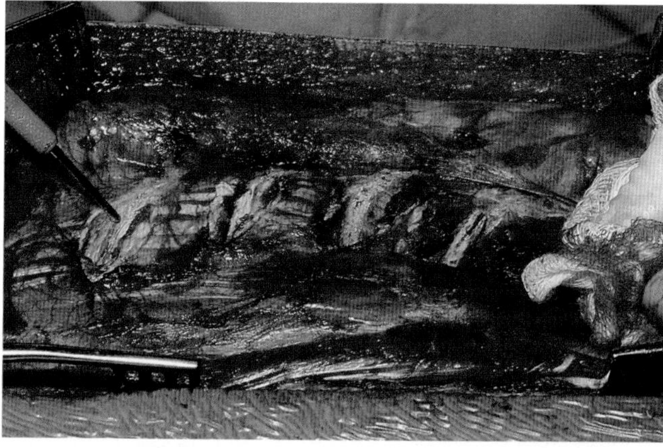

Figure 9. Starting at the center of the rib deformity, the rib is marked and then incision performed by alternating one rib proximal, one rib distal, and then proximal and distal; generally four to six ribs must be incised to correct a rib deformity adequately.

Starting at the center of the deformity, the rib is marked with electrocautery and outlined. Palpating the rib with the fingers, a midline incision is cut into the paraspinal muscles medially. When the four to six ribs are outlined for the periosteal cut, an Alexander elevator is used to pull the periosteum point off the surface of the rib to the lateral edge (Fig. 10). It is very important to pull only on the periosteum and never push with the Alexander elevator, as one would ordinarily do during periosteal stripping. This is to prevent inadvertently slipping off the rib and plunging through the pleura. Once the periosteum is stripped to the side of the rib, the opposite end of the Alexander elevator is used to strip the periosteum and muscle around the inferior edge of the rib (Fig. 11).

Using a Cobb elevator, the periosteum is stripped underneath the rib. It should be done with smooth strokes, medial to lateral, to gain slack on the periosteum before trying to progress underneath the rib. This is the most important time to

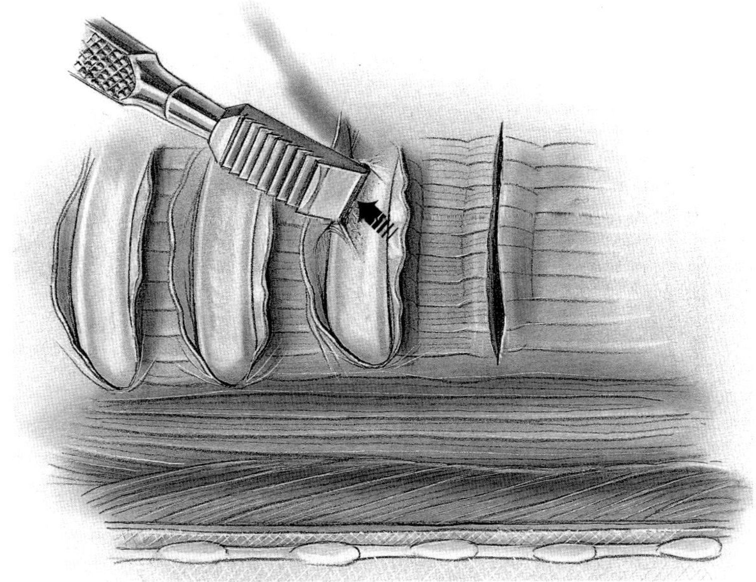

A

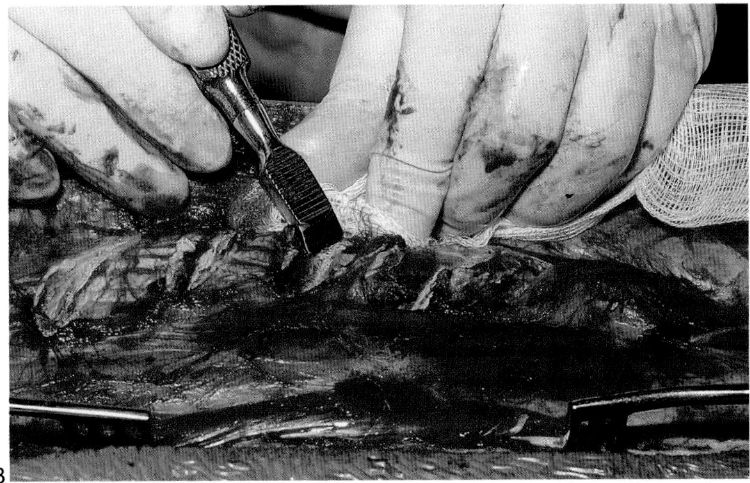

B

Figure 10. A,B: After the ribs are outlined with a Bovie electrosurgical cautery unit, an Alexander elevator is used to pull the periosteum off the rib. It is *very important* to pull the periosteum off the rib (*arrow*) and not to push the periosteum, as with ordinary periosteal stripping. This is to prevent slipping off the rib inadvertently and plunging through the pleura.

be extremely careful to avoid puncturing the pleura. Cobb elevators are used from both sides of the rib: when they finally meet in the middle, a Doyen elevator is passed circumferentially and medial to lateral on the exposed rib (Figs. 12 and 13).

Next, two right-angled retractors are placed on the medial aspect of the rib, pulling back the paraspinal muscle. Using electrocautery and a Cobb elevator, more periosteum is stripped until the medial-most attachment of the rib to the transverse process is identified (Fig. 14). A rib cutter is then passed around the rib and pushed as far medially as possible, right up against the transverse process.

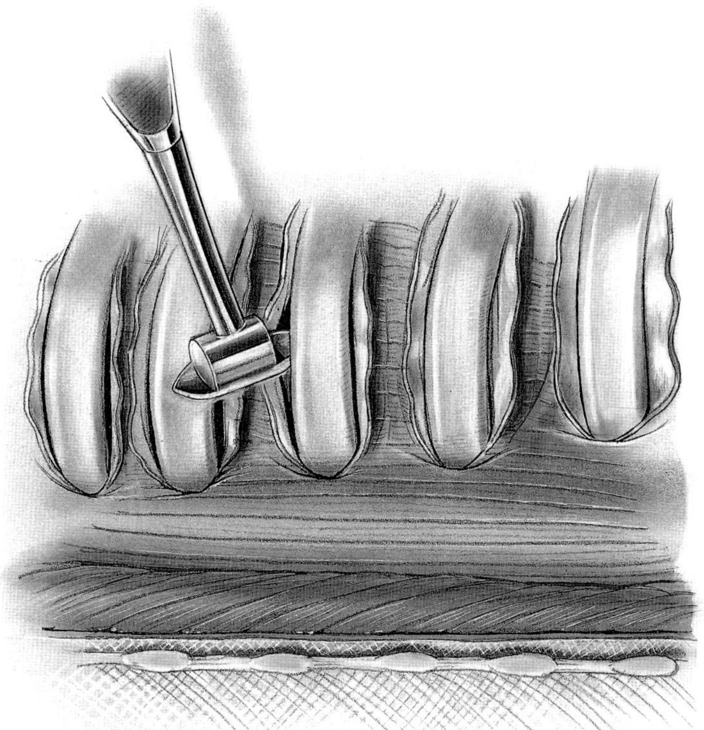

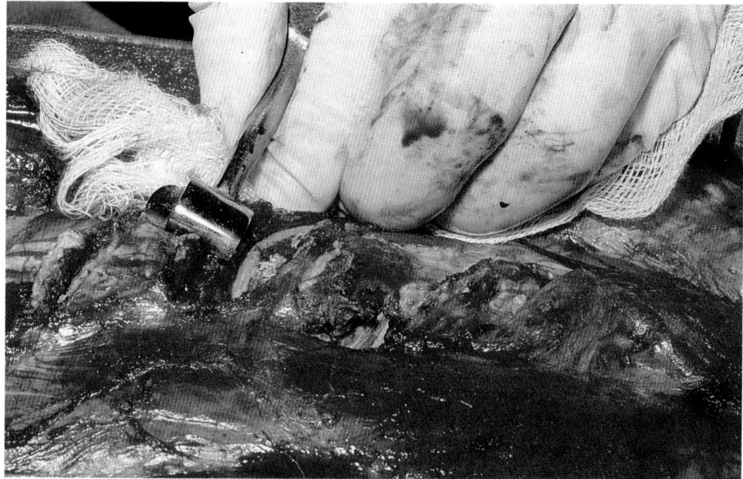

Figure 11. A,B: Once the periosteum is stripped off to the side of the rib, the opposite end of the Alexander elevator is used to strip further the periosteum and muscle around the inferior and superior edge of the rib.

The rib is grabbed with a towel clip or a Kocher clamp to prevent it from plunging through the pleura when it is cut. The rib is then cut medially (Fig. 15), with the plane of the cut as parallel to the floor as possible. (Important note: In Figs. 15 and 16, the camera is now on the opposite side of the patient.)

The rib cutter is now moved so it is at the lateral aspect of the rib. For a standard rib resection with a 55-degree right thoracic curve, 2 cm of rib should be cut for a start (Fig. 16). This is where judgment again comes into play, keeping in mind that it is easy to keep trimming more rib but impossible to put back. Start with 2 cm, come back to that rib, and cut more if it appears necessary. Keep in mind

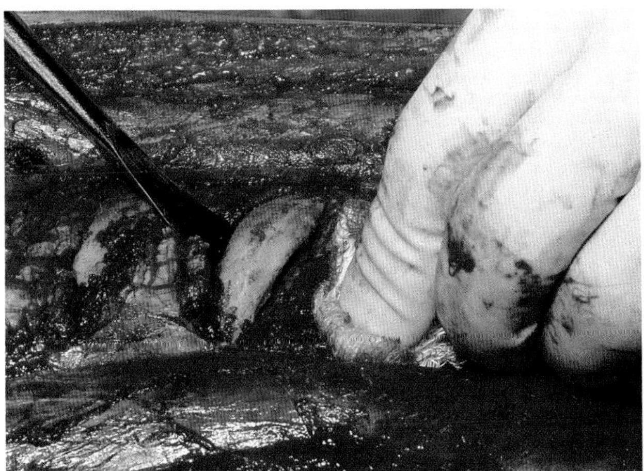

Figure 12. Using a Cobb elevator, the periosteum is stripped underneath the rib. This procedure should be performed in smooth strokes back and forth to gain length on the periosteum. If not, the operator could plunge into one small area.

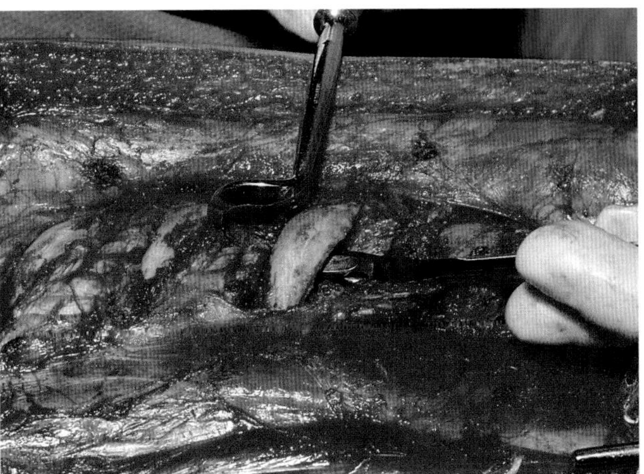

Figure 13. Once the periosteum is stripped, a Doyen elevator is passed with the assistance of a Cobb elevator to guide it. When this is passed circumferentially around the rib, the Doyen elevator is then passed proximally and distally on the rib that is exposed.

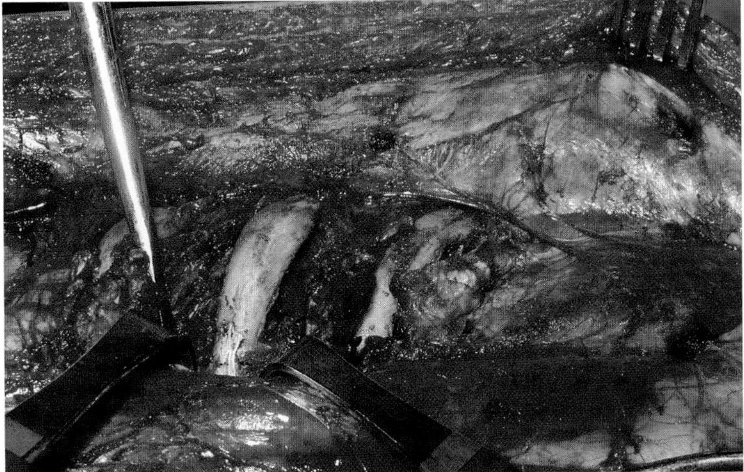

Figure 14. Next, two right-angled retractors are placed on the medial side of the rib and then, using a Cobb elevator, the periosteum is further stripped until the most medial attachment of the rib is identified.

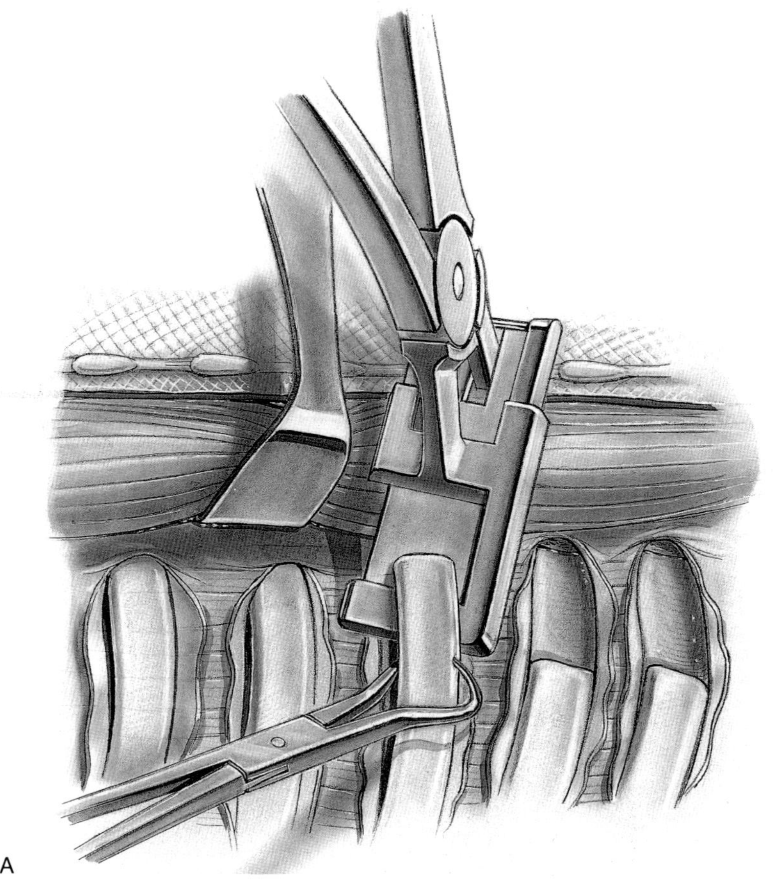

A

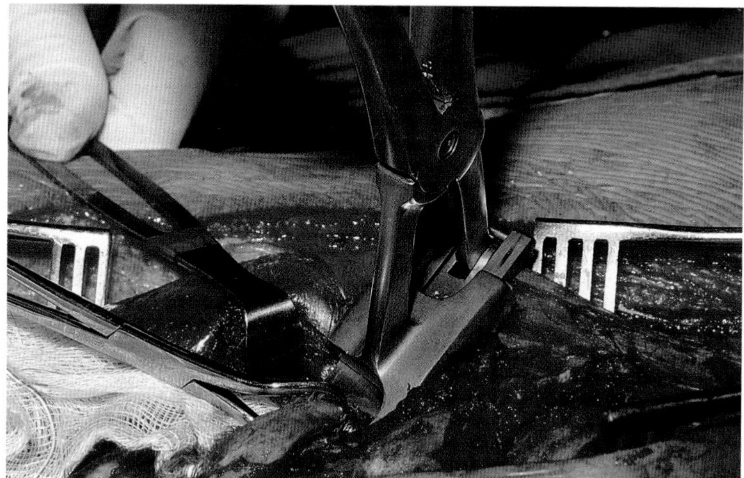

B

Figure 15. A,B: In Figures 15 and 16, the photographer has switched sides to facilitate visualization of rib cutting. A rib cutter is passed around the rib and pushed medially as far as possible. The cut is then made as parallel to the floor as possible and a towel clip used to protect the cut end of the rib from plunging back through the pleura.

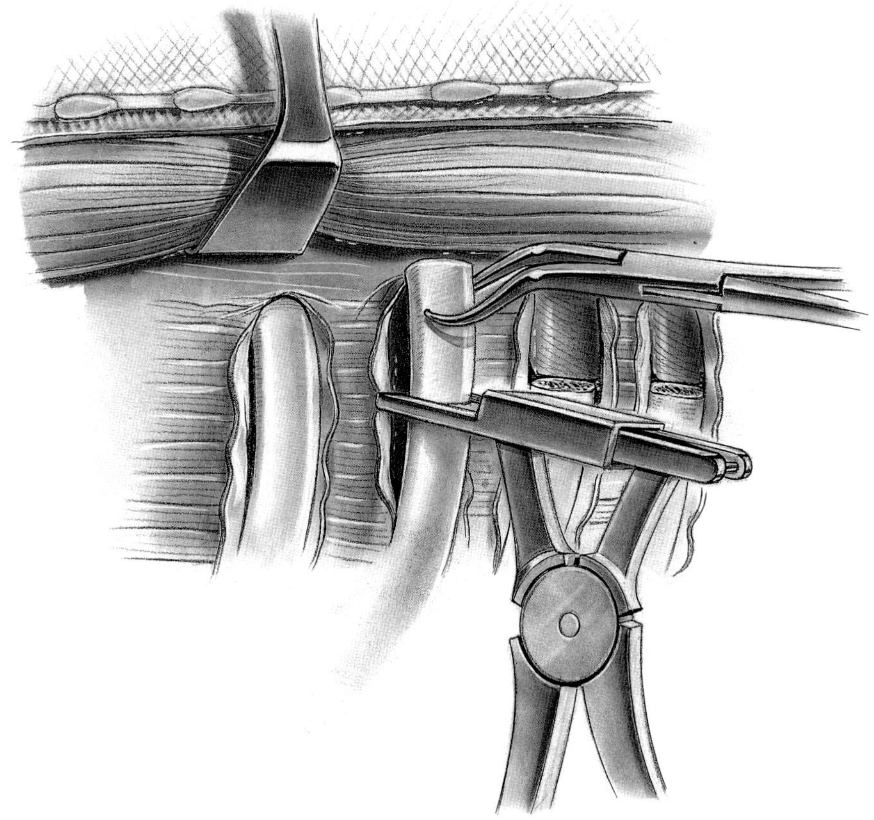

A

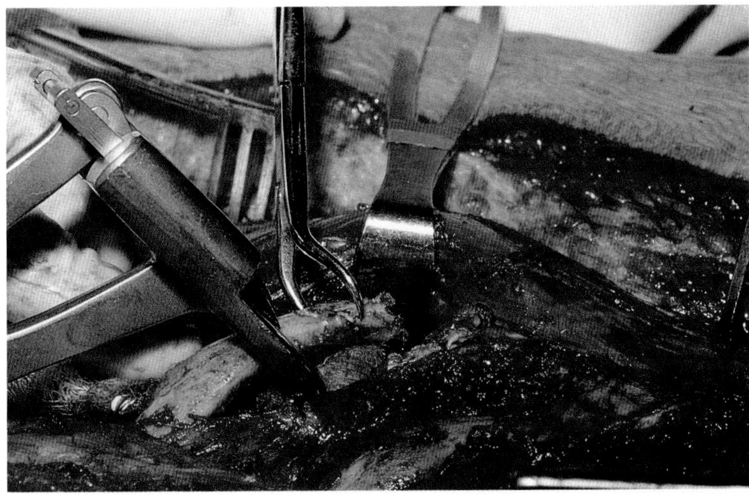

B

Figure 16. A,B: Then the rib cutter is moved so that it can now cut the lateral aspect of the rib. At first, 2 cm of rib is cut. This is where judgment comes into play; as a general philosophy, it is much easier to keep trimming the rib to improve the deformity than to put it back once it has been cut. The biggest fear in taking too much rib is creating a concavity where the original rib deformity was.

that the apex of the curve will translate to the midline of the spine, ultimately leaving a much larger gap than is apparent at the time of the rib resection (Figs. 17 and 18). (This does not apply when the spine is already fused and the operation is a secondary procedure, or if the procedure is done following insertion of the instrumentation.) Bone wax is then applied to the ends of the rib, and Gelfoam is packed into the periosteal bed to assist with hemostasis (Fig. 19). Bone wax is used to seal the ends of bone because of bleeding; it should be remembered that the rib regenerates through the periosteum and not from the ends of the bones, so the bone wax has no inhibitory effect on regeneration of the rib. The additional ribs are then cut in identical fashion; generally, as one goes proximally and distally, less rib is cut. For example, if 2 cm are taken at the apex, then only ½ cm would be taken at the most proximal and distal ribs.

Once the entire resection has been completed, the operating room table is rotated and the edges of the wound carefully lifted so a small pocket is created (Fig.

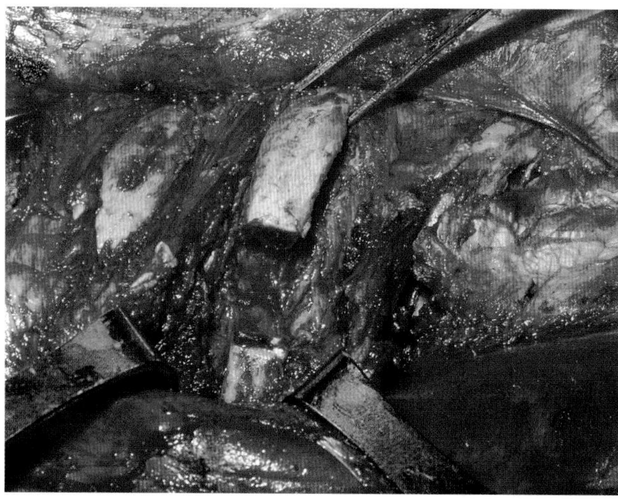

Figure 17. A resected portion of the rib showing the small piece removed. It should be remembered that during instrumentation of the spine, translation of the apex of the curve will displace medially away from the cut edge of the rib, so that in actuality the rib gap is approximately 3 to 4 cm after the spine is corrected.

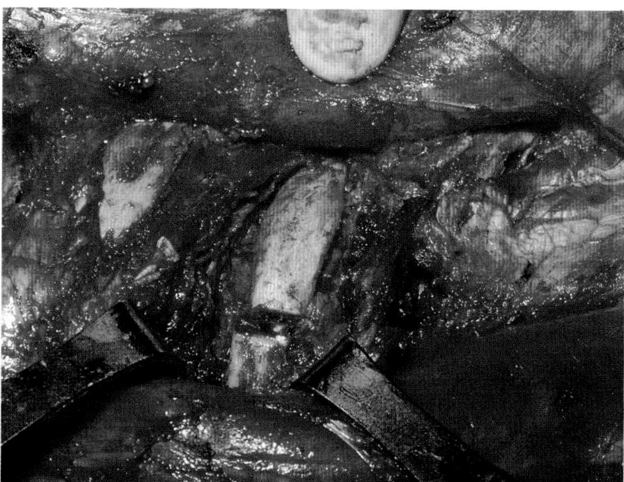

Figure 18. With finger pressure on the thoracic wall, the cut ends of the rib sometimes come together when the spine wound is closed.

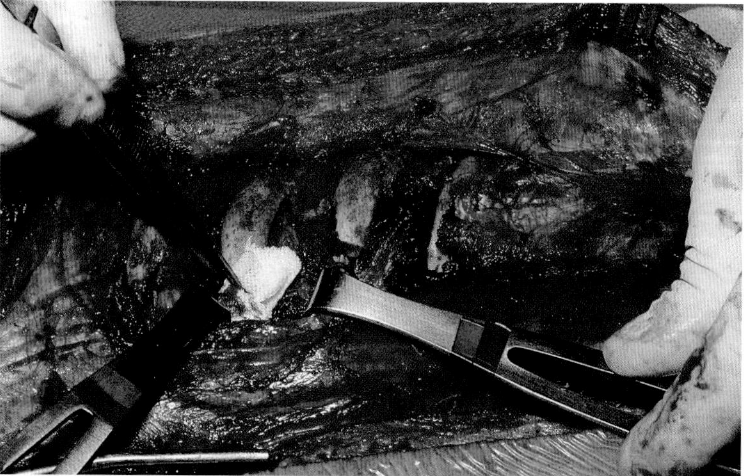

Figure 19. Small pieces of Gelfoam are packed into the rib bed to help with hemostasis.

20). Using a small pitcher (not the bulb syringe), saline is poured into the wound carefully so as not to create any additional air bubbles. The anesthesiologist does a Valsalva maneuver three times to look for a leak in the pleura. (For what to do if a leak is found, see "Complications.")

A Hemovac drain is placed over the resected rib bed. It is important not to suck on the pleura; a hole can easily be made by suction. Using long-acting, absorbable suture, the thoracolumbar fascia is closed with a running suture starting at the distal aspect of the wound (Fig. 21). It may be necessary to incise additional paraspinal muscle fascia off the spinous process to make sure the suture has a hold on the fascia. When closing the incision at the end of the case, a double closure of this area is thus created. It is necessary to close the fascia now so that debris from decortication does not fall into the rib resection area and cause an inflammation. The removed pieces of rib can then be cut into small pieces for use as autogenous graft in the spinal fusion (Figs. 22 and 23). The instruments used

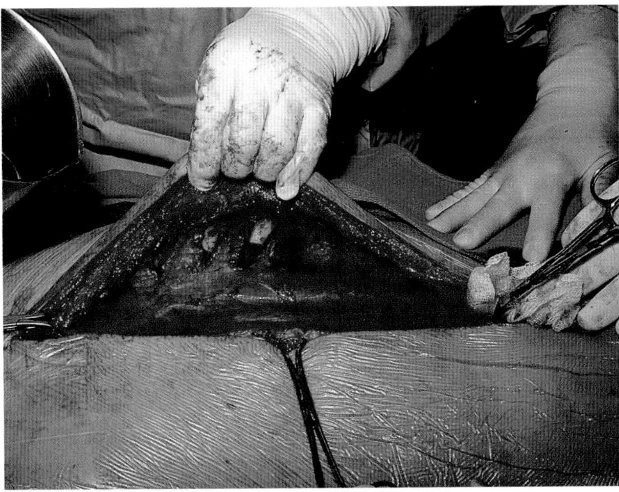

Figure 20. A water test is performed to make absolutely sure the pleura is still intact. To do this, towel clips are placed in order to pull upward on the wound edges. The operating room table is rotated so that a pool of saline in the rib resection area can be sustained. Using a small pitcher, saline is poured into the wound carefully so as not to create any air bubbles. The anesthesiologist does a Valsalva maneuver three times to look for a leak in the pleura. See section entitled "Complications" for what to do if a tear is observed.

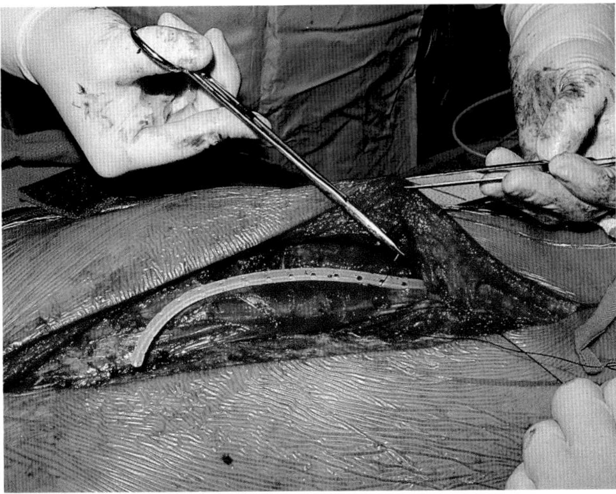

Figure 21. A Hemovac drain is placed over the rib bed, exiting lateral to the spine. Then, using a long-acting absorbable suture, the thoracolumbar fascia is closed with a running stitch, starting at the distal aspect of the wound.

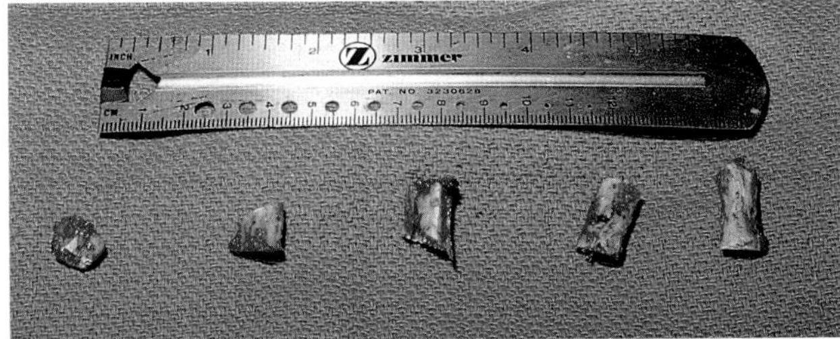

Figure 22. The cut pieces of rib. In this particular case, five small pieces were removed.

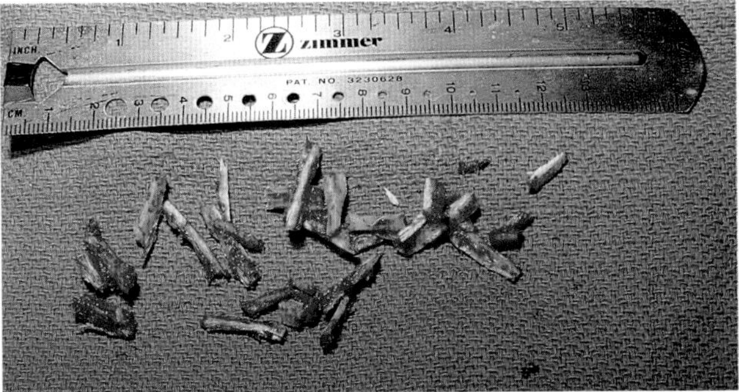

Figure 23. The rib graft is then cut up into small pieces to be used as an autogenous graft for the spine wound.

are shown in Fig. 24, and the postoperative appearance of the wound is shown in Fig. 25.

POSTOPERATIVE MANAGEMENT

Following skin closure and dressing application, a small protective shell is applied over the rib resection area. This shell is essential. It helps avoid a postoperative flail chest and, more importantly, minimizes motion of the cut ribs on top of the pleura and prevents pleural effusion. Historically, in 1985 when we switched from Harrington to Cotrel-Dubousset instrumentation, we briefly stopped utilizing the shell postoperatively. With the Harrington instrumentation, the shell was thought to help prevent dislodgment of the rod while rolling the patient until a cast could be applied. When the shell was eliminated, the first five patients with rib resections and Cotrel-Dubousset instrumentation developed large pleural effusions. We then went back to using the posterior shell for the first 48 hours postoper-

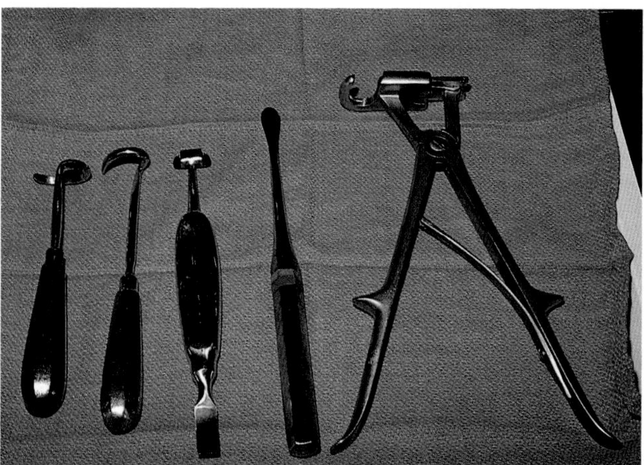

Figure 24. The basic instruments needed for a thoracoplasty, including (from left to right) two Doyen elevators going in opposite directions, an Alexander elevator, a Cobb elevator, and a rib cutter.

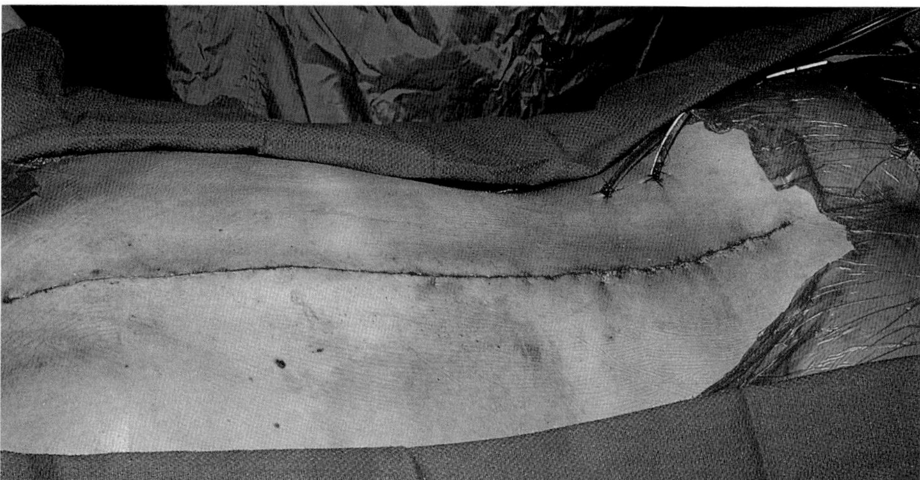

Figure 25. Postoperative appearance of the wound and reduction of the thoracic deformity on the table.

atively, and the problem was eliminated, suggesting that the shell reduces the pleural irritation from the movement of the cut ribs.

The shell can be made of plaster, with foam underneath to protect the skin. The mold is made while the patient is prone on the table but is not applied until the patient is in the recovery room, to prevent a severe plaster burn (which the author has experienced in one case). After a chest radiograph is obtained to rule out pneumothorax and the shell has cooled, it can be applied, wrapping it on with 6-inch Ace wraps (Fig. 26). As an alternative, the posterior shell of a spinal orthosis that was custom made preoperatively can be recycled with Velcro straps and used postoperatively (Fig. 27).

To determine long-term postoperative management, the patient's back is carefully examined 2 days after surgery. If no evidence of flail chest is seen and the rib resection gap is thought to measure less than the width of the palm of the hand, then no prolonged postoperative immobilization is needed. If a larger gap or a flail chest are seen, a postoperative rib protector (posterolateral half of a thoracolumbosacral orthosis) is ordered. The rib protector is worn for 3 months by adolescents and 6 months by adults, generally the amount of time needed for the ribs to heal (8).

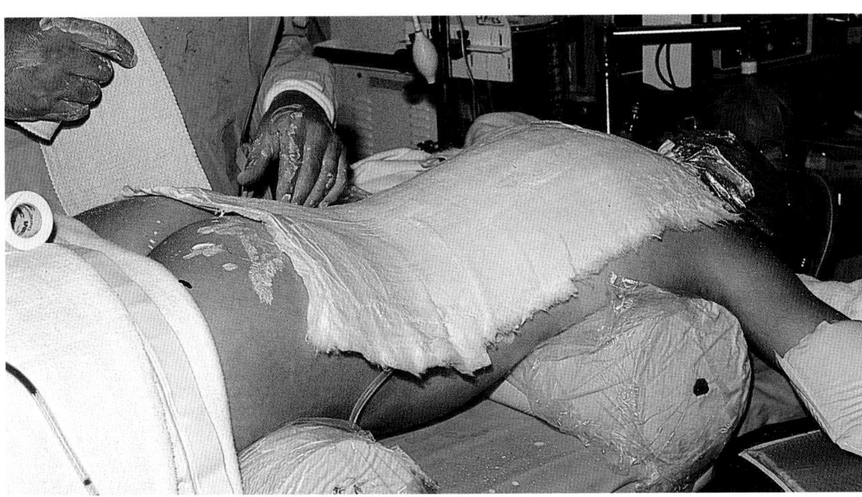

Figure 26. Plaster shell molded to patient, to be held in place with Ace wraps.

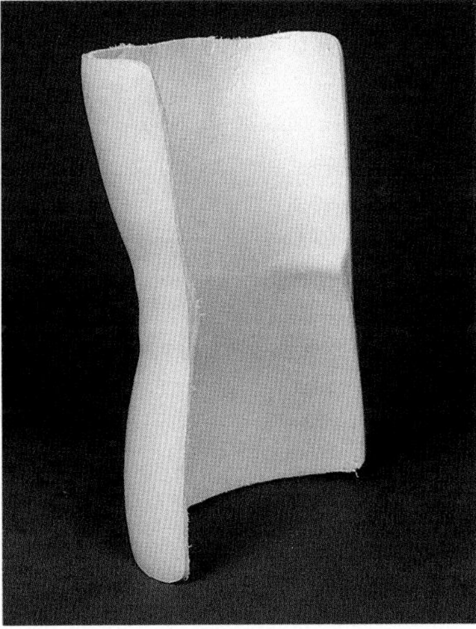

Figure 27. Shell made from used spinal orthosis to be held in place with Velcro straps.

Expectations

The rib prominence should decrease in all patients. It may not be possible to eliminate a large rib prominence completely during the first procedure for fear of producing a concavity (see ''Complications''), and a second rib thoracoplasty may be necessary in the future. Objectively, the postoperative results can be evaluated by obtaining a postoperative rib prominence radiograph; for our studies we score them good, fair, and poor, as seen in Fig. 28. It has been our experience that the rib resection does not increase the pain or prolong the postoperative course following spinal fusion with instrumentation.

COMPLICATIONS

Hole in the Pleura

A hole in the pleura occurs during the rib resection in 5% of patients. *It is extremely important not to attempt to repair the pleura itself.* The hole in the rib bed should be gently packed with Gelfoam and the intercostal muscle sewn in a running suture from the most medial to lateral aspect. As the last sutures are tightened, the anesthesiologist expands the patient's lungs, expressing as much air from the pleural cavity as possible, and the final sutures are tied. The purpose of closing the hole is to prevent blood from seeping into the pleural cavity. An expanding pneumothorax should not occur, as only the parietal pleura is violated and usually not the visceral pleura. Hemovac drains are routinely used. If there is a large hole in the pleura, two Hemovac drains should be placed in the rib resection area and two large drains in the spine fusion area. Of the patients with pleural holes, less than one-half subsequently require chest tubes, so we do not

A
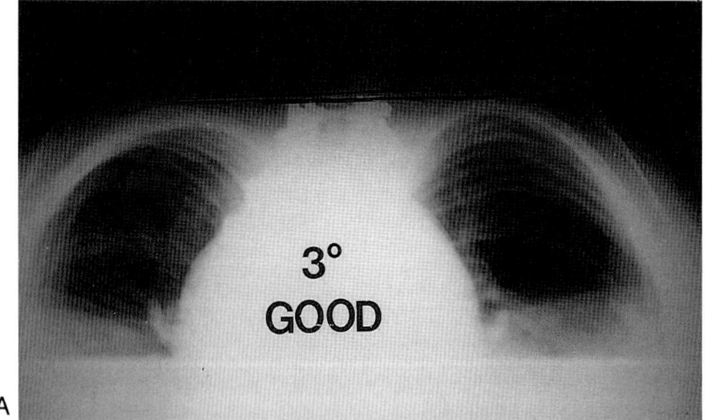

B
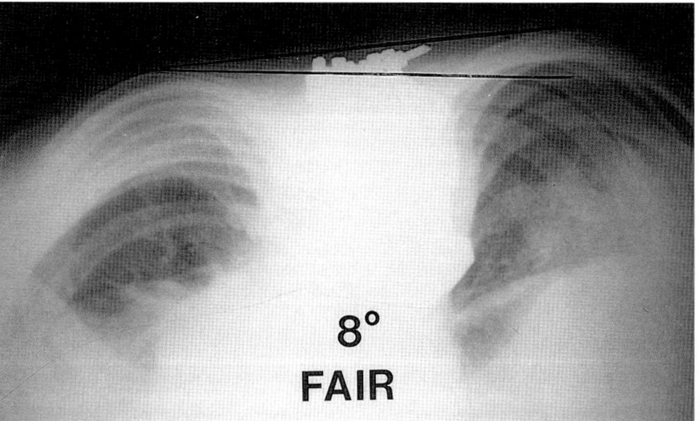

C
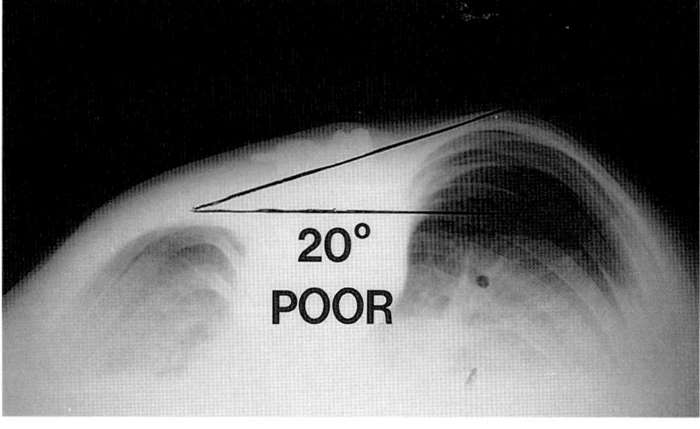

Figure 28. A–C: Examples of good, fair, and poor postoperative results.

routinely place a chest tube for a pleural hole. The patients are observed with daily semierect and lateral decubitus radiographs for 3 days. If fluid accumulates persistently and the patient is symptomatic, then a thoracentesis is performed. If the fluid reaccumulates and a second thoracentesis is necessary, then a chest tube is considered.

Pleural Effusion

On occasion, even without evidence of a pleural hole at the time of surgery, a pleural effusion may develop, most commonly when patients have not worn a protective shell postoperatively. The patient is observed with semierect and lateral decubitus radiographs. For expanding, symptomatic effusion, a thoracentesis is performed and, if it occurs a second time, a chest tube is inserted.

Rib Concavity from too Much Rib Resection

Fortunately, with experience, rib concavity from excess resection rarely occurs. This complication must be prevented at the time of surgery. It is better to do too little rib resection and come back later than to do too much. Eight or 9 ribs should be the maximum taken if resecting less than 2 cm. We try not to resect more than 8 cm in length of any one rib.

Residual Rib Prominence

Residual rib prominence occurs in two scenarios. In the first, a long rib deformity exists, requiring resection of six, seven, or eight ribs; the risk of causing a rib concavity is high. In this situation, it is better to decide that second procedure will be performed later. When the original rib resection area is healing well, a subsequent rib resection is planned for approximately 10 months later. This is really not a complication; it can usually be determined preoperatively and definitely intraoperatively, and the family and patient may be told ahead of time that a second rib resection might be necessary.

In the second scenario, the medial portion of the ribs is prominent and the spine is severely rotated, so that a secondary procedure must be planned. We generally wait 2 years after the original spinal fusion so that the convex rod can be removed from the spine. At this point, the transverse process area of the fusion and the entire medial portion of the rib down to the attachment of the vertebral body can be removed.

Prominent Scapula

In the authors' experience, the inferior medial portion of a prominent scapula (up to 50%) has been removed without causing any functional deficits.

Decreased Pulmonary Function

Although thoracoplasty is a safe and effective method of obtaining cosmetic correction as well as a substantial bone graft source, a consistent decrease in pulmonary function is seen in the early postoperative period, which mandates proper patient selection. In one study, over 6 months average declines of 22% forced vital capacity, 24% forced expiratory volume in 1 second, and 25% total lung capacity were found (L. G. Lenke, personal communication). According to this study, although pulmonary function tests are diminished in the early postoperative period, the results return to near normal at 2-year follow-up.

ILLUSTRATIVE CASE FOR TECHNIQUE

A 13-year-old girl presented with a 57-degree right thoracic curve that was progressive despite bracing (Fig. 29A). On forward bending she had a 17-degree rib

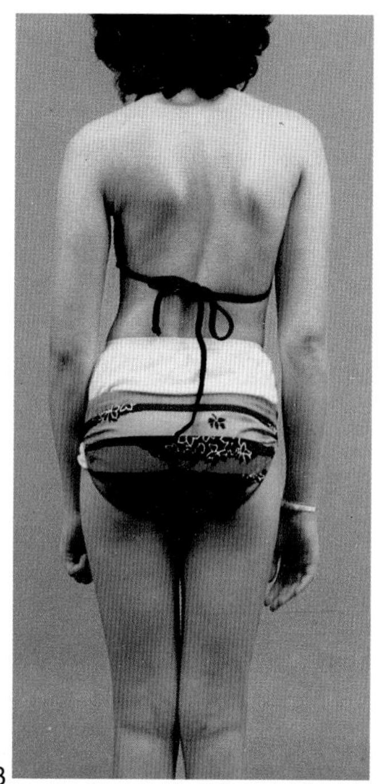
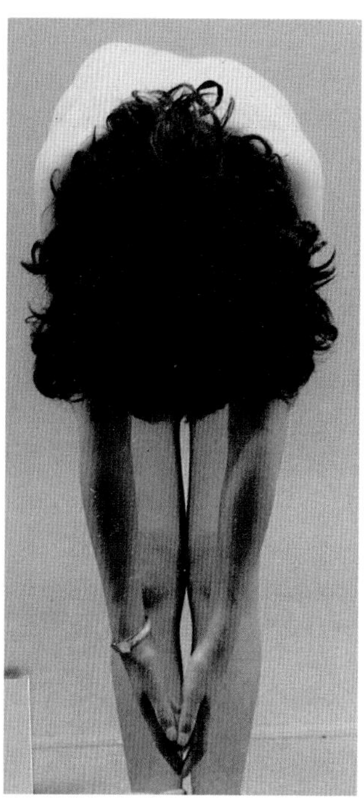
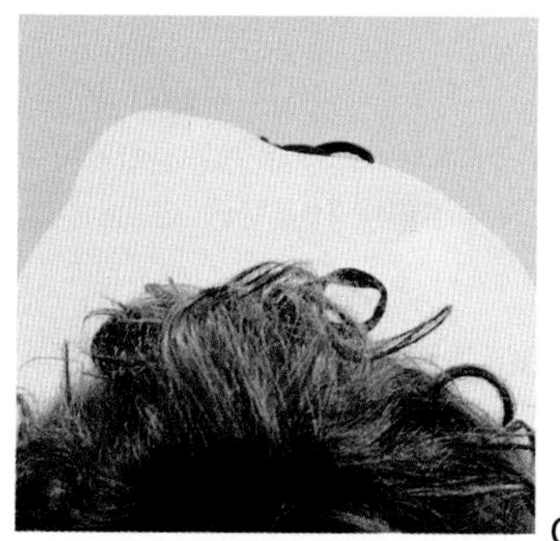
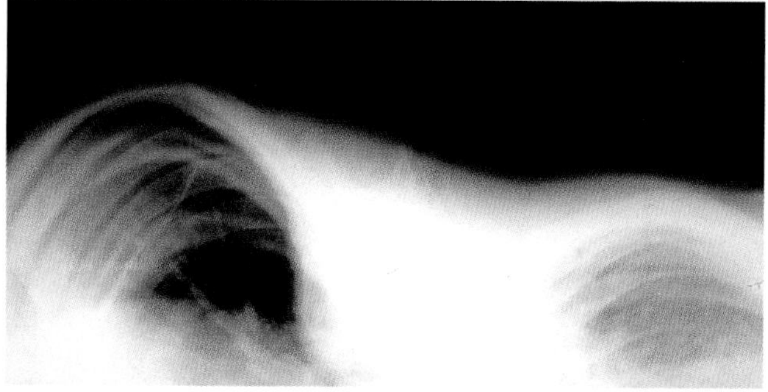

A,B C D

Figure 29. Preoperative photographs **(A–C)** and radiographs **(D)** of illustrative case.

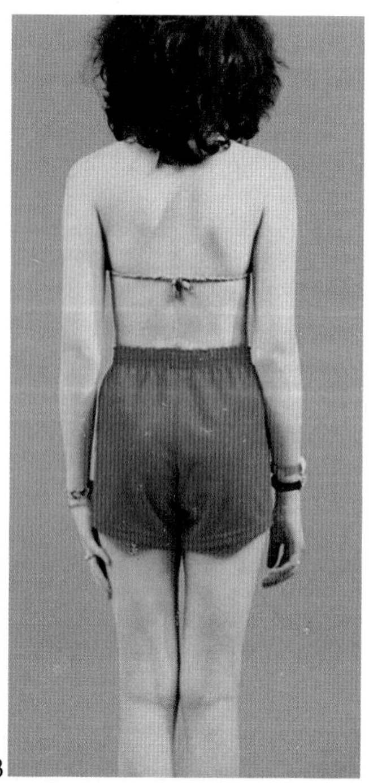
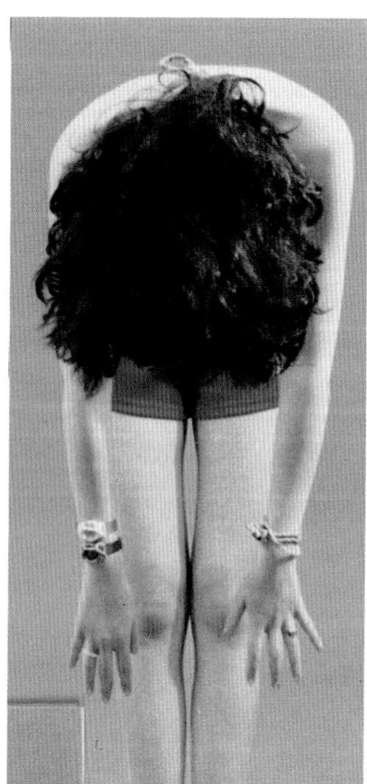
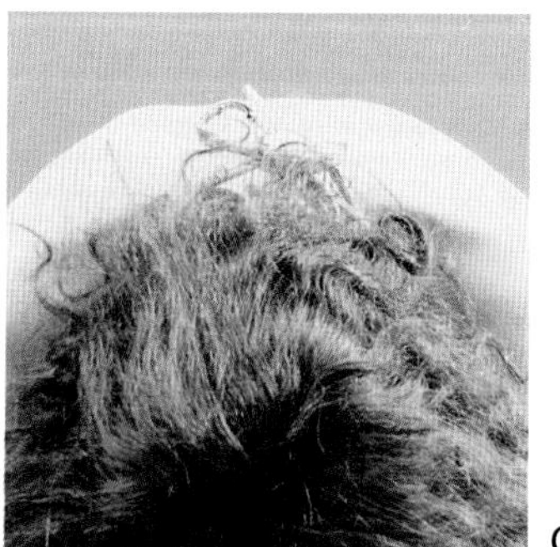
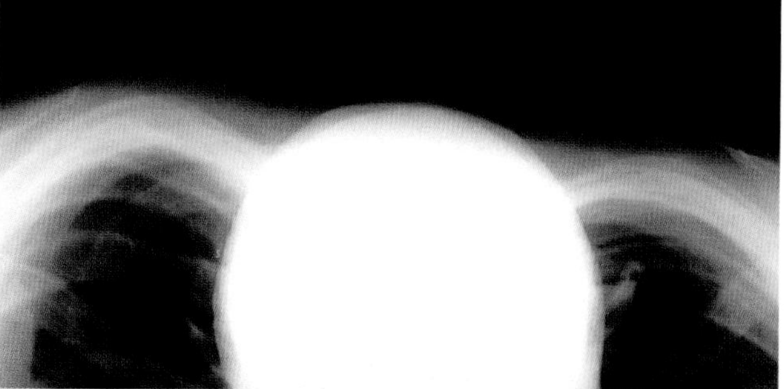

A,B C D

Figure 30. Postoperative photographs **(A–C)** and radiographs **(D)** of illustrative case.

prominence confirmed on both clinical examination (Fig. 29B,C) and radiographic evaluation (Fig. 29D). She underwent a standard posterior spinal fusion with Cotrel-Dubousset instrumentation. At the time of surgery she had five apical ribs resected through a single incision, as described above. Figure 30A–C shows the reduced rib deformity clinically after surgery, along with the radiographic improvement (Fig. 30D). This patient was extremely satisfied and her result was rated as good according to objective and subjective criteria.

Acknowledgment The authors gratefully thank Kathy Goodstein for all the photographs in this chapter, and to Carolyn Hendrix for editorial assistance.

RECOMMENDED READING

1. Barnes, J.: Rib resection in infantile idiopathic scoliosis. *J. Bone Joint Surg.*, 61B: 31–35, 1979.
2. Boachie-Adjei, O., and Bradford D. S.: Vertebral column resection and arthrodesis for complex spinal deformities. *J. Spinal Disord.*, 4: 193–202, 1991.
3. Flinchum, D.: Rib resection in the treatment of scoliosis. *South. Med. J.*, 36: 1378–1380, 1963.
4. Halsall, A. P., James, D. F., Kostuik, J. P., and Fernie, G. R.: An experimental evaluation of spinal flexibility with respect to scoliosis surgery. *Spine*, 8: 482–488, 1983.
5. Harvey, C. J. Jr., Betz, R. R., Clements, D. H., Huss, G. K., and Clancy, M.: Are there indications for partial rib resection in patients with adolescent idiopathic scoliosis treated with Cotrel-Dubousset instrumentation? *Spine* 18(12):1593–1598, 1993.
6. Heisel, J., and Schmitt, E.: Technic and results of rib hump resection in thoracic scoliosis. *Z. Orthop.*, 124: 606–612, 1986.
7. Manning, C. W., Prime, F. J., and Zorab, P. A.: Partial costectomy as a cosmetic operation in scoliosis. *J. Bone Joint Surg.*, 55B: 521–527, 1973.
8. Steel, H. H.: Rib resection and spine fusion in correction of convex deformity in scoliosis. *J. Bone Joint Surg.*, 65A: 920–925, 1983.
9. Thulbourne, T., and Gillespie, R.: The rib hump in idiopathic scoliosis: measurement, analysis, and response to treatment. *J. Bone Joint Surg.*, 56B: 64–71, 1976.

Master Techniques in Orthopaedic Surgery,
THE SPINE, edited by D. S. Bradford,
Lippincott-Raven Publishers, Philadelphia, © 1997.

14

Osteotomy of the Thoracic/ Lumbar Spine

Ronald L. DeWald

INDICATIONS/CONTRAINDICATIONS

Osteotomy by definition is cutting of bone. Cutting the spine bone may be indicated in selective conditions and really implies reestablishing the motion segments of the spine. A motion segment is two vertebrae joined together at the disc bond and the facet joints. The vertebrae have 6 degrees of motion in relation to each other. Osteotomy of the spine implies that this motion segment or multiple motion segments are cut apart to allow motion to recur.

Osteotomy may be indicated anteriorly and/or posteriorly in patients with major spinal deformity with or without severe pain resulting from either acquired conditions (as in scoliosis, kyphosis, trauma, tumor, or infection) or autofusion secondary to ankylosing spondylitis. Congenital scoliosis is a rigid defect, is difficult to correct, and may carry a high risk of neurologic complication. Following osteotomy a patient with idiopathic scoliosis usually has an excellent prognosis after revision surgery. Patients with paralytic scoliosis associated with amyotonia, hypotonia, cerebral palsy, or muscular dystrophy may not be good candidates for revision surgery.

Patients who have minimal deformity and/or little pain as well as those with severe osteoporosis would be contraindicated for revision surgery with osteotomy.

PREOPERATIVE PLANNING

Before assessing spinal deformity that requires osteotomy, the surgeon must understand normal three-dimensional spinal anatomy. Normal coronal alignment

R. L. DeWald, M.D.: Division of Spinal Surgery, Department of Orthopaedic Surgery, Rush Medical College, Chicago, Illinois 60612.

is straight. The stable zone in the coronal plane extends superiorly from the two lumbosacral facets. Sagittal alignment follows the sagittal vertical axis line. This line falls from C2, in front of T7, behind L3, and across S2. The individual vertebrae are neutral or they are ventrally or dorsally oriented. In the lumbar spine L4 and 5 are ventrally oriented, L3 is neutral, and L1 and 2 are dorsally oriented (Fig. 1). In the lumbar spine it is important to note factors such as the maximum lordosis, which is usually measured from the superior end plate of L1 to the superior end plate of S1, and ranges from 32 to 84 degrees with an average 50 degrees, and the sacral slope, which is measured from the superior S1 end plate to the horizontal, ranges from 18 to 66 degrees, and averages approximately 40 degrees. Disc contribution to the maximum lordosis is generally 80% (Fig. 2).

After reviewing normal anatomy, study the patient and the radiographs. Anteroposterior (AP) and lateral standing radiographs of the entire spine are examined for balance, orientation of vertebrae, pseudarthrosis, and degenerative changes. The stable zone is inspected and the sagittal vertical axis line is drawn. The side-bending, flexion-extension, spine, and prone films are all studied to analyze how each vertebra is to be restored to normal spatial alignment (Fig. 3).

The problem requiring correction is usually one of balance. Coronal balance is not as severe a problem as sagittal balance, nor is it as noticeable. The surgeon must devise a surgical plan with a goal of balancing the spine, taking in consideration the following:

Same-day, staged, or simultaneous surgery: This judgment must be made during a planning session. If osteotomy and intercurrent traction are required, staged surgery is necessary. Same-day surgery is preferable to staged surgery because the recovery is faster and the patient's nutrition better. On occasion, simultaneous surgery is needed, if both columns are to be osteotomized and fused. Generally this procedure is used when the spine is in kyphus and the desire is to place the lumbar segments into lordosis. The patient is placed in the lateral decubitus position to allow the surgeons to work simultaneously both anteriorly and posteriorly.

Predicted blood loss: Significant blood loss can be expected, and replacement with the patient's own blood is preferred. Correct positioning on a four-poster frame or the knee-chest position with a free abdomen is valuable for control of blood loss as well as for correction of the osteotomized spine. We routinely use a cell saver. We always reinfuse the patient's cells as well as the patient's own fresh-frozen plasma.

Length of time of surgery: The length of time required for surgery must be considered in planning the number of operations to be done. Surgical team fatigue is a consideration. Same-day surgery is preferred, but to start a second stage after 6 to 7 hours of surgery is not in the patient's best interest.

Rigidity of deformity: By review of all the previous radiographs, the surgeon will be able to sense the rigidity of the deformity and to determine what can be accomplished by revision surgery. Although the surgeon will probably not be able to make the patient better than the improvement seen on the original side-bending films, sagittal plane balance may be improved regardless of the rigidity of the deformity.

Bone quality and bone graft availability: Osteoporosis limits the amount of force that a surgeon can apply to correct the deformity. Autogenous bone is preferred; however, if it is unavailable, irradiated allograft bone is suitable for spinal fusion.

Age and health: Special attention must be paid to the age and health of the patient. Some chronic pain patients are chemically dependent, addicted, and have poor nutrition. It is better to rehabilitate these patients physically, mentally, and nutritionally before undertaking revision spinal surgery. In some cases, concurrent medical problems can rule out spinal surgery.

Once the plan is devised, the patient must be adequately counseled about risks, hazards, and expected results. Clearly the benefits to be gained must outweigh

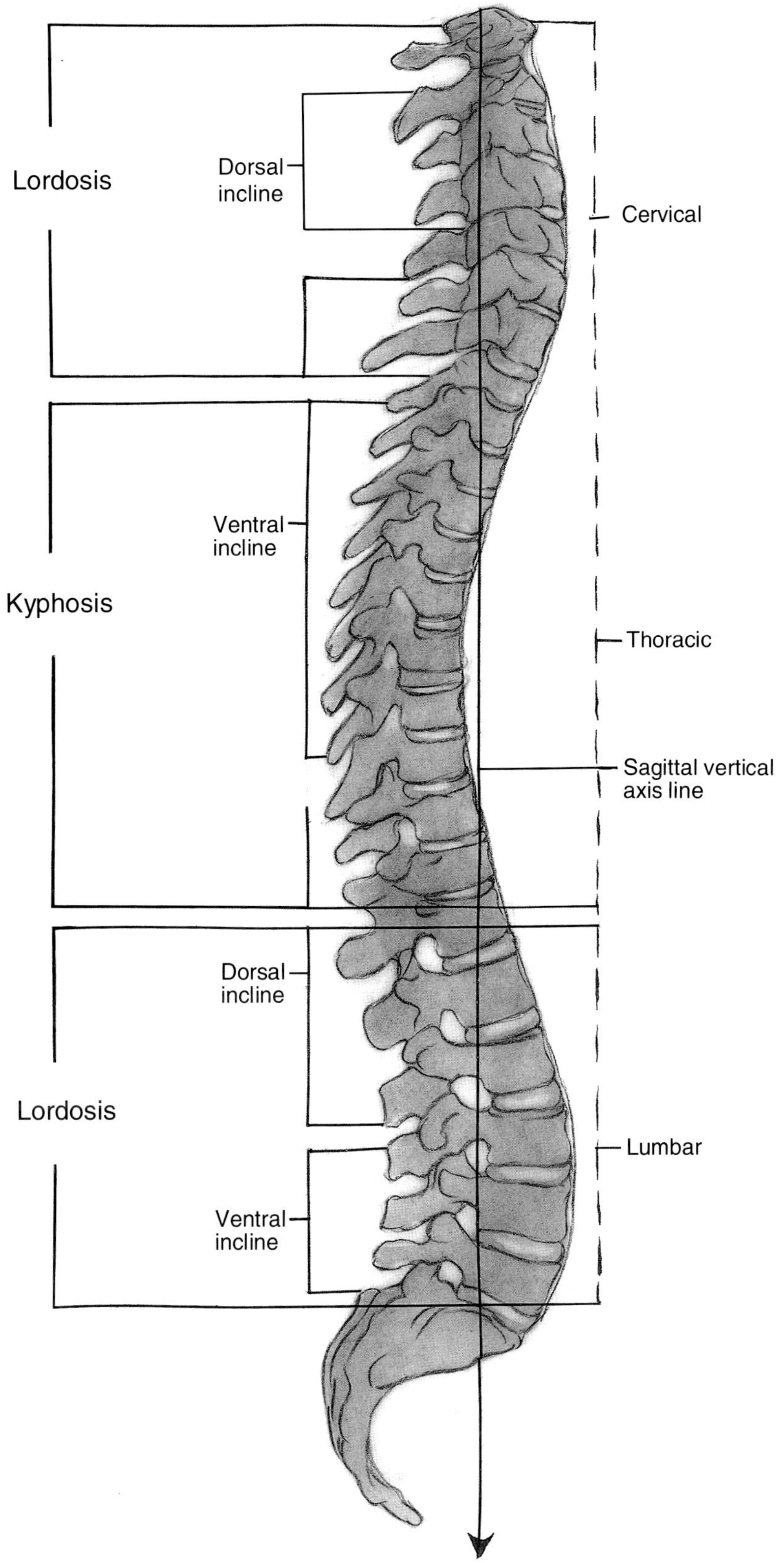

Figure 1. Sagittal alignment of the spine and the sagittal vertical axis line that falls from C2, in front of T7, behind L3, and across S2. The inclination of each vertebra (dorsal or ventral) is also shown. Note that L3 is neutral.

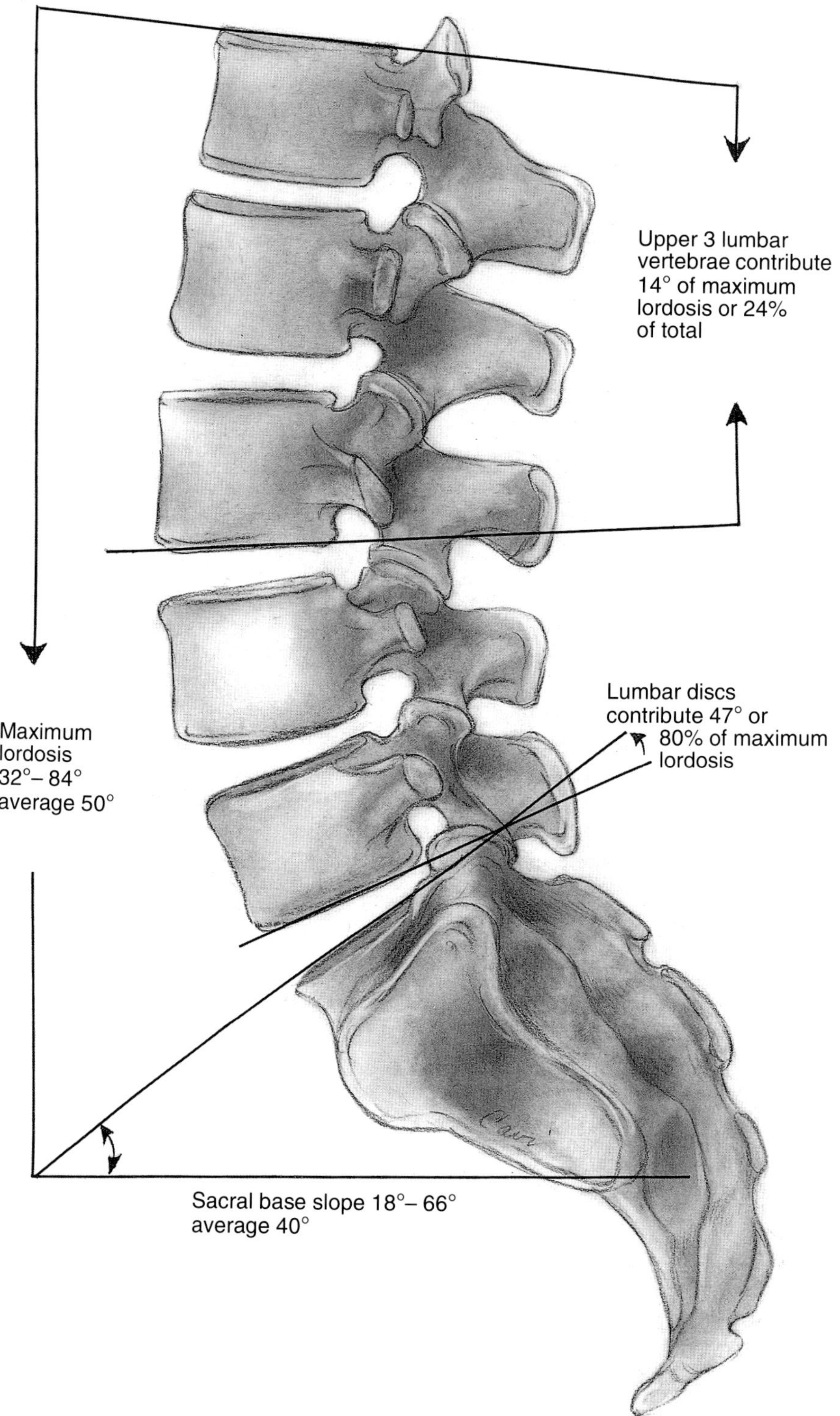

Figure 2. Extension of the previous illustration, showing maximum lordosis and its range. Maximum lordosis is measured from superior L1 to superior S1. The sacral slope is measured from superior S1 to the horizontal. Note how much the discs contribute to the overall lumbar lordosis. The upper three lumbar vertebrae of the disc constitute only 24% of the maximum lordosis.

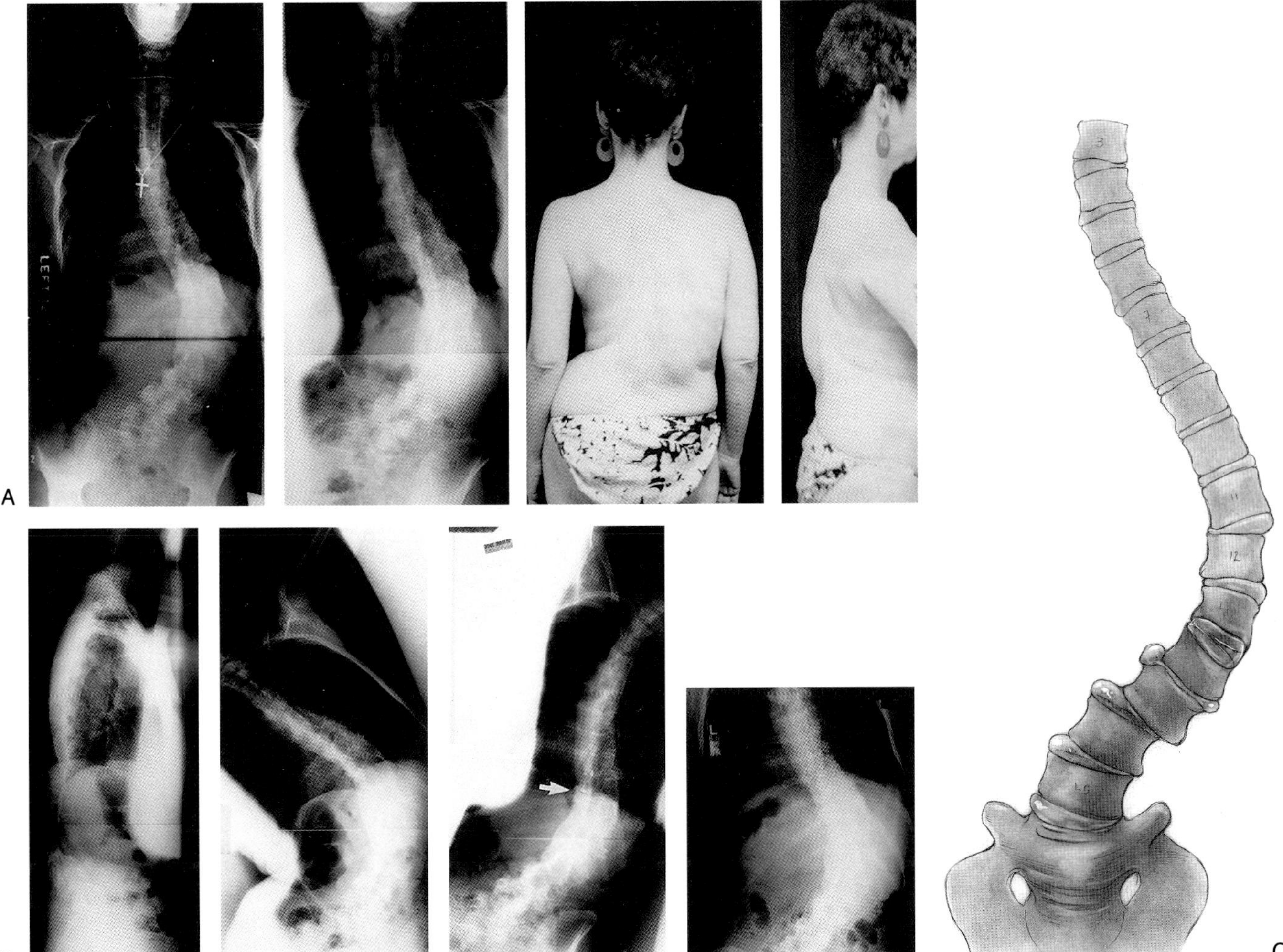

Figure 3. Photographs and radiographs from an obviously very deformed scoliotic patient. The most evident problem is coronal balance. Note the change that has taken place between the 1985 **(A)** and 1992 **(B)** AP radiographs. Note the staircase effect of the lateral subluxation of L3 on L4 and L4 on L5. Note the distance between L3 and the iliac crest in 1985 and in 1992 and also the staircase effect, representing the lateral subluxation. The area that had been fused can be easily identified (T9–L2). An obvious pseudarthrosis can be identified at T10 and T11. A not-so-obvious pseudarthrosis is present at L2–L3 and L3–L4. By comparing bending and upright radiographs, the surgeon can judge the mobility of the lumbar spine. The bending films indicate the degree of mobility as well as where and how many osteotomies must be performed. T11, T12, and L1 are in a fairly straight line. If the ends of the fusion are osteotomized the balance of this patient may be improved. A cognitive plan must be developed.

the risks and hazards encountered in performing the surgical treatment. This is especially true if the surgery would be a two- or three-part staged procedures.

SURGERY

Somatosensory evoked potential (SSEP) monitoring is employed. On occasion neuromotor evoked potentials (NMEP) may be utilized. Controlled hypotensive anesthesia is used along with a cell saver. It is important to know the hematocrit of the cell saver aliquot to judge red blood cell replacement. We routinely use autologous blood and autologous fresh-frozen plasma. The fresh-frozen plasma helps to correct any coagulopathy that may occur using cell saver.

Posterior Osteotomy of the Lumbar Spine

Whether it is acquired or developmental, a previously fused spine may be osteotomized; the procedure is similar in the thoracic or lumbar spine. The acquired fused spine is much more difficult to osteotomize than the developmental fused spine because all the previous anatomic landmarks are gone. The surgeon must use all senses to become and stay oriented.

I prefer the patient positioned in the knee-chest position (Fig. 4). This allows the pelvis to rest on the femoral heads, and, if necessary, the pelvis-spine relationship can be altered by pivoting the pelvis on the femoral heads. In essence, you will be changing the sacral slope, which is defined as the angle between the superior end plate of the sacrum to the horizontal.

Surgical Procedure. The approach is always midline and the spine and previous fusion are exposed from the tip of the transverse process to the tip of the transverse process. The telltale transverse process and any previous implants help to identify levels and the area for osteotomy. If hooks, screws, wires, or rods are present, they will help to identify the vertebral level and often the old intralaminar space also. Frequently a pseudarthrosis is found, which will usually follow through the old facet joint. In scoliosis, the rotation of the spine must be respected as well as the adaptive changes of the vertebrae. Complete exposure is essential.

The next step is to find the spinal canal (Fig. 5). Again, previous implants can help. The implant is removed, and the canal can be located. Using gentle dissection, the dura can be mobilized and the bone removed using a Kerrison rongeur. The osteotomy line is in the shape of a chevron, with the base inferior and the ends going across the old inferior facet to the intervertebral foramen. Sometimes

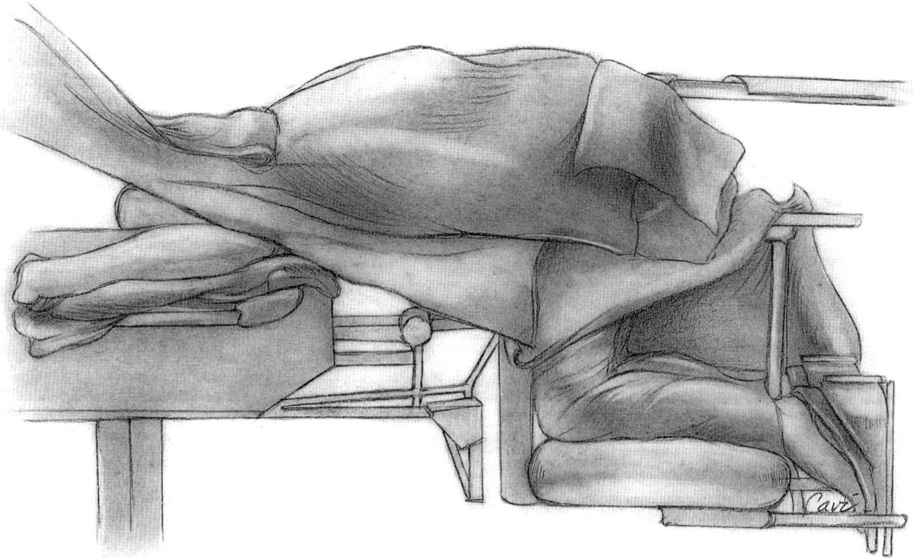

Figure 4. A patient in the knee-chest position. Note that the hips are flexed to 95 to 100 degrees. The chest is on the torso support, and the sternal notch can be palpated. The foot and ankle are held with positioners that allow pressure to be distributed across the length of the tibia. The pelvis is held with a trochanteric clamp. The tibial rest can be adjusted to increase or decrease the lumbar lordosis.

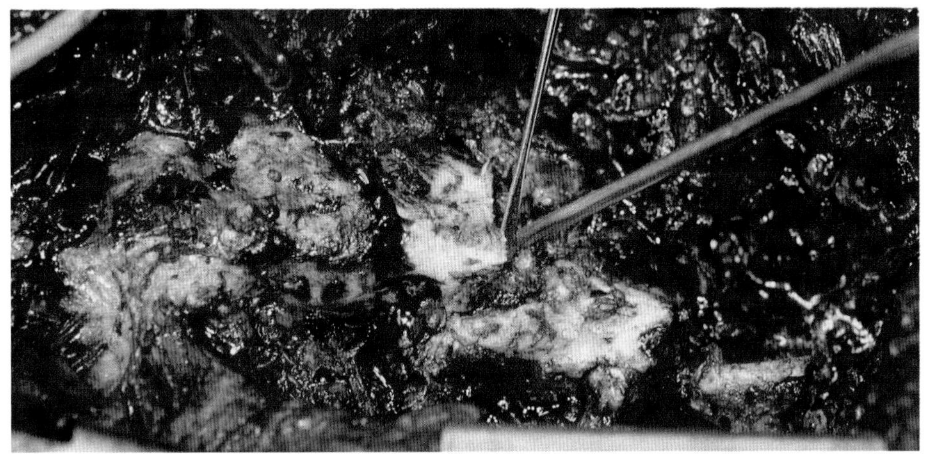

A

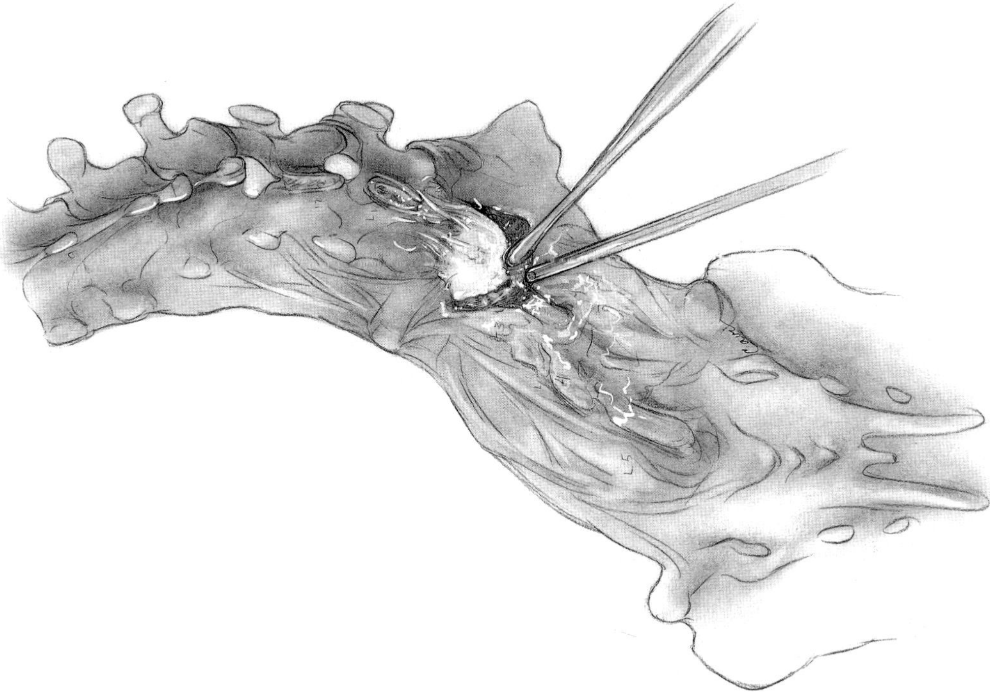

B

Figure 5. A: Operative field of the patient seen in Fig. 3. The patient is prone in the knee-chest position on the previously illustrated table. The head is to the left and the feet are to the right. A large thick fusion mass is seen on the left side of the picture. The Penfield probe is in the midline of the neural canal between L2 and L3. The photographer is standing just above the surgeon's left shoulder so the view is almost identical view to that of the surgeon. The same position is maintained throughout this series of photographs. **B:** Illustration showing the Penfield probe and the suction tip. Note that previously operated spines are very difficult to recognize. The surgeon must use every effort to become and stay oriented.

a bur is needed. (Fig. 6) If no deformity is present, the procedure moves rapidly; on occasion the surgeon can identify the neural foramen laterally and work both sides of the fusion (Fig. 7).

In a deformity case, the procedure is more difficult, since the vertebra is rotated and the pedicles are at different positions. The key here is to know which transverse process belongs to which transverse process and to be sure your osteotomy

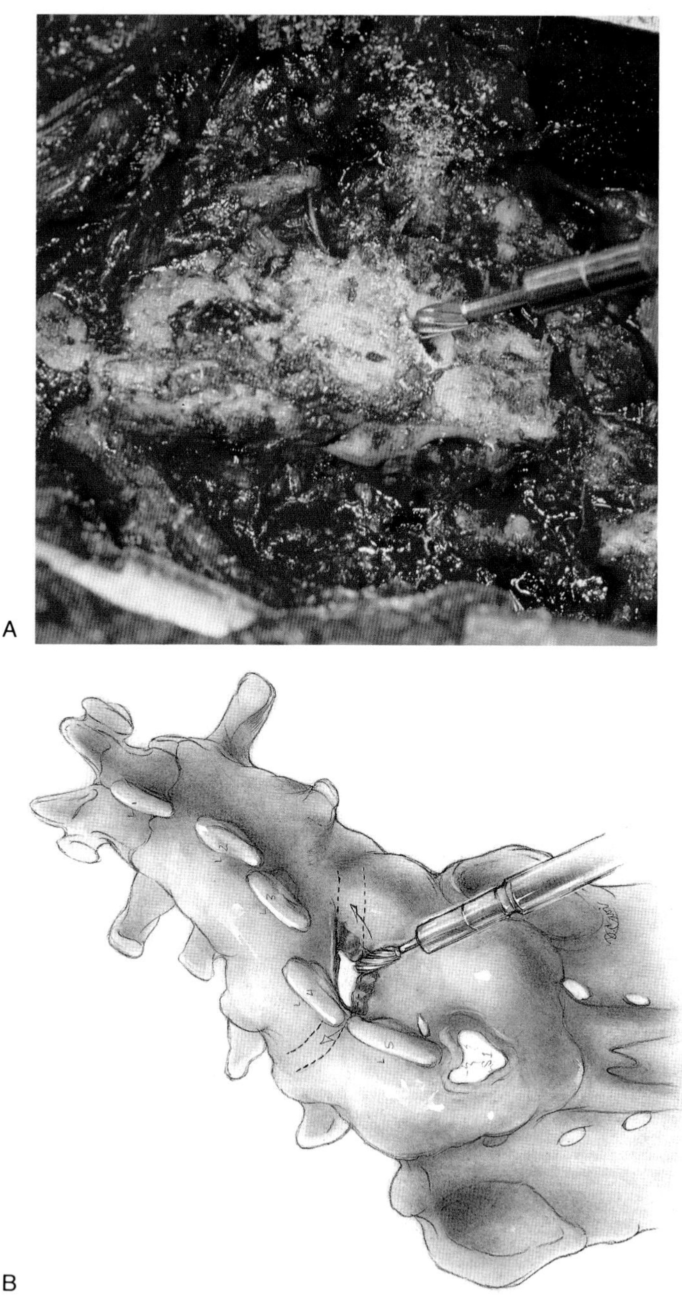

Figure 6. A,B: The beginning of the osteotomy using the Midas Rex bur. The tips of the transverse processes are identified and the osteotomy is shaped like a chevron. It should be about 7 mm wide. The osteotomy must be between the correct transverse processes. Note how the previously operated spine distorts the anatomy.

is at the correct level. The midline canal is identified. The neural foramen can be found.

If the lumbar spine is flat as you perform the osteotomy, the spine will fall into lordosis. For this reason we perform the procedure unilaterally and then do the opposite side secondarily. We use a vertebral spreader to maintain the position of the vertebrae until the osteotomy is complete (Fig. 8). We undercut the osteotomy before we allow it to fall into lordosis to prevent nerve crush. Sometimes (if using pedicle fixation) it may be easier to place the pedicle screw before the spine falls into lordosis. If a scoliotic component exists, it is necessary to place the convex screw first, use a bent rod, and roll the spine into lordosis. The concave screws

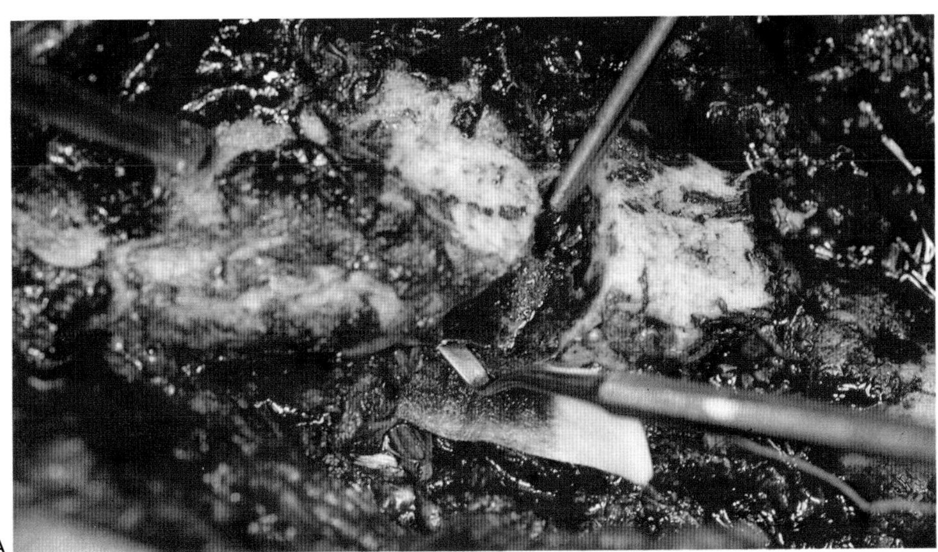

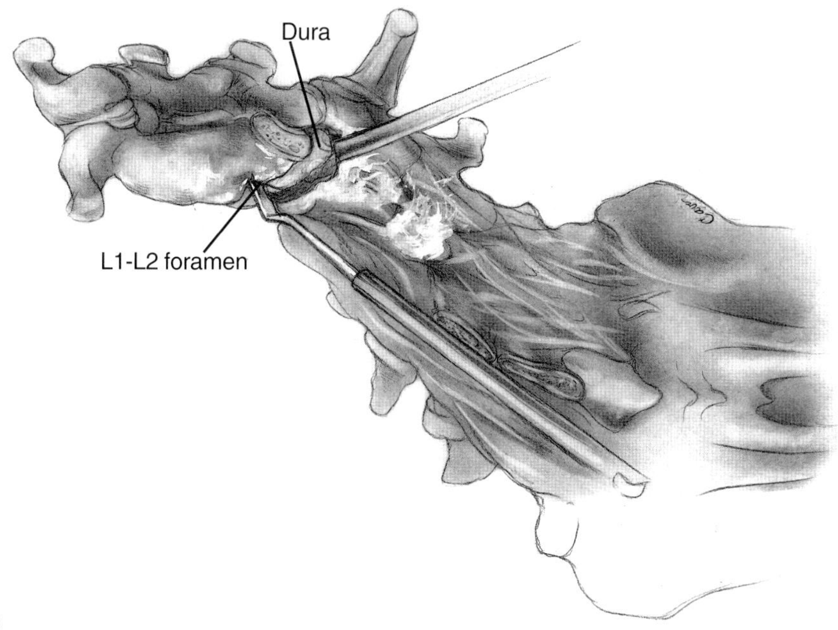

Figure 7. Surgical view **(A)** and illustration **(B)** of the location of the intervertebral foramen by the Woodson dissector. It is now possible to work from the midline out to the intervertebral foramen or the other way around.

can then be placed with greater ease since the insertional angle of the screw will not be as great (Fig. 9).

Once the location of the cut is identified and the canal located, it is possible to sense the thickness of the fusion mass and its maturity. Sometimes it may be necessary to use a Midas Rex bur. Great care must be taken to avoid damage to the neural structures. The use of the Midas Rex bur down to the opposite cortex is frequently helpful. The opposite cortex can be identified as a white bone compared with the red cancellous bone. Once this is found the Kerrison rongeur is used to remove the remaining thin piece of bone. The dura must be gently teased away before proceeding. This may be difficult if a wire or hook has been in the canal previously. Frequently many adhesions are present. The surgeon must be prepared at all times to repair or patch a dural leak. The Midas Rex bur does not allow you to save the bone for graft. Otherwise all bone removed during the osteotomy is saved for use later as autogenous graft. Once the osteotomies have been performed and the spine falls into lordosis, coronal plane correction can be performed.

A

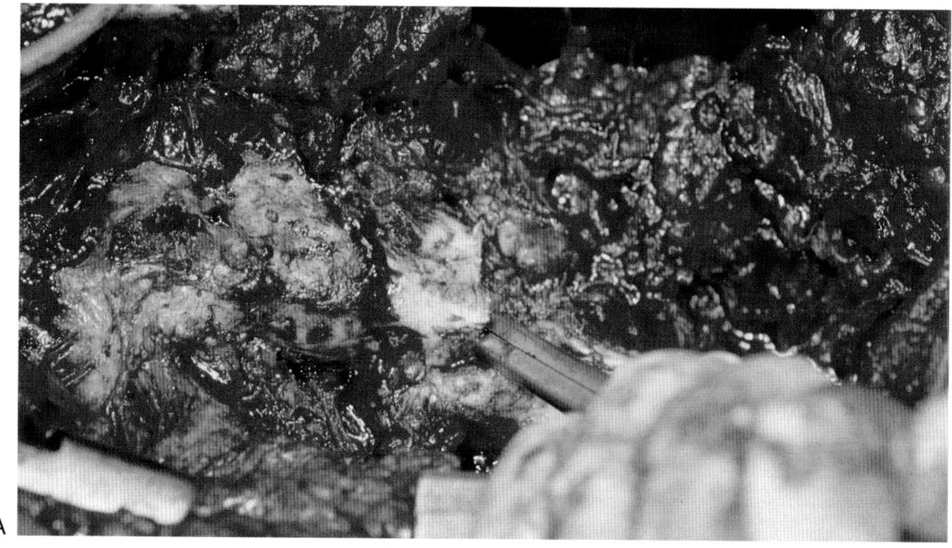

B

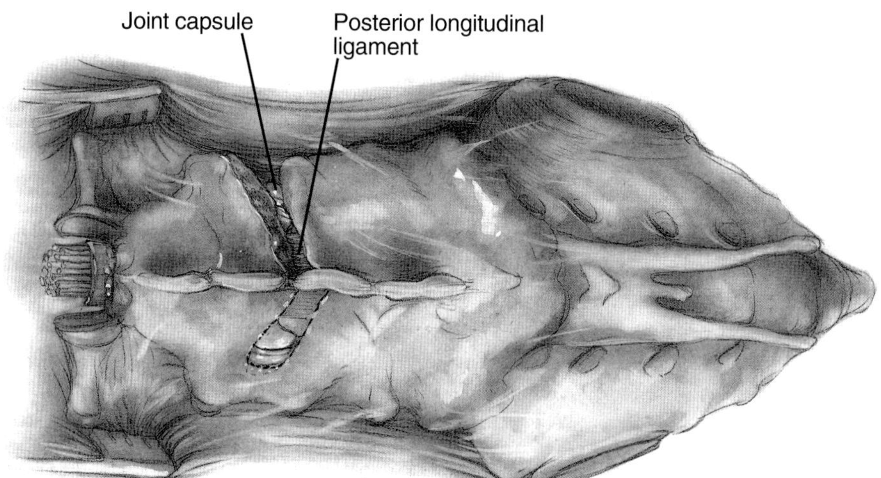

Figure 8. A: The Kerrison rongeur is used to complete the osteotomy. It is also used to undercut the osteotomy to prevent nerve crush when the spine falls into lordosis. The illustration **(B)** demonstrates the osteotomy in better detail.

Posterior Osteotomy of the Thoracic Spine

Osteotomy of the thoracic spine is identical to that of the lumbar spine except that there is less room to work so great care must be exercised in removing bone. Again, the message is the same. The osteotomies must be between the transverse processes and must exit through the neural foramen (Fig. 10).

Anterior Thoracic Osteotomy for Coronal Deformity

The patient is positioned in the lateral decubitus position with the convex side of the deformity up and held with a Seimen's positioner at the sacrum and at the

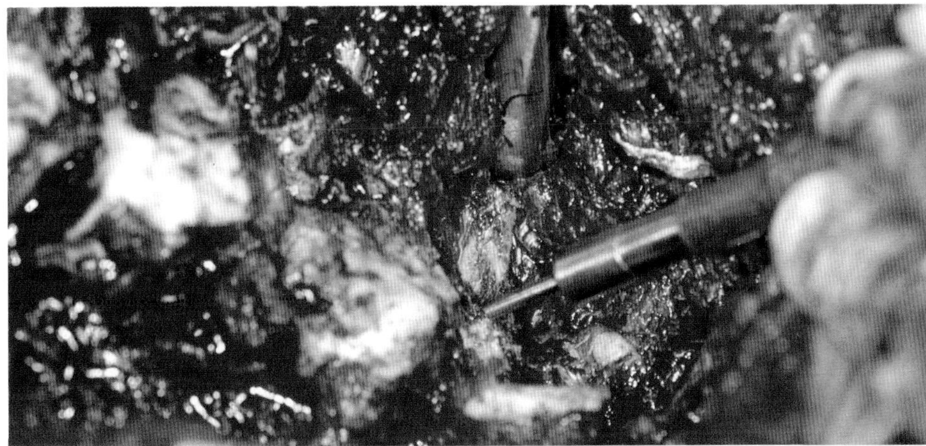

A

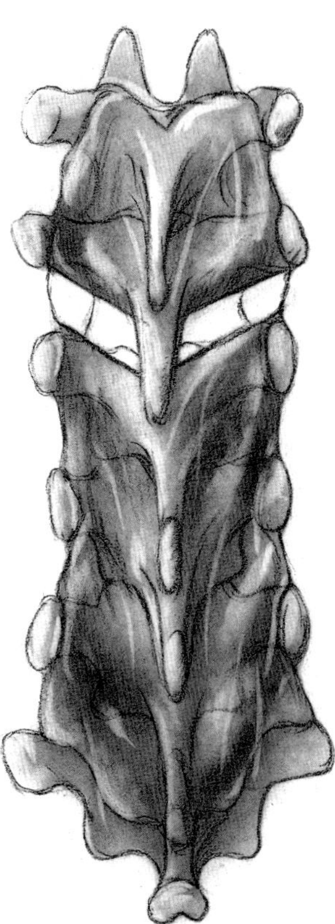

Figure 10. A posterior spine fusion on a thoracic spine. The osteotomy is outlined. Always note which transverse process goes with which transverse process.

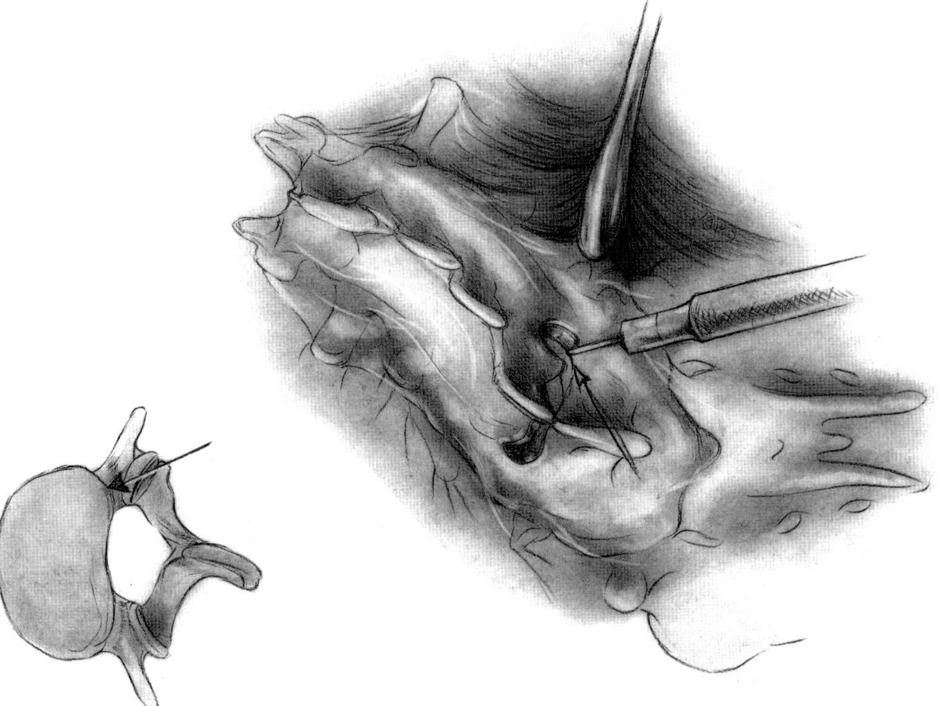

B

Figure 9. Surgical view **(A)** and illustration **(B)** of the transverse process of L4. The Midas Rex bur is opening the dense cortical bone in order to locate the pedicle. Previous fusion, which makes the outer cortical bone very dense, must be burred before trying to locate the pedicle.

pubis. A 10-pound sandbag supports the abdomen and another Seimen's positioner is high on the dorsal spine. The patient's spine is as close to the edge of the operating table as possible. The surgeon will stand at the back of the patient. The prep and drape is always from the shoulder to below the iliac crest and from umbilicus to the spinous processes. The iliac crest is always included in case a bone graft is needed.

Surgical Procedures. The anterior approach to the spine is used. It is important to stop the incision 4 cm from the midline posteriorly to prevent possible skin ischemia if a posterior approach is planned (Fig. 11).

If more than five osteotomies are contemplated, the chest will have to be opened through two ribs, for example, ribs 5 and 10. The same skin incision can be utilized. The surgeon must be able to see directly down the disc space between the end plates. On occasion it is possible and preferable to remove some or all of the

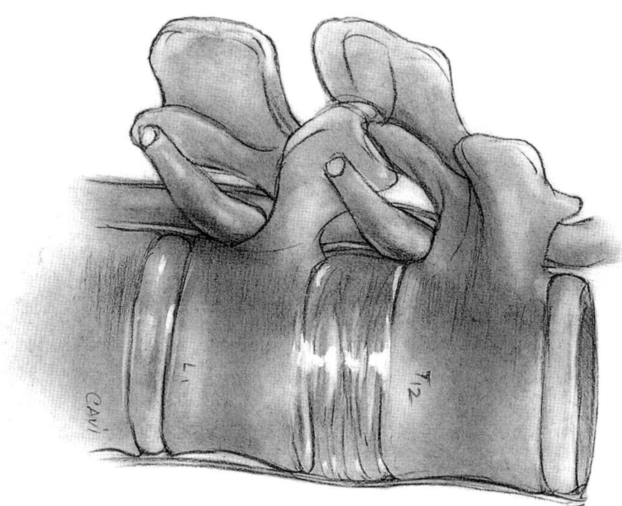

Figure 11. T12–L1 motion segment fused anteriorly.

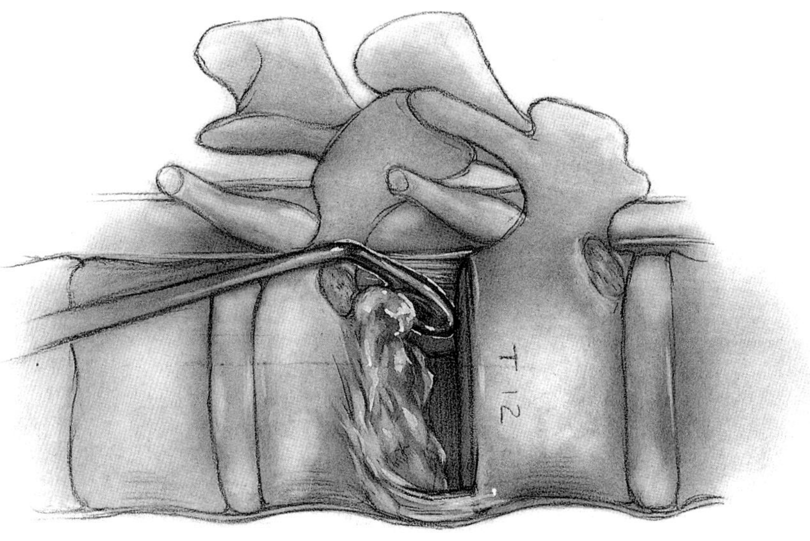

Figure 12. The osteotomy is begun using either an osteotome or rongeur. Angle curettes are now useful to continue the osteotomy.

vertebral body when doing an osteotomy. Which rib to remove for the approach should be decided in the planning conference. If this is a revision surgery the old rib bed can be utilized, and frequently some of the rib will have regenerated from periosteal bone growth.

If the spine has been previously fused or if there are anterior instruments, dissection to the vertebral bodies can be direct, since the segmental vessels will have been previously ligated. If the vessels are to be ligated, they should be ligated in the midbody line to preserve the collateral circulation at the intervertebral foramen. The spine must be exposed from the neuroforamen without disturbing the collateral circulation.

The location of the previous disc is usually easily discernible and removal can be performed with ronguers, osteotomy, or Midas Rex bur (Fig. 12). It is unusual for bone fusion to be complete to the posterior longitudinal ligament. The surgeon can generally recognize this ligament. If the ligament is ossified as in ankylosing spondylitis, the dura may be adherent and will tear and may be impossible to repair (Fig. 13). Extreme care must be taken in performing osteotomy at the cord level. Small tools and good vision are vital. These are high-anxiety, exhausting procedures and must be undertaken only by the most experienced surgeon. The rewards are small, since correction of the coronal plane deformity is less than that for sagittal plane deformity.

Anterior Thoracic Osteotomy for Sagittal Deformity

Anterior osteotomy of the thoracic spine for kyphoses deformity is a slightly different procedure and is best described as an anterolateral decompression. Gibbus is a severe kyphus at one, two, or three levels. The spine and spinal cord are very posterior and attempting to reach them through a typical thoracotomy can be disappointing. It is better to do a three-level costotransversectomy and find the lamina and pedicles of the spine.

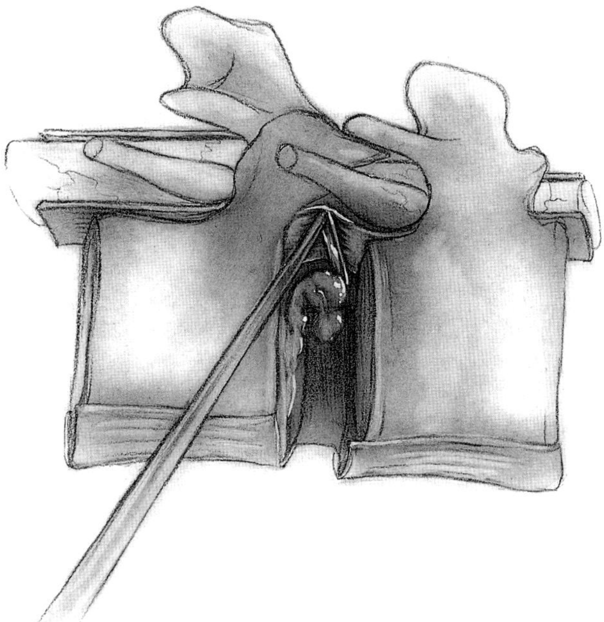

Figure 13. A fine, small, strong curette is now used for dissection to the posterior longitudinal ligament and to depress the bone into the cavity that has been created. A spreader may be used to facilitate this dissection.

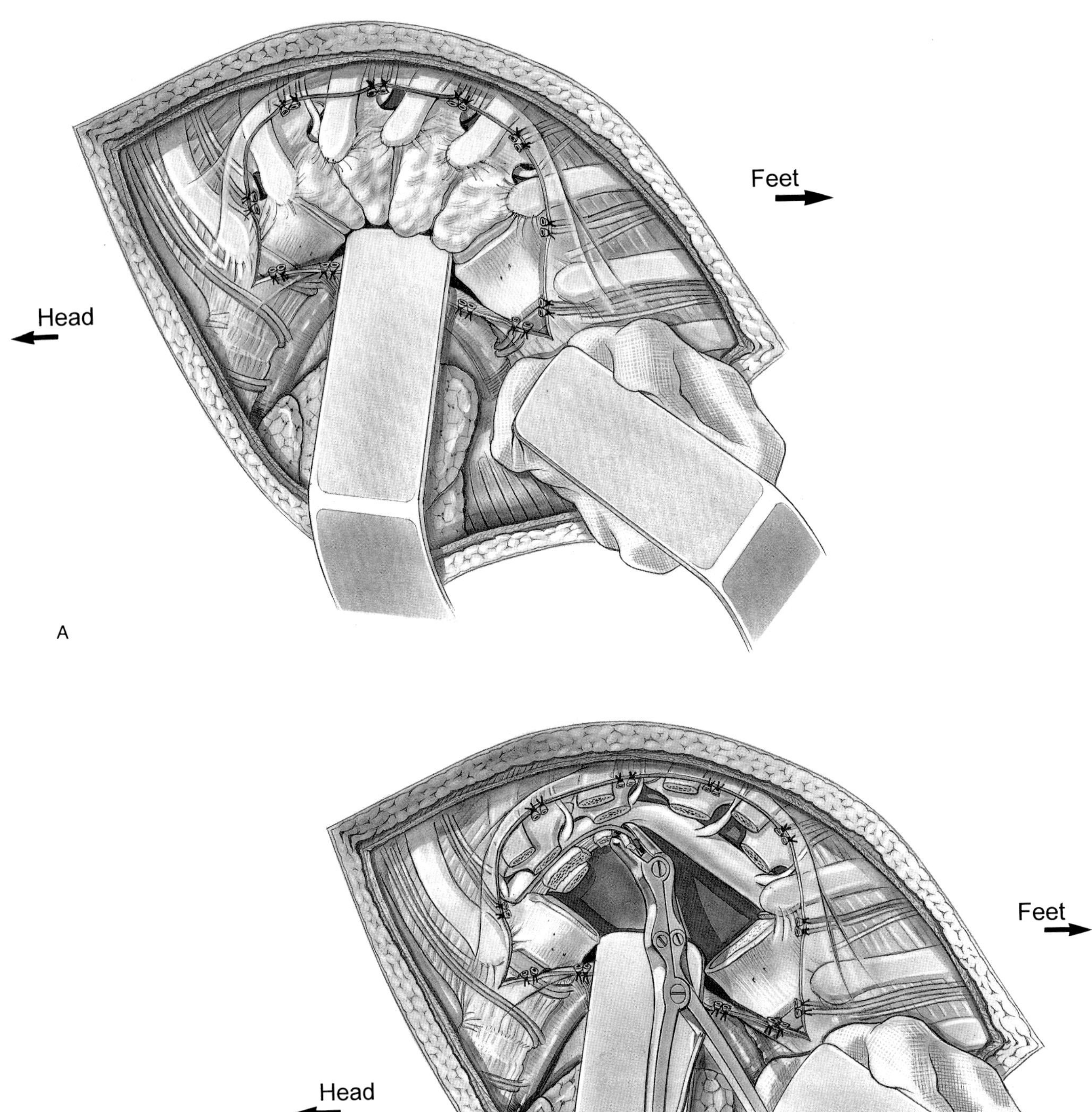

Figure 14. Drawings illustrate the gibbus usually seen in late tuberculosis spondylitis. It is easier to perform an anterolateral osteotomy because the spine is so posterior. **A:** Before decompression. **B:** During decompression.

The segmental nerve can be found entering the neuroforamen and the pedicles identified. The pedicles are osteotomized. After the vessels are ligated, the bodies are removed back to a thin shell of bone beneath the posterior longitudinal ligament. The remaining bone and posterior longitudinal ligament can then be depressed away from the spinal cord and removed. In tuberculosis gibbus the infection usually does the dissection and a complete debridement is usually accomplished easily. The approach is really an anterolateral approach (Fig. 14).

Anterior Lumbar Osteotomy

Lumbar anterior osteotomy is identical to the thoracic procedure. The same incision can be continued to expose the spine to the sacrum. The diaphragm must be divided and the psoas muscle retracted. We use a Taylor retractor and place it in the intervertebral foramen anterior to the spinal nerve. The osteotomy technique is similar to that described for the thoracic spine. If the posterior aspect of the spine has been instrumented and fused, the anterior portion may not move significantly after the osteotomy. In selected conditions either simultaneous surgery is indicated or else anterior surgery followed by posterior surgery followed by anterior surgery. If possible, the surgeon should devise plans to turn the patient as few times as needed.

POSTOPERATIVE MANAGEMENT

Postoperative management begins in the operating room. A good neurologic examination is performed before leaving the operating room. The patient spends approximately 24 hours in the surgical intensive care unit. This time is important for blood and fluid management and frequent neurologic examinations. Patient-controlled analgesia is used but should not mask any severe pain, which would represent nerve root crush or ischemia. We rarely exceed 20 to 30 mg morphine/4-hr period via this route, depending on the size and weight of the patient.

The patient's spine must be very well fixed during surgery. This allows us to dangle the patient's legs on postoperative day 2 and stand the patient on postoperative day 3. Patient-controlled analgesia is cut in half on day 3 and discontinued on day 4 or 5. Oral medication is then used for pain control. Pain control may be a problem for a patient who has had multiple low back surgeries. Reorienting the spine will often cause a neuropraxia of a root for a period of time.

We follow specific rules for immobilizing the patient from the bed to prevent excessive forces on any sacral screws in our construct. The patient side-lies, elevates the head off the bed, and pushes up sideways as the legs dangle to the floor. At the time of discharge from the hospital the patient will be ambulating independently and taking care of most personal hygiene needs. Whereas no skilled nursing care is required at home, someone should be with the patient for the first few days to aid in homebound activities. Following discharge, the patient is instructed to increase activity with a walking program. Walking will be increased as tolerated. A postoperative follow-up visit is scheduled for 3 weeks after discharge to assess the patient's progress. Activity levels will be increased to include driving, shopping, and meal preparation. If, however, the patient is still requiring significant pain medication and came to the surgical procedure debilitated, an additional 2 to 3 weeks may be required to resume the above activities.

Each patient is managed on an individual basis, and specific instructions are given. The patient would be expected to be able to return to sedentary work activities within 3 months from surgery. Those patients whose jobs require heavy lifting or significant movement would be restricted until the fusion is deemed solid.

COMPLICATIONS

Generally the fused lumbar spine is not in lordosis. It is usually in a relative kyphosis if we accept the idea that normal lumbar lordosis is about 35 to 40 degrees. As the osteotomy is performed the spine will fall into lordosis. Here it is important to remember the orientation of the vertebrae and try to reestablish the norm. It is important to fix each segment and to compress across the lumbar spine after osteotomy and segmental fixation so that the posterior column will be shortened and the anterior column lengthened. The key is to make L3 neutral and orient L4 and L5 ventrally and L1 and L2 dorsally. Most of the lordosis must occur at L4, L5, and the sacrum. Also, in this position, the abdomen is free, and no pressure will be applied to the abdomen or to the vena cava, to allow the epidural venous plexus to fill. As the lumbar spine falls into lordosis after the osteotomies, the anterior longitudinal ligament acts as a check rein. If this has been removed by previous anterior osteotomy, the spine may translate if it is not fixed as you perform the posterior osteotomy.

The most severe complication in this type of spinal surgery is paraplegia. How common is it? This is a difficult question to answer. No two revision spinal surgeries are similar. It is safe to assume that large corrections at the cord level are more prone to neurologic complications than lesser corrections below the cord level. Anterior and posterior surgery in the thoracic spine may interrupt the important medullary blood supply to the spinal cord. For this reason we prefer to stage thoracic surgery. Of course SSEPs or NMEPs are used. Blood pressure must be kept at a reasonable level for cord perfusion, especially when altering the anatomy of the spine. Clearly if the SSEPs or NMEPs show problems, the deformity must be allowed to recur by adjusting the correcting instrumentation. If no return of motor function occurs, all instruments are removed, blood pressure raised, and a large amount of cortisone given intravenously.

Other complications are minor compared with paraplegia. Bone failure may occur postoperatively and must be recognized. The patient should be reoperated early. We generally use a longer construct to disperse the forces that caused the bone to fail. Late problems are pseudarthroses and instrument failure, which generally result in having a poorly-balanced spine or some metabolic bone problem.

ILLUSTRATIVE CASE FOR TECHNIQUE

K.K. is a 46-year-old white woman first diagnosed with scoliosis at age 9. At age 13 (1958) she underwent surgical treatment. A tibial graft was used. The exact attempted fusion levels are unknown. The patient had few complaints until 1977, when she began to experience back and leg pain. She was first seen and evaluated by the spine reconstruction team in 1991. Her chief complaint was severe back and right leg pain. Inspection of the patient revealed severe imbalance of the spine in both the coronal and sagittal planes (Fig. 15), progressing over a period of 4 years. The goal of revision surgery is to correct the imbalance of the spine. To accomplish this, it is important to:

1. select the end vertebrae of the construct
2. select where and how many osteotomies are needed
3. decide if an anterior release is necessary
4. plan how to improve the sagittal balance
5. plan how to locate L3, L4, and L5 in the sagittal plane
6. determine the steps for the surgery
7. determine the advantage of the three-rod technique in this situation

Since the major deformity is in the coronal plane, the three-rod technique is ideal because it allows the center of the scoliotic spine to be translated to the midline. The T3 vertebra is in the correct coronal-sagittal alignment. The L5 vertebra is in good coronal alignment, but the sagittal alignment is 20 to 40 degrees too dorsal and needs to be corrected. The scoliosis seems mobile except for the fused sections. The bending radiograph allows the lumbar spine to become perpendicular to the pelvis. Anterior release is not needed, as the segments are not solidly fused and are mobile. The center portion of the spine is straight until L2. Therefore the L2 vertebra needs to be separated (osteotomized) from the fused segment. The pseudarthrosis at T10–T11 can be mobilized slightly.

The considerations for surgery now include:

1. no anterior surgery
2. osteotomy at L1–L2 for coronal correction

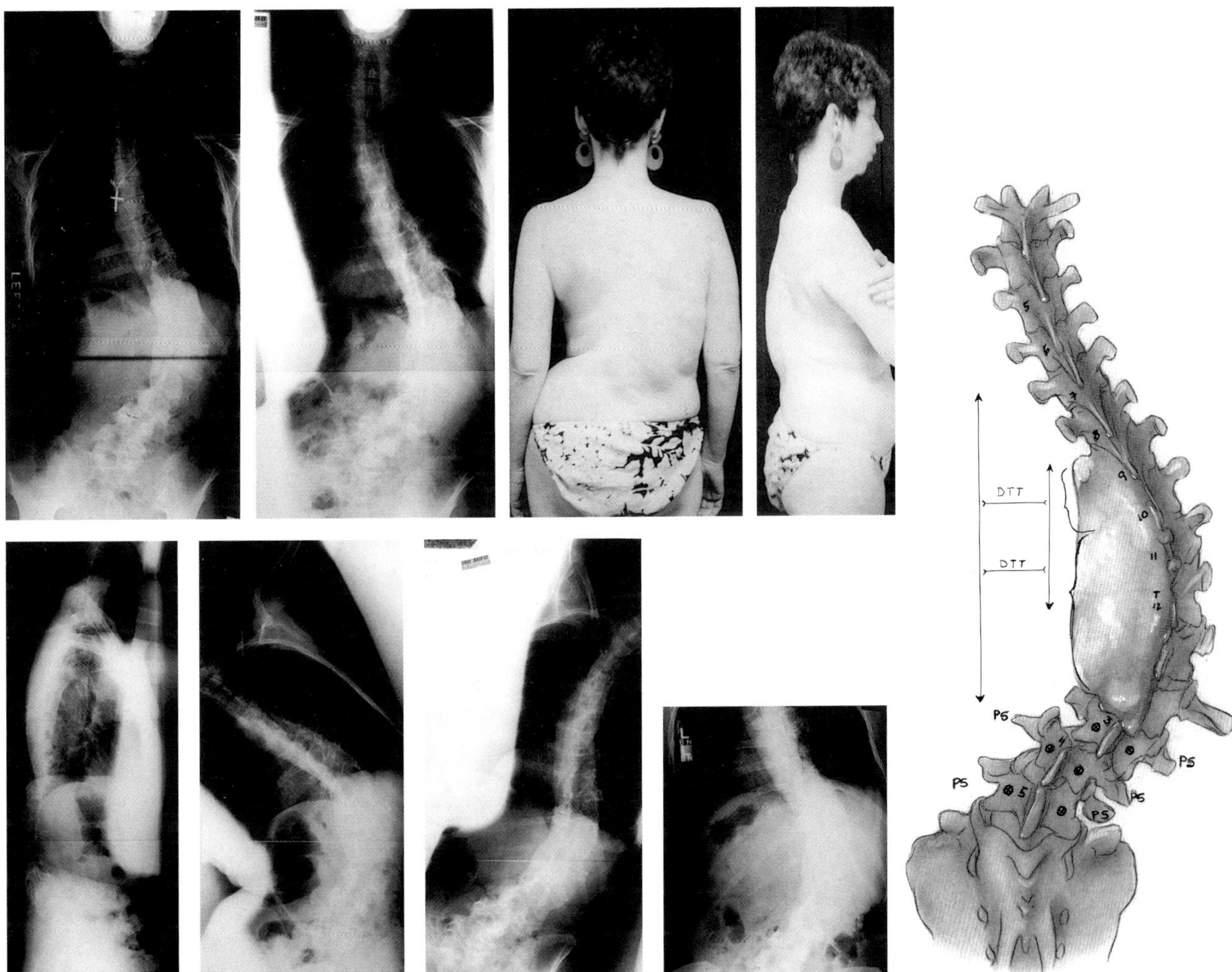

Figure 15. Photograph of patient, radiographs, and planning diagram. Note the increase in the scoliosis, the mobility of the lumbar spine even though it was fused, the solid arthrodesis at T11–L2, and the pseudarthrosis at T10–T11. The staircase effect of lateral subluxation is seen on the AP radiograph. The lateral radiographs reveal the orientation of the vertebrae. The bending film demonstrates the mobility of the spine above and below the obvious fusion. A pseudarthrosis is obvious cephalad at T10–T11. Pseudarthroses are present caudally. The lumbosacral disc space seems normal. The fused segment is straight from T11 to L1.

3. osteotomy of the previously attempted fusion, at L2–L3, L3–L4, and L4–L5 for coronal and sagittal correction.
4. proper alignment of L3, L4, and L5 with T4
5. estimated length of surgery, 6 to 8 hours
6. estimated blood loss, 6 units
7. seemingly strong bone quality

The inferior facet joints between L2–L3, L3–L4, and L4–L5 were identified and generously removed, which was difficult because of the distorted anatomy. The cartilage of the superior facets was removed. The pedicles were identified and screws placed on the right side (Fig. 16). The L1–L2 area was osteotomized (Fig. 17). The spine was manually pushed straight and screws placed on the left side (Fig. 18).

Sagittal alignment was attempted by rolling the rod on the right. The superior portion of the spine was then exposed. A transverse pedicle claw was placed at T3 (left). The T10–T11 pseudarthrosis was opened (Fig. 19). A cold rolled rod was placed from the transverse pedicle claw at T3 to L3–L4–L5 screws and re-

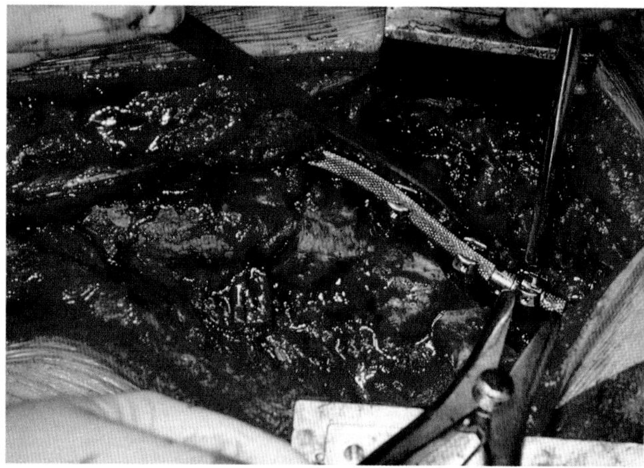

Figure 16. The lower lumbar spine, which was previously fused. The fusion was not solid, as was seen on the bending radiographs. The pseudarthroses were opened, facets generously removed, and screws placed on the right side.

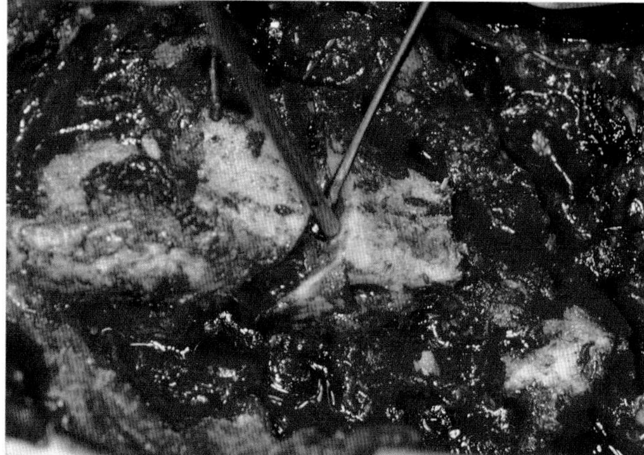

Figure 17. Osteotomy at L1–L2 of the classic type. It is important to undercut the osteotomy. This motion segment will move even though it has been fused for years. Thoracic vertebrae, however, do not enjoy as much motion as lumbar vertebrae after osteotomy.

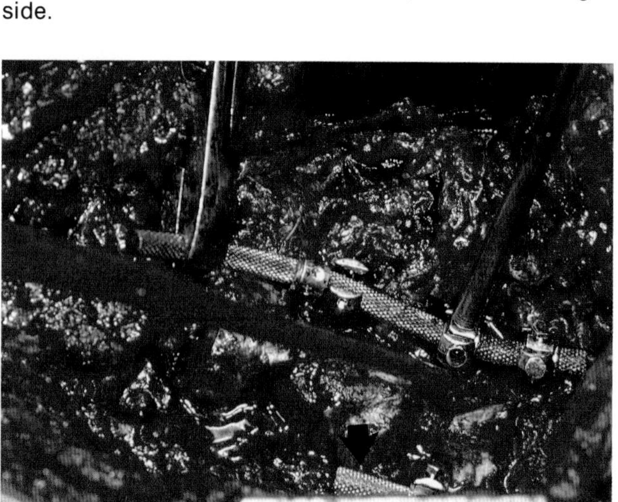

Figure 18. The photograph now illustrates the right rod reducing the coronal imbalance; the *arrow* points to a short rod on the left side that allows the pedicle screws to become aligned.

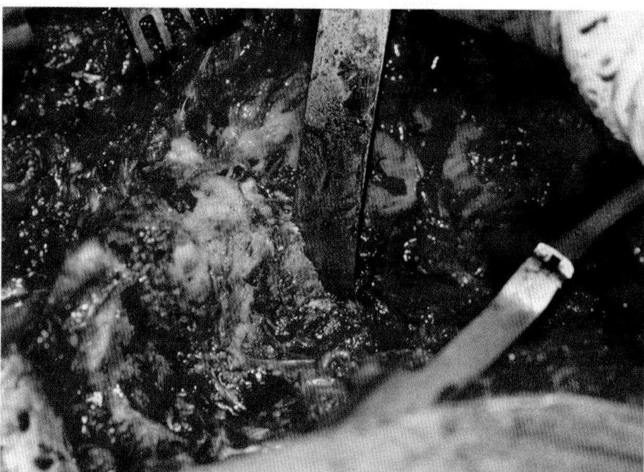

Figure 19. The obvious pseudarthrosis at T10–T11 is opened, although not much motion is expected here.

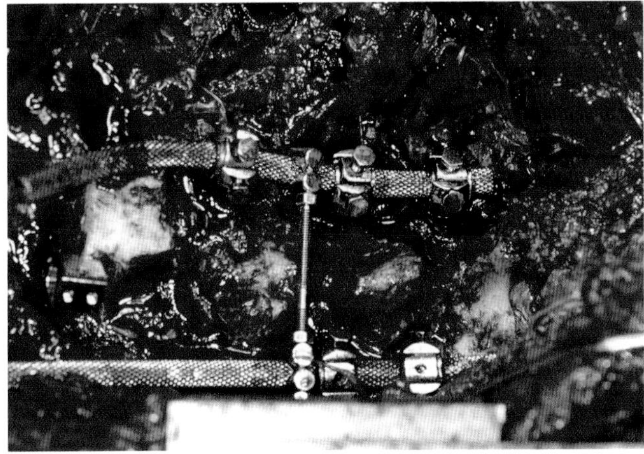

Figure 20. The long left rod and the short right rod now rolled into lordosis. A down hook in the osteotomy site at L2 is visualized. The inner rod can be placed and drawn to the long rod through dynamic transverse traction device.

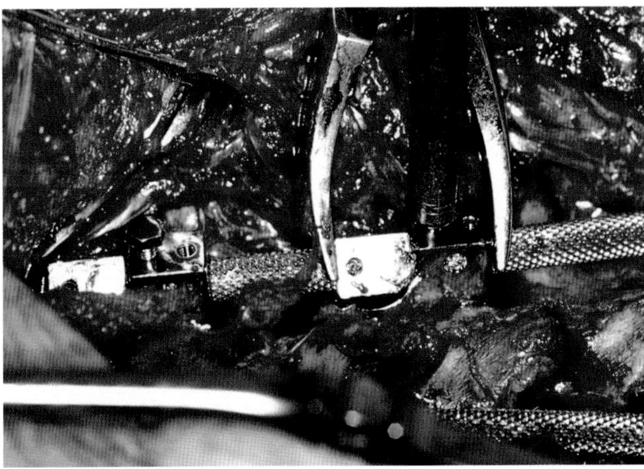

Figure 21. Two pedicle transverse claws are applied at T3 and T5 and connected to the lower rod by a domino connector.

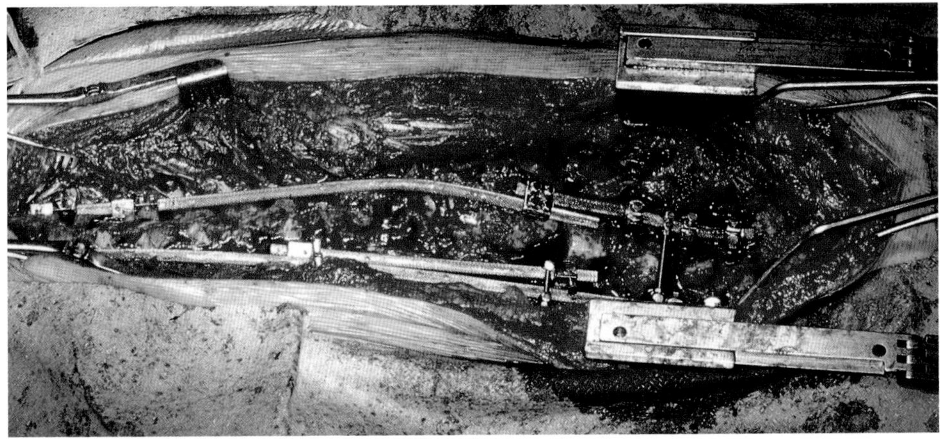

Figure 22. The final construct.

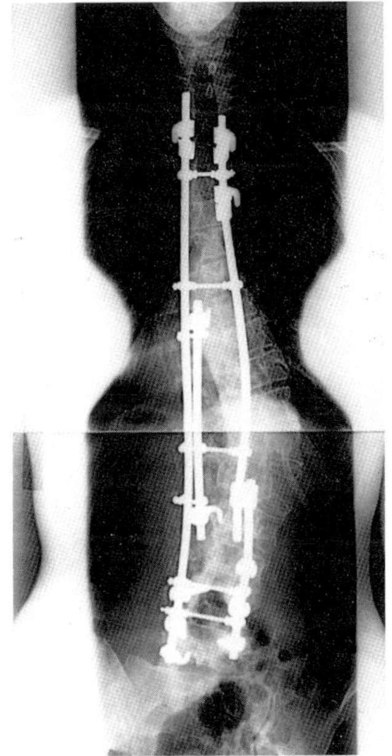

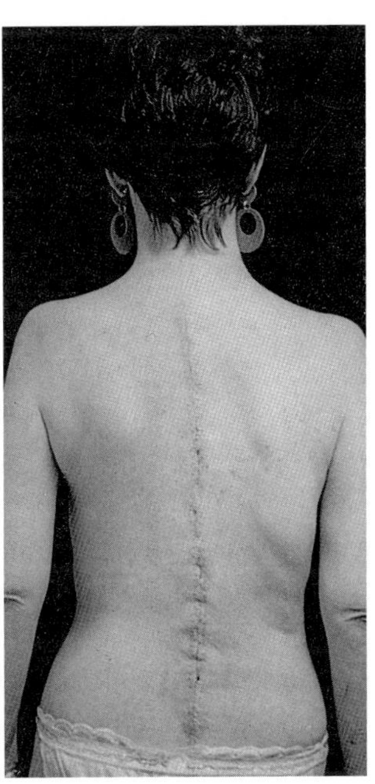

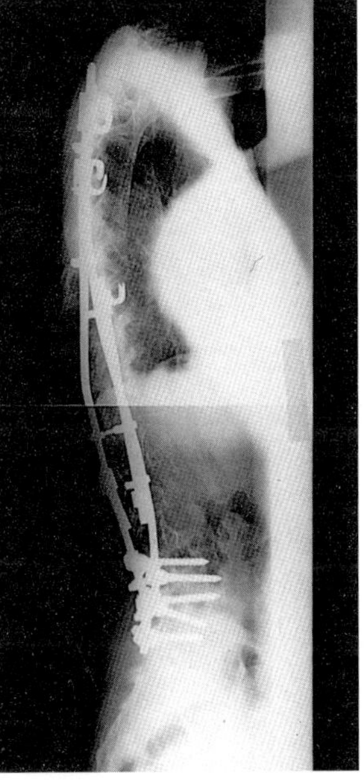

Figure 23. Final standing radiographs and the patient are illustrated. Constructive statements may be made concerning this result: (a) no infralaminar hook is seen at L5 on the right; the last screw in a construct needs to be protected with an infralaminar hook; (b) the lumbosacral junction has been left open, but may degenerate in the future; and (c) the right long rod is now almost across the midline and if placed in too much compression through the domino may actually increase the scoliosis.

mained rigid while the middle of the spine was drawn to it. A regular rod will deform, pulling the center rod to it (Fig. 20).

The middle rod was placed. The hooks at T8 and L2 were intracanal and distracted. Two DTTs were placed and the middle segment drawn to the long rod. Once the middle rod was brought to the long rod, the stabilizing convex rod was placed with two transverse pedicle claws at T4 and T6 on the right (Fig. 21) and brought to a domino connector to the inferior rod already in L3–L4–L5 (Fig. 22). The domino connector was used for compression (Fig. 23).

RECOMMENDED READING

1. Goel, M. K.: Vertebral osteotomy for correction of fixed flexion deformity of the spine. *J Bone Joint Surg* (AM) 50: 287, 1968.
2. LaChapelle, E. H.: Osteotomy of the lumbar spine for correction of kyphosis in a case of ankylosing spondylarthritis. *J Bone Joint Surg* 28: 851, 1946.
3. Law, W. A.: Surgical treatment of the rheumatic diseases. *J Bone Joint Surg* (Br) 34: 215, 1952.
4. Law, W. A.: Lumbar spinal osteotomy. *J Bone Joint Surg* (BR) 41: 270, 1959.
5. Law, W. A.: Osteotomy of the cervical spine. *J Bone Joint Surg* 41: 640, 1959.
6. Law, W. A.: Osteotomy of the cervical spine. *J Bone Joint Surg* (AM) 44: 1199, 1962.
7. Law, W. A.: Osteotomy of the spine. *Clin Orthop* 66: 70, 1969.
8. Leatherman, K. D.: Resection of vertebral bodies. *J Bone Joint Surg* 51A: 206, 1969.
9. Leatherman, K. D.: The management of rigid spinal curves. *Clin Orthop* 92: 215, 1973.
10. Leatherman, K. D., Dickson, A.: Spinal deformity in myelodysplasia–surgical treatment. 11th Annual Meeting of the American Scoliosis Research Society, Ottawa, Canada, 1976.
11. Roy-Camille, R., Demeulenaere, C.: Ostesynthese due rachis dorsal lumbaire et lambo-sacre par plaques metalliques vissees dans les pedicules vertebraux et les apophyses articulaires. *Presse Med* 78: 1447, 1970.
12. Simmons, E. H.: The surgical correction of flexion deformity of the cervical spine in ankylosing spondylitis. *Clin Orthop* 86: 132, 1972.
13. Simmons, E. H.: Kyphotic deformity of the spine in ankylosing spondylitis. *Clin Orthop* 128: 65, 1977.

Master Techniques in Orthopaedic Surgery,
THE SPINE, edited by D. S. Bradford,
Lippincott-Raven Publishers, Philadelphia, © 1997.

15

Lumbar Discectomy

Dan M. Spengler

INDICATIONS/CONTRAINDICATIONS

Patient selection for elective lumbar discectomy represents the most important step in achieving a good outcome. Although I will review the essentials for patient selection in this chapter, I highly recommend that the reader pursue the references at the end of the chapter for more in-depth coverage of this important decision-analysis step.

All authors agree that the patient who presents with a progressive neurologic deficit secondary to lumbar disc herniation should be rapidly evaluated and taken to the operating room for definitive treatment. However, the number of patients who qualify for lumbar discectomy based on neurologic progression is indeed small and represents at most one or two patients a year in my practice. The vast majority of patients are considered for elective lumbar discectomy based on their subjective complaints of pain. Thus a comprehensive objective analysis of these patients is essential to differentiate between those who have true lumbar disc herniations and those who have similar symptoms but do not have a surgically remedial lesion.

Nonoperative approaches that I employ include the use of salicylates and the nonsteroidal antiinflammatory drugs for short periods of time. Bed rest is used but only for short periods of time, usually not to exceed 48 hours. Most patients will begin to respond to short-term bed rest and antiinflammatories, thus avoiding the necessity for surgical intervention. Patients who have recurrent symptoms and those who do not improve with these nonoperative strategies can be considered for epidural steroid injections. This modality is reserved for patients who prefer to

D. M. Spengler, M.D.: Department of Orthopaedics and Rehabilitation, Vanderbilt University Medical Center, Nashville, Tennessee 37232-2550.

avoid surgery. The published literature does not support the effectiveness of epidural steroid injections. Nevertheless, a percentage of patients do respond to them, and surgical intervention is thereby avoided.

Although most patients who present with lumbar radicular pain and evidence of a herniated disc will exhibit mild forms of neurologic involvement, a significant percentage of patients with disc herniations will not exhibit any neurologic signs (approximately 22%). This observation reaffirms the need to evaluate all four of the categories listed above. Neurologic findings are of course dependent on the observer's evaluation. A truly comprehensive neurologic evaluation is essential to identify the most subtle of findings. For example, many examiners overlook weakness of the extensor hallucis longus muscle, since they do not specifically evaluate the patient with respect to this muscle. A patient with an L5 radiculopathy may have no neurologic findings other than weakness of the extensor hallucis longus muscle. The strength of all muscle groups of the lower extremities should be carefully evaluated in patients who present with lumbar radicular syndromes. The gluteus medius muscle can also be weak in patients with an L5 radiculopathy. Likewise, one would expect some weakness in the quadriceps muscle with upper lumbar disc herniations (L3–L4). In a patient with an S1 radiculopathy, the strength of the triceps surae group should be carefully assessed. Patients with S1 radiculopathy may be able to stand on their toes, but they do not have the strength for repeated pushoff that they would on the normal asymptomatic side. Thus having the patient hop on tiptoes is a good way to identify modest weakness in the S1 innervated structures.

Occasionally a discrete mapping of a dermatome may be possible on sensory examination. In general, a patient with an L4 radiculopathy will have evidence of decreased sensation to pinprick over the medial portion of the leg. The patient with an L5 radiculopathy will often manifest decreased sensation in the web space between the great and second toe. S1 deficits are present on the lateral border of the foot. Electromyography is often a worthwhile diagnostic study for patients in whom the diagnosis is unclear. Documenting electrical evidence of fibrillation in specific nerve root distributions can often reaffirm nerve root irritation, consistent with radiculopathy.

Sciatic tension signs are positive in most individuals who present with true lumbar disc herniations. In my experience, the problem with sciatic tension signs revolves around the overinterpretation of these findings by the unsophisticated examiner. Distracting tests must also be employed to differentiate symptom amplifiers from patients who truly have sciatic tension. I refer the reader to the classic article by Waddell for further elucidation of this point (18). Suffice it to say that the patient who has no evidence of back or leg pain while extending the knee in the seated position but who complains of severe pain with slight elevation of the straight leg off the examining table only 5 to 10 degrees probably represents a symptom amplifier as opposed to a patient with true sciatic tension (18). Consistency of response throughout the evaluation must be included as a part of the evaluation.

Crossed straight-leg raising, although not present in all patients with disc herniations, does represent a highly specific finding when present. When the examiner picks up the asymptomatic lower extremity and the patient complains of pain on the side opposite, the crossed straight-leg raising test is positive. This finding virtually seals the diagnosis of a lumbar disc herniation. The other sciatic tension that I believe is important to identify is best described as *dysrhythmia* with lumbar spinal flexion-extension. When the patient is standing and is asked to touch the toes, the examiner stands behind the patient and observes the paraspinal muscle mass. When the left and right paraspinous muscle masses contract asymmetrically, dysrhythmia is present. This observation cannot be simulated by patients who do not have nerve root irritation. The finding can be positive in a patient who has sustained direct trauma to the paraspinous muscle masses, but this does not pose a difficult diagnostic dilemma. In a patient who had no direct trauma to the paraspinal muscle area, dysrhythmia is indeed a highly objective finding and constitutes evidence of nerve root irritation, consistent with a disc herniation.

Psychological information can be gleaned from patients by using formal psychological testing or more readily through the pain drawing (10). Psychological testing using instruments such as the Minnesota Multiphasic Personality Inventory can be reserved for the patient who is borderline with regard to indications or for the patient with a failed spinal surgery. My previous work has reaffirmed the importance of psychosocial parameters by noting that the outcome of lumbar discectomy procedures is more closely predicted by the preoperative psychological composition of the patient than by the operative findings (15,17).

Imaging studies represent the basis on which the anatomy of the lumbar spinal canal is defined. At present, magnetic resonance imaging (MRI) can often delineate this anatomy without the need for myelography or postmyelogram computed tomography (CT) scans. The problem with MRI alone is its sensitivity. In many patients, MRI studies will reveal "disc herniations," at multiple levels of the spine, that are clearly inconsistent with clinical findings. In these situations, I insist on a lumbar myelogram with a postmyelogram CT scan to define the anatomy of the canal more clearly. In patients who have classic lumbar radicular syndromes with specific neurologic findings and an MRI scan consistent with a disc herniation at a single level, the myelogram-CT scan is not warranted. A CT scan without contrast material is not useful for the assessment of patients with lumbar radicular syndromes. The CT scan alone does not differentiate a double nerve root exit from a disc herniation, and in fact this finding can be misinterpreted as a disc herniation. Likewise, a conus level lesion cannot be excluded by CT scan alone. Thus I do not recommend the CT scan without associated contrast material following myelography.

Once the patient has been thoroughly assessed in each of the four categories (neurologic signs, sciatic tension signs, psychological factors, and imaging studies), the data are synthesized and a recommendation advanced (17). Lumbar discectomy is recommended to patients who have not responded to appropriate nonoperative treatment and who believe that their quality of life has been sufficiently adversely impacted to justify a surgical approach. In addition, I rarely recommend surgical intervention for any patient who does not have 50 or more points on our Objective Patient Evaluation Score (OPES) (15,17). Indeed, the clinical outcome correlates quite well with the preoperative OPES. Patients who have fewer than 50 points on the OPES are unlikely to benefit from surgical intervention (15,17). Continued nonoperative management with a return to work focus is recommended.

Contraindications to the procedure can be minimized by using an objective patient evaluation scoring mechanism (15,17). Additional contraindications for elective lumbar disc surgery are contingent on the surgeon. In my opinion, elective discectomy procedures are not indicated for patients who are drug dependent or who are involved in active litigation with no motivation to exhibit well behavior. In addition, in these litigious times, I personally would not perform elective lumbar disc surgery when I perceive poor motivation or have inadequate rapport with the patient (or both). Such patients can be referred to colleagues who may develop better rapport. Surgery is clearly contraindicated when the patient does not have nerve root irritation or a lumbar disc herniation. Too many lumbar discectomy procedures are performed in the United States. The false-positive rate of most of our imaging studies is in excess of 25%. Therefore based on imaging studies alone, a great many patients would be subjected to surgical intervention even though their imaging studies do not correlate with clinical findings.

PREOPERATIVE PLANNING

To be as accurate as possible with regard to patient selection, the following four general categories need to be carefully analyzed: neurologic evaluation, sciatic tension signs, psychological assessment, and imaging studies. Preoperative planning optimizes the likelihood for an excellent outcome from lumbar disc surgery. The surgeon must review the imaging studies carefully to identify the surgical level or levels to be addressed with the discectomy. Most patients will require intervention at only one level. In my experience, fewer than 5% require discectomy at two levels.[15,17] If the patient has a pericentral disc herniation, the surgeon may elect to expose the epidural space on both the left and right sides. Anulotomies can then be performed on the left and right sides to reduce the likelihood that the patient will develop a contralateral pain syndrome following surgery. For example, if the surgeon performs a pericentral discectomy through a single unilateral anulotomy, disc material may be displaced to the opposite side, resulting in contralateral symptoms after surgery. I prefer to perform bilateral anulotomies for all central disc herniations and most pericentral herniations. In patients who have very large extradural defects, the surgeon should carefully review the surgical approach. In these situations, a hemilaminectomy may be essential to afford proper longitudinal decompression prior to retracting the nerve root. Patients who have very large extradural herniations often have extremely tight nerve roots. Any excessive root retraction may risk a neural deficit. Partial discectomy may be performed prior to manipulation of neural tissue, but only if adequate lateral visualization is afforded. Planning also allows the surgeon to determine in advance whether a foraminotomy will be necessary and on rare occasions whether a stabilization procedure will be necessary. Essentially, I rarely recommend a surgical stabilization procedure if the patient has a soft disc herniation unless the patient has measurable hypermobility of the involved motion segment (≥4 mm translation, ≥20-degree angular deformity). The other exception would be the patient with multiple recurrences (more than two) at the same level or a patient with evidence of a degenerative spondylolisthesis associated with a disc herniation.

In addition to focusing on the pathologic processes inherent in the spinal canal, preoperative planning should also involve a thorough evaluation of the patient with regard to any possible complications that might be anticipated. If the patient has a history of a bleeding diasthesis, this information must be resolved. Allergies to specific medications and/or tape likewise should be determined. Any risk factors that may adversely impact on the anesthetic or postoperative management must be identified beforehand, to provide the opportunity for appropriate properative consultation as well as intraoperative management.

SURGERY

Patients who undergo elective lumbar discectomy should receive intravenous antibiotics in the operating room prior to beginning the incision. Once the patient has been anesthetized, careful positioning is essential. I use the Roger Anderson (Tower) table (Fig. 1). After the patient has been positioned on this table, blood loss is lessened because of the decreased venous pressure on Batson's plexus. The surgeon must pay careful attention to detail during positioning. Careful inspection must include the eyes, ulnar nerves, genitalia in males, and breasts in females to ensure that excessive pressure does not exist. Once the patient has been positioned, the lower back is prepped with an antiseptic solution. I recommend the use of loupe magnification (2.5 to 3.5×) plus a fiberoptic headlight (Fig. 2). Loupe magnification facilitates exposure and improves tissue handling. Higher magnifications can be used but are not necessary.

Once the patient has been properly draped, a vertical midline incision is made overlying the interlaminar space of choice (Fig. 3). The well-centered incision is approximately 6 cm in length. Dissection is carried through the skin and subcutaneous tissue to the level of the lumbar fascia. Hemostasis is obtained and self-retaining retractors inserted. The lumbar fascia is opened directly over the spinous processes of the motion segment of interest. Thus, if the L4–L5 interspace is being approached, the incision using electrocautery occurs directly on top of the spinous process of L4 and then of L5. A continuation between L4 and L5 is then extended using cautery, and dissection is carried down to the laminae. I usually expose the lamina bilaterally, on both left and right sides, which facilitates dissection and visualization. In addition, a midline entry into the canal is ensured, which, in my opinion, lessens the likelihood of nerve root injury.

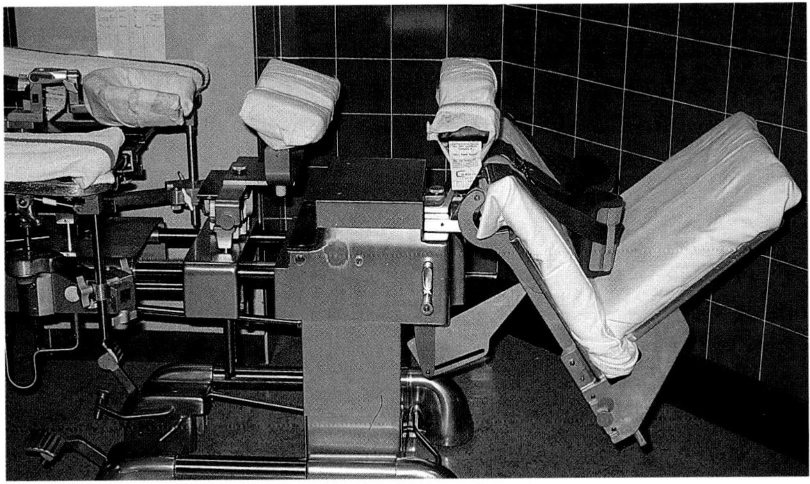

Figure 1. I prefer the use of the Tower table when performing lumbar discectomy. This table has many adjustments and ensures proper decompression of the abdominal viscera.

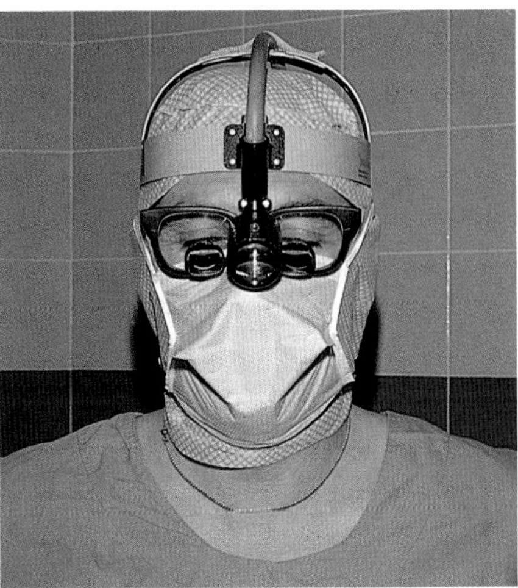

Figure 2. Magnification (×2.5 to 3.5) and a fiberoptic headlight are used during standard discectomy to facilitate visualization.

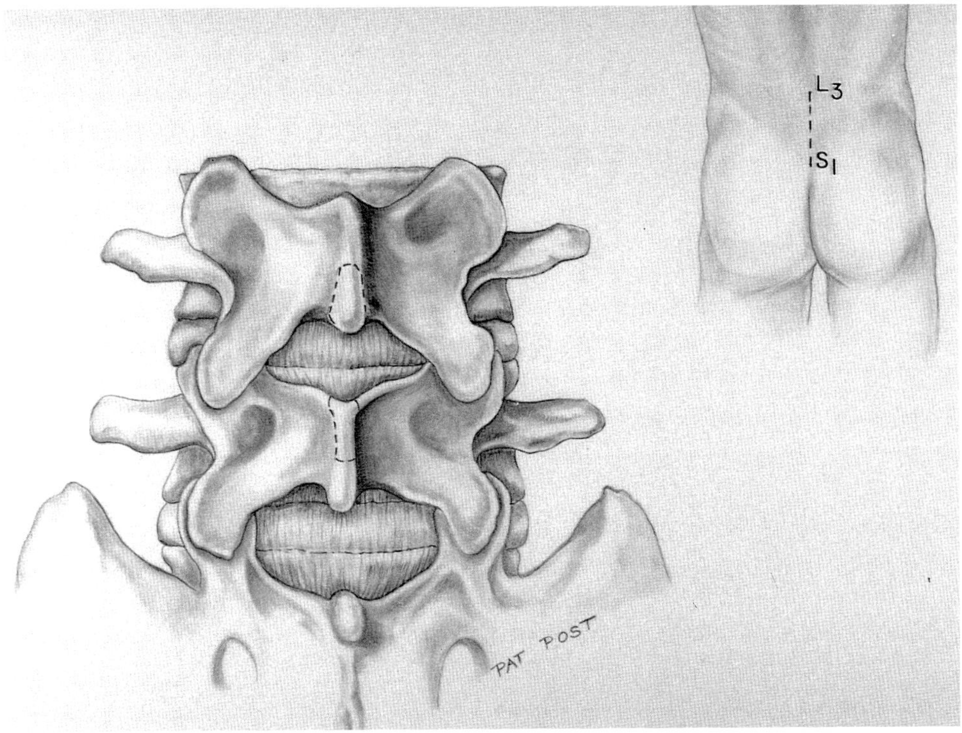

Figure 3. A vertical midline incision is made centered over the appropriate interspace.

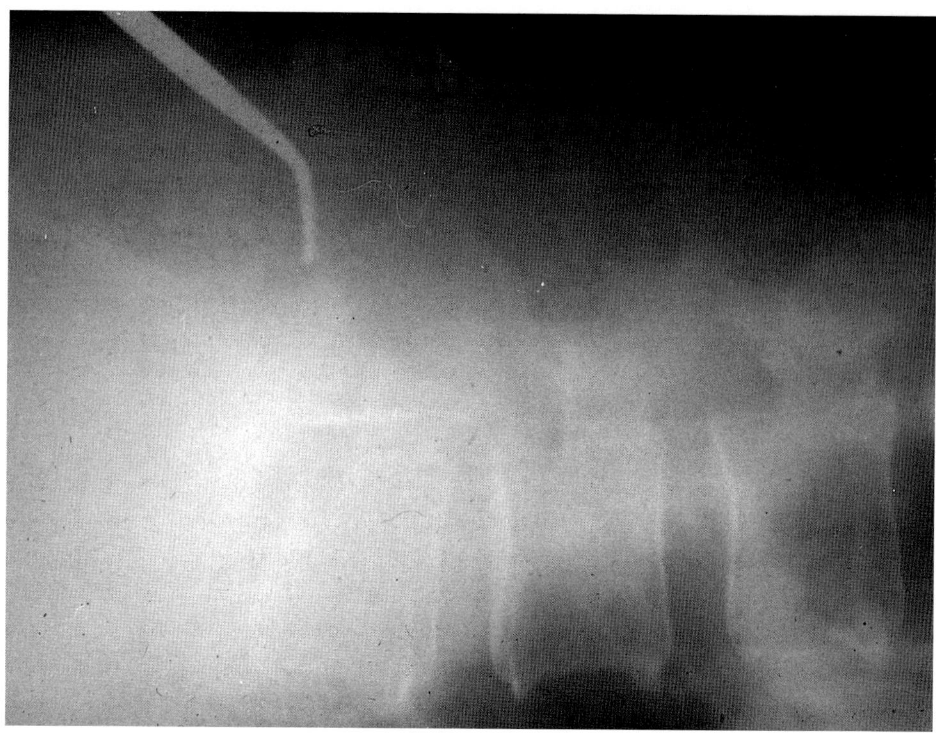

Figure 4. A lateral radiograph is obtained immediately after exposing a spinous process so that the appropriate vertebral disc level can be clearly identified.

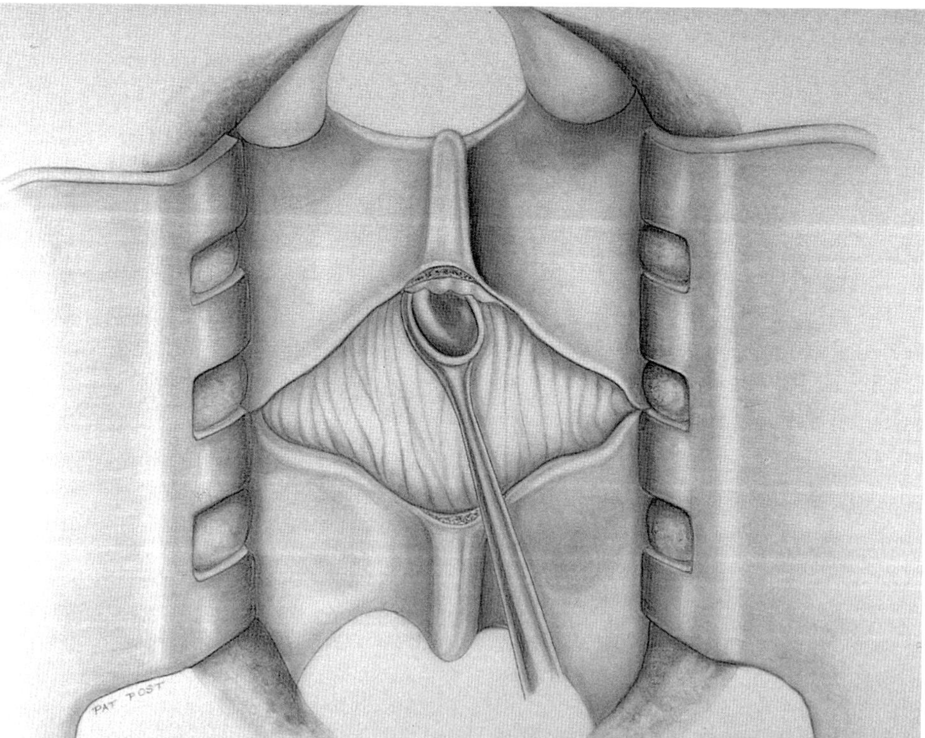

Figure 5. Although this exposure depicts a complete removal of the supraspinous and interspinous ligaments in younger patients, a smaller unilateral approach may well be used. The importance in this dissection is to ensure safe entry into the epidural space without injuring a posteriorly displaced nerve root. This illustration depicts the use of a Penfield #1 probe to detach the superior portion of the ligamentum flavum from the anterior attachment to the lamina.

Once the lamina has been exposed, a towel clip is placed on the spinous processes and a lateral intraoperative radiograph obtained (Fig. 4). Radiographic localization is important to minimize wrong-level procedures. After the appropriate level has been verified, the interlaminar space is exposed. A larger, self-retaining retractor is inserted and a Penfield #1 elevator used to dissect the ligamentum flavum gently from the anterior surface of the lamina from the midline toward the side of the herniation (Fig. 5). The 45-degree angled Kerrison rongeur is used to enhance visualization in the midline (Fig. 6). The raphe of the ligamentum flavum is identified. With the use of a Penfield #4 elevator, followed by a Penfield #3, the midline of the flavum is exposed. A #15 blade on a long-handled scalpel is used to divide the flavum using the Penfield elevator to protect the underlying dura (Fig. 7). The ligamentum flavum is excised from the side of the herniation using upbiting rongeurs and/or curettes (Fig. 8). After the flavum has been excised, attention is turned laterally to the lateral reflection of the flavum. This tissue is carefully removed to expose the dural sac and nerve root (Fig. 9). A midline entry into the epidural space lessens the likelihood of neural injury. Once the dura and nerve root are fully visualized, Penfield #4 and Freer elevators are used to mobilize the nerve root and dura gently.

Care must be taken during this portion of the dissection to handle the nerve root gently. In my experience, approximately one-third of patients who undergo surgery for a herniated lumbar disc also have a degree of lateral recess stenosis. Proper preoperative planning through a careful assessment of the CT scan will usually identify these patients prior to the procedure. Once the lateral recess stenosis is recognized by the decrease in normal nerve root mobility (<1 cm), the upbiting Kerrison rongeurs will be required to enlarge the recess and the neural foramina to free the nerve root completely. Although by definition a portion of the zygoapophyseal joint is resected in this situation, the amount of joint removed

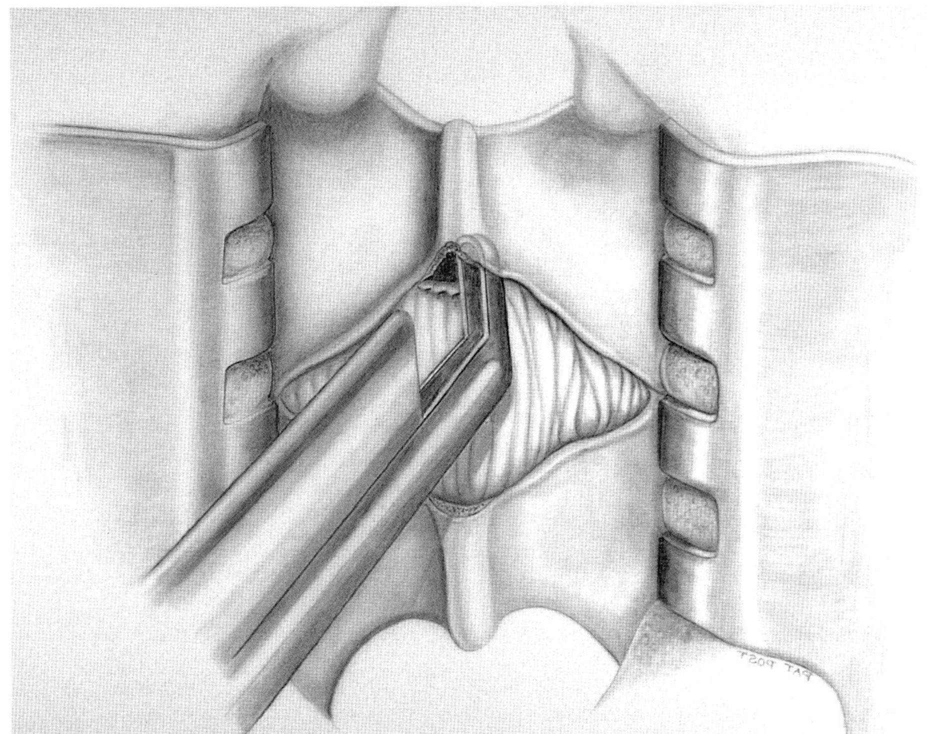

Figure 6. A small upbiting Kerrison rongeur is used to develop the midline dissection. Once epidural fat and the midline raphe of the ligamentum flavum is identified, dissection of further superior dissection is seldom necessary.

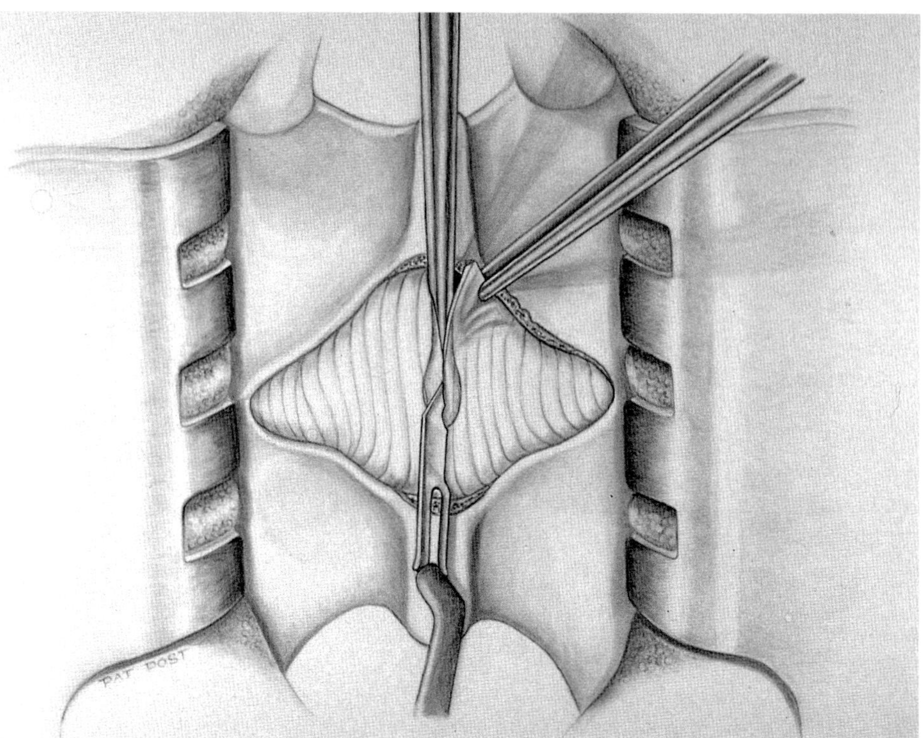

Figure 7. A Penfield #3 or possibly #4 elevator is placed under the dura, and a #5 blade is used to divide the dura in the midline using the elevators as protectors.

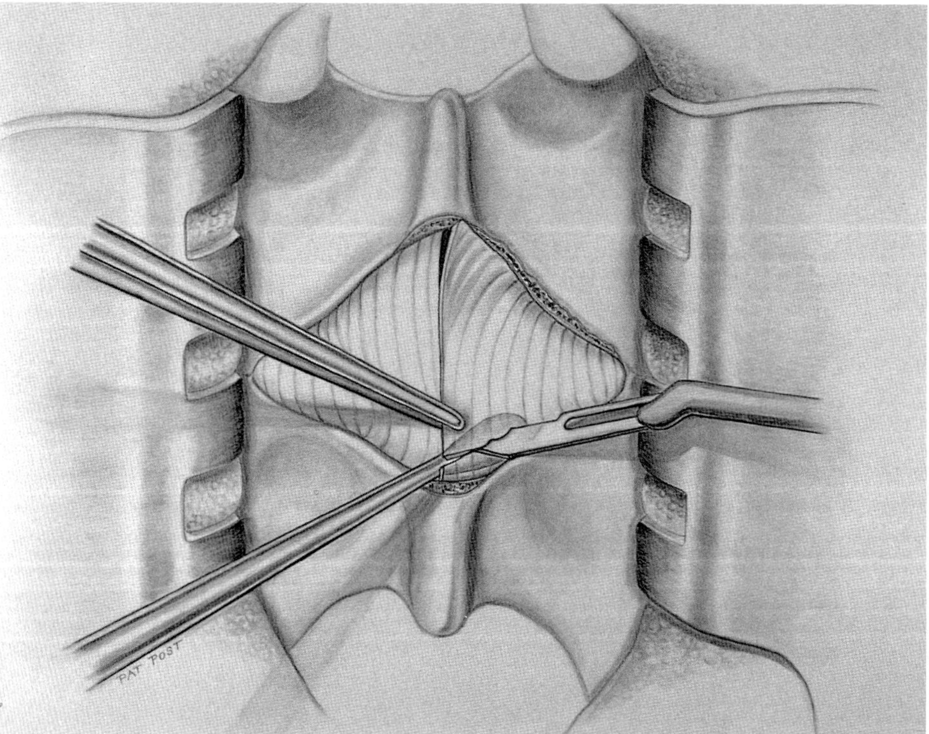

Figure 8. Either sharp or curette dissection can be used to resect the ligamentum flavum from the attachments to the lamina both superiorly and posteriorly. Another option is to ensure that no adhesions exist on the interior surface of the flavum, where an upbiting rongeur can also be used to remove the flavum in a piecemeal fashion under direct vision. When performing a central discectomy, I resect the flavum on both sides and perform anulotomies on both sides to ensure appropriate complete discectomy.

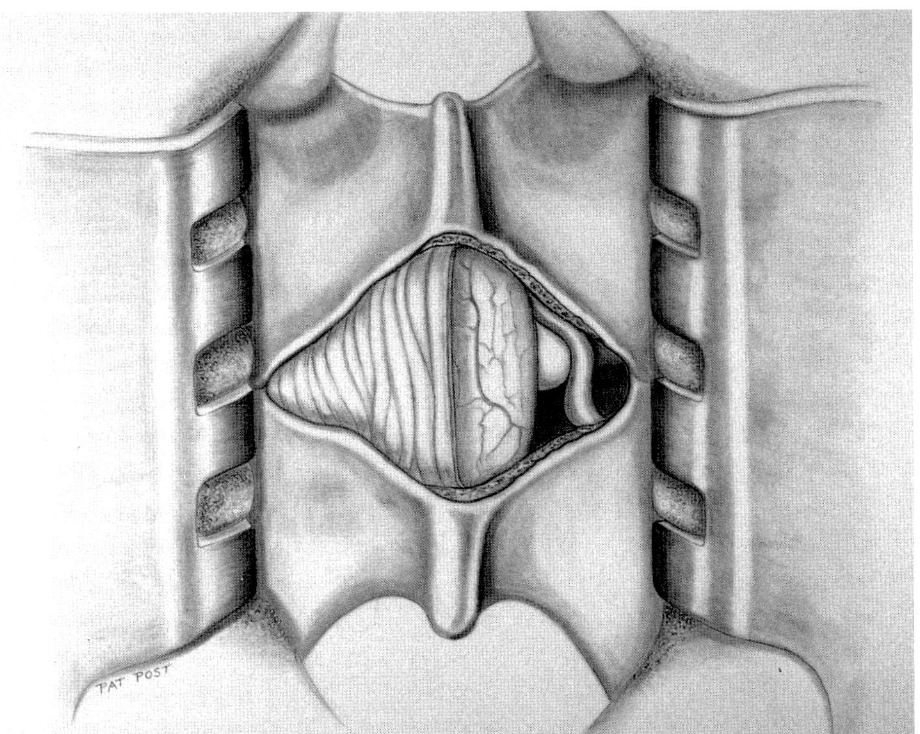

Figure 9. An axillary disc herniation with the root lateral to the disc. This is not the most common presentation but is perhaps the riskier presentation with respect to potential injury to the nerve root. The lateral portion of the dura often appears to be the lateral border of the nerve root. When this anatomic information is misinterpreted, injury to the nerve root can certainly occur. The importance here is to perform the dissection lateral enough to identify the existing nerve root clearly.

is usually insufficient to warrant stabilization. Failure to recognize lateral recess stenosis is certainly a cause for failed lumbar spine surgery. Usually the nerve root can be easily displaced medially to expose the disc herniation. Once the disc herniation has been observed, pituitary rongeurs are used to remove the offending extrusion (Fig. 10). A Love nerve root retractor protects the nerve root from injury. The initial incision into the anulus should be in the direction of the nerve root, so that the likelihood of major damage will be lessened in the event of a root entry.

I perform a limited discectomy and make no attempt to remove the entire intervertebral disc. This technique has no higher recurrence rate than the more formal and complete discectomy procedures advocated by others (13). In addition, patients who have limited discectomy are less likely to complain of low back pain on long-term follow-up. Once the disc has been removed with pituitary rongeurs, the nerve root is mobilized to ensure that at least 1 cm of medial displacement is possible (Fig. 11). When this objective has been reached, the wound is irrigated and an interposition membrane of Gelfoam is put in place. The wound is then closed in layers over a drain. Blood loss seldom exceeds 150 ml.

Other surgical options to consider include microscopic discectomy using an operating microscope and percutaneous discectomy using automated devices, lasers, and/or microrongeurs. Chemonucleolysis is still used in other countries but not often in the United States. Outcome expectations from traditional open discectomy and microdiscectomy are similar. Both techniques have their proponents. Complication rates with microdiscectomy procedures are higher, at least during the "learning curve" (8). Nevertheless, either procedure is a reasonable option as long as the objective of safely decompressing the neural elements is achieved

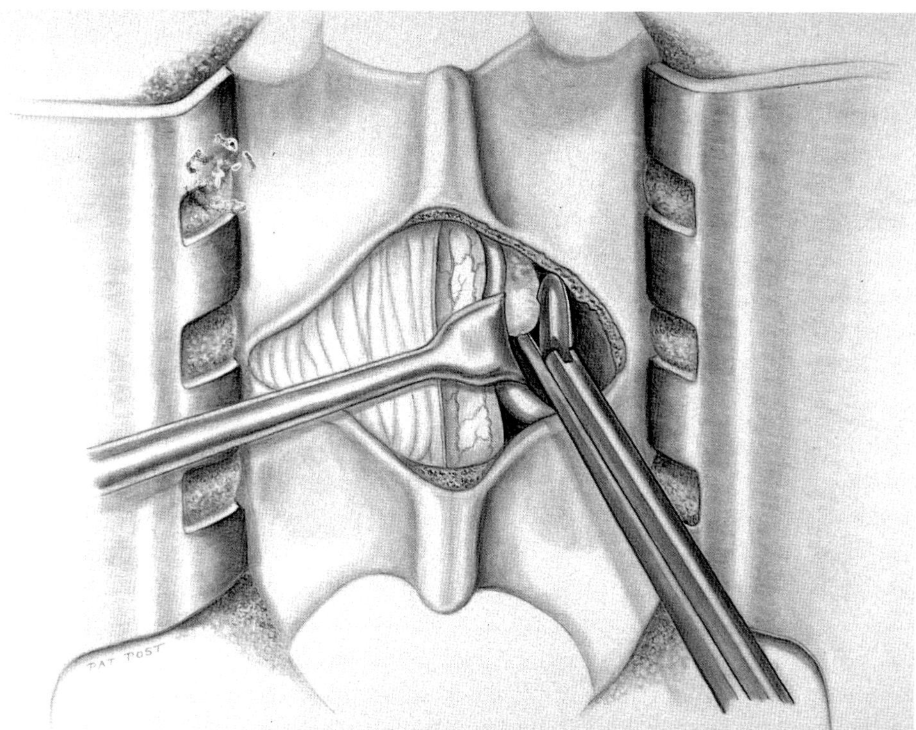

Figure 10. Two options exist for the surgeon. The nerve root may be gently elevated and displaced medially to the herniated disc. At that point, the disc can be easily removed using a pituitary rongeur. Another option is to debulk the disc herniation through the axilla in the junctional zone between the dural sac medially and nerve root laterally. This requires caution and careful knowledge of the precise location of all structures.

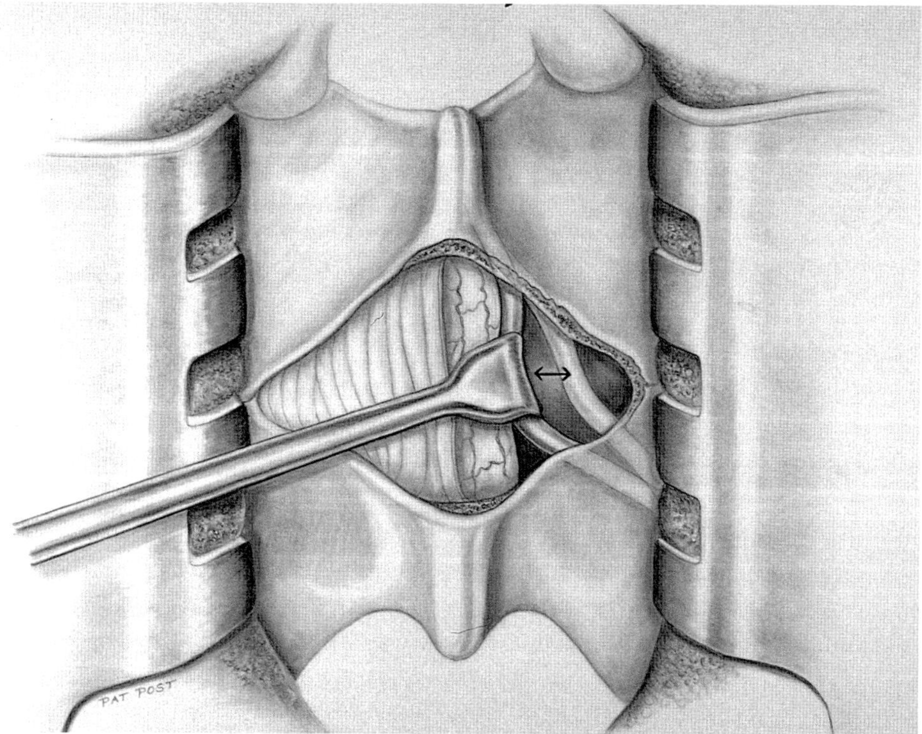

Figure 11. When the disc has been removed, the section is completed when the nerve root can be easily displaced 1 cm medially. Careful inspection is carried out to ensure that no other sequestered or extruded disc material is present; at this point, the wound is irrigated and closed.

(8,17). Using valid patient selection techniques, the expected outcome at 1 year of follow-up will be in the 85% to 90% good/excellent range (8,17). Fusion of the motion segment is not warranted in patients who have a primary lumbar disc herniation, unless segmental hypermobility of the involved motion segment is objectively documented. More controversy exists with regard to the value of percutaneous discectomy procedures. In a prospective study in France that compared chemonucleolysis with percutaneous discectomy, only 40% of the patients who had percutaneous discectomy improved, compared with 60% of the chemonucleolysis group (11). Both of these outcomes are below traditional discectomy or microdiscectomy standards. Although the minimally invasive nature and lower costs of the percutaneous procedures are attractive, the ultimate proof has to be a clinical outcome close to the gold standard discectomy procedure. More compelling to me is the use of spinal endoscopy with direct removal of the herniated disc tissue, as advocated by Kambin (6). Preliminary results in well-selected patients are good (80% or better) (6). This technique is evolving, and final judgment awaits the ability of others to duplicate these initial results. Chemonucleolysis still has a hard-core group of supporters, but the vast majority of American surgeons have stopped using this technique probably because of concern over infrequent catastrophic complications such as transverse myelitis.

POSTOPERATIVE MANAGEMENT

Once the surgical procedure has been performed, the patient is placed in a lumbosacral binder for 1 month. Patients generally comply with the use of a binder since abdominal support is provided. Thirty days after discectomy, patients begin an aggressive trunk-strengthening program involving both flexion and extension exercises with resistive equipment. Progress can be monitored by a multiaxis dynamometer. Motivated patients with high physical demands on the job are released for full duty approximately 4 months after surgery. Patients who have office-type jobs may be released to work within the first 10 days.

Nearly 90% of well-selected patients can be expected to do well following lumbar discectomy. In the event that a patient does not respond, a thorough reevaluation should be undertaken to exclude the multiple possible causes for low back symptoms. In addition, the surgeon should carefully reaffirm that the proper intervertebral disc level was addressed at the time of surgery. Although they are difficult to interpret in the first days to weeks following surgery, imaging studies should be repeated. Imaging studies often do not change substantially, even in those individuals who have extruded disc herniations and marked clinical improvement. Additional studies could be useful to provide further data.

COMPLICATIONS

Proper localization of the intervertebral disc level is essential to lessen the likelihood of a wrong-level procedure. Counting mobile spinous processes is not completely accurate and should not represent the sole method of localizing a spinal level. Gentle technique is required during exposure and manipulation of the dura and nerve roots to lessen the likelihood of a neural injury. The exposure must be adequate, which implies that the lateral extension of the exposure must be fully developed. In the event an axillary disc herniation is identified, the surgeon must be especially careful that the laterally displaced nerve root is not injured. All the potential hidden zones for disc herniation should be inspected and the nerve root mobilized to ensure at least 1 cm of mobility. Nerve root foramina can be probed using a Penfield #3 elevator to ensure that no lateral disc herniation is present. I seldom use electrocautery within the vertebral canal, since I believe nerve root injury can occur through electrical stimulation. I am also concerned about increased scar formation with the use of electrocautery within the canal. I obtain hemostasis by using small squares of thrombin-soaked Gelfoam and cottonoids tamping.

As with any surgical procedure, a list of potential complications that might occur would be exhaustive. Dural tears may occur during an initial discectomy procedure but are more commonly encountered during repeat surgery. These tears usually occur when adhesions are being separated from the dura. Repair of the dura should be carefully performed using magnification to avoid small rootlets. Generally a 6–0 nonabsorbable suture works well. Cauda equina syndrome can develop during the recovery phase. Such an event is usually related to an epidural hematoma. Close monitoring of the patient's neurologic status in the recovery room and hospital room will permit early recognition of this uncommon but potentially devastating complication. Early surgical reexploration represents the optimal choice to manage this complication.

Injuries to the iliac arteries and veins and visceral injuries to virtually every structure from the appendix to the ureter have been reported in association with a lumbar discectomy procedure. Errors in diagnosis may also occur, so that a patient may have symptoms suggestive of a lumbar disc herniation that in fact are related to other problems such as referred pain from intraabdominal pathologic processes such as aneurysms or malignancies. By developing a thorough diagnostic assessment and using judicious intraoperative technique, these extraordinary complications will be minimized.

ILLUSTRATIVE CASE FOR TECHNIQUE

R.M.B. is a 36-year-old physician who presented with an 8-month history of low back pain and right sciatica. His symptoms increased greatly 1 month before

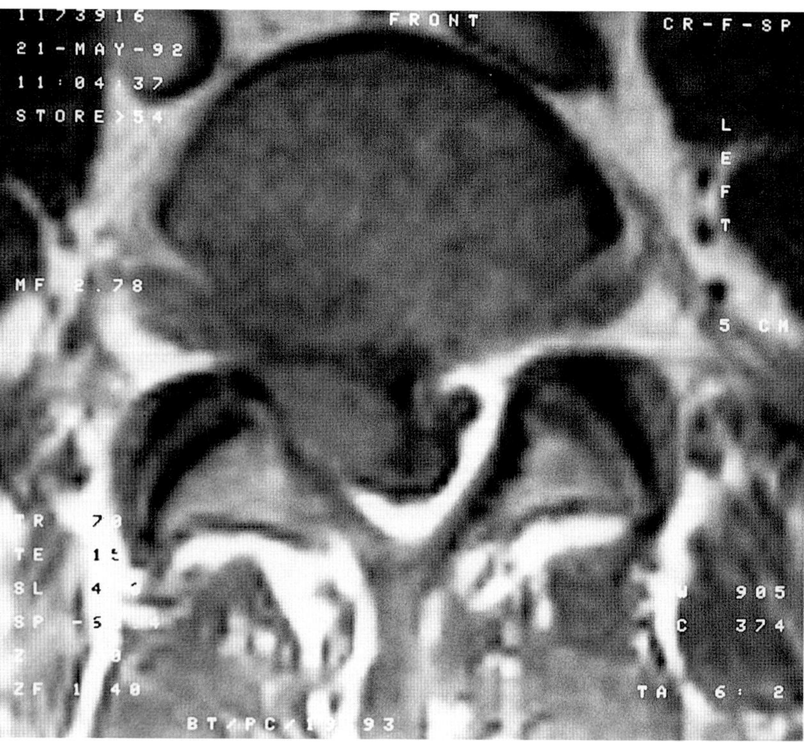

Figure 12. Axial image depicting a large extruded disc fragment immediately anterior to the S1 roots, displacing both the root and dural sac.

his orthopaedic evaluation. Nonoperative treatment had been ineffective. Because of his adverse quality of life, he wished to consider surgical treatment.

Physical examination revealed marked dysrhythmia with flexion. He had a dramatic positive crossed straight-leg test left to right. His right ankle jerk was diminished, and no motor weakness was observed. His preoperative OPES was 90. The preoperative MRI is shown in Fig. 12. At the time of discectomy, a large 1 × 3-cm extruded fragment was removed anterior to the S1 nerve root.

His postoperative course was uneventful; rehabiliation was implemented at 1 month, and he has an excellent result 20 months after discectomy.

RECOMMENDED READING

1. Abdullah, A. F., Wolber, P. G., Warfield, J. R., and Gunadi, I. K.: Surgical management of extreme lateral lumbar disc herniations: review of 138 cases. *Neurosurgery*, 22: 648–653, 1988.
2. Dandy, W. E.: Serious complications of ruptured intervertebral disks. *JAMA*, 119: 474–477, 1942.
3. Hakelius, A., and Hindmarsh, J.: The comparative reliability of preoperative diagnostic methods in lumbar disc surgery. *Acta Orthop. Scand.*, 43: 234–238, 1972.
4. Holmes, H. E., and Rothman, R. H.: Technique of lumbar laminectomy. In: *American Academy of Orthopaedic Surgeons Instructional Course Lectures*, Vol. 28. pp. 200–207.
5. Kane, W.: Incidence of lumbar discectomy. Presented at the 6th Annual Meeting of the International Society for the Study of the Lumbar Spine, New Orleans, Louisiana.
6. Kambin, P.: Arthroscopic Microdiscectomy. *Arthroscopy*, 8: 287–295, 1992.
7. Kostuik, J. P., Harrington, I., Alexander, D., Rand, W., and Evans, D.: Cauda equina syndrome and lumbar disc herniation. *J. Bone Joint Surg.*, 68A: 386–391, 1986.
8. McCulloch, J. A.: *Principles of Microsurgery for Lumbar Disc Disease*. Raven Press, New York, 1989.
9. O'Connell, J. E.: Protrusions of the lumbar intervertebral discs. A clinical review based on five hundred cases treated by excision of the protrusion. *J. Bone Joint Surg.*, 33B: 8–30, 1951.
10. Ransford, A. O., Cairns, D., and Mooney, V.: The pain drawing as an aid to the psychological evaluation of patients with low-back pain. *Spine*, 1: 127–134, 1976.
11. Revel, M., Payan, C., Vallee, C., et al.: Percutaneous lumbar discectomy versus chemonucleolysis in the treatment of sciatica: a randomized multicenter trial. *Spine*, 18: 1–7, 1993.
12. Spangfort, E. V.: The lumbar disc herniation: A computer-aided analysis of 2,504 operations. *Acta Orthop. Scand. Suppl.*, 142: 1–95, 1972.
13. Spengler, D. M.: *Low Back Pain*. Grune & Stratton, New York, 1982.
14. Spengler, D. M.: Lumbar discectomy. In: *Operative Orthopaedics*, Vol. 3, pp. 2055–2064. J. B. Lippincott, Philadelphia, 1988.
15. Spengler, D. M., and Freeman, C. W.: Patient selection for lumbar discectomy. *Spine*, 4: 129–134, 1979.
16. Spengler, D. M., Freeman, D., Westbrook, R., and Miller, J. W.: Low-back pain following multiple lumbar spine procedures. *Spine*, 5: 356–360, 1980.
17. Spengler, D. M., Ouellette, E., Battie, M., and Zeh, J.: Elective discectomy for herniation of a lumbar disc. *J. Bone Joint Surg.*, 72: 230–237, 1990.
18. Waddell, G., McCullough, J. A., Kummel, E., et al.: Nonorganic physical signs in low back pain. *Spine*, 5: 117–125, 1980.
19. Weber, H.: Lumbar disc herniation: a controlled, prospective study with ten years of observation. *Spine*, 8: 131–140, 1983.
20. Wiesel, S. W., Tsourmas, N., Feffer, H. L., et al.: A study of computer-assisted tomography. *Spine*, 9: 549–551, 1984.
21. Wiltse, L. L.: In: *Lumbar Discectomy and Laminectomy*, edited by R. G. Watkins and J. C. Collis. Aspen, Rockville, Maryland, 1987.

Master Techniques in Orthopaedic Surgery,
THE SPINE, edited by D. S. Bradford,
Lippincott-Raven Publishers, Philadelphia, © 1997.

16

Disc Excision by Thoracoscopy

John J. Regan

INDICATIONS/CONTRAINDICATIONS

Thoracic disc herniation is an uncommon but important cause of severe, incapacitating local or radicular pain. It presents with a variety of nonspecific symptoms, leading to wrong or delayed diagnosis (8,12,14,15,24). Although the incidence has been reported at 1 in 100,000 persons/year using computed tomography (CT) scan, current studies using magnetic resonance imaging (MRI) put this number at 14.5% of all disc herniations (26). Improved methods of early detection have led to controversy on the appropriate management of this disease (2,5). Diagnosis of clinically significant thoracic disc disease (TDD) is established by a history of central or radicular thoracic pain that is sometimes accompanied by paresthesias in a dermatomal distribution. This pain is usually aggravated by activity. Lumbar radicular symptoms may accompany thoracic pain, but occasionally lower extremity symptoms may be the only manifestation of TDD. In fact, TDD has been called the great imitator and is often misdiagnosed as angina, cholecystitis, pleurisy, renal colic, lumbar disc disease, and intrabdominal pathology. In the elderly patient, TDD may present as progressively unstable gait resulting from myelopathy without thoracic pain. Myelopathy and paralysis are also presenting complaints in the younger population as a result of large disc herniations or acute herniations arising from trauma. Severe pain is usually an accompanying complaint in these middle-aged and younger patients who present with myelopathy.

Once a diagnosis of clinically significant thoracic disc herniation is made, a period of conservative management of up to 6 months is indicated. Surgery is warranted in patients with signs of myelopathy and in those with intractable thoracic mechanical or radicular pain failing to respond to nonsurgical management. An MRI evaluation or CT-myelography must demonstrate a thoracic disc that indents the spinal cord.

J. J. Regan, M.D.: Department of Orthopaedic Surgery, University of Texas Southwestern Medical Center; Texas Back Institute, Plano, Texas 75093.

Video-assisted spinal surgery has several advantages over conventional transthoracic open procedures in the treatment of TDD. Video-monitored visualization of the procedure is provided to the entire operating team, including anesthesiologist, which results in more interest and participation. Two surgeons may work side by side, allowing standard instruments to be inserted while enhanced magnified visualization is preserved, in spite of minimal incisions. Extensive visualization of the thoracic spine anatomy exceeding that possible with an open incision is provided by the 30-degree angled scope. The result is that less vertebral body excision is required to visualize and excise the disc herniation. Rib resection or spreading of ribs associated with open thoracotomy is avoided with video-assisted thoracic surgery (VATS), resulting in less incisional pain, less chest tub drainage, fewer respiratory problems, and little shoulder girdle dysfunction—problems commonly associated with open procedures (9,11,16). Decreased blood loss and decreased potential for infection result from the minimal incisions made in a relatively closed body cavity, as opposed to the large incisions required with rib distraction and its associated trauma. Reduced postoperative pain leads to improved perioperative ventilation, decreased intensive care unit time, decreased blood loss, shorter hospitalization, and shorter rehabilitation time, with a resultant decrease in overall medical cost (2,3,21). The major obstacle is the technical skill that must be acquired to master this technique. In many ways, the technique is similar to those of microsurgery and arthroscopy. In our experience, surgeons familiar with the basic principles of endoscopy and those with previous experience in arthroscopy quickly adapt to thorascopic spinal surgery. We believe that a period of practice in the in vivo and cadaver laboratory, as well as assistance from an endoscopic qualified thoracic surgeon for a period of time, is essential to a safe outcome.

In general, thoracoscopic discectomy is indicated if the above conditions of special training are met (Table 1). Patients at high risk for thoracotomy, such as the elderly, may be better candidates for thoracoscopy. Thoracotomy produces many physiologic sequelae, which are detrimental to high-risk patients. These include decrease in functional residual capacity as well as documented incidence of postoperative atelectasis, secondary to chest wall splinting from pain (Table 2) (10,13,25). Patients with chronic obstructive pulmonary disease or patients with interstitial fibrosis, who have abnormal pulmonary function, obviously fit the high-risk category. Cardiac patients who require medication for hypertension or mild congestive heart failure are considered high risk for the postoperative sequelae of thoracotomy and may be more suitable candidates for thoracoscopy.

TABLE 1. *Thoracoscopic spinal reconstructive procedures*[a]

Procedure	No. of patients
Thoracic discectomy	41
Multilevel anterior discectomy for correction of scoliosis	20
Anterior release for kyphosis	4
Excision of hemivertebrae	3
Vertebral corpectomy for neurologic decompression	8
Pyogenic vertebral osteomyelitis decompression	2
Total	78
Anterior laparoscopic interbody stabilization and fusion procedures: L4–L5 or L5–S1	22

From ref. 27.

[a] In two recent reports of 28 patients undergoing thoracoscopic discectomy and a larger series of 100 patients who underwent endoscopic thoracic and lumbar spinal reconstructive procedures, a total of seven cases of atelectasis was reported with no major pulmonary sequelae.

Degenerative disc disease from T4–T5 to T12–L1 can be approached from the left or right side depending on the location of the pathology (3). Patients who have undergone previous thoracotomy or costotransversectomy with retained disc herniation may be approached from the contralateral side. The endoscope provides a clear view across to the contralateral disc, which may be excised without going through scar tissue from previous surgery. Clarified disc herniations can be approached endoscopically using modified Penfield probes and ball-tipped probes to dissect adherent disc away from the dura.

Thoracoscopic discectomy is contraindicated in patients with inability to tolerate one-lung ventilation, severe or acute respiratory insufficiency, high airway pressures with positive pressure ventilation, and pleural symphysis. Patients with a history of empyema, previous thoracotomy, or tube thoracostomy are relatively contraindicated depending on the degree of pleural adhesions.

PREOPERATIVE PLANNING

Patients with thoracic disc herniation often present with central or radicular thoracic pain aggravated by activity. Physical examination may reveal sensory abnormalities in the appropriate dermatomal distribution. Patients with spinal cord involvement may present with gait disturbance or bowel and bladder incontinence. Spastic gait may be identified on examination, as well as hyper-reflexia that results from upper motor neuron pathology. Motor weakness, sensory disturbance, and paralysis are found in the more severe cases of spinal cord compression. In the rare situation of acute paresis from thoracic disc herniation, administration of high-dose steroids is recommended prior to emergency spinal cord decompression.

The most sensitive method for diagnosis of TDD is high-resolution MRI. This allows extensive scanning of the entire thoracic spine with a high degree of sensitivity and specificity. This improved method of early detection has led to contro-

TABLE 2. *Complications*

Complication[a]	No. of patients
Thoracoscopic	
Intercostal neuralgia (all transient)	6 p
Atelectasis	5 p
Excessive epidural blood loss, 2,500 ml	2 p
Conversion to open thoracotomy due to previous costotransversectomy	1 p
Penetration of right hemidiaphragm from thoracoport in patient with prior empyema	1 p
Transient paraplegia related to spinal stenosis at a different vertebral level and operative positioning	1 p
Laparoscopic	
Conversion to open laparotomy for repair of left common iliac vein	1 p
Bone graft donor site infection	2 p
Postoperative upper GI bleed in patient anticoagulated with Coumadin up to 2 weeks prior to surgery	1 p

From ref. 27.

[a] No cases of permanent iatrogenic neurologic deficit and no cases of spinal wound infection were reported.

versy in the appropriate management of the disease (5,12). Williams et al. (26) reported a 14.5% incidence of all disc herniations in asymptomatic oncology patients undergoing screening examinations. The use of CT-myelography, especially when MRI has localized the appropriated level, can sometimes add information to the preoperative planning of the procedure. Magnetic resonance images obtained in obese patients, low-resolution MRI scans, or scans with motion artifact may not give detailed information on the location of the herniation, the indentation on the spinal cord, or calcification of the disc material. However, CT-myelography can provide this vital information, which is important in deciding whether surgery is indicated as well as the appropriate approach.

One of the most important aspects of preoperative planning is the identification of the correct disc to be excised. In our experience of 28 consecutive thoracoscopic discectomies, mostly physician-referred cases, five cases were inaccurately identified on the radiologist's report. This resulted from anomalies in the number of lumbar vertebrae and ribs. We recommend counting from C1 in MRI scans and from T1 for CT-myelograms. Prior to surgery, we obtain an anteroposterior (AP) thoracic and lumbar roentgenogram to count the number of thoracic and lumbar vertebrae. Confirmation at the time of surgery is obtained by cross-table AP thoracolumbar radiograph, counting up from the last rib.

SURGERY

Setup and Equipment

Spinal VATS should be performed in a standard operating room that has monitors for assessing patients receiving general anesthesia and equipment available

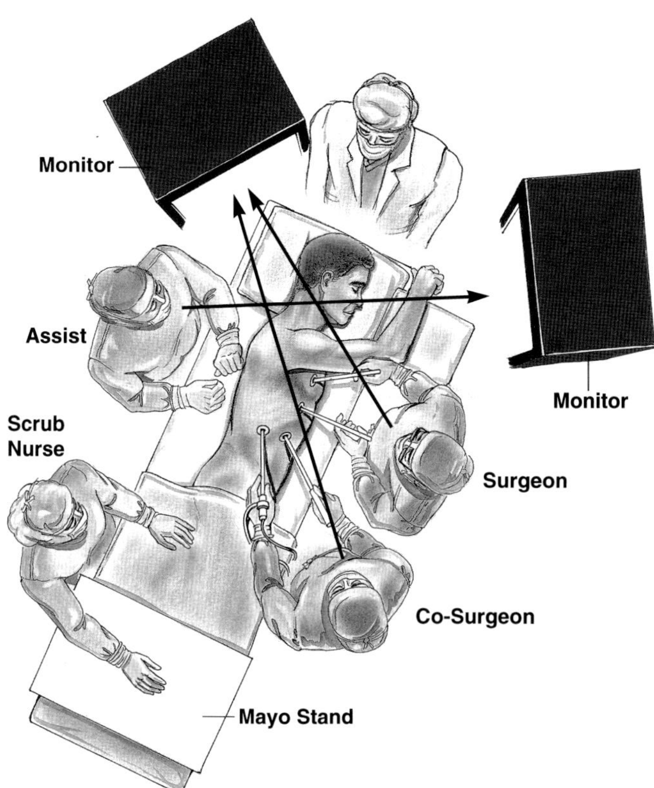

Figure 1. Operating room setup with surgeon and cosurgeon on abdominal side of patient.

for open thoracotomy. Some modifications of the standard thoracoscopy setup are necessary for spinal procedures. After the anesthesiologist has set in place a double-lumen endotracheal tube, the patient is positioned in a straight lateral decubitus position and held securely in an Olympic positioner (Fig. 1). The hips and lower extremities may be gently brought down, but the extreme jack-knife position should be avoided, as this may stretch an already compromised spinal cord. The patient should be fully prepared for a standard posterolateral thoracotomy with the iliac crest available, if additional bone graft is needed. For approaches to the upper thoracic spine, the arm should be flexed slightly above 90 degrees and the axilla draped out. The anesthesiologist must be prepared to set the table in an anterior tilt (Fig. 2) and apply Trendelenburg or reverse Trendelenburg positions as needed to permit the deflated lung to fall away from the dorsal spine.

In addition to the standard operating room setup, two video monitors are optimal. The surgeon and first assistant stand on the same side of the operating table, the abdominal side of the patient, viewing the monitor on the opposite side of the table when performing spinal VATS. Because two-hand control of the orthopedic instruments is essential, a third assistant is necessary, especially when continuous fan retraction on the lung is required. The third assistant stands at the back side of the patient facing the opposing monitor. Dual monitors are placed at the head of the table in cases involving the mid and upper thoracic spine (Fig. 1). For surgery of the lower thoracic spine, in proximity to the diaphragm, a monitor is placed at the foot of the table so the surgeon can look toward the lower thoracic spine directly facing the monitor. This orientation of camera and monitor in the same general direction is the most comfortable working setup for the surgeon.

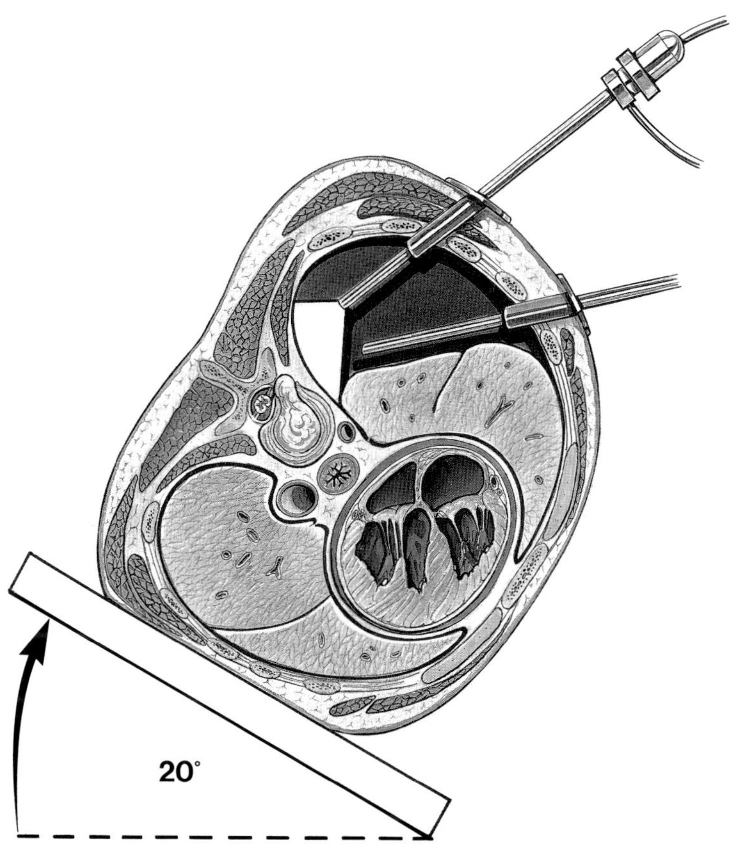

Figure 2. Cross-sectional view demonstrating anterior tilt to the table allowing ipsilateral collapsed lung to fall away from dorsal spine.

Extra personnel are usually required for spinal thoracoscopy. The spinal surgeon is usually assisted by a thoracic surgeon with experience in thoracoscopy until the spine surgeon has gained considerable experience. The thoracic surgeon provides and maintains the exposure, holding the camera and operating the suction-irrigator or grasper. The spine surgeon in many cases must use two hands to control the orthopaedic instruments safely. The third assistant may be called on to hold the camera, retract the lung, or assist in the suction or removal of disc or bony debris. When working in the spinal canal, close-up camera work is required without obstructing the path of the instruments. Often the individual holding the camera must gently zoom out to view an incoming instrument and then follow it in close to the spinal canal without changing camera angle.

The equipment required for spinal thoracoscopy is similar to general thoracoscopy with a few exceptions. The basic equipment required for thoracoscopy includes telescopes, light sources, cameras, monitors, video records, and insufflators. The 30-degree angled telescope is almost exclusively used for spinal procedures. The vast array of instruments designed for use in general thoracoscopy may also be needed in spinal VATS procedures. Endoscopic gastrointestinal anastomosis (GIA) stapling devices, lung clamps, grasper, trocars, scissors, retractors, suction irrigation systems, and endoscopic vascular clipping devices must be available to complete the procedure. In addition to this, modified thoracospinal instruments have been developed to assist in removal of discs and infusion (Fig. 3). Endoscopic bipolar cautery devices and drill systems adapted for endoscopic use have recently become available.

Technique

The procedure is performed under general anesthesia. A double-lumen tube is placed for unilateral ventilation, and an arterial line is inserted for monitoring. Somatosensory and motor evoked potentials are also monitored during the procedure. The patient is approached from the side of the herniation, although the right side is preferred in central disc herniations.

A three- or four-portal approach is employed starting with the initial trocar placement in the sixth or seventh intercostal space toward the anterior axillary

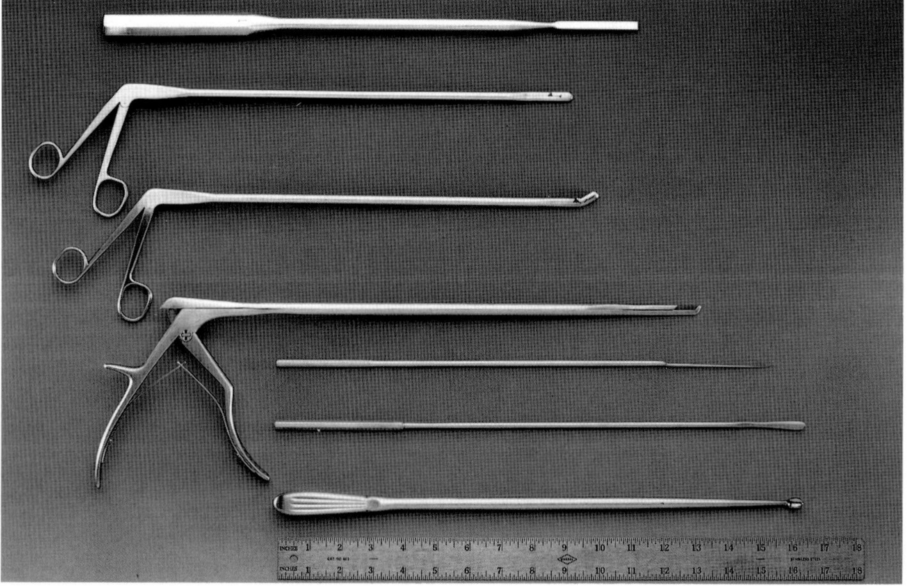

Figure 3. Modified thoracospinal instruments include: (a) Cobb elevator, (b) pituitary rongeurs, (c) Kerrison rongeur, (d) nerve and Penfield probes, and (e) angled curette.

line after the lung has been collapsed. The initial trocar placement is without direct visualization of the thoracic cavity and must be performed after digital palpation of the portal site to avoid injury to the lung, which may occur if pleural adhesions are present. This initial site is chosen to ensure insertion above the diaphragm. After a 30-degree angled rigid endoscope is inserted, following resorptive atelectasis of the lung, two or three additional trocars are placed under monitored vision, with one or two in the anterior axillary line and one toward the posterior axillary line just below the appropriate disc space (Figs. 4 and 5). A three-portal approach can be employed if successful atelectasis and patient positioning allows the lung to fall away from the dorsal spine, eliminating the need for a fan retractor. The ribs are then counted endoscopically until the appropriate level is identified (Figs. 6 and 7). A Verees needle is placed into the disc space anterior to the rib head and a cross-table AP radiograph is obtained to confirm the appropriate level (Fig. 8). The rib articulates at the disc space and corresponds to the vertebra below the disc space.

After radiographic confirmation, the rib head overlying the appropriate level is rejected after divining the radiated and costotransverse ligaments (Fig. 9) and then sectioning the rib 2 cm distal to the rib head using an osteotome or drill (Fig. 10). This step is not necessary below T9, where the rib articulates below the disc space.

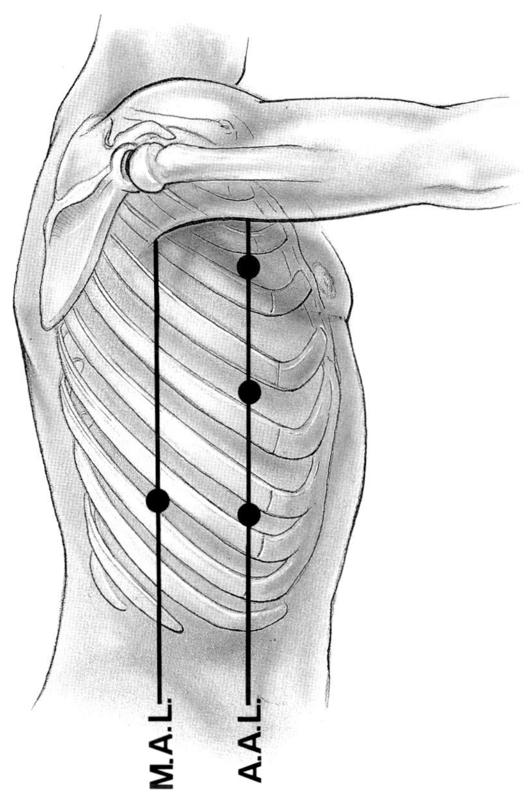

Figure 4. Four-trocar strategy for standard approach to mid-dorsal spine. *A.A.L.*, anterior axillary line; *M.A.L.*, midaxillary line.

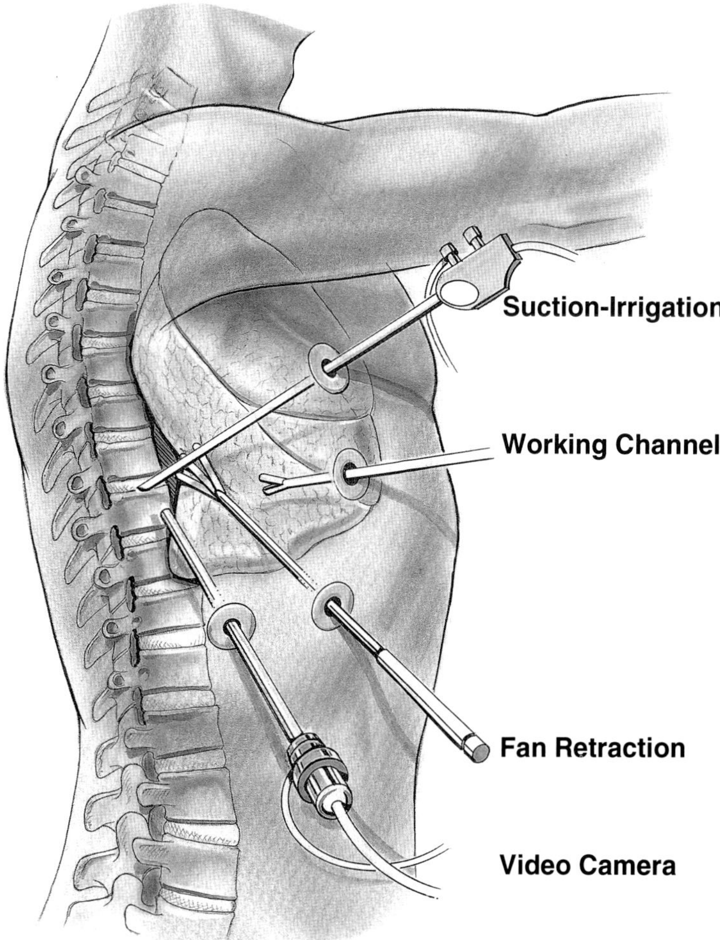

Figure 5. Four-trocar technique with instruments in place. A 30-degree telescope is brought in from below in the midaxillary line. Working channel (rongeur) is positioned directly opposite the disc space.

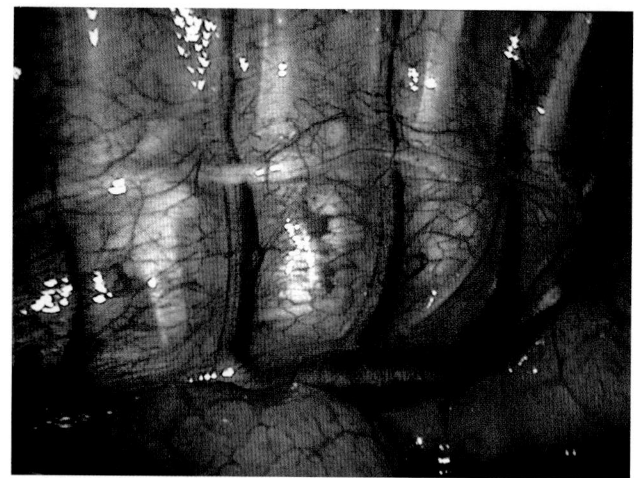

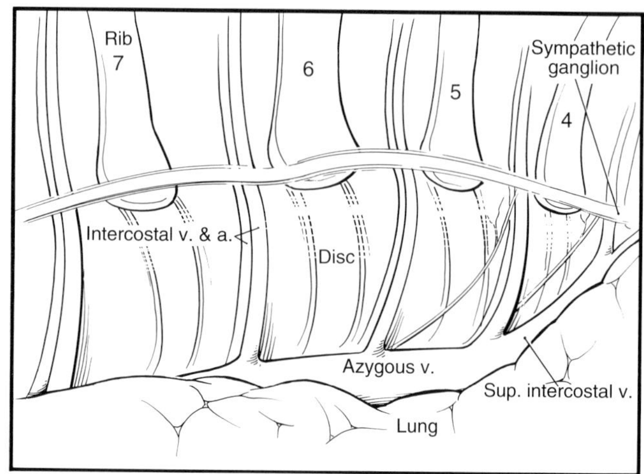

Figure 6. Surgical **(A)** and schematic **(B)** views of right mid-dorsal spine.

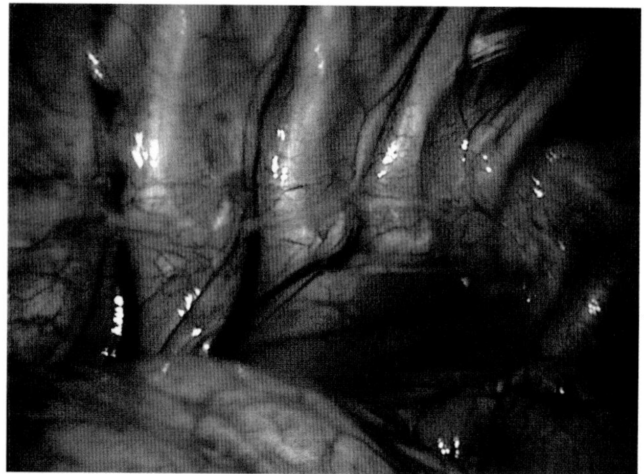

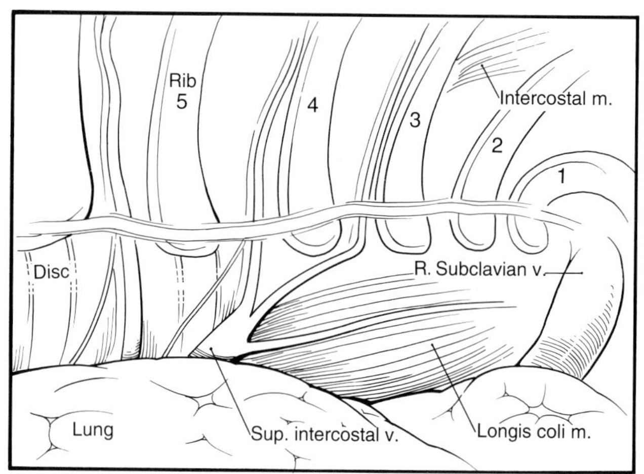

Figure 7. Surgical **(A)** and schematic **(B)** views of the upper thoracic spine with first rib obscured by fat. Rib count for correct level is initiated by this view.

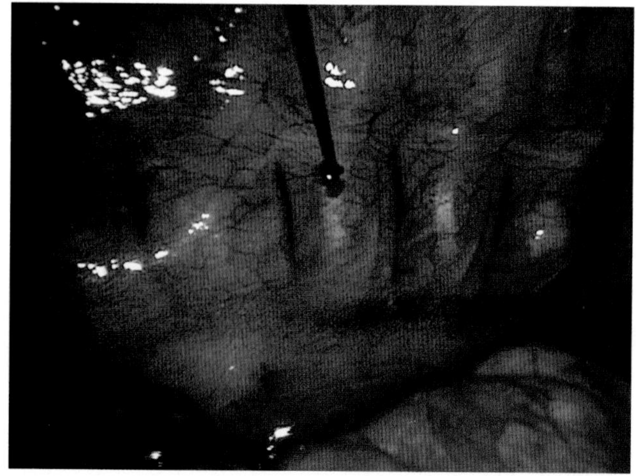

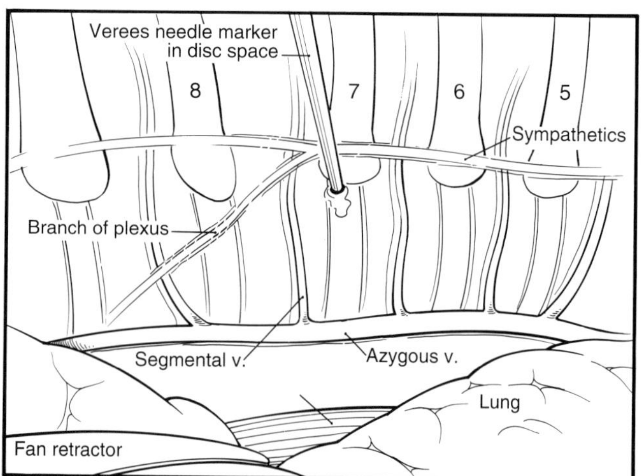

Figure 8. Surgical **(A)** and schematic **(B)** views of a Verees needle marker in T6–T7 disc space anterior to the seventh rib.

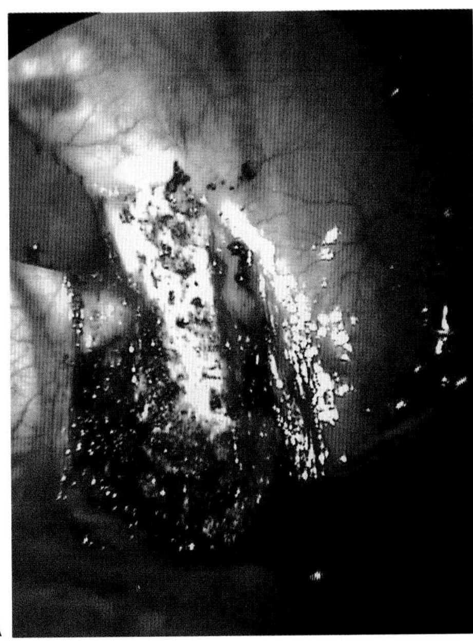

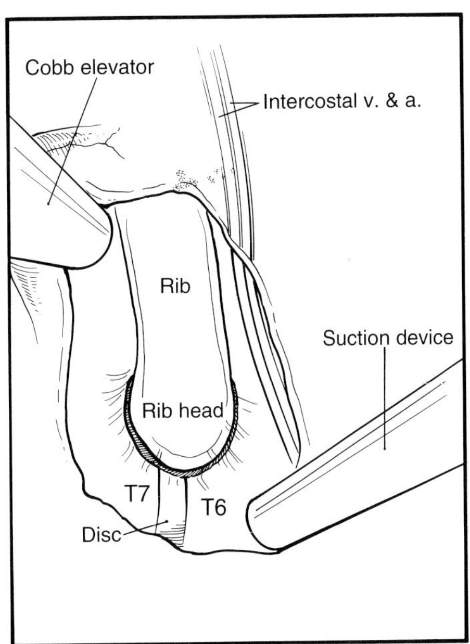

Figure 9. A,B: Surgical **(A)** and schematic **(B)** views of a periosteal elevator used to separate rib head from radiate and costotransverse ligaments.

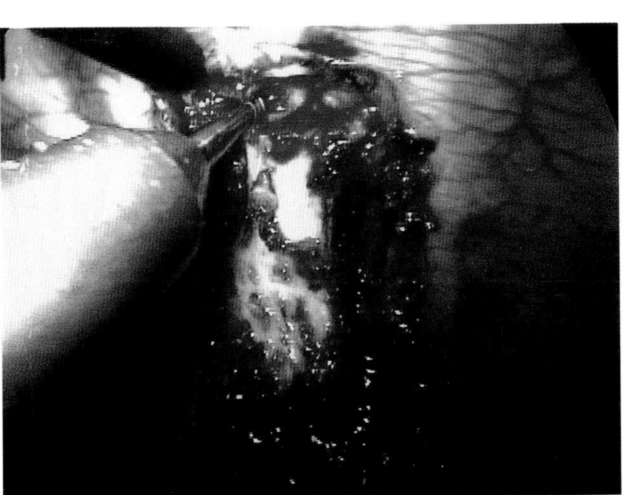

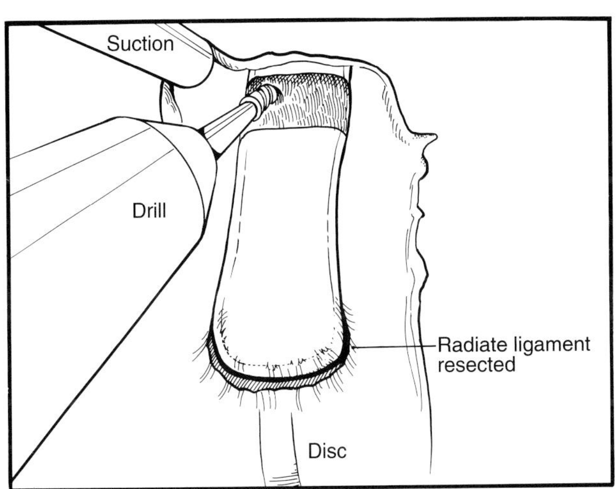

Figure 10. A,B: A high-speed side-cutting bur is used to section the rib before removal.

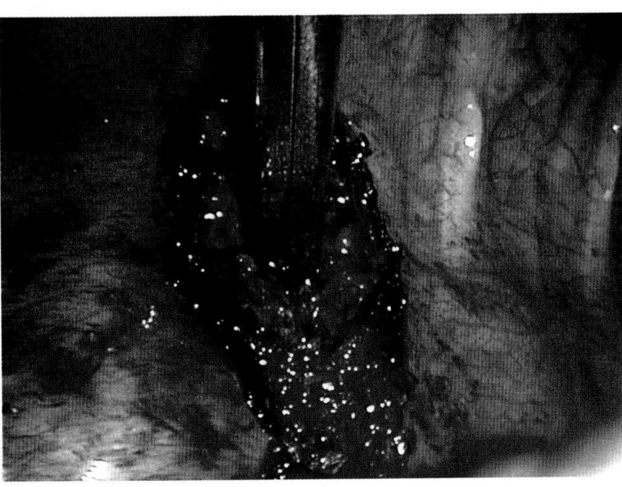

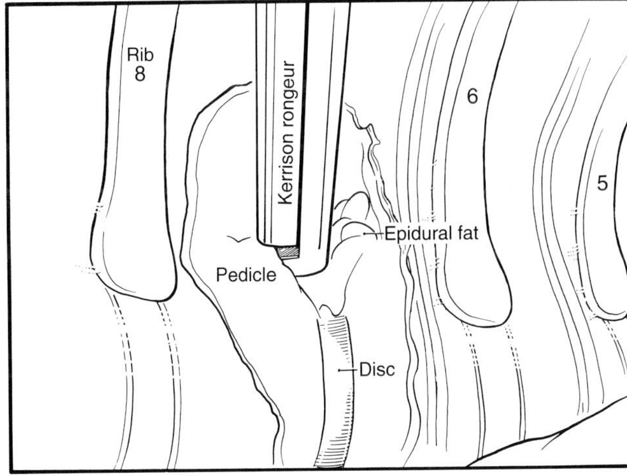

Figure 11. A,B: Kerrison ronguer is used to remove the superior edge of the pedicle once it is clearly defined.

Access to the spinal canal is gained by resecting the superior portion of the pedicle. The disc herniation is found by tracing the superior edge of the pedicle to the vertebral body and disc space. Once the dura is identified after partial pedicle resection using a modified Kerrison rongeur (Fig. 11), the disc herniation may be removed using a small angled curette directed away from the dura (Fig. 12). A small Penfield probe or nerve probe may be used to separate the herniation from the posterior longitudinal ligament and dura (Fig. 13). Once it is felt that adequate decompression has occurred (Fig. 14), a Penfield probe is placed in the intervertebral defect and a roentgenogram obtained to ensure that decompression has extended past the midline. Epidural bleeding can be controlled using endoscopic bipolar cautery or endoscopically applied Avitene. It is rarely necessary to sacrifice segmental vessels unless a fusion is done, in which case endoscopic vascular clips are used. A #24 Fr chest tube is inserted prior to lung expansion and wound closure. Marcaine blocks are also used to minimize postoperative pain.

If a fusion is to be performed, segmental vessels are ligated and divided above and below the disc space. A drill modified for endoscopic use is used to create a

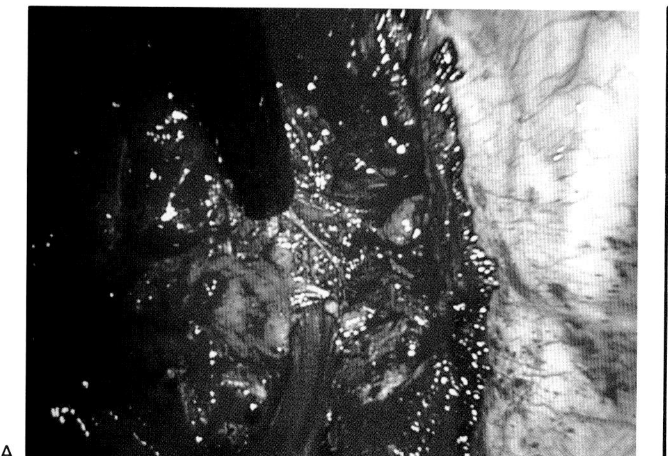

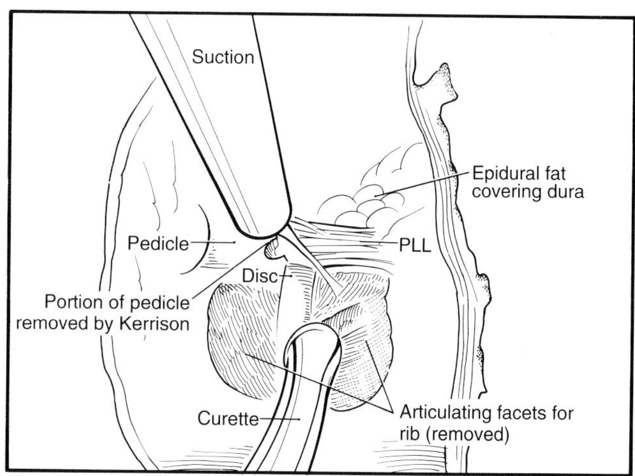

Figure 12. A,B: Angle curette is used for removing disc and end plate after the dura is visualized.

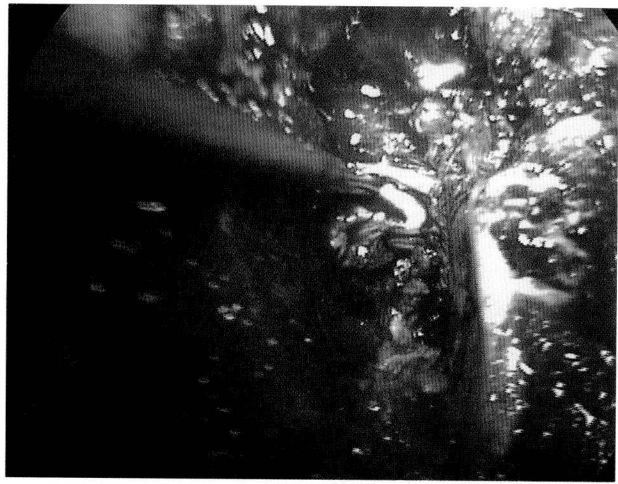

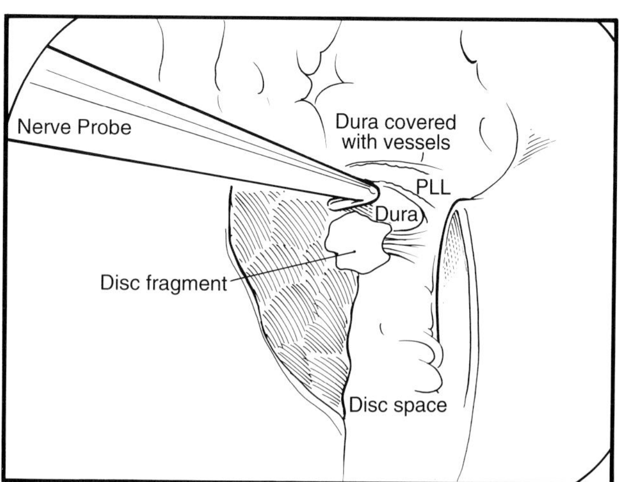

Figure 13. A,B: A nerve probe is used to remove a disc fragment from behind the posterior longitudinal ligament (*P.L.L.*).

trough above and below the disc space. A section of rib harvested during the discectomy is introduced endoscopically and secured using a bone tamp (Fig. 15). A suture is tied to the graft during insertion to prevent loss of the graft in the thoracic cavity.

POSTOPERATIVE MANAGEMENT

Patients early in our series were monitored in the intensive care unit, but we feel this is no longer necessary. The chest tube is usually removed on the first postoperative day unless drainage exceeds 50 ml in an 8-hour shift. Patients are also mobilized on the first postoperative day. Deep breathing exercises and mobilization of the upper extremities are encouraged. Patient-administered intravenous narcotics are used for 1 to 2 days, after which the patient is switched to oral medication.

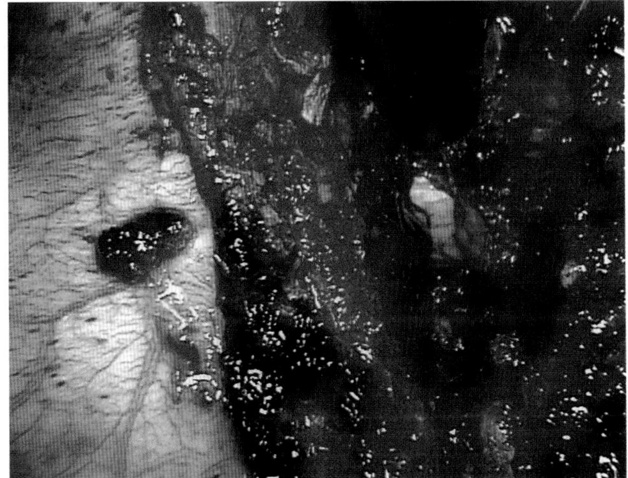

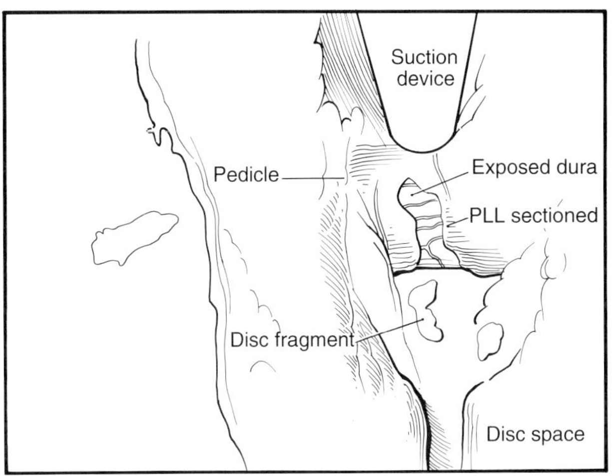

Figure 14. A,B: The dura is clearly viewed after removing the P.L.L. to ensure successful removal of herniated disc.

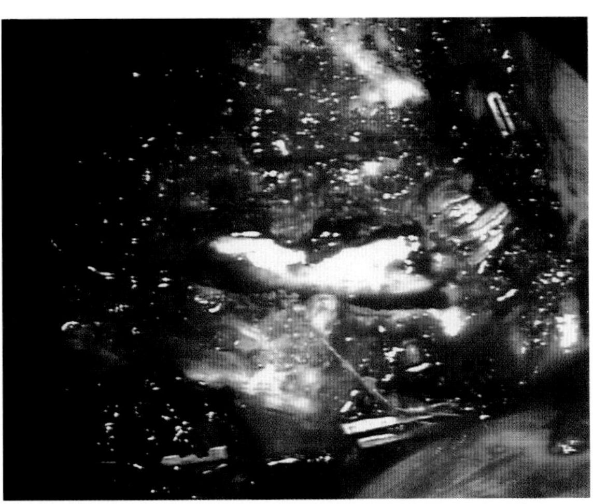

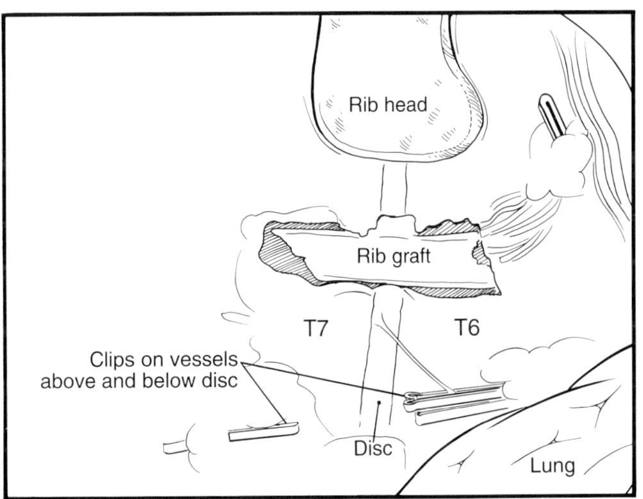

Figure 15. A,B: A rib strut graft is inserted into a trough created above and below disc space for interbody fusion.

TABLE 3. *Mean results of thoracoscopic (VATS) discectomy (28 patients)*

Parameter	Mean	Range
Age of patient	42 years	23–84 years
Operative time	2:44 hours	1:23–5:10 hours
Chest tube	21.6 days	0–3 days
Intraoperative estimated blood loss	494 ml	25–2500 ml
Postoperative length of stay	5 days	3–9 days
Return to work		
Non-workers' compensation (16 patients)	5.3 weeks	1–16 weeks
Workers' compensation (3 patients)[a]	10 weeks	6–13 weeks

From ref. 28, with permission.

[a] Seven workers' compensation patients were not working at minimum 6-month follow-up. Two patients were not working before the surgery.

Hospitalization in our series of 28 ranged from 3 to 9 days, with a mean of 5 days (Table 3). Sixteen non-workers' compensation patients returned to work at a mean interval of 5 weeks (range, 1 to 16 weeks). At a mean 1-year follow-up, 43% of our patients reported complete relief of primary symptoms, 43% reported improvement, and 14% remained unchanged, with no cases of worsening (Table 4). In a combined series of 93 patients undergoing open anterior transthoracic surgery or costotransversectomy for disc herniation [Albrand and Corkill (1), 7 patients; Bohlman and Zdeblick (4), 22 patients; Otani et al. (19), 23 patients; Simpson et al. (24), 23 patients; and Currier et al. (6), 8 patients 6], two patients developed transient paraparesis following open surgery with no infections. Improvement or resolution of symptoms varied from 66% to 89%. In our series, 86% of patients reported improvement or resolution of their primary symptoms with no neurologic deterioration (Table 4).

COMPLICATIONS

The most common problem is intercostal neuralgia, which is thought to occur from compression of the intercostal nerve by rigid trocars and levering against the nerve with instruments. This can be decreased by strategic positioning of the trocar, atraumatic manipulation of the instruments, and use of flexible trocars.

Postoperative atelectasis is the second most common complication significant enough to prolong the hospitalization in three patients. Loculated pleural effusions can be managed by thoracoscopic techniques if surgical lysis of adhesions is felt to be necessary. Diaphragm penetration, which may occur as a result of blind

TABLE 4. *Clinical results according to presenting classification*

Patient group	No. of patients	Complete	Improved	Same	Worse
I Mechanical pain	6	2	3	1	0
II Mechanical/radicular pain	11	4	6	1	0
III Radicular pain	6	2	2	2	0
IV Myelopathic symptoms	3	2	1	0	0
V Paralytic state	2	1	1	0	0
Total	28	12	12	4	0
Relief of primary symptoms at mean 9 months' follow-up:		43%	43%	14%	0%

insertion below the ninth rib, can be avoided by reviewing the chest radiograph for the position of the diaphragm before surgery and placing the initial trocar at the sixth or seventh intercostal space using digital palpation.

The patient must be informed that conversion to open thoracotomy is a possibility and the necessary equipment must be readily available in the operating room. We currently recommend using the cell-saver and endoscopic Avitene, bipolar cautery, vascular clips, and a period of tamponade with endoscopically inserted cottonoids and sponges to control epidural bleeding.

Transient paraparesis seldom occurs. We recommend spinal cord monitoring and, most importantly, meticulous dissection and adherence to the techniques set forth early in this chapter.

ILLUSTRATIVE CASE FOR TECHNIQUE

A 34-year-old grade school teacher presented with 13 months of thoracic radicular pain aggravated by leaning forward, increased activity, and Valsalva maneuver. The problem began after a motor vehicle accident that resulted in a twisting injury to the thorax. She complained of dysesthesias radiating under the right breast. She had little relief with a trial of physical therapy and nonsteroidal antiinflammatory medication. An epidural steroid injection resulted in only temporary relief. An MRI of the thoracic spine demonstrates a right paracentral disc herniation at T6–T7 (Fig. 16). A CT-myelogram demonstrates indentation of the spinal cord and calcification of the anulus lateral to the herniation in the neural foramen (Fig. 17). The patient underwent thoracoscopic discectomy as illustrated (see Figs. 6–15). An intraoperative cross-table AP radiograph was obtained after identification of the T6–T7 disc and marking with a Verees needle (Fig. 18). When the procedure was completed, a Penfield probe was carefully positioned in the disc

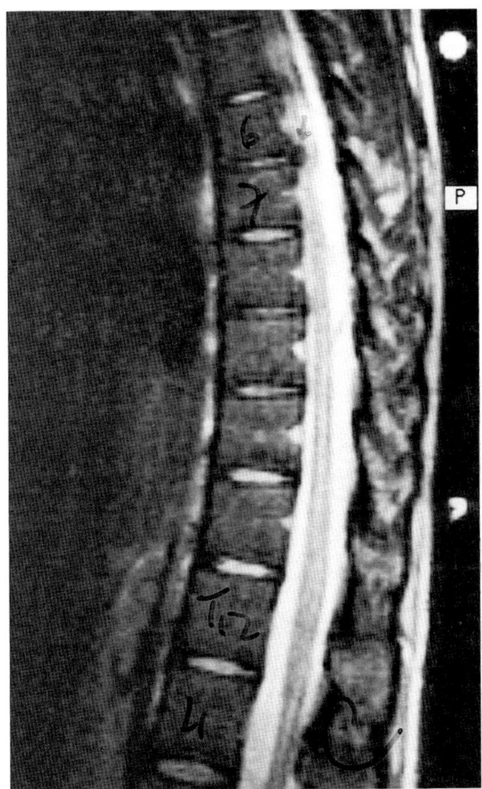

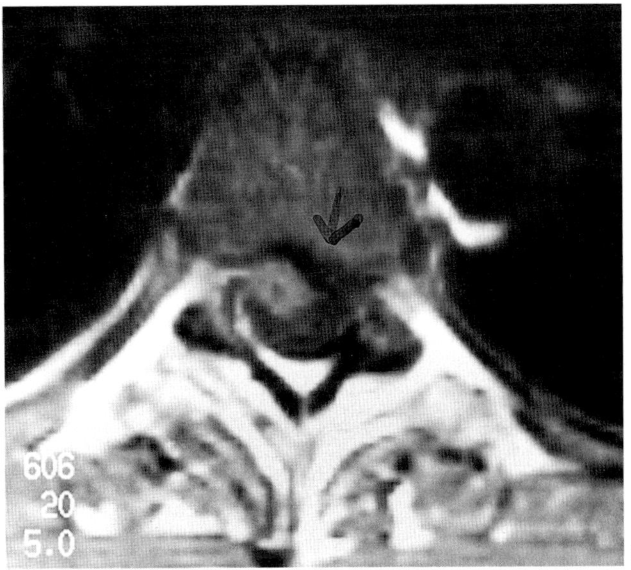

Figure 16. Lateral MRI scan **(A)** demonstrating central disc herniation at T6–T7. Axial image **(B)** confirms right paracentral herniation with cord effacement.

space and a radiograph obtained to confirm that decompression had extended past the midline (Fig. 19). A chest tube inserted at the end of the procedure was removed the next morning when drainage was noted to be less than 50 ml. A chest radiograph was obtained after removal to check for pneumothorax. The patient was admitted to the floor after the procedure and discharged on the third postoperative day with a Darvocet prescription. At that time the patient was given instructions to ambulate as tolerated and perform gentle range-of-motion exercises of the shoulder girdle. She noted resolution of the preoperative pain by the time of discharge. Her only complaint was tenderness around the portal sites and intercostal paresthesias that resolved over 2 weeks. The patient returned 1 week after surgery, at which time a chest radiograph was obtained to check for loculated effusion, atelectasis, or pneumothorax. She returned to her job teaching 10 days after surgery. Exercise therapy was progressed as tolerated.

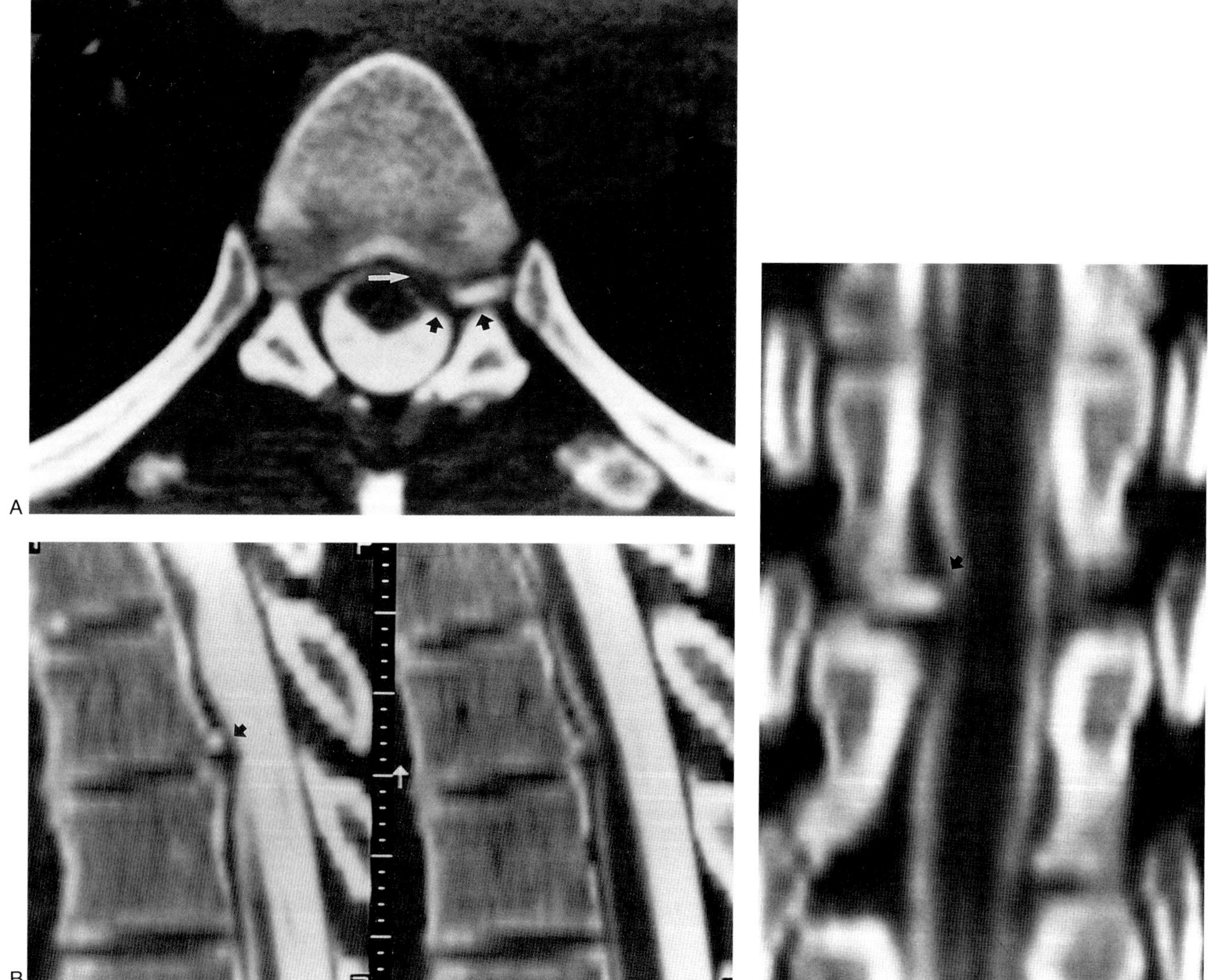

Figure 17. A CT-myelogram demonstrates calcified lateral disc herniation indenting spinal cord on axial **(A)**, sagittal **(B)**, and coronal **(C)** reconstructed images.

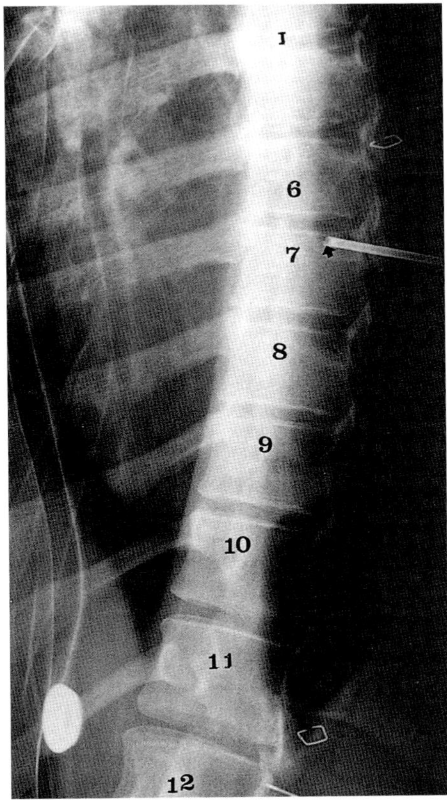

Figure 18. Intraoperative cross-table AP radiograph with Verees needle at T6–T7 disc (*arrow*).

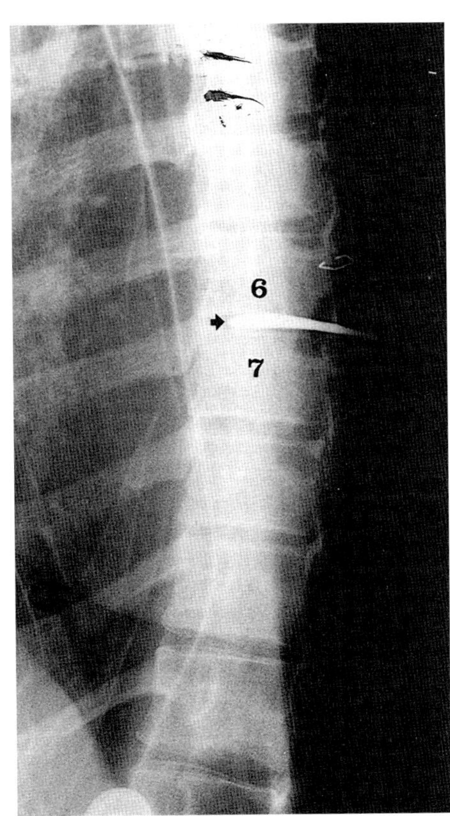

Figure 19. Intraoperative cross-table AP radiograph following discectomy demonstrating Penfield elevator across the midline (*arrow*).

RECOMMENDED READING

1. Albrand, O. W., and Corkill, G.: Thoracic disc herniation: Treatment and prognosis. *Spine*, 4: 41–46, 1979.
2. Awward, E. E., Martin, D. S., Smith, K. R., and Baker, B. K.: Asymptomatic versus symptomatic herniated thoracic discs: Their frequency and characteristics as detected by computed tomography after myelography. *Neurosurgery*, 28: 180–186, 1991.
3. Ben-Yishay, A., Regan, J. J., and McAfee, P.: Early results of excision of herniated thoracic disc utilizing video-assisted thoracoscopy. Presented at the Twenty-ninth Annual Meeting of the Scoliosis Research Society, Portland, Oregon, September 21–24, 1994.
4. Bohlman, H. H., and Zdeblick, T. A.: Anterior excision of herniated thoracic discs. *J. Bone Joint Surg. [Am.]*, 70A: 1038–1047, 1988.
5. Brown, C. W., Deffer, P. A., Jr, Akmakjian, J., Donaldson, D. H., and Brugman, J. L.: The natural history of thoracic disc herniation. *Spine*, 17 [Suppl 6] 97–102, 1992.
6. Currier, B. L., Eismont, F. J., and Green, B. A.: Transthoracic disc excision and fusion for herniated thoracic discs. *Spine*, 19: 323–328, 1994.
7. Dekutowski, M. B., Transfeldt, E. E., Cohen, M. A., et al.: Treatment of thoracic disc disease: Clinical spectrum, classification and recommendations. Presented at the Annual Meeting of the North American Spine Society, San Diego, CA, 1993.
8. Feiring, E. H.: Extruded thoracic intervertebral disc. *Arch. Surg.*, 95: 135, 1967.
9. Ferson, P. F., Landreneau, R. J., and Dowling, R. D.: Comparison of open versus thoracic biopsy for diffuse infiltrative pulmonary disease. *J. Thorac. Cardiovasc. Surg.*, 106:2, 194–199, 1994.
10. Harmon, E., and Lillington, G.: Pulmonary risk factors in surgery. *Med. Clin. North Am.*, 63: 1289–1298, 1979.
11. Landreneau, R. J., Mack, M. J., Hazelrigg, S. R., et al.: Video-assisted thoracic surgery: Basic technical concepts and intercostal approach strategies. *Ann. Thorac. Surg.*, 54: 800–807, 1992.
12. Lesoin, F., Rousseaux, M., Autricque, A., et al.: Thoracic disc herniations: Evolutions in the approach and indications. *Acta Neurochir. (Wien)*, 80: 30–34, 1986.

13. Logas, W. G., El-Baz, N., El-Ganzouri, A., et al.: Continuous thoracic epidural analgesia for postoperative pain relief following thoracotomy: A randomized prospective study. *Anesthesiology*, 67: 787–791, 1987.
14. Love, J. G., and Schorn, V. G.: Thoracic disc protrusions. *JAMA*, 191: 627–631, 1965.
15. Love, J. G., and Schorn, V. G.: Thoracic disc protrusion. *Rheumatism*, 23: 2–10, 1967.
16. Mack, M. J., Regan, J. J., Bobechko, W. P., and Acutt, T. E.,: Application of thoracoscopy for diseases of the spine. *Ann. Thorac. Surg.*, 56: 736–738, 1993.
17. McAfee, P., Regan, J. J., and Picetti, G. D.: The incidence of complications in endoscopic anterior thoracic spinal reconstructive surgery: A prospective multicenter study comprising the first fifty consecutive cases. Presented at the 29th Annual Meeting of the Scoliosis Research Society, Portland, Oregon, September 21–24, 1994.
18. Otani, K., Nakai, S., Fujimura, Y., Manzoku, S., and Shibasaki, K.: Surgical treatment of thoracic disc herniation using the anterior approach *J. Bone Joint Surg.*, 64B: 340–343, 1982.
19. Otani, K., Yoshida, M., Fujii, E., et al.: Thoracic disc herniation: Surgical treatment in 23 patients. *Spine*, 13: 1262–1267, 1988.
20. Regan, J. J., Mack, M. J., and Picetti, G. D.: A technical report on video-assisted thoracoscopic surgery (VATS) of the thoracic spine. *Spine*, 20:831–837, 1995.
21. Regan, J. J., Mack, M. J., Picetti, G. D., Guyer, R. D., Hochschuler S. H., Rashbaum, R. F. A comparison of video-assisted thoracoscopic surgery (VATS) with open thoracotomy in thoracic spinal surgery. *Todays Ther. Trends*, 11: 203–218, 1994.
22. Reif, J., Gilsbach, J., and Ostheim-Dzerowycz, W.: Differential diagnosis and therapy of herniated thoracic disc: Discussion of six cases. *Acta Neurochir. (Wien)*, 67: 255–265, 1983.
23. Russell, T.: Thoracic intervertebral disc protusion: Experience of 67 cases and review of the literature. *Br. J. Neurosurg.*, 3: 153–160, 1989.
24. Simpson, J. M., Silveri, C. D., Simeone, F. A., Balderston, R. A., and An, H. S.: Thoracic disc herniation: A Reevaluation of the posterior approach using a modified costotransversectomy. *Spine*, 18:1872–1877, 1993.
25. Tarhan, S., Moffitt, E. A., and Sesson, A. D.: Risks of anesthesia and surgery in patients with chronic bronchitis and COPD. *Surgery*, 74: 720–726, 1973.
26. Williams, M. P., Cherryman, G. R., and Husband, J. E.: Significance of thoracic disc herniation demonstrated by MR imaging. *J. Comput. Assist. Tomogr.*, 13: 211, 1989.
27. McAfee, P., Regan, J. J., and Picetti, G. D.: The incidence of complications in endosopic anterior thoracic spinal reconstructive surgery: A prospective multicenter study comprising the first 100 consecutive cases. *Spine*, J. B. Lippincott, Philadelphia, 1995.
28. Ben-Yishay, A., Regan, J. J., and McAfee, P: Early results of excision of herniated thoracic disc utilizing video-assisted thoracoscopy. Presented at the 29th Annual Meeting of the Scoliosis Research Society, Portland, Oregon, September 21–24, 1994.

Master Techniques in Orthopaedic Surgery,
THE SPINE, edited by D. S. Bradford,
Lippincott-Raven Publishers, Philadelphia, © 1997.

17

Thoracic Discectomy

Ensor Transfeldt

INDICATIONS/CONTRAINDICATIONS

The incidence of symptomatic thoracic disc herniations is much more uncommon than herniations occurring in the cervical and lumbar spines. A wide variety of presenting symptoms is associated with thoracic disc syndrome. However, there is characteristic clinical presentation of this condition, which may in fact mimic other disorders such as spinal tumors, infections, spinal cord lesions, intercostal neuralgias, herpes zoster lesions of the thoracic and abdominal viscera, breast neoplasms, and costal chondritis.

Recent studies have shown a high incidence of thoracic disc lesions in asymptomatic patients. Furthermore, the clinical presentation may involve neurologic symptoms alone, pain alone, or a combination of the two. The lack of a clear definition of thoracic disc syndrome, the difficulties in attributing radiographic abnormalities to patient symptoms, and the difficulties in differentiating the patient's symptoms from other causes make management of thoracic disc herniations a challenge.

Because the natural history of thoracic disc herniations is not well understood and also because these lesions may be asymptomatic or mildly symptomatic, it is difficult to provide a clear list of indications. No prospective controlled studies have compared treatment methods. Most patients presenting with acute thoracic spine pain and positive magnetic resonance imaging (MRI) will not require surgical treatment because they are unlikely to improve. The most common presenting symptoms of thoracic disc herniation are local pain, weakness, sensory loss, bowel and bladder dysfunction, and radicular symptoms including pain and paresthesia. If examination shows no neurologic deficit, then severity of clinical symptoms, pain in particular, will determine the need for surgery. Before surgery is planned, the patient must first have been placed on a comprehensive program of nonoperative treatment including nonsteroidal antiinflammatory agents, decreased level

E. Transfeldt, M.D.: Twin Cities Scoliosis Spine Center, Minneapolis, Minnesota 55407.

of activity and/or rest, and physical therapy and exercise (in particular, trunk strengthening and postural training, patient education, electrical nerve stimulation, or other modalities of physical therapy). The chronologic progression of weakness and bowel and bladder function or sensory loss, together with corresponding positive radiographic findings correlating with these symptoms, is also an indication for surgery. The psychosocial makeup of the patient and the patient's expectations must also be considered when surgery is being recommended in the absence of clear objective neurologic deficits. Individualizing the treatment to suit the patient and making sure that the patient fully understands the risks and complications together with the possible outcomes of surgery is most important in the management of thoracic disc herniation.

Myelopathic findings that are progressive should be considered an absolute and more urgent indication. The cause of long-standing myelopathy may be more difficult to determine, particularly in the elderly patient. Other causes of myelopathy or other levels of spinal cord compression in cervical and thoracic spine must be excluded. Under these circumstances, a myelopathy with a clear-cut sensory level correlating with the level of the thoracic disc herniation is also an absolute indication for surgery. There is, however, no clear relationship between the size of the thoracic disc herniation and the severity of the clinical picture or myelopathy.

Radicular pain and paresthesia are not in themselves absolute indications for surgery. However, if these symptoms are present together with thoracic spine pain (and conservative treatment has failed), one can predict a better outcome for a thoracic discectomy.

The surgical treatment for unisegmental thoracic disc degeneration and/or herniation with mechanical-type thoracic spine pain alone without neurologic findings is highly controversial. If, however, the patient has tried a prolonged period of conservative treatment (6 months to 1 year) and continues to have severe and disabling pain even for menial activities of daily living, then surgery may be of benefit. Thoracic discography for these patients may be helpful in localizing the exact source of the pain. The failure to demonstrate a radiographic compressive lesion that correlates with the patient's clinical symptoms and signs is a contraindication for surgery. The patient with a poor psychosocial profile and unreasonable expectations in the absence of objective neurologic findings should also not be offered surgery.

PREOPERATIVE PLANNING

The preoperative workup of the patient should include a detailed physical examination including the motor and sensory evaluation of all extremities and the torso as well as examination of all deep tendon reflexes and spinal cord reflexes including the Babinski response. These findings need to be clearly correlated with abnormal radiographic findings, particularly with regard to the level of spinal cord compression. A global sensory loss of the trunk and lower extremities below the level of the spinal cord compression is useful in making such a correlation. However, there is no good correlation between lateral thoracic disc herniations and radicular sensory loss of the intercostal nerves.

If there is no clear-cut neurologic orientation of the symptoms and the patient is having a thoracic discectomy mainly for pain, evaluation by a internist to exclude cardiac, pulmonary, or other visceral causes of the pain is of value. Routine investigations such as a chest radiograph and electrocardiogram may also be useful.

The general medical condition of the patient, as well as the pulmonary status as measured by pulmonary function studies and arterial blood gasses, may help in the planning of pre- and postoperative patient care. If there are any indications for the evaluation of the cardiovascular system, appropriate investigation might also decrease the risk of postoperative complications.

Good quality plain radiographs of the thoracic spine should be obtained before surgery. They may demonstrate calcified intracanal protrusions, which would require a greater exposure as well as a more careful dissection from an adherent dura. Plain radiographs should also be evaluated for the number of thoracic vertebrae containing normal ribs and correlated with MRI or computed tomography (CT) studies to ensure that the decompression will be done at the correct level. Intraoperative localizing radiographs will be easier to interpret if they can be compared with good quality preoperative routine films.

The radiographic diagnosis of a thoracic disc herniation will already have been made if one has reached the preoperative planning stage. However, it is important to have good quality MRIs or CT scans or myelo-CT scans to evaluate the level of disc herniation, the side that the lesion is located on, and the sequestration or migration of disc fragments behind the vertebral body.

In the event that surgery is recommended, and the surgeon plans to perform a fusion for mechanical thoracic spine pain associated with a thoracic disc herniation, then discography may be of help. It is useful if the patient's typical pain is reproduced at the level of the disc degeneration and adjoining normal discs do not have any pain provocation.

Some centers recommend preoperative angiography to determine the presence and location of the artery of Adamkiewicz or other major spinal cord segmental vessels. We do not recommend that this be done routinely. We do feel, however, that it is important to avoid potential damage to the radiculomedullary feeder vessels to the spinal cord during the surgical dissection. This is done by avoiding dissection in the neural foramina because of the rich collateral circulation in this region providing blood flow to the spinal cord. If it becomes necessary to ligate these segmental vessels, we feel it should be done in front of the vertebral bodies.

Routine evoked potentials and electromyography are generally not helpful in the evaluation of patients with thoracic disc herniations. Cystometrograms, however, should be used if there is a history of bowel and bladder incontinence; they should be combined with urodynamic studies.

SURGERY

I strongly recommend the anterolateral approach. The disc herniation occurs in the anterior and anterolateral part of the spinal canal and with this approach, manipulation of the spinal cord and nerve roots is minimized. This allows for an effective versatile and low-risk approach. The anterolateral retropleural approach using a small incision over the posterior angle of the rib allows for minimal dissection without the need for a chest tube and facilitates early postoperative recovery. However, previous experience and familiarity with a normal transthoracic approach is important and makes this procedure considerably easier and safer.

Posterior-Transpedicular Approach

The patient is placed in a prone position with a routine straight midline incision and subperiosteal muscle stripping of the posterior laminae. This is done on the side of the disc herniation. The facet and pedicle inferior to the disc herniation is identified and, after initially removing a major part of the facet with a high-speed bur or drill, the pedicle itself is drilled. Some authors recommend complete removal of the pedicle and hence visualization of the cord as well as the exiting nerve root, thus allowing exposure of the nerve roots. A modification of this technique is to preserve as much of the pedicle as possible but to remove the superior portion of the pedicle more anteriorly, allowing visualization of the exiting nerve root as well as the disc space. The protruding disc is pushed anteriorly into an empty space, which has already been created with the bur in the end plate and disc space. This is performed with downbiting curettes. Because of the limited exposure, a microscope is recommended. A flexible endoscope may also be used to confirm the degree of decompression.

Technically this procedure is extremely demanding and even with a microscope visualization may be extremely limited. If there is a large calcified fragment or sequestration and migration of disc material, this approach is grossly inadequate. This approach may be valuable for lateral disc herniations alone, but it does not provide satisfactory visualization for central disc herniations. If more aggressive removal of the pedicle and facets is carried out and a significant amount of disc and bone is removed anteriorly, instability may be produced. Under such circumstances, an anterior interbody strut stabilizing graft cannot be placed through this approach.

Posterolateral-Costotransversectomy Approach

The patient can be placed either in the prone or lateral decubitus position, and the incision is either a straight midline skin incision with a lateral muscle splitting approach to the spine or a longitudinal paraspinous or transverse incision. Subperiosteal elevation of the muscles may be performed either from the midline or from a paraspinal muscle splitting approach. The facet joint and costotransverse joints are identified. The costotransverse joint is removed with a rongeur together with the proximal portion of the rib. The intercostal nerve with the neurovascular bundle is identified and will guide the surgeon to the neural foramen. The remaining portion of the rib is then disarticulated from its attachment to the vertebral body. The lateral edge of the transverse process is then incised (Fig. 1). This allows exposure of the lateral border of the pedicle, the vertebral body, and the disc space. It is important that when removing the proximal portion of the rib a periosteal elevator be used to dissect soft tissues from anterior to the rib and thus avoid penetration of the pleura.

This procedure is indicated only in pure lateral disc herniations. It does not allow good visualization across the midline or the opposite side of the spinal canal.

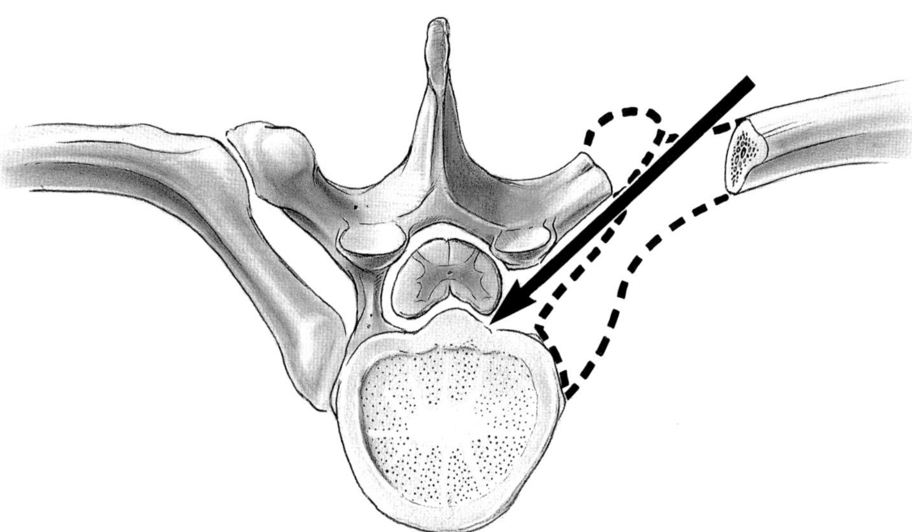

Figure 1. Schematic drawing of costotransversectomy approach to lateral spinal canal.

This approach may also be more useful in the upper thoracic spine, where routine anterolateral exposures may be more difficult. It is important to recognize a pleural leak if it occurs.

Anterior-Trans-sternal Approach

Extensive dissection is involved in the anterior-trans-sternal approach and thus this approach is not routinely recommended. It may be indicated in significant spinal canal stenosis of the upper thoracic (T2–T4) spine requiring extensive bone removal. A cardiothoracic surgeon should assist the spine surgeon with this approach.

I believe that in the future, thoracoscopic procedures for disc removal will become routine. At the present time, however, this is a developing and evolving technique. Thoracoscopy offers the advantage of minimizing the dissection but at the same time providing adequate visualization and illumination in the area where decompression is needed.

Anterolateral-Transthoracic Thoracotomy Approach

The standard transthoracic thoracotomy approach can be used safely for exposure of the disc from T2 to T12. The use of a double-lumen endotracheal tube with collapse of the ipsilateral lung during surgery will improve the interoperative exposure.

The side of the exposure is determined primarily by the side of the disc herniation. If a disc herniation is more central, a left-sided approach is preferable, since it is safer and easier to deal with the aorta and segmental vessels from this side. However, the spine can be approached safely and easily from either side.

The patient is placed in the lateral decubitus position and the midthoracic region is centered over the break in the table (Fig. 2). Pillows are placed between the legs, and the torso can be stabilized with sandbags on either side with a strap or broad tape to hold the pelvis securely on the table. The patient is placed in a lateral decubitus position in the upper extremity and the side of the surgical approach is supported on a padded elevated arm rest or on pillows and draped out of the field. It is advisable to place a soft gel pad or a rolled sheet under the axilla on the dependent side to protect the brachial plexus and axillary nerves. It is also important to ensure that the head is well supported on a pillow, providing a horizontal relationship of the cervical and thoracic spines. Lateral flexion of the cervical spine for prolonged periods of time, particularly if the table is divided in the thoracic region, may produce a brachial plexus palsy.

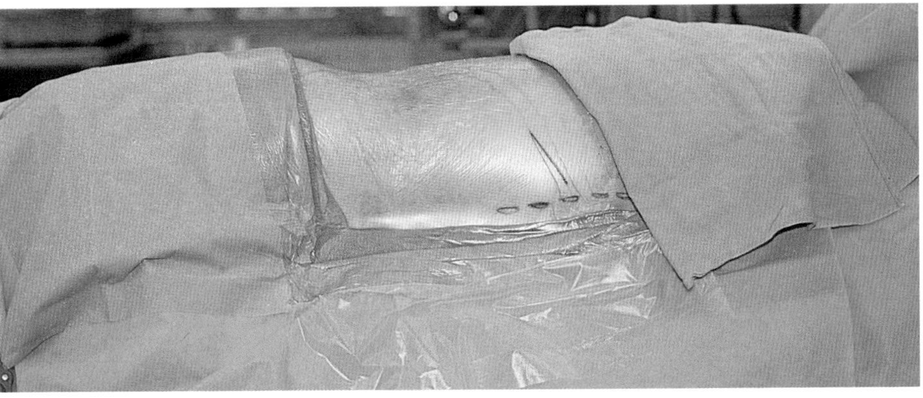

Figure 2. Lateral decubitus position on operating table.

The level of incision will depend on the level of the disc involved as well as the amount of exposure required. If the surgeon requires a wide exposure, it is generally recommended that the incision be made following the rib two levels above the vertebral level. The obliquity of the ribs, however, should also be taken into consideration when making this analysis. If this wider exposure is selected, the incision runs from the posterior angle from the rib and as far anteriorly as needed. The author prefers a more limited exposure over the posterolateral margins of the thoracic cage. The rib selected in this approach is the one leading directly to the disc space involved. For example, the ninth rib is removed for a T8–T9 disc herniation. In this approach only a short segment of rib will be removed from approximately 2 inches lateral to the posterior angle of the rib to the costal transverse joint. It is important to be sure that one is removing the correct rib. An intraoperative radiograph should be taken prior to rib resection if one is unable to count the ribs by soft tissue palpation.

The skin incision is made from the lateral border of the paraspinal muscles extending along the line of the rib for approximately 3 to 4 inches (Fig. 3), but it can be extended if further exposure is required. Self-retaining retractors are then placed in the wound, and, using electrocautery, the incision is deepened down through the muscle layers to the rib that is to be resected. Depending on the level of the disc herniation, it may be necessary to divide all the muscles with electrocautery including the latissimus dorsi and trapezius muscles. Rarely are the rhomboids divided for upper thoracic exposures. Frequently, however, it may be possible to mobilize these muscles, particularly in the mid to lower thoracic spine and retract them with a blunt retractor. For more medial exposure of the rib it is necessary to mobilize and retract the paraspinous muscles toward the midline. In muscular individuals, it may be necessary to divide the lateral margins of these muscles.

The outer periosteum of the rib is then cut along the line of the rib with an electrocautery and the periosteum is elevated first off of the outer surface (Fig. 4) and then, using a curved tip elevator, off the superior and inferior borders of the rib (Fig. 5). It is important to maintain contact between the elevator and the rib on the inferior margins to avoid damaging the intercostal or subcostal neurovascular bundle. Using a curved-tip elevator or a Doyen, the periosteum on the undersurface of the rib is then elevated (Fig. 5). Strict contact between the periosteum elevator and the bone will prevent penetration of the pleura and lung. The rib is then cut as far posteriorly as possible and as far anteriorly as is necessary (Fig. 6). The remaining bone edges should be smoothed off with a regular rongeur.

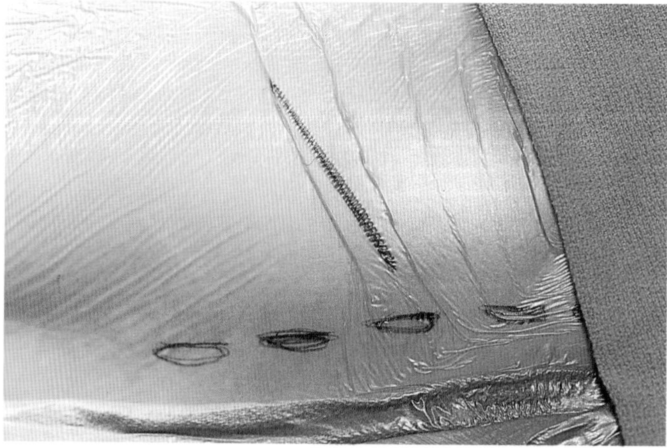

Figure 3. Proposed skin incision along medial border of rib.

The rib head is now exposed (Fig. 7). The resected rib is saved in the event an interbody strut graft is performed. The pleural space is entered by incising the bed of the rib and dividing the periosteum and parietal pleura along the line of the rib. The lung is retracted medially, and a self-retaining chest retractor is inserted to improve the view further. If a wide exposure has been used, a Feochetti retractor can be used, but for smaller exposures, a narrower firm instrument such as a Toutier retractor is used. If a double-lumen endotracheal tube has been used, the lung can be collapsed, and retraction is frequently much easier. It is important to release lung retraction regularly throughout the procedure to prevent subsequent atelectasis.

The parietal pleura overlying the vertebral body is then incised with long scissors and forceps, exposing the soft elevated disc space as well as the segmental vessels lying in the valleys or hollows of the vertebral bodies. The cut edges of the parietal pleura are reflected anteriorly and posteriorly, and the segmental vessels are ligated anterior to the neural foramen to avoid disturbing the important collateral supply to the spinal cord feeder vessels. The soft tissue over the posterior part of the vertebral body and disc is then elevated with the ligated vessel using a Cobb

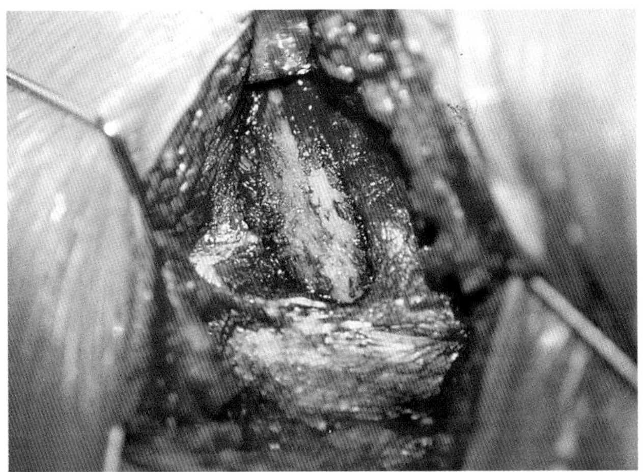

Figure 4. Exposure of rib with retraction of posterior chest wall muscles and paraspinal muscles traversing at right angles to the rib.

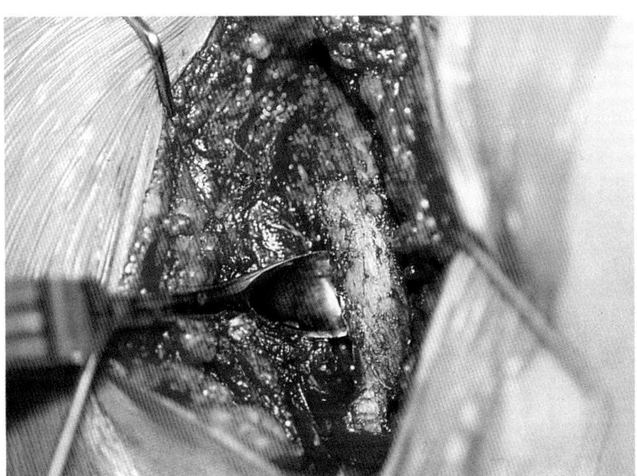

Figure 5. Elevation of inferior rib margin with curved elevator or Doyen.

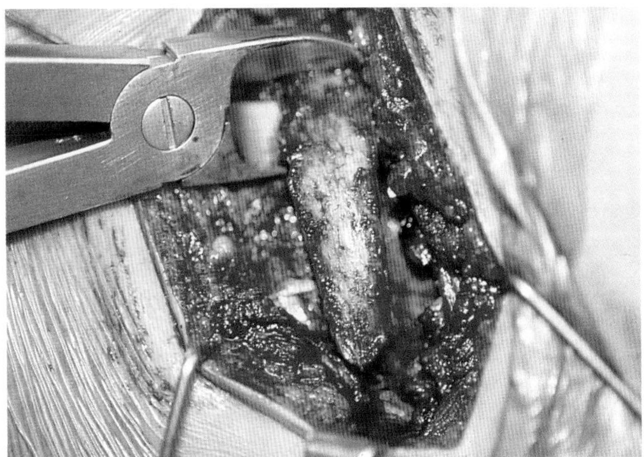

Figure 6. Incising cut end of rib anteriorly.

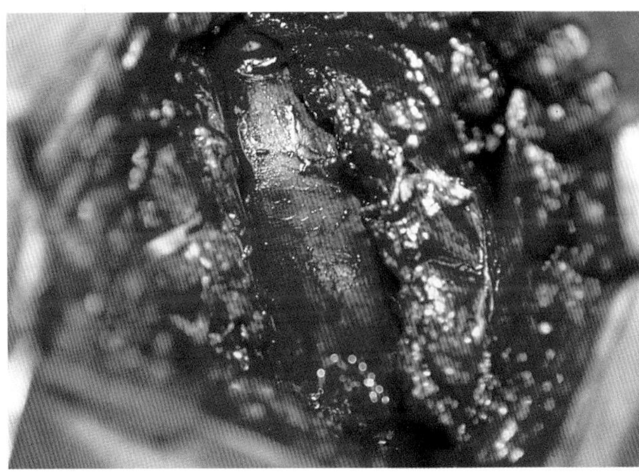

Figure 7. Bed of rib with rib excised.

elevator. If a long lateral or anterolateral transthoracic approach has been used, this exposure is adequate to proceed with discectomy (Fig. 8). If a short posterolateral approach is used, then the parietal pleura over the head of the rib is also incised, exposing the proximal end of the rib. The remaining portion of the resected rib is elevated from the costotransverse and costovertebral articulations. This maneuver is made easier by incising the ligaments around the respective joints and elevating the rib head with a large curette. This will allow improved exposure of the posterolateral disc as well as the posterior margins of the vertebral body and the pedicle (Fig. 9). The neurovascular bundle will be seen entering the intervertebral foramen. Some authors recommend that the intervertebral foramen be identified by following the thoracic nerve root into the foramen. Following the nerve root directly into the foramen, however, may interfere with the segmental blood supply to the spinal cord, since bleeding is frequently encountered. It should

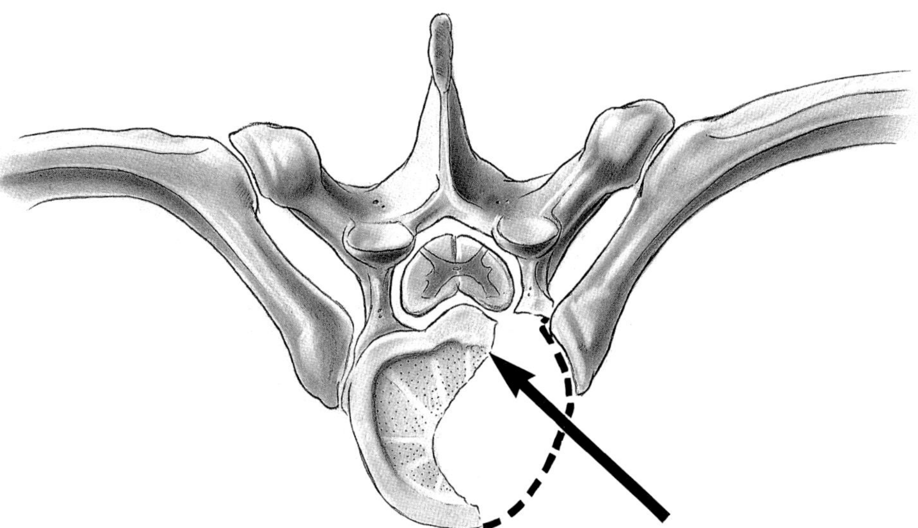

Figure 8. Schematic drawing of transthoracic direct approach to anterior spinal canal without rib head resection.

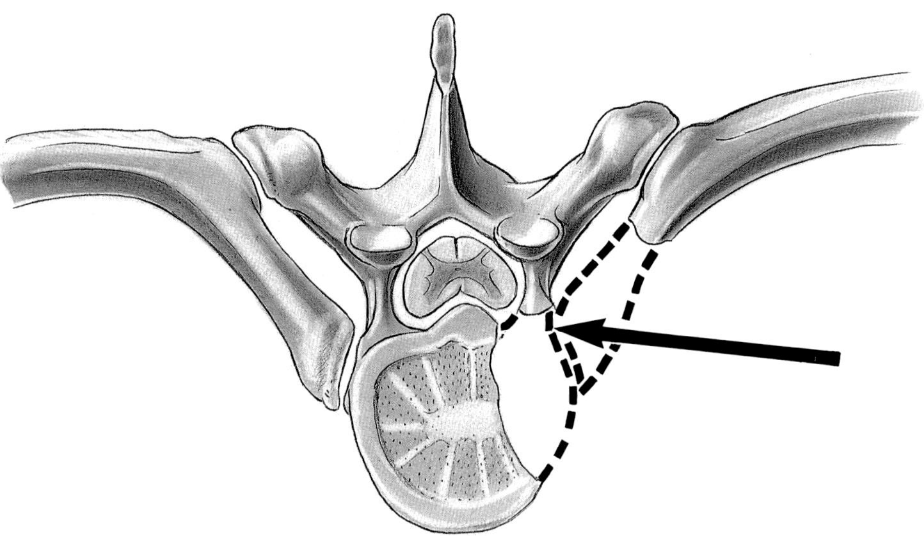

Figure 9. Oblique transthoracic or retropleural approach with resection of rib head and discectomy or partial corpectomy.

be noted that the thoracic nerve root leaves the spinal sac posteriorly and does not have a close relationship to the intervertebral disc itself.

Orientation to the position and location of the spinal cord is best obtained by identifying the pedicle as well as the posterior margins of the vertebral body and the intervening discs. The tip of a malleable retractor is then placed against the anterior portions of the disc space and held against the lateral margins of the spine incision, improving the exposure. It is not necessary to remove the anterior intervertebral disc. The sympathetic trunk should be preserved and retracted if possible.

The disc is then incised and removed immediately anterior to the area of prolapse. Disc material is removed with small and large pituitary-type ronguers. It is further removed from the end plate with a curette, and this dissection is then carried posteriorly until the posterior margins of the end plate are reached. This then creates a space into which herniated disc material can be delivered with a reverse-angle curette. The reverse angle allows the surgeon to cut away from the spinal cord into the space created. The disc is removed sequentially with a curette and the pituitary forceps and ronguers by following the posterior margins of the vertebral body all the way across the midline. The disc space in the thoracic spine may be very narrow, and the exposure can be improved by removing more disc material anteriorly as well as by removing the bony end plates of the adjacent vertebrae. It is important that the posterior longitudinal ligament be removed together with the posterior anulus to allow adequate exposure of the dura and thus confirm that an adequate decompression has been obtained. It is possible through this technique to expose the entire anterior half of the spinal canal to the opposite side.

If a large defect has been produced, the resected rib can be used to fill this space. These resected ribs are placed in troughs cut out of the body end plates. The parietal pleura over the spine is then closed with a running suture. The intercostal nerve and foraminal area are infiltrated with a long-acting local anesthetic. A chest tube is inserted through the intercostal space one or two levels above in the mid- or anterior axillary lines. Closure of the enlarged intercostal space is facilitated by using a rib approximator and one or two large pericostal sutures. The parietal pleura and intercostal musculature are closed with a running suture. If muscles are divided, they are closed in layers.

This approach provides good exposure of the intervertebral disc, including midline lesions. It is not necessary to remove the pedicle or a portion thereof. The view of the spinal canal through the intervertebral foramen allows direct decompression under vision. Bone graft and fusion can be adequately achieved. If the short posterior incision is used, a headlight and loops is recommended. An operating microscope may also be helpful but is not necessary.

Retropleural Extracavity Approach

The retropleural extracavity approach also provides direct visualization of the posterior vertebral bodies and disc margins and allows decompression of the spinal cord under direct vision. It has all the advantages of a transthoracic approach without the need for chest tube placement.

The patient is placed in a lateral decubitus position, and the surgical exposure of the rib is similar to that outlined in the transthoracic approach. A short posterior incision with removal of the posterior portion of the rib is strongly recommended in this approach.

Following removal of the rib extraperiosteally, the parietal pleura is separated from the undersurface from the adjacent ribs as well as the remaining portion of the proximal rib and vertebral body using blunt finger dissection or cottonoid swabs placed at the end of an instrument (Fig. 10). The pleura and adjacent tissue appear firmer more posteriorly, and it is therefore preferable to start this blunt dissection more posteriorly. It is important to remove the remaining portion of the rib, especially the rib head, to allow satisfactory exposure of the spinal canal and the posterior vertebral body (Fig. 9). Retraction with chest retractors and the malleable retractor are used to provide the same exposure as described in the transthoracic approach (Figs. 11 and 12). Closure for this approach is the same, and an extra pleural drain should be used. It is important, however, prior to closure of the intercostal muscles and chest muscles to ensure that a pleural leak has not inadvertently been caused. The wound should be filled with water and respirations observed; continuous bubbling would indicate a pleural leak.

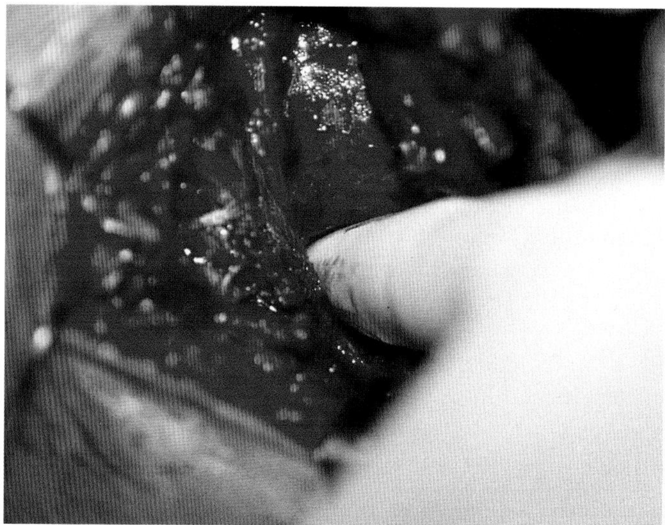

Figure 10. Blunt dissection and elevation of pleural space by sweeping the finger underneath the adjacent ribs and elevating the parietal pleura forward.

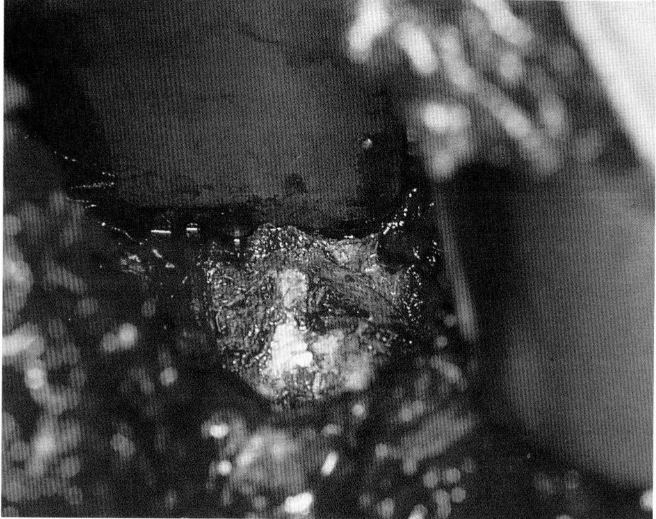

Figure 11. Malleable retractor placed over anterior aspect of spine exposing disc space.

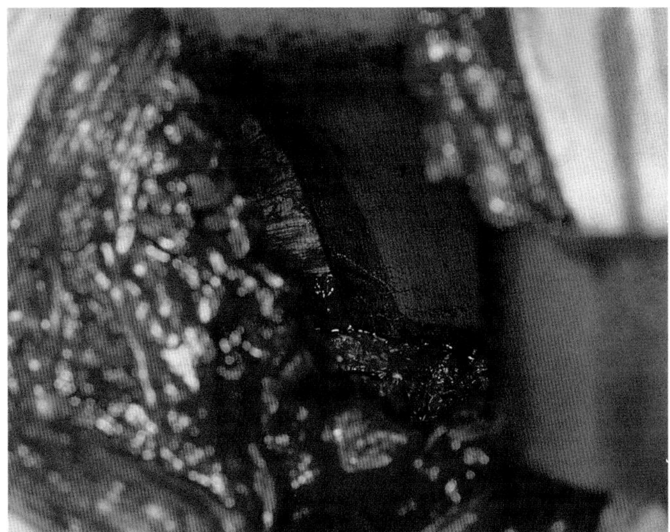

Figure 12. Spinal exposure with discectomy.

POSTOPERATIVE MANAGEMENT

If a chest tube is used, it is connected to an underwater seal and removed when the 24-hour drainage is less than 150 ml. If a retropleural approach is used, the drain is usually removed at 24 hours since the expanded lung provides a tamponade effect, creating hemostasis. The use of long-acting local anesthetic in the wound decreases the need for pain control postoperatively, but rib resection can frequently cause severe pain, and it may be necessary to use intravenous or intramuscular narcotic analgesics for 2 to 3 days. We recommend the use of a self-administered pain control device.

The patient is allowed free activity immediately after the operation. We recommend that the patient stand and walk the evening of the surgery and be encouraged to mobilize the following day. When the short posterolateral incision with a retropleural exposure is used, patients may be discharged from the hospital 1 to 4 days after the surgery. However, if a longer thoracotomy incision is used with chest tubes, patients may need to stay in the hospital for 3 to 6 days postoperatively. The use of braces is confined to those patients in whom the discectomies have been performed below T10, where the spine is more mobile and less protected by the thoracic cage. The use of subarticular skin sutures makes postoperative wound care easier. The patient should be examined by a nurse or physician within the first 10 days after discharge to ensure that the wound is healing normally without signs of infection. A chest radiograph should be taken postoperatively if the retropleural exposure is used and after chest tube removal if a transthoracic approach is used.

Routine follow-up of the patient in a clinic should be performed at 1 month and again at 4 months after the surgery. Spine radiographs should be taken if a bone graft and strut graft were performed to ensure that grafts have not been displaced. The patient should be able to return to normal daily routine activities within 2 to 3 days and to more exertional activities by 3 to 4 months. Trunk strengthening and thoracic extension exercises are begun at 3 to 4 months after the surgery.

COMPLICATIONS

Complications related specifically to thoracic discectomy include neurologic deficit of the spinal cord due to compression or ischaemia. The latter is extremely unlikely to occur in this procedure because of the limited exposure; refraining from coagulation in the neuroforamen will certainly decrease this even more. Tears in large vessels are unlikely to occur, but if segmental vessels are ligated, it is important that this be done securely, since clips and sutures may be displaced, resulting in large amounts of blood loss even after closure. Postoperative atelectasis can be prevented by frequent expansion of the lung during the procedure and ensuring prior to closure that the lung is fully expanded with positive pressure ventilation. Atelectasis in the opposite lung, that is, on the dependent side, has also been described due to poor mechanical ventilation during surgery. Post-thoracotomy pain and intercostal neuralgias may occur and may be due to prolonged retraction or incorporation of the intercostal nerve in the closing sutures.

ILLUSTRATIVE CASE FOR TECHNIQUE

A 46-year-old man presented with interscapular pain following a lifting injury. The pain was made worse by coughing, sneezing, and straining and was associated with a radiating pain around the chest wall on the left side. He had no neurologic deficit. There were no long track signs. Plain radiographs of his thoracic spine were normal. An MRI of his spine showed a T7–T8 disc herniation (Fig. 13).

He was initially placed on conservative treatment with bed rest and anti-inflammatories. He failed to show any improvement, and his pain become progressively worse. After 3 months of treatment, his pain had reached the point of disablement, and he was severely restricted. A decision was made to proceed with surgery.

A transthoracic discectomy through an anterolateral approach was performed. A short incision over the posterolateral angle of the rib was performed. A discectomy was carried out. The resected rib was used as a strut graft together with morcelized bone at the T7–T8 level. The postoperative MRI showed an excellent decompression of the cord with restoration of the spinal cord to its normal shape after successful removal of the herniated disc (Fig. 14). The sagittal MRI showed the fibula strut in place at the T7–T8 level (Fig. 15).

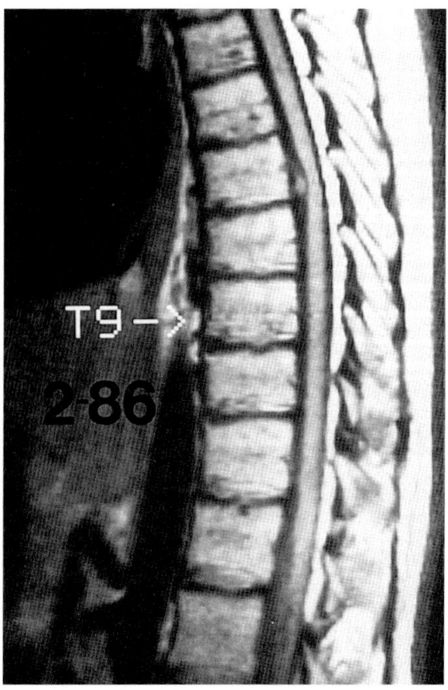

A

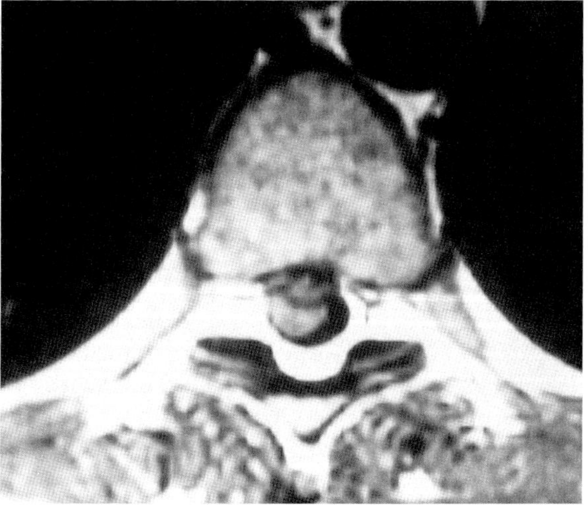

B

Figure 13. Preoperative sagittal **(A)** and axial **(B)** MR images showing T7–T8 disc herniation.

Postoperatively this patient had immediate relief of his pain. The chest tube was removed 24 hours after surgery, and the patient was discharged from the hospital on the third postoperative day. He made an excellent recovery and by 5 months was back to work and performing normal activities of daily living. His follow-up 6 years after the surgery revealed a normal examination, and the patient stated that he was not having any thoracic spine pain at all. The follow-up radiographs show that the rib strut graft is still in place at the T7–T8 level and that the alignment of the thoracic spine has remained satisfactory (Fig. 15).

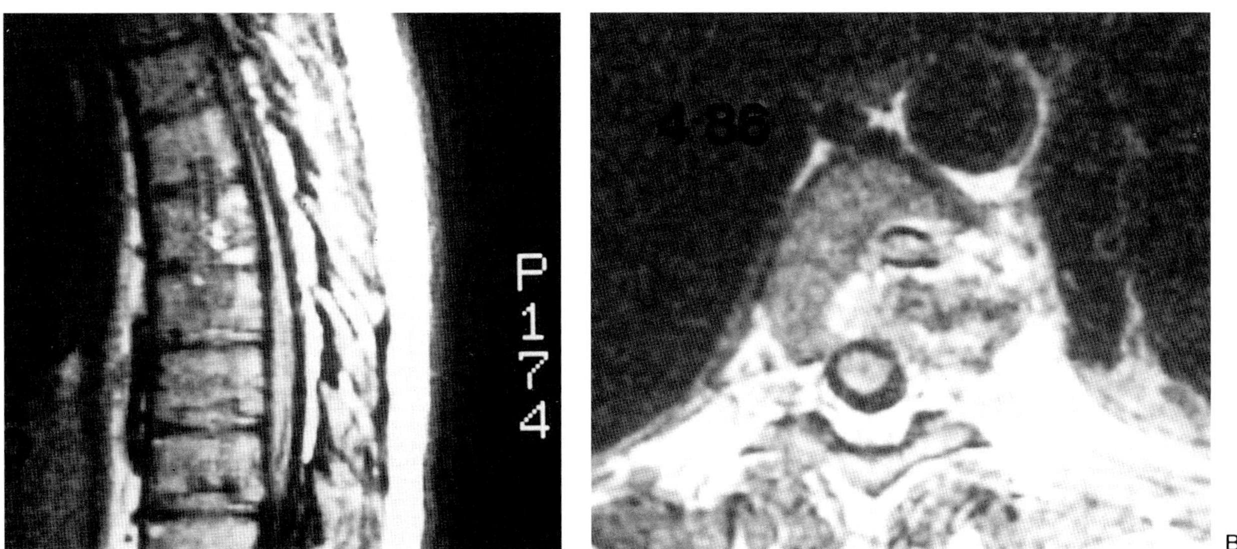

Figure 14. Postoperative sagittal **(A)** and axial **(B)** MR images showing the spinal cord restored to its normal shape.

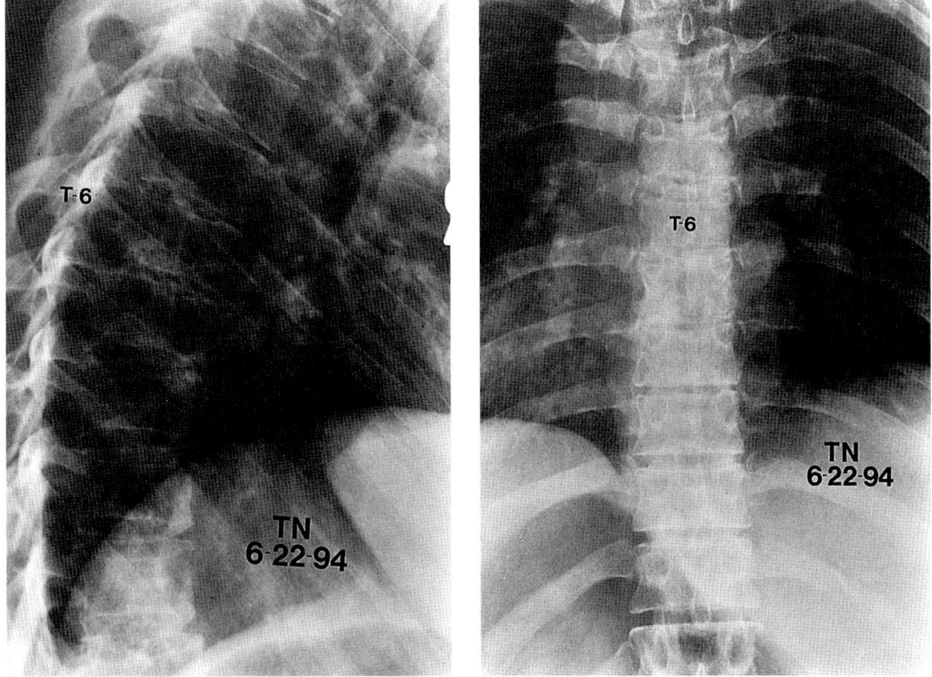

Figure 15. Lateral **(A)** and AP **(B)** radiographs 6 years after surgery show the rib graft in place at the T7–T8 level and satisfactory alignment of the spine.

RECOMMENDED READING

1. Anderson, T. M., Kamal, A. M., and Miller, J. I.: Thoracic approaches to anterior spinal operations: Anterior thoracic approaches. *Ann. Thorac. Surg.*, 55: 1447–1552, 1993.
2. Currier, B. L., Eismont, F. J., and Green, B. A.: Thoracic disc disease. In: *Spine*, vol. I, edited by R. H. Rothman, and C. A. Simeone. W. B. Saunders, Philadelphia, 1992.
3. Hulme, A.: The surgical approach to thoracic intervertebral disc protrusions. *J. Neurol. Neurosurg. Psychiatry*, 23: 133–137, 1960.
4. Le Roux, P. D., Haglund, M. M., and Haris, A. B.: Thoracic disc disease with the transpedicular approach in twenty consecutive patients. *Neurosurgery*, 33: 58–66, 1993.
5. Maiman, D. J., Larson, S. J., Luck, E., and El-Ghatit, A.: Lateral extracavitary approach to the spine for thoracic disc herniation: Report of 23 cases. *Neurosurgery*, 14: 178–182, 1984.
6. Moskovich, R., Benson, D., Zhang, Z., and Kabins, M.: Extracoelomic approach to the spine. *J. Bone Joint Surg. [Br.]*, 75-B: 886–893, 1993.
7. Ogilvie, J. W.: Thoracic disc herniation. In: *Textbook of Spinal Surgery*, vol. 2, edited by K. Bridwell and R. Dewald. J. B. Lippincott, Philadelphia, 1991.
8. Otani, K., Nakai, S., Fujimjura, Y., Shunichi, M., and Shibasaki, K.: Surgical treatment of thoracic disc herniation using the anterior approach, *J. Bone Joint Surg. [Br.]*, 64B: 1982.
9. Otani, K., Yoshida, M., Fuji, E., Nakai, S., and Shibasaki, K.: Thoracic disc herniation. Surgical treatment in 23 patients. *Spine*, 13: 1262–1267, 1988.
10. Patterson, R. H., and Arbit, E.: A surgical approach through the pedicle to protruded thoracic discs. *J. Neurosurg.*, 48: 768–772, 1978.
11. Rossitti, S., Stephensen, H., Ekholm, S., and Von Essen, C.: The anterior approach to high thoracic (T1–T2) disc herniation. *Br. J. Neurosurg.*, 7: 189–192, 1993.
12. Simpson, J. M., Silveri, C. P., Simeone, F. A., Balderston, R. A., and An, H. S.: Thoracic disc herniation. *Spine*, 18: 1872–1877, 1993.
13. Stillerman, C. B., and Weiss, M. H.: Management of thoracic disc disease. *Clin. Neurosurg.*, 38: 325–352, 1992.
14. Watkins, R. G.: Thoracotomy approach. In: *Surgical Approaches to the Spine*, edited by R. G. Watkins. Springer-Verlag, New York.

Master Techniques in Orthopaedic Surgery,
THE SPINE, edited by D. S. Bradford,
Lippincott-Raven Publishers, Philadelphia, © 1997.

18

Anterior and Posterior Spinal Cord Decompression

John P. Kostuik

INDICATIONS/CONTRAINDICATIONS

The goals of spinal cord decompression, regardless of the route used, depend on the degree of spinal cord compression. In the absence of neurological deficit, the goal may be to preserve function, while in the presence of neurological deficit, the goal may be to restore and preserve function.

The approach indicated for spinal cord decompression depends on the type and the site of pathology. Anterior or anterolateral approaches are reserved for anterior pathology and posterior approaches for posterior pathology. Occasionally, both approaches are necessary, especially for primary tumors of both the anterior and posterior columns and in some cases of metastatic diseases of the spine. Posterolateral decompression of the spine can be performed for anterior pathology, for example, in cases of angular kyphosis or when the patient's general health status renders an anterior approach, particularly at the thoracolumbar junction, medically dangerous.

Thoracic Disc Herniation

The neurological morbidity for an anterior approach and decompression for thoracic disc herniation with associated myelopathy or radiculopathy is considerably less than for a posterior approach, and it is the preferred technique (Fig. 1). A posterolateral approach may be used, but it is more difficult than the anterior approach because of problems with visualization and hemorrhage. For thoracic pain syndromes of a discogenic nature with pain reproduction via discography, the anterior approach is preferred. If discography does not reproduce the patient's

J. P. Kostuik, M.D.: Departments of Orthopaedics and Neurosurgery, The Johns Hopkins University Medical Center, Baltimore, Maryland 21287–0882.

symptoms but facet blocks alleviate the pain, a posterior or posterolateral approach is preferred.

Infections

In infection, most disease involves the anterior middle columns of the spine. Removal of a vertebral body is indicated if there is significant bone destruction,

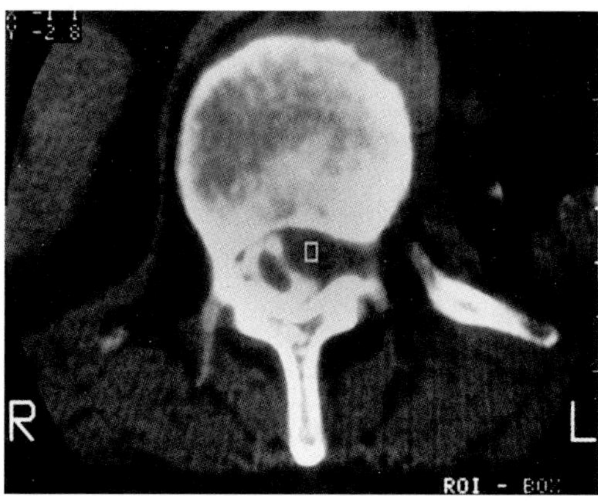

Figure 1. Thoracic disc herniation, CT myelogram. An MRI is as effective. An anterior decompression was done together with a fusion.

A 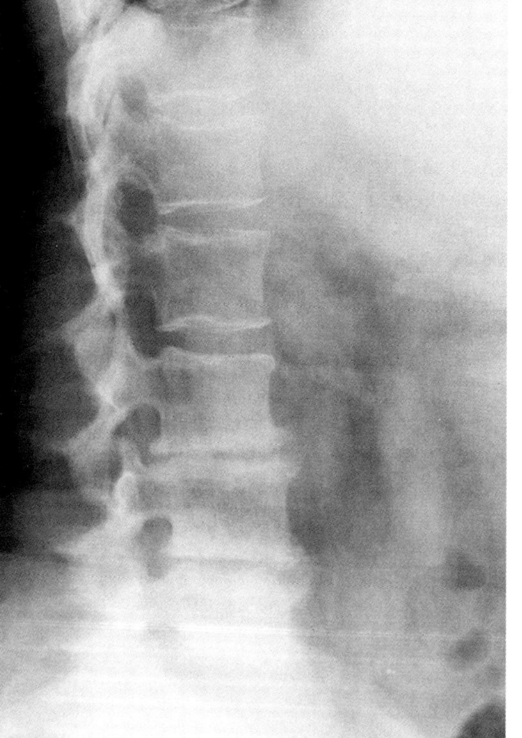

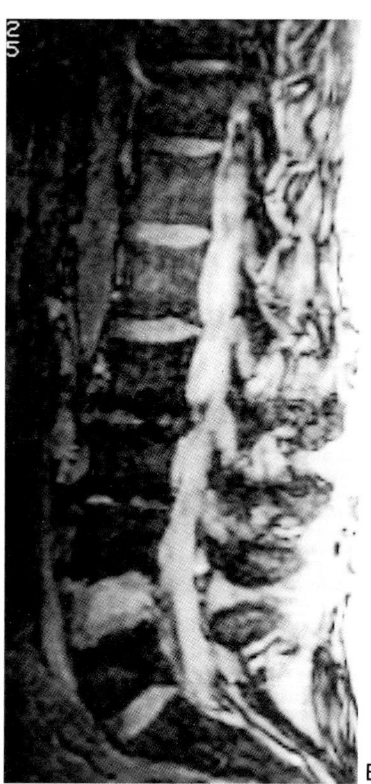 B

Figure 2. Infection. A 62-year-old diabetic woman presented with back pain. A possible infection was suspected. Following referral, a successful anterior decompression debridement and autogenous iliac crest grafting were performed. Frequently, in the elderly, a second-stage posterior stabilization is recommended. **A:** Lateral view of the spine demonstrates early changes in the anterior metaphysis under the anterior longitudinal ligament typical of pyogenic osteomyelitis of the spine and confirmed on MRI **(B)**. **C,D:** Late changes with collapse and neurological changes. **E:** Anterior debridement. Bone grafting was performed followed by a second-stage stabilization.

neurological compromise, or failure to respond to appropriate antibiotics, which may be the case if significant bone destruction has occurred. This is best analyzed by computed tomography (CT) scanning in the both the axial and sagittal planes (Fig. 2).

An anterior approach is preferred for both pyogenic and granulomatous infections since the disease process usually involves the anterior column. Cord or cauda equina decompression is required if there is direct anterior compression with or without neurological compromise. Epidural abscesses are usually best dealt with by posterior decompression, especially if they involve more than one level.

Tumors

Metastatic Tumors. Indications for surgery include neurological compromise, pain, impending fracture, or pathologic fracture. Most tumors involving the anterior column are amenable to the anterior approach. Cord or cauda equina decompression is warranted if there is neurological impingement and/or signs and symptoms related to neurological compromise.

If the disease is widespread or involves the posterior elements, or if skip lesions exist, a posterior approach is preferable. Decompression of anterior tumors in the lumbar spine can be accomplished from a posterior approach by going between the nerve roots and scooping out the tumor. In the thoracic spine, nerve roots

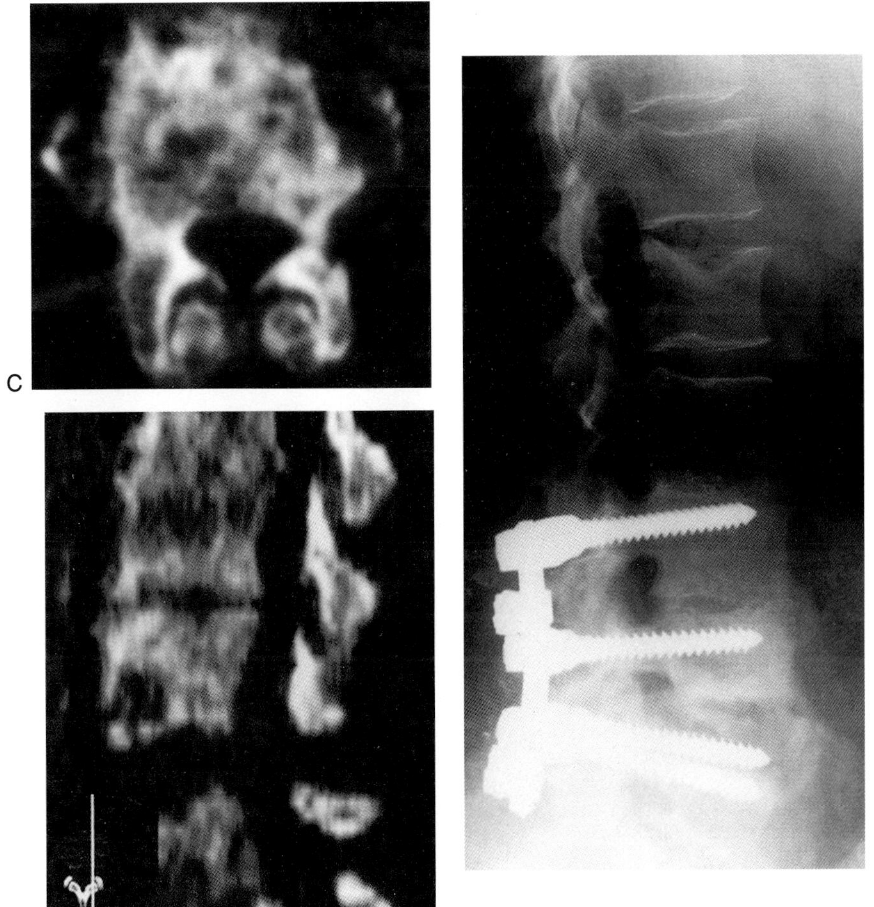

Figure 2. *Continued.*

sacrificed if need be, to remove tumor masses lying anteriorly through a posterior approach. In all situations, stabilization will be required (Figs. 3 to 5).

Primary Tumors. Most primary tumors, with the exception of osteoid osteomas and some blastomas, involve the vertebral body. Malignant tumors, which also tend to involve the anterior column, are best treated by en bloc resection via anterior and posterior approaches (Fig. 6), followed by reconstruction. Benign tumors can be safely approached either anteriorly or posteriorly.

Fractures

Burst Fractures. Anterior approaches are reserved for acute burst fractures with significant neural damage (Frankel grades A, B, and C, with some D), canal compromise 70% or greater, and late (greater than 5 to 7 days) fracture (Fig. 7; see also Fig. 18). Posterior approaches will not reduce a late burst fracture, since the fracture is through cancellous bone and healing has already commenced, making posterior reduction difficult. Posterolateral approaches for cauda equina decompression have been described for burst injuries with or without neurological compromise. However, decompression may be incomplete from this approach due to difficulties in visualization of the anterior pathology. This approach is also more dangerous because of the necessity to manipulate the dorsal sac to remove most of the fragments.

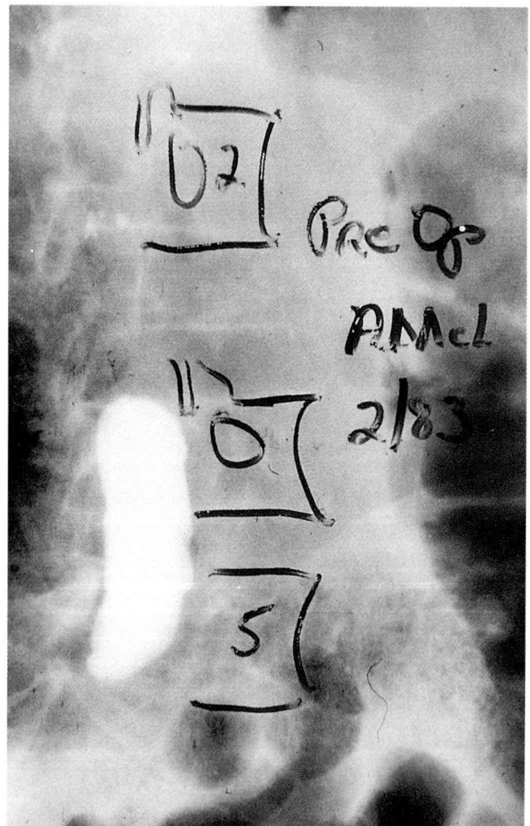

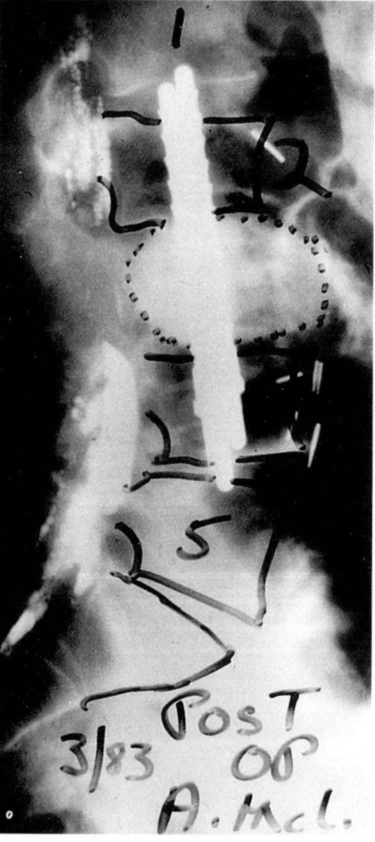

Figure 3. A,B: Renal cell carcinoma demonstrating anterior decompression with cement-reinforced polymethylmethacrylate (PMMA).

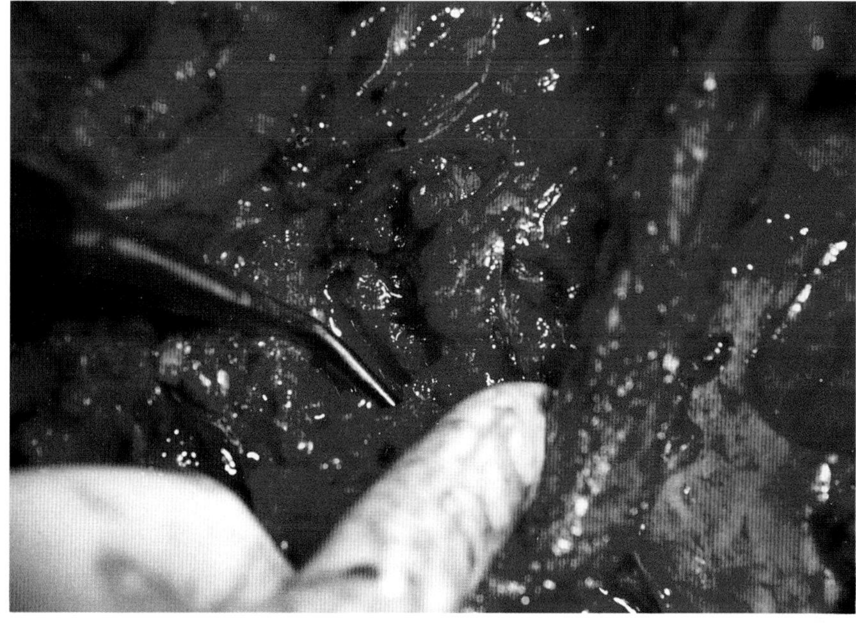
A

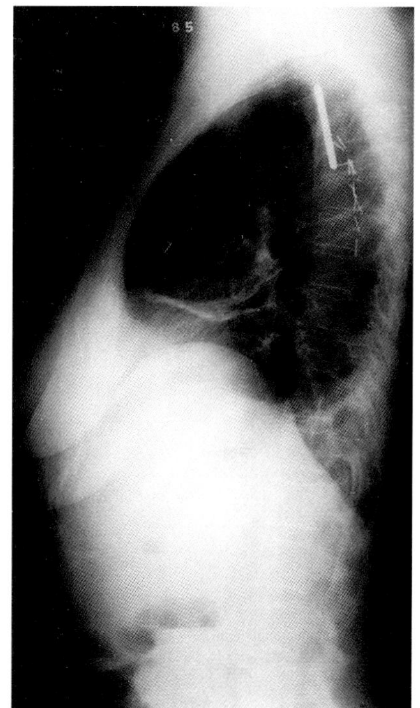
C

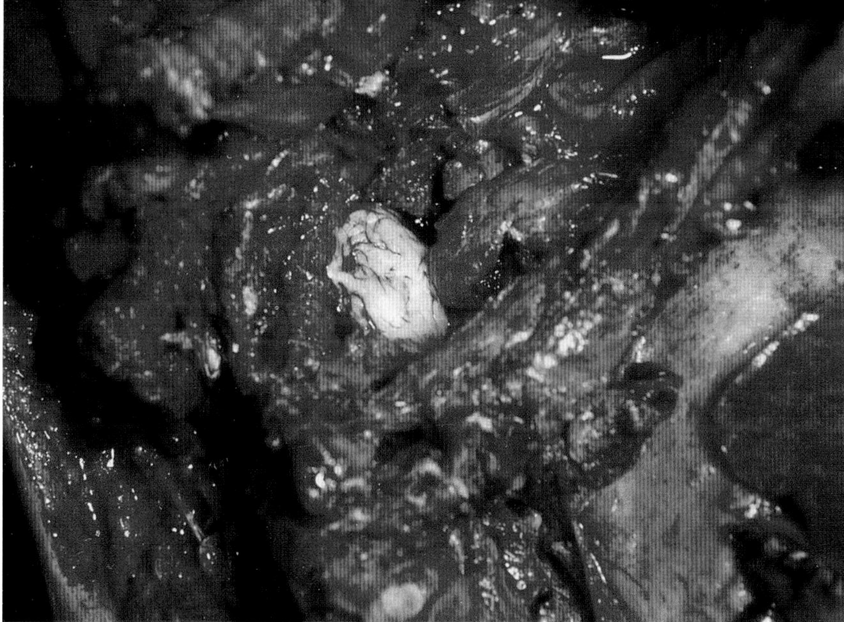
B

Figure 4. A–C: Technique of anterior decompression and stabilization. In metastatic disease, following decompression, the proximal and distal vertebral bodies are partially evacuated. They are then filled with soft PMMA, the precut and sized metal rod(s) are inserted, and more PMMA is added. The vertebral body has been resected. The spinal cord is decompressed. The bodies proximal and distal are evacuated with curettes. The body is replaced with metal-reinforced PMMA.

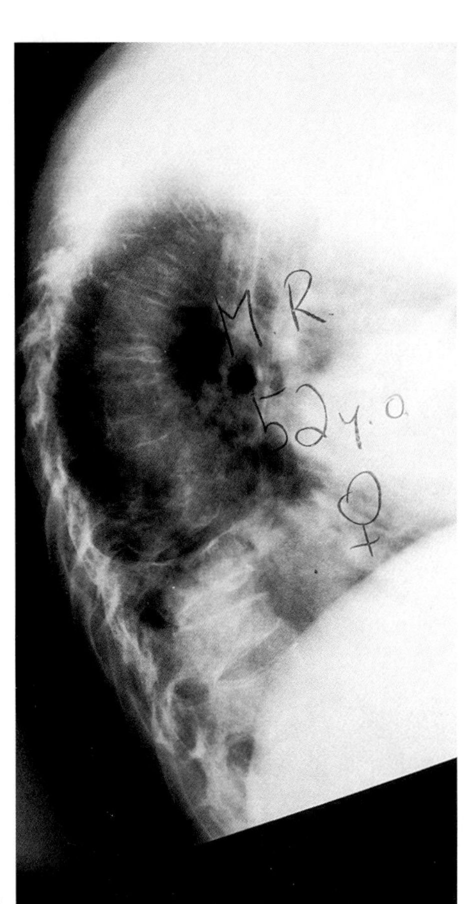

A

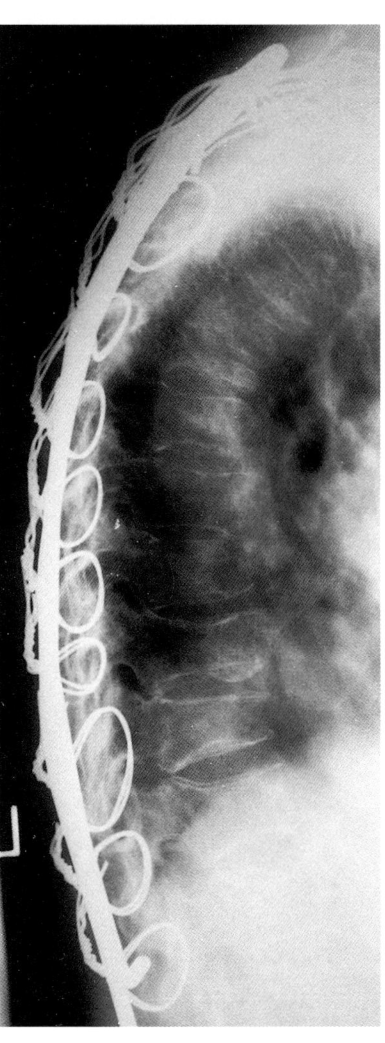

B

Figure 5. A: Metastatic breast carcinoma with widespread disease and myelopathy. **B:** Stabilization following posterior and posterolateral decompression was done with Luque rods and wires supplemented with PMMA.

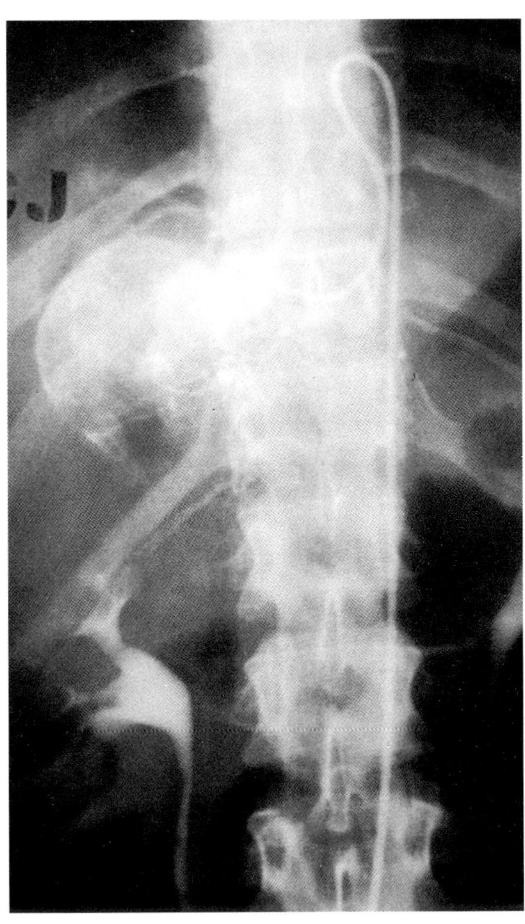

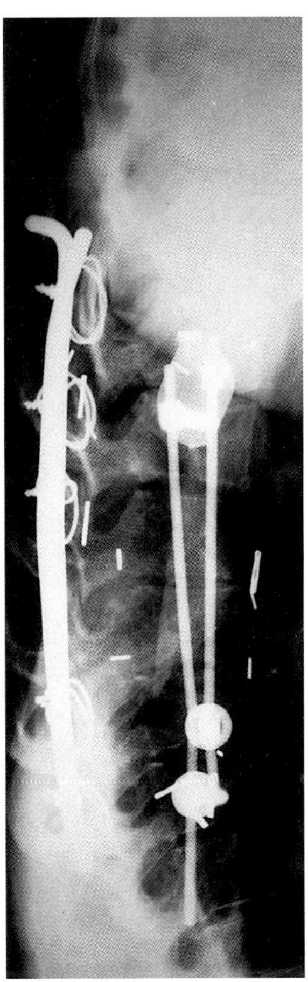

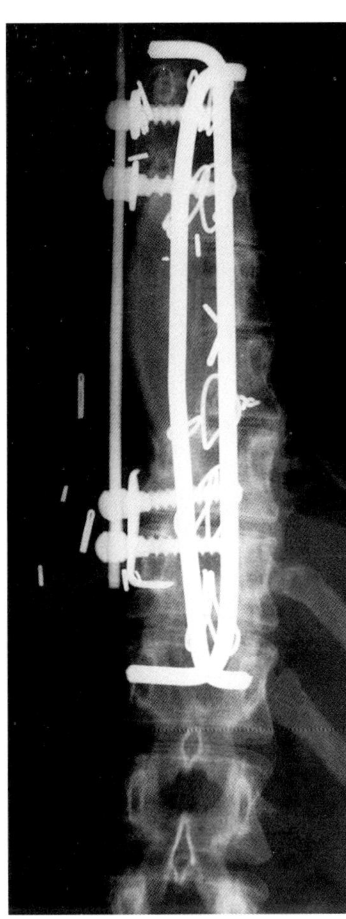

A B,C

Figure 6. A: Malignant ganglioneuroma. **B,C:** En bloc resection was done with anterior and posterior stabilization in 1981. The patient is alive and well today. Pedicle screw construction posteriorly and plate fixation anteriorly would be the preferable form of stabilization.

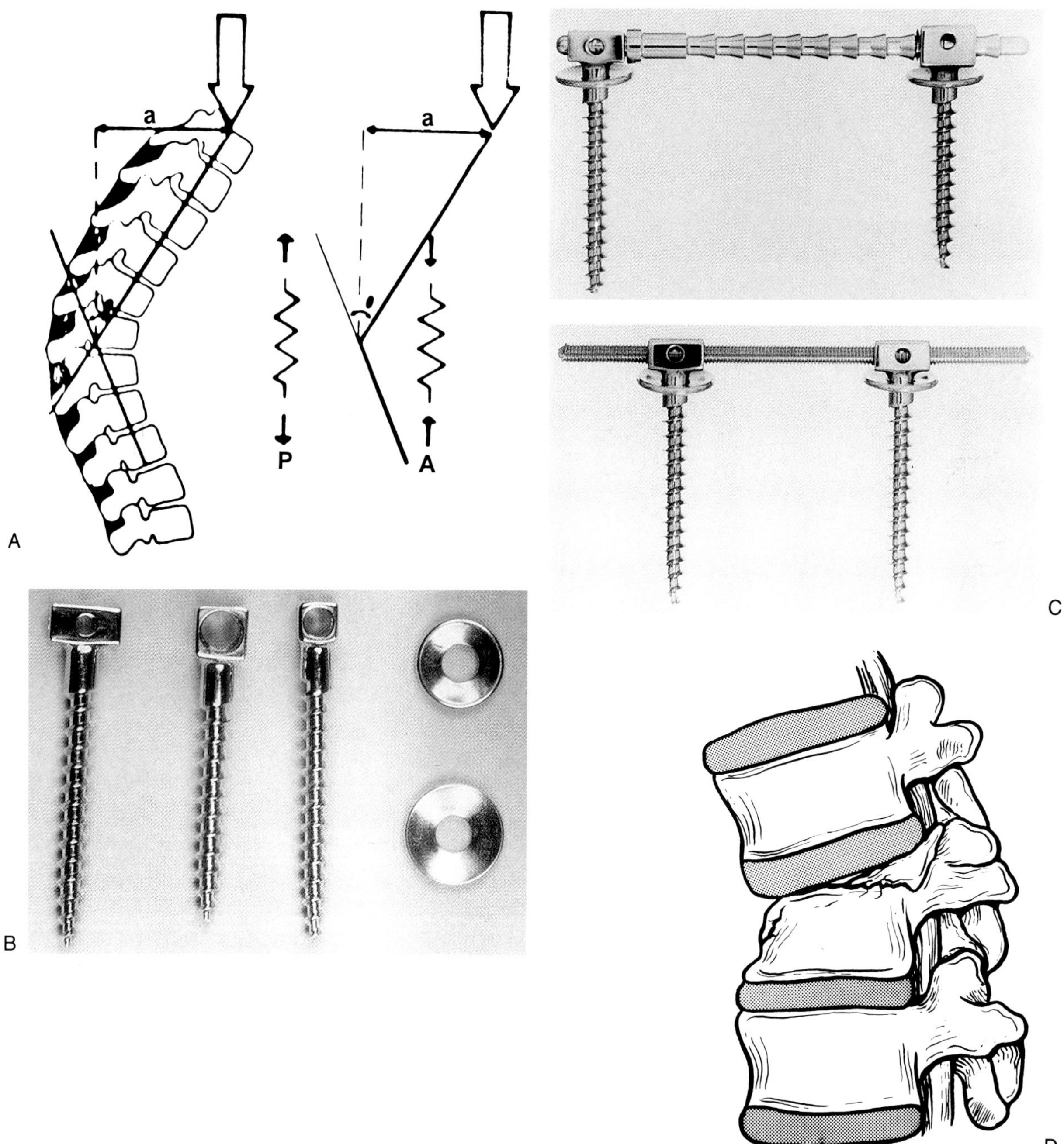

Figure 7. A: Biomechanics of kyphosis. *Left:* Kyphotic deformity showing a Cobb angle of 58 degrees. Vertical directed physiological forces (*large arrow*) work at a moment arm at length (A). *Right:* Schematic depiction of deformity showing that the posterior elements (P) resist tensile loading. The anterior elements (A) resist compressive loading. Factors contributing to kyphosis include increase in physiological load (*white arrow*), increase in moment arm (A), weakening of posterior elements, and weakening of anterior elements. **B:** Kostuik screws. Distraction screw (ratchet end) and collar-ended screw

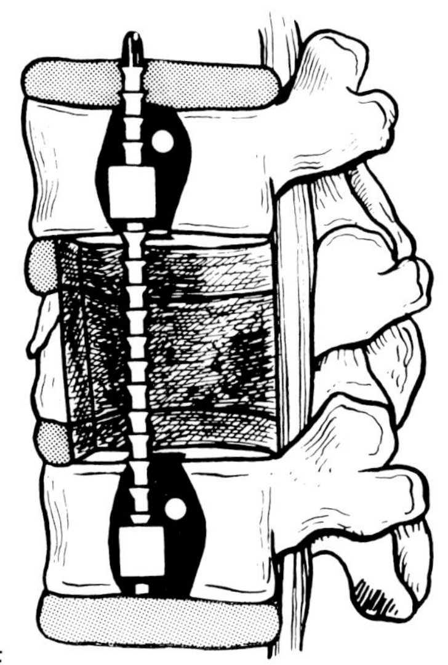

E

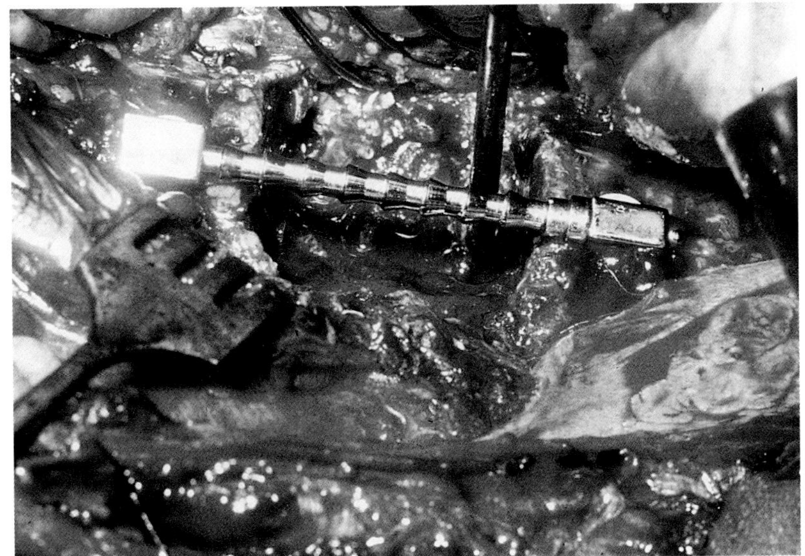

F

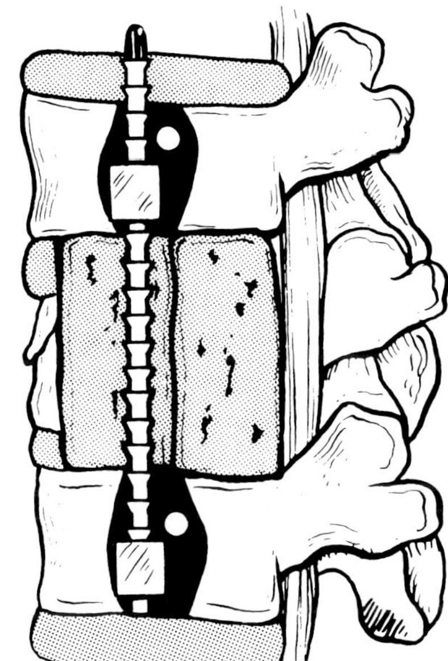

G

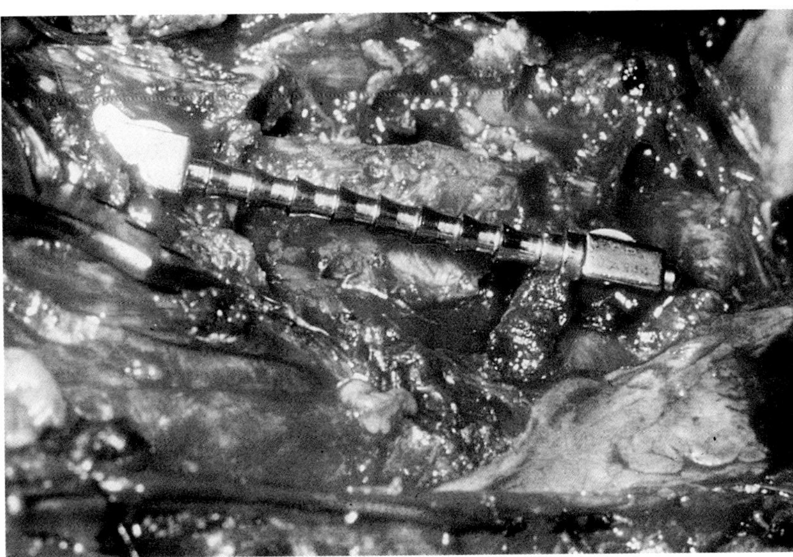

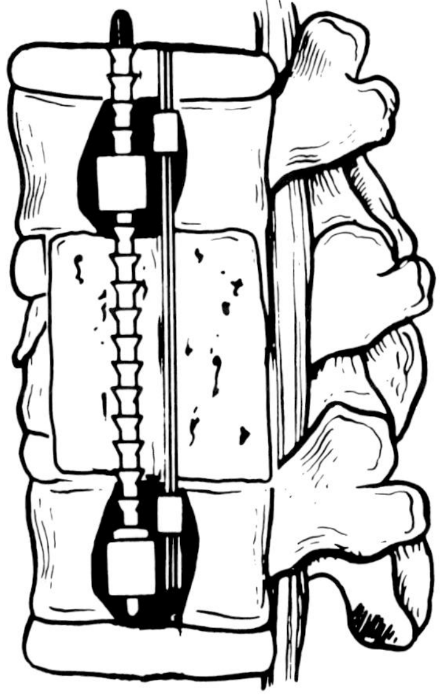

H

(for compression rods and end of distraction rod). **C:** *Top:* Kostuik-Harrington system. Round-ended Harrington rod distraction screw (ratchet end), collar-ended screw, washers. *Bottom:* Heavy compression Harrington rod. **D:** Burst fracture. **E,F:** Dura decompressed; anterior one-fourth of body is left as graft. Kyphosis is reduced with Kostuik-Harrington distraction device. **G:** 1 and 2, Anterior lateral rod is inserted to reduce kyphosis, and bone graft (iliac crest) is added. **H:** Second heavy Harrington compression rod is added to increase stability. Slight compression is applied. Collar-ended screw heads are crimped.

Compression Fractures. Compression fractures in osteoporosis may occasionally lead to dural compression and neurological compromise and are best dealt with by an anterior approach rather than the general posterior approach. In these elderly patients, an extrapleural approach is preferred to a transpleural approach in the thoracic region because there is less respiratory morbidity postoperatively. An anterior approach is contraindicated in medically unwell patients who have a painful compression fracture with neurological problems. The eggshell posterior approach may be performed, although there is greater neurological risk than with the anterior approach.

Post-Traumatic Kyphosis. Post-traumatic kyphosis requires an anterior correction decompression when indicated (neural compromise), because the grafts will then be under compression (Fig. 8 and 9). Posterior approaches do not solve the problems of residual pain, neural compromise, or deformity. Posterior surgery to restore alignment is rarely successful, with the exception of the eggshell procedure. An anterior approach consisting of removal of multiple level discs in the area of pathology and/or corpectomy together with anterior instrumentation can easily achieve this goal. An alternative is anterior decompression and/or releases followed by posterior instrumentation.

Deformity

Most deformities requiring anterior decompression are kyphotic in nature. These are often congenital or infective (old tuberculosis) in origin. Where there

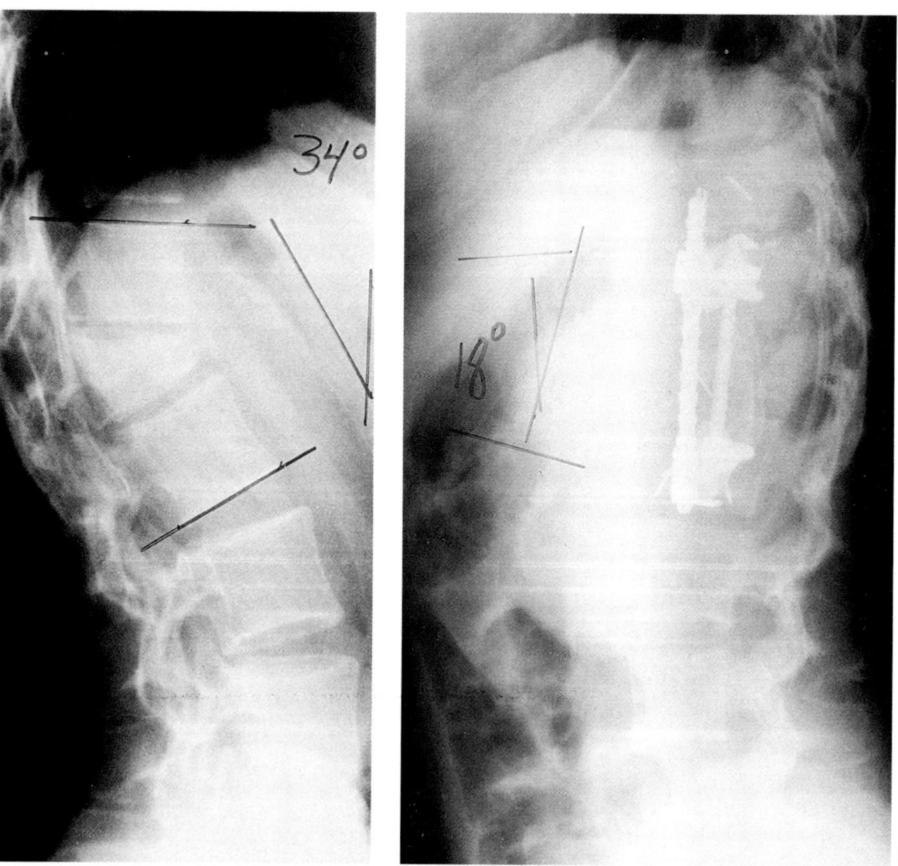

Figure 8. A: Post-traumatic kyphosis at L1 with increasing neurological signs 1 year after accident. **B:** Anterior decompression grafting and stabilization was done with a successful outcome. The technique is the same as that used for burst injuries.

is dural impingement, correction of a kyphotic or kyphoscoliotic deformity must first consist of an anterior decompression. This is often followed by a posterior release and a period of dependent traction following a posterior stabilization.

PREOPERATIVE PLANNING

Decision making in spinal surgery is primarily based on a careful and comprehensive history. An accurate neurological history is paramount in a patient who may require decompression of neural elements. The degree of disability as well as the general ergonomics of the problem (i.e., age, sex, family, general health, degree of disability vis-à-vis occupation, activities of daily living, and extracurricular activities) must be assessed. It is imperative to know how significantly disabled the patient is by the pain and/or neurological deficit.

Pain

A thorough knowledge of the type of pain, its referral pattern or radiation, what provokes it, and what alleviates it must be obtained. Pain of a mechanical nature due to instability is aggravated by motion and alleviated by rest, whereas pain

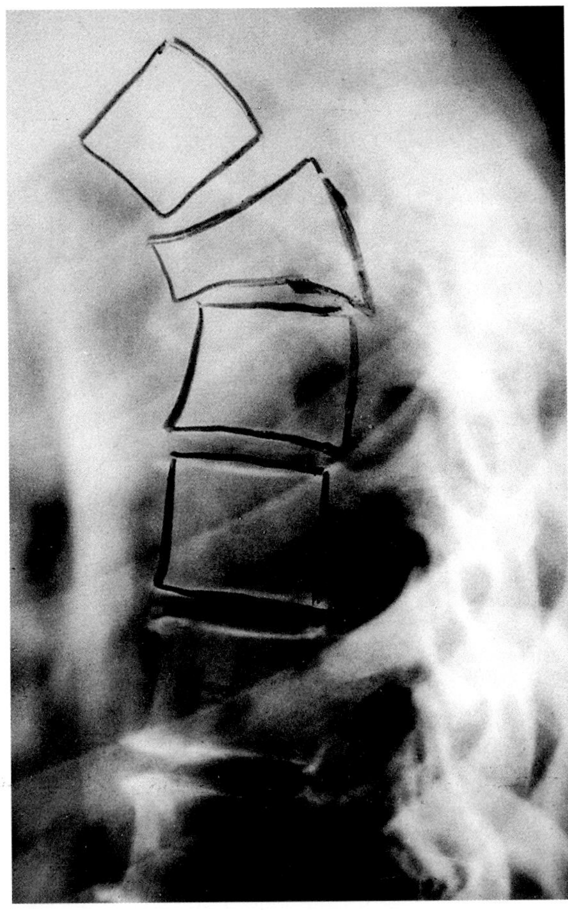

A

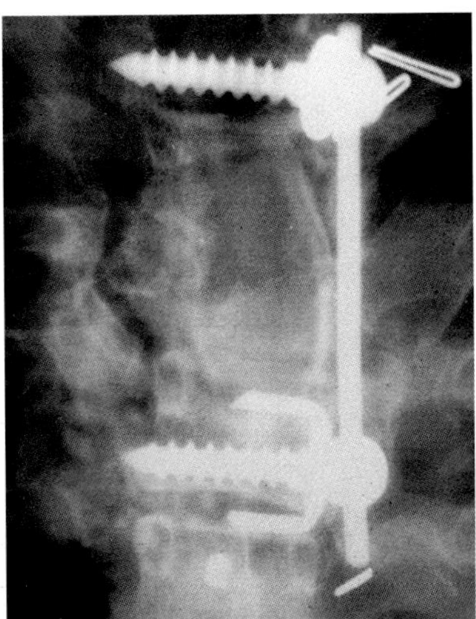

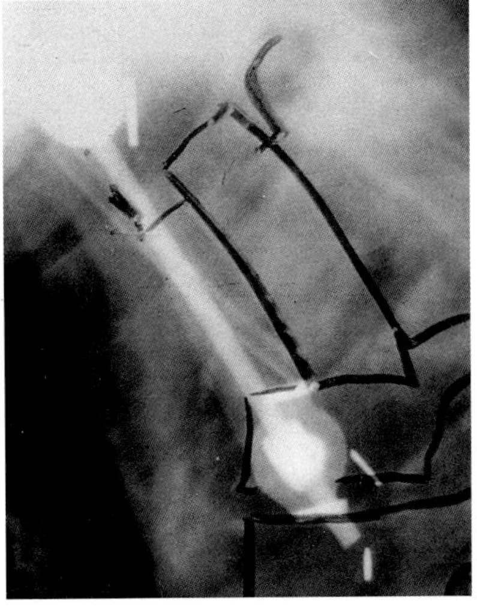

B

Figure 9. A problem similar to the one shown in Figure 8 in the upper thoracic spine. **A:** A previously performed laminectomy aggravated a pre-existing myelopathy. **B:** This was relieved following anterior decompression and stabilization.

secondary to tumor is generally not alleviated by rest. Musculoskeletal pain is generally aching in nature, whereas neurological pain may vary from a burning dysesthetic pain to a sharp pain to an ache.

The ability of the patient to ambulate must be thoroughly examined in terms of distance and the factors that limit ambulation. For example, limitation of ambulation due to neurogenic claudication is of a more gradual onset, is alleviated by forward flexion, and disappears more slowly on stopping or sitting than the pain of vascular claudication.

Gait disturbance is often the first manifestation of myelopathy, particularly for problems arising from the cervical thoracic spine. Patients may have concurrent symptoms of upper and lower motor neuron lesions.

Bowel or bladder function history is very important. Stress incontinence in the elderly female has often been attributed to childbearing and the effects of aging, whereas a frequent cause is neural compression, particularly in lumbar stenosis.

It is important to assess the degree of disability vis-à-vis daily function. A compression fracture producing mild neurological complaints in a housebound patient is not as serious as it is for a patient who is fully ambulatory and involved in community affairs.

Physical Examination

The spine should be observed for deformity such as loss of lumbar lordosis, the presence or absence of a kyphosis or lateral deformities, a rib hump, waist asymmetry, or exaggerated cervical lordosis secondary to thoracic kyphosis. It is important that the hips be examined. Not uncommonly, people are referred for anterior thigh pain, but the pathology is related to their hip and not their spine. Leg length and the girth of the calves and thighs should be determined.

Peripheral pulses must be palpated. The presence of peripheral pulses or good hair growth on the foot eliminates problems due to vascular claudication.

Neurological examination is generally divided into two parts and consists of tests that indicate nerve root irritation (straight leg raising, femoral stretch, and bowstring stretch) and tests that indicate impaired nerve conduction (reflexes, motor power, and sensation, including deep pain, light touch, position sense, temperature, and vibration). Careful examination for signs of upper motor neuron lesions must be made and should include tests for gait disturbance, clonus, Babinski response, and sensory disturbance. Patients with evidence of upper motor neuron lesions in the lower extremities should be examined for evidence of problems in their upper extremities. Examination of abdominal reflexes and cremasteric responses in the male are important. Rectal examination for tone, voluntary contraction, perianal sensation, and anal wink are important.

Radiological Imaging

Plain radiographs are paramount. Not only do they provide insight into pathology, but they are necessary for preoperative planning of degree of resection and insertion of implants, particularly pedicle screws.

Magnetic resonance imaging (MRI) has become the image of choice for most conditions requiring decompression of the spinal cord and is of particular value in assessing soft tissue. In the cauda equina, CT myelography and MRI may be of comparable value, depending on the institution and technique used. In the region of the spinal cord, however, MRI is preferred over CT myelography to assess cord compression. CT myelography increases in value in cases of repeat surgery.

For assessment of bony elements, CT is preferred. Axial and sagittal reconstructive cuts should be obtained. Occasionally three-dimensional CT imaging is of value. Quite frequently, in cases of metastatic disease, both MRI and CT scanning aid significantly in preoperative planning of the extent of the resection because MRI can assess soft tissues and CT the bony structures. For patients with post-traumatic kyphosis, assessment should include CT scanning, metrizamide myelography, discography above and below the fracture (four levels), and facet blocks if there has been no previous fusion. Discograms and facet blocks are done to make sure all painful levels are incorporated in the subsequent surgery.

SURGERY

The choice of approach is dictated by the site of primary pathology. Anterior approaches through the thorax, abdomen, or flank are best for pathology involving the vertebral bodies, whereas problems involving the posterior elements are best approached posteriorly through a vertical midline approach. Posterior lateral structures may be approached either through a midline posterior approach or posterior lateral muscle spinning approach. Approaches should be planned so they can be extensile at the time of surgery, if necessary.

Anterior Corpectomy

Burst fractures and metastatic disease are the two most common indications for corpectomy. The technique for both conditions is similar.

After having approached the area of pathology, it is important to mobilize great vessels by ligating segmental vessels, preferably two levels proximal and two levels distal to the site of pathology. This permits retraction of the great vessels and a safe approach to the contralateral side. The great vessels should be protected by a malleable retractor.

To minimize blood loss, discs at the level above and the level distal to the corpectomy should first be removed. The most proximal and distal end plates on the normal vertebral bodies should be left intact at this point.

In the case of a burst injury (Fig. 17), the part of the body most opposite the side of the approach may be preserved; essentially about one-fourth of the body can be osteotomized and left attached to the soft tissues. Most of the body is then removed with sharp chisels, taking progressively thinner slices. As one approaches the posterior aspect of the body, these slices should be approximately 1 mm in thickness. Use of rongeurs or high speed burs may also be helpful. Once the epidural space is entered, antral punches of various angles will aid in increasing exposure of the underlying dura.

Sharp dissection of the disc with the use of a scalpel will aid in removing any fracture fragments that may remain attached to the disc. The use of a small sharp chisel on the superior/inferior end plate of the uninvolved vertebral bodies can also help to detach fragments. Undermining on the up side can be carried out with antral punches. On the contralateral side, it is our technique to remove a piece of bone, leaving 2 to 3 mm intact against the dorsal sac. After the trough has been established to the depth of 3 to 4 mm, the ridge closest to the dural sac may be removed, completing decompression. Next the end plates of the intact superior and inferior vertebral bodies are removed. Bleeding is controlled by bipolar cautery. If significant bleeding occurs, it may be necessary to stop the procedure for a short period and to compress at the dural veins with large pieces of thrombin-soaked Gelfoam with overlying gauze.

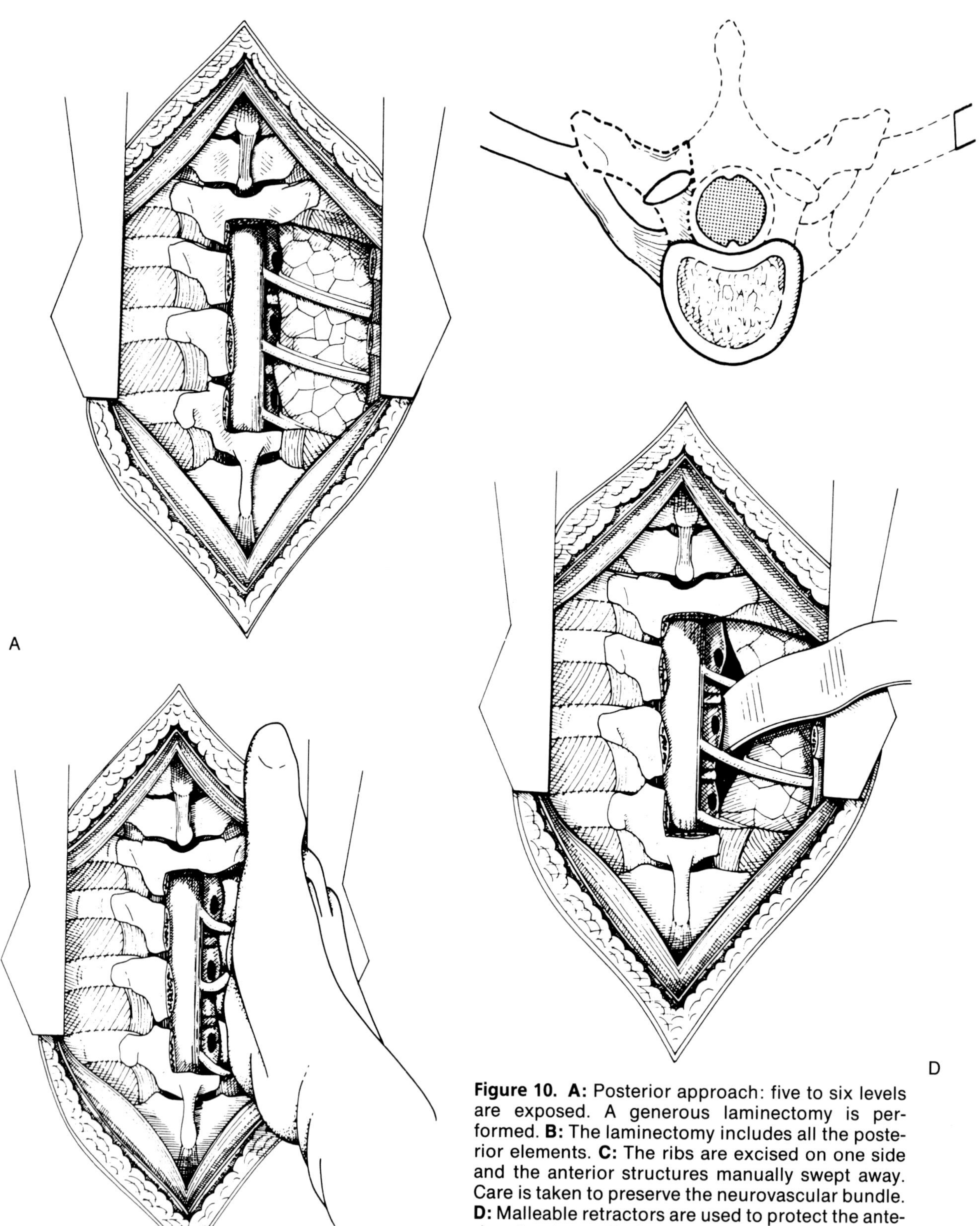

Figure 10. A: Posterior approach: five to six levels are exposed. A generous laminectomy is performed. **B:** The laminectomy includes all the posterior elements. **C:** The ribs are excised on one side and the anterior structures manually swept away. Care is taken to preserve the neurovascular bundle. **D:** Malleable retractors are used to protect the anterior structures. **E:** Complete posterior decompression and rib resection bilaterally has been performed. **F:** All structures are protected. **G:** The tumor (T) is fully exposed. **H:** Partial posterior stabilization has been achieved.

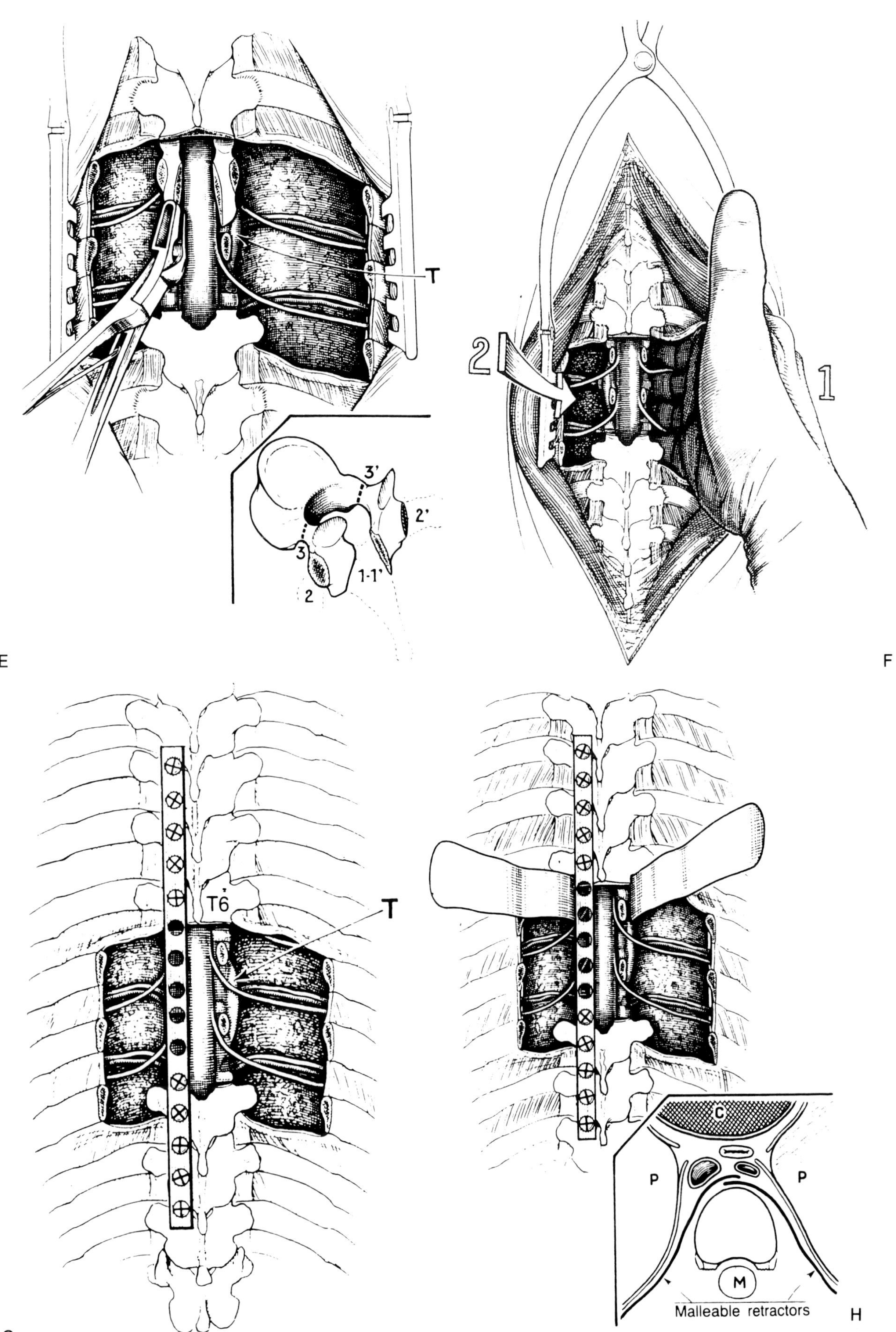

E

F

G

H

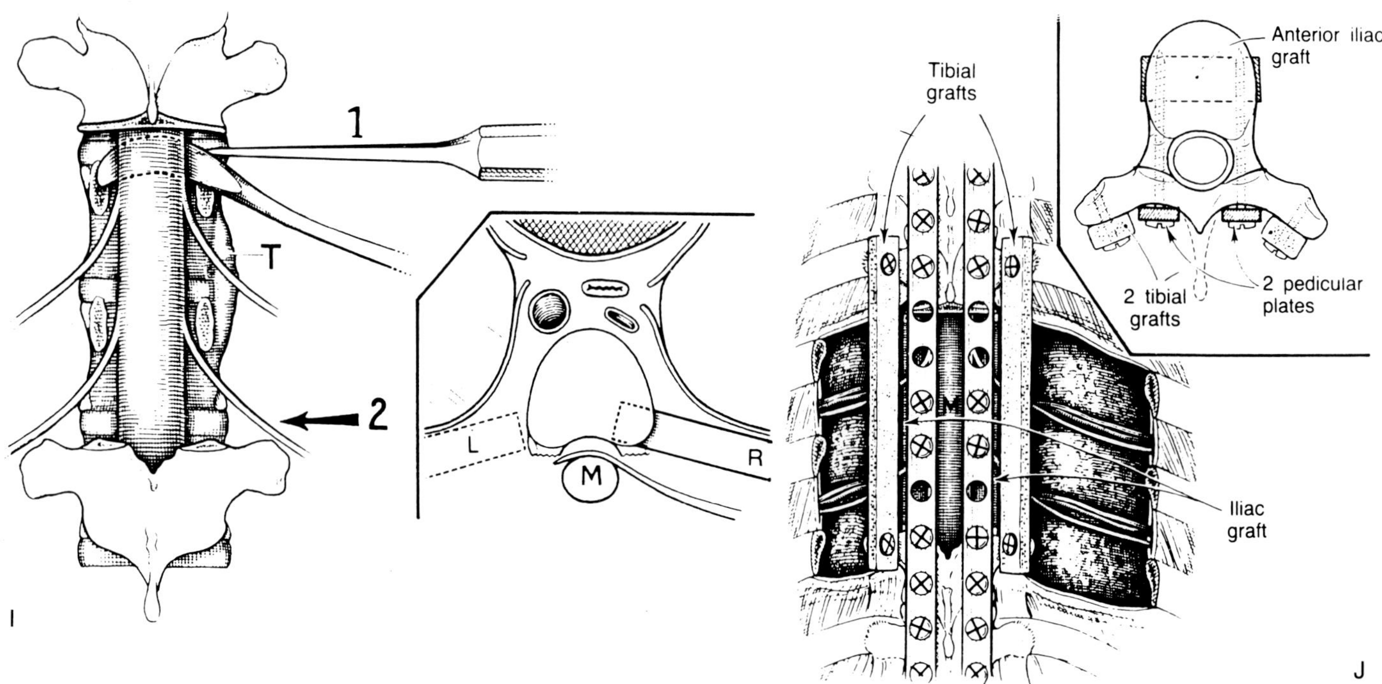

Figure 10. *Continued.* **I:** Vertebral body resection proximal and distal to the tumor (T) is begun. **J:** The tumor has been resected and the spine fully stabilized and grafted.

In the case of tumor (Figs. 3 to 5), segmental vessels should be similarly ligated. If the tumor is suspected of being vascular, especially secondary to renal cell carcinoma, preoperative embolization will significantly decrease blood flow and may safely be carried out up to 24 hours prior to surgery. Since treatment of cases of metastatic disease is not curative, tumor spill is not important. After isolating the disc space above and below, rongeurs and curettes are usually the instruments most valuable in achieving the corpectomy. Alternatively, a Cavitron may be used. Any remaining tumor attached to the dural sac should be removed by finding a plane between the dura and tumor either by sharp dissection using a scalpel or by a small elevator.

Extended Anterior Posterior Approach

Used primarily for tumors, the extended anterior posterior approach gives access to the entire spine, including the contents of the spinal canal; allows for the combined exposure of both the posterior and anterior structures of the spine; and may be unilateral or bilateral. Total vertebrectomies can be performed in the thoracic spine with one procedure. Because the approach is so extensive, the risk of neurological complications from direct damage to neurological structures or interruption of the blood supply in the watershed area of the thoracic spine, is high.

The patient is placed in the prone position on a frame to prevent compression of the thoracic and abdominal contents. A midline posterior incision is used to permit complete visualization of the posterior vertebral arch and the posterior aspect of the ribs for at least 5 cm. The incision must be three to four levels proximal and distal to the area of resection to allow sufficient retraction. In some cases, exposure is facilitated by dividing the paravertebral muscles transversely (Fig. 10A).

A complete laminectomy of the desired number of vertebral levels is performed

(Fig. 10B), thus permitting the spinal canal and its contents to be visualized. Usually, a minimum of three levels is necessary. The ribs are divided 3 cm lateral to the costotransverse joints. The neurovascular pedicles may or may not be ligated. The posterior mediastinum can then be entered. Ideally, resection of the ribs is done extrapleurally, but in most adults the pleura is very thin and tenuous and may be torn, necessitating insertion of a chest tube at completion of the procedure. The articular processes and the pedicles are resected. The posterior mediastinal structures are swept away from the vertebral body, preferably by hand with the use of swabs. Mobilizing the vascular structures requires the segmental vessels to be ligated. A malleable retractor is inserted to protect and displace the anterior structures (Fig. 10C,D). The vertebral bodies are excised, generally through the disc space above and below the pathology. Less blood loss usually occurs with this procedure, but the length of resection is greater. Alternatively, vertebral bodies may be sectioned with a Gigli saw, starting anteriorly and extending through vertebral bodies, from anterior to posterior, through the anterior two-thirds of the vertebral body. The osteotomy is then completed in the remaining posterior one-third of the vertebral body from either side with a thin osteotome. The posterior longitudinal ligament is then easily cut with a knife.

Prior to this anterior resection, the posterior part of the spine should be stabilized. Otherwise, the spine is temporarily completely destabilized and at even greater risk of neurological compromise (Fig. 10E–J). Following resection of the vertebral bodies, posterior stabilization and grafting can be added. The extended posterior approach is often long, laborious, and tedious and must be done with great care.

Posterior Decompressions

Posterior decompressions are generally reserved for pathology involving the posterior bony elements (e.g., an osteoid osteoma) or for decompression of the spinal cord when the pathology is posterior.

While the patient is appropriately monitored using spinal and motor evoked potentials (after suitably preparing the skin and infiltration of the skin and subcutaneous tissues and deeper tissues with a solution of 1:500,000 adrenalin solution), exposure is carried out in a standard fashion. In the older adult, we prefer to use electrocautery to expose the posterior bony elements; in the younger individual and adolescent, a sharp dissection is carried out with the use of a knife. Following exposure of the spinous processes, the laminae are cleansed with the aid of Cobb elevators, packing off the paravertebral muscles to decrease blood loss. In the upper thoracic spine in particular, large venous plexuses must be cauterized.

In the presence of any posterior decompression when there is felt to be some loss of integrity of the anterior supporting column, posterior stabilization should be carried out. In a long decompression, this may require the use of pedicle screws. The pedicles are preserved to provide segmental fixation. In a shorter two- to four-level decompression, fixation for two levels proximal to the decompression and two levels distal to the decompression may suffice. A wide decompression leaves only the transverse process to fuse to if a fusion is indicated; careful decortication of the transverse process is important. In cases of metastatic disease, we reinforce the posterior internal fixation with methylmethacrylate (Figs. 3 to 5).

Transpedical Approaches

Transpedicular approaches or ''eggshell procedures'' are used for the treatment of kyphotic deformities, particularly of a congenital nature, for biopsy through the pedical to prevent spread of tumor cells in cases of potential malignancy, and in elderly patients who require an anterior decompression. The transpedicular approach allows for anterior decompression and posterior stabilization (Fig. 11). The spinal column may be operated on from both sides, permitting access to the anterior part of the spine through a single posterior approach. Since this technique is used to address both sides of the neural tube, it is usually prudent to use intraoperative evoked potentials.

The posterior spine is exposed. The cortical bone over the pedicle is removed. The pedicle hole is enlarged, using progressively larger curettes to allow access to the vertebral body (Fig. 12A–C). To gain greater access to the vertebral body, the lateral wall of the pedicle is fractured and refracted laterally. A curette may then be directed in a more lateral to medial direction to permit removal of the bone directly anterior to the spinal canal (Fig. 12D,E). The pedicle on the contralateral side is approached in a similar manner. The contents of the spinal canal are still protected by the laminae, medial walls of the pedicle, and posterior wall of

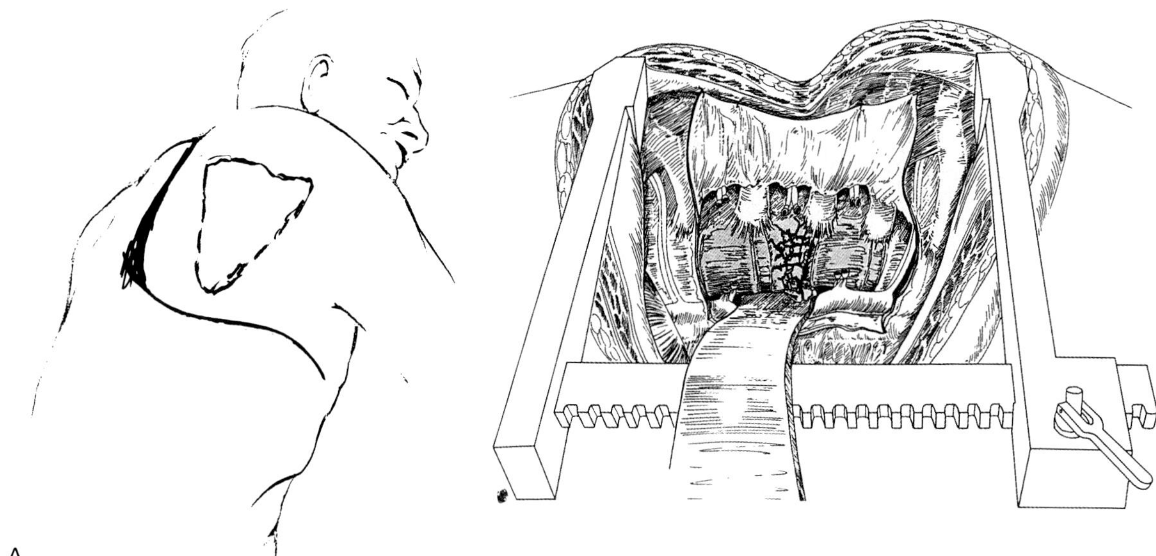

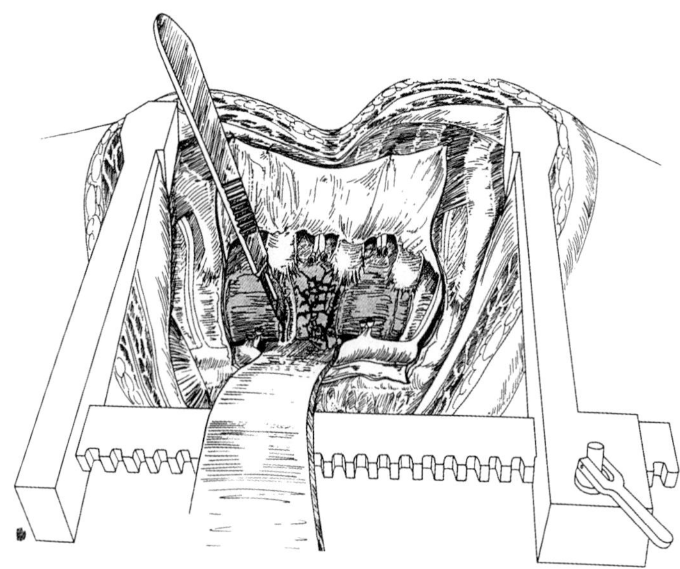

Figure 11. A: Place the patient in the lateral decubitus position with the left side up. Prep the entire extremity. Drape it out of the sterile operative field. Incise the skin and subcutaneous tissue from the lateral paraspinous area of C7 under the scapula to the costal margin of the third rib. **B:** After the thoracic cavity has been entered, the self-retaining chest retractor is inserted. The parietal pleura is incised half-way between the anterior great vessels and the posterior neural foramina, and the segmental vessels are ligated at this same level. The vertebra to be excised as well as one vertebra above and one vertebra below is exposed. Extraperiosteal dissection provides the best plane. A malleable retractor is then placed on the opposite side of the spine and connected to the self-retaining chest retractor with a clamp. This malleable retractor serves to protect the great vessels during the vertebral corpectomy. Scalpel and rongeur are used to remove the discs above and below the level of the vertebral fracture.

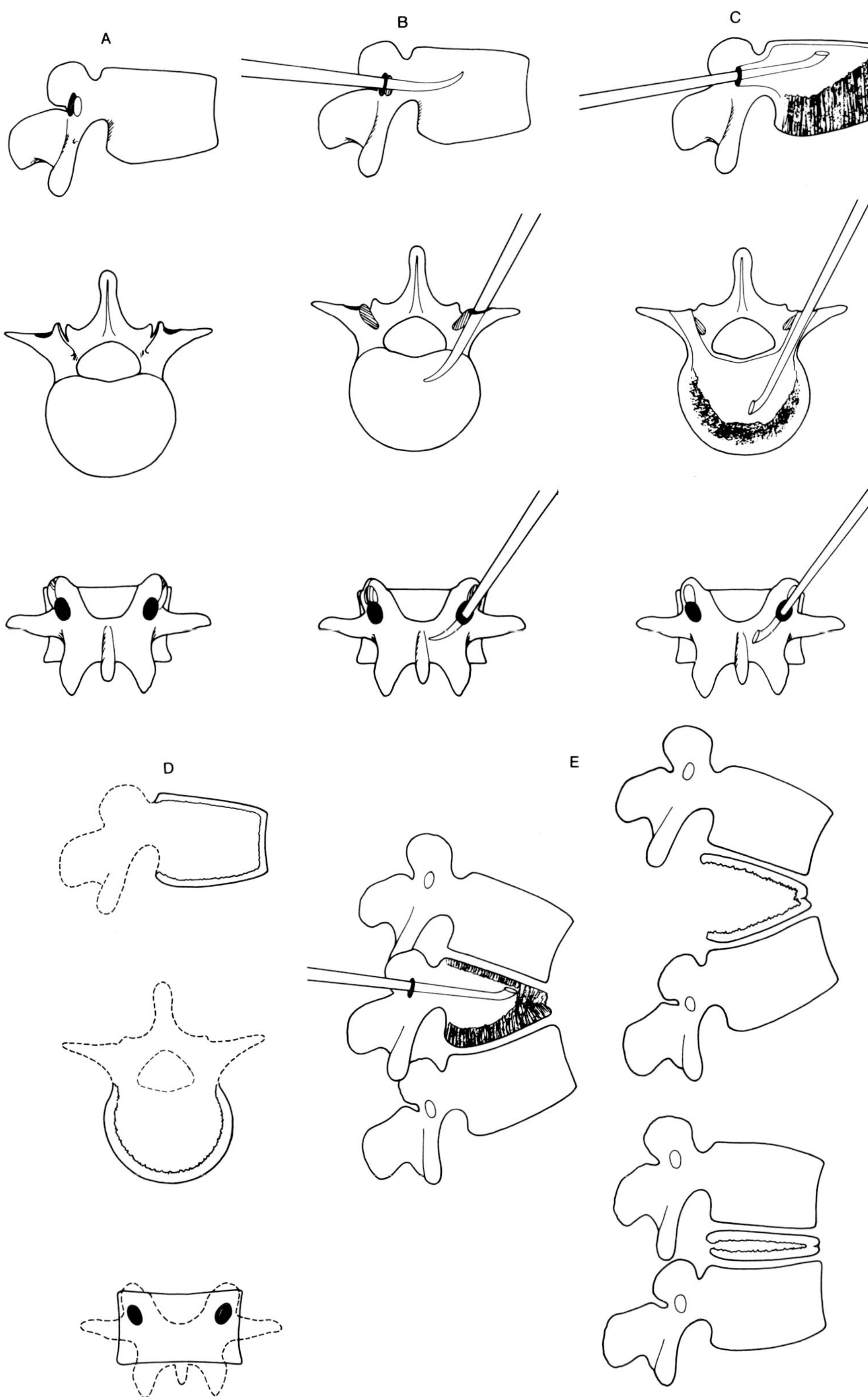

Figure 12. A–E: Eggshell procedure. Anterior decompression is done via the pedicle. Posterior stabilization can be added.

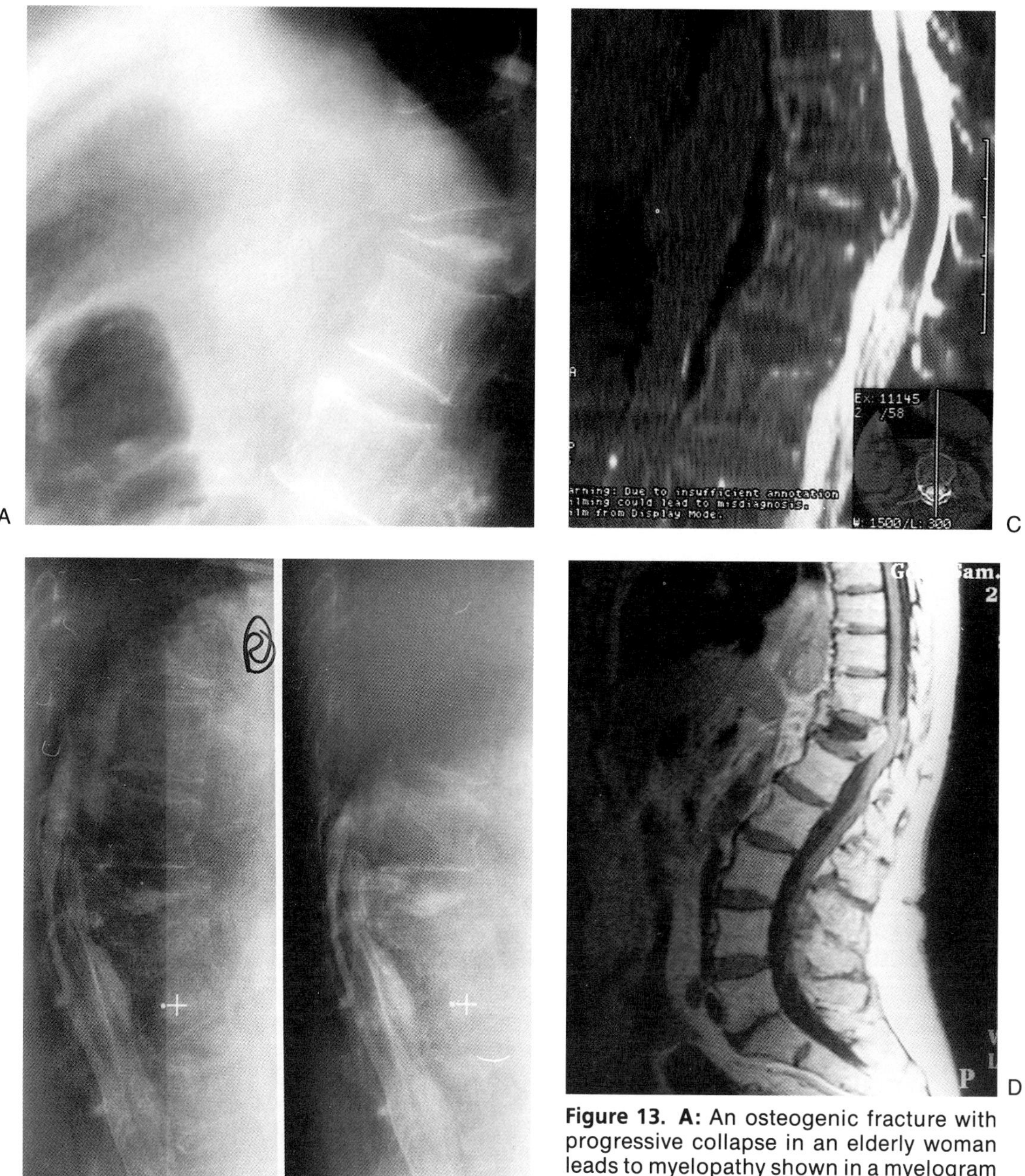

Figure 13. A: An osteogenic fracture with progressive collapse in an elderly woman leads to myelopathy shown in a myelogram **(B)** and MRI **(C,D)**.

the vertebral body. If there is anterior impingement of the dural sack by retropulsed bone, an elevator placed between the dura and the fragment will allow the retropulsed bone to be forced anteriorly into the vertebral body. Then internal fixation and transpedicular bone grafting can be used if desired (Fig. 13).

If an osteotomy is to be performed instead, the entire posterior arch of the pedicle and the posterior wall of the vertebral segment must be removed. The retropulsed fragments are removed as well. Increased mobility may be obtained by disc removal. Greater correction may also be obtained by fracturing the lateral vertebral body walls of the involved segment. This can be accomplished by the use of an osteotome to cut the side of the cortical shell. With this degree of mobility, severe fixed flexion deformities of the spine can be corrected. During the process of correction of the kyphotic deformities, it is necessary to ensure that no bony impingement of the neural elements occur by the posterior laminae that may require partial removal.

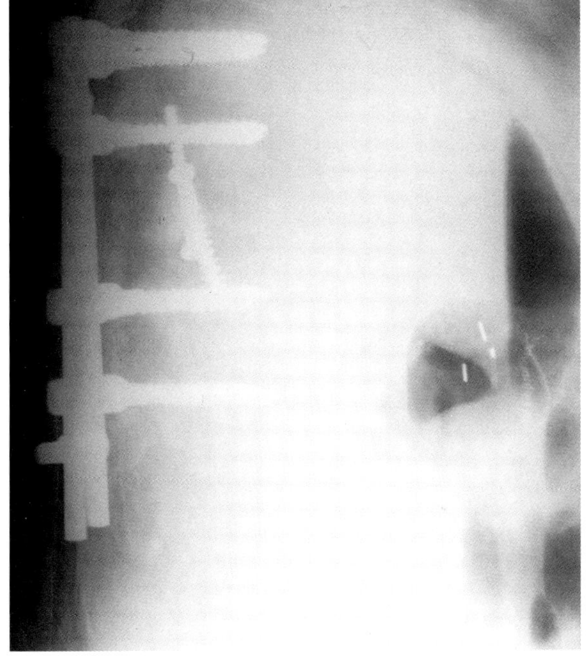

E

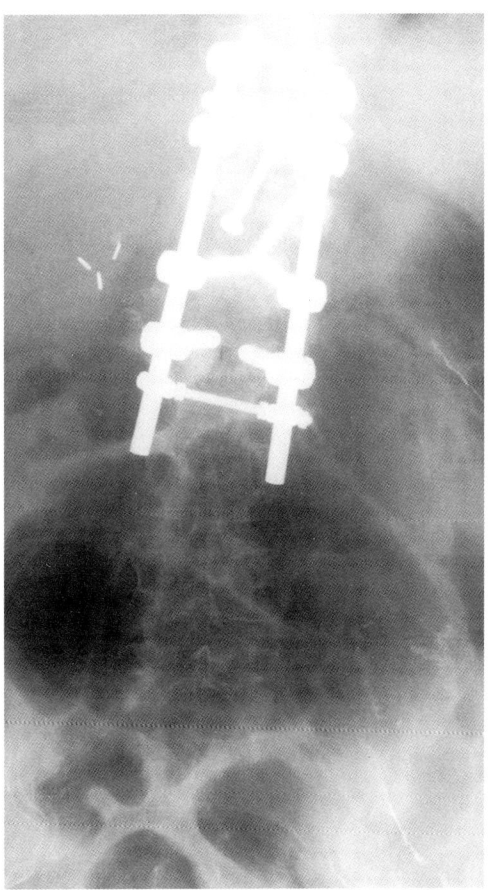

F

Figure 13. (*Continued.*) **E,F:** Because her health precluded an anterior procedure, an eggshell procedure was performed together with posterior stabilization.

Laminoplasty

A circumferential decompression of the thoracic cord may be achieved through a single posterior approach. The posterior elements medial to the facet joints and medial two-thirds of the pedicle are removed (Fig. 14). The lateral third of the pedicle is preserved for reconstruction. The vertebral body is deepened with the use of an air drill, to gain access to the anterior central one-third of the vertebral body immediately beneath or attached to the dura. The base of the remaining bony masses is removed, leaving untouched the part of bone in contact with the anterior dura. The remaining portion of bone may then be gently freed or resected. If the dural tube is ossified, it is opened and expanded with a fascial patch. Reconstruction of the posterior elements may be accomplished using a thin cortical cancellous graft taken from the other aspect of the iliac crest and bent into a semicircle (Fig. 14). Posterior instrumentation may be used to supplement stabilization above or below the level of decompression.

Lobster Shell Technique

The lobster shell is an alternative technique to standard laminectomy that some believe is faster and less traumatic to the neural elements. It is advocated for two- to four-level decompressions. In the first step, the posterior arch is resected with the use of an oscillating saw or a high-speed microbur (Fig. 15). The cut is usually made about 3 mm from the inferior articular process and about 5 mm from the

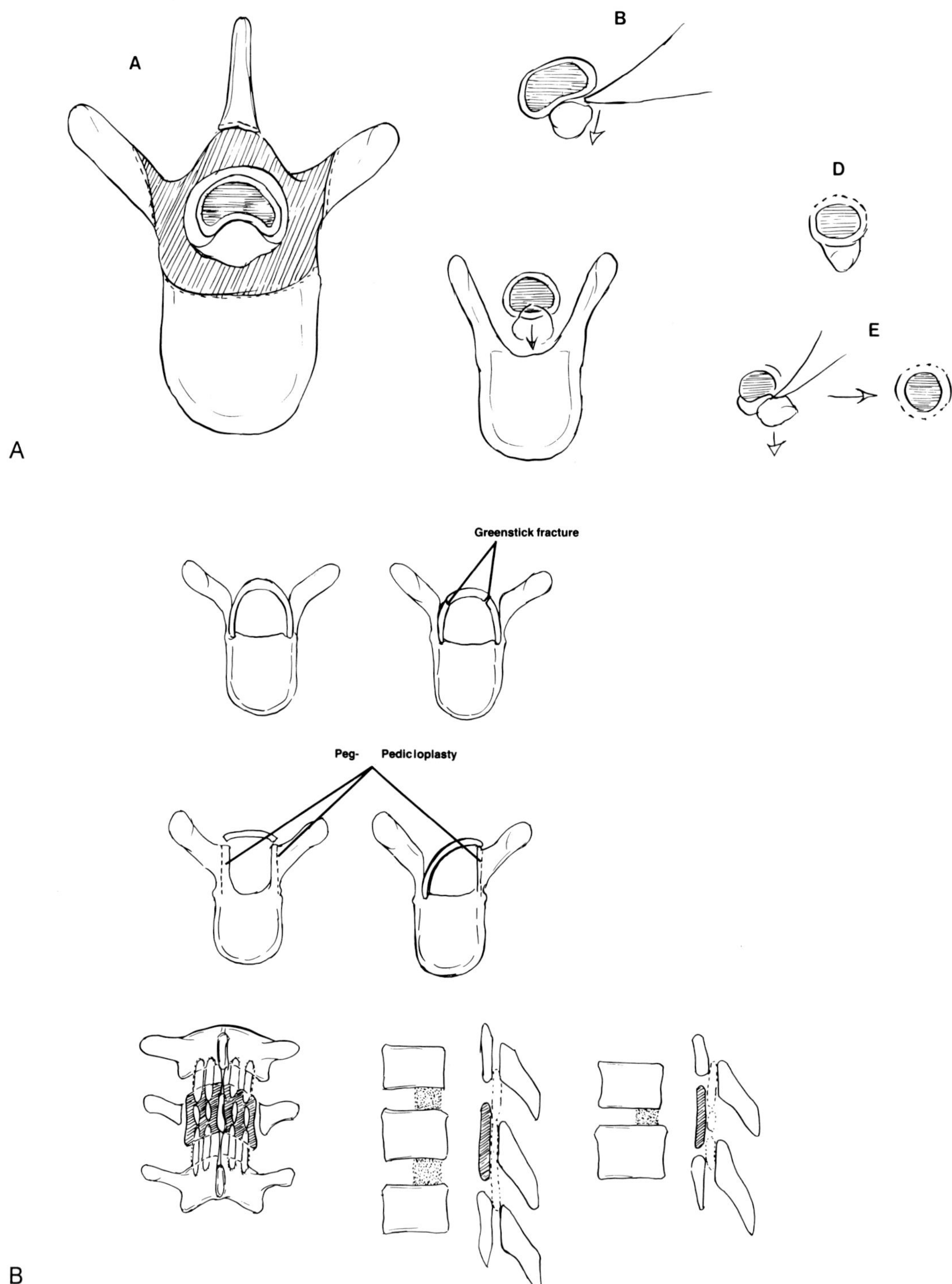

Figure 14. A,B: Tsuzuki technique of thoracic anterior-posterior laminoplasty.

facet joint. Following exposure of the ligamentum flavum, this is cut with a sharp scalpel. The posterior arch is removed en bloc by grasping the spinal process distally and pulling the laminae cranially. A small elevator can be used to divide adhesions between the dura and posterior arch and the ligamentum flavum laterally. We prefer to replace this en bloc resection with intralaminar screw fixation.

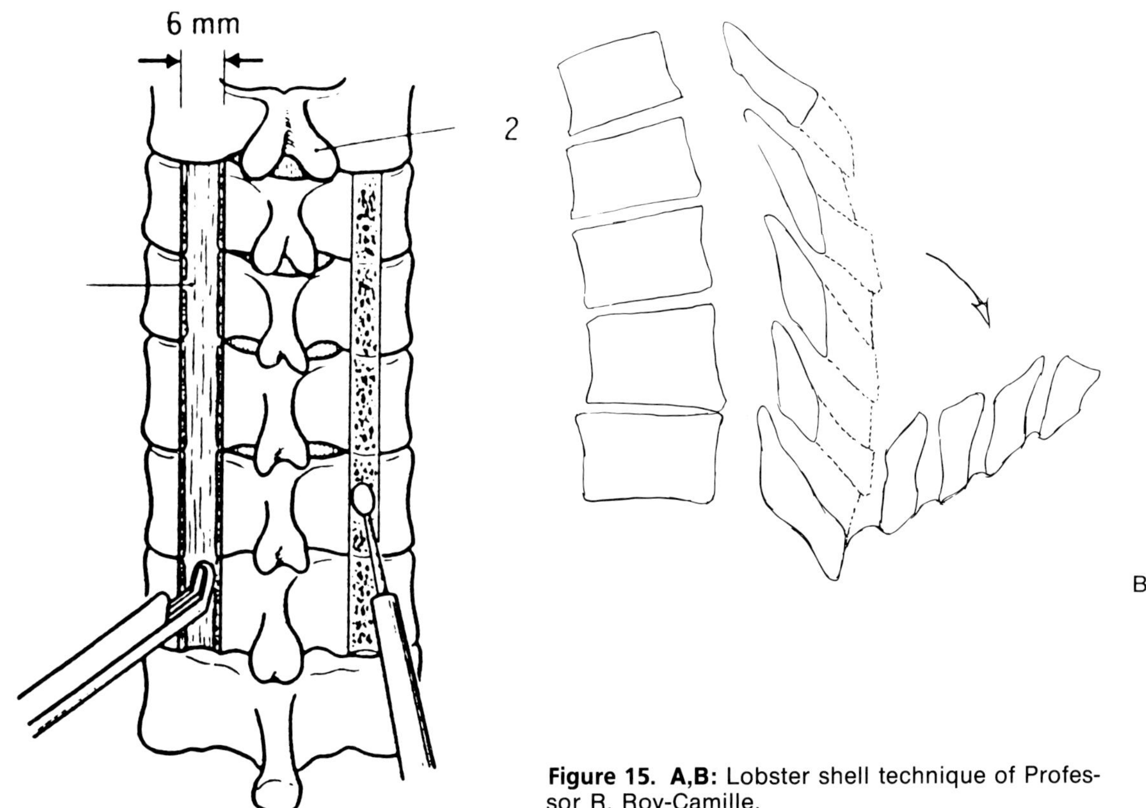

Figure 15. A,B: Lobster shell technique of Professor R. Roy-Camille.

Pars Interarticularis Osteotomy

An osteotomy through the pars interarticularis into the neural foramina may be performed to provide a form of laminoplasty. The ligamentum flavum is divided proximally and distally. The facet capsules are divided and the neural arch can be removed en bloc and preserved. This can be done bilaterally or unilaterally. If it is done unilaterally, then the spinous process must be split as well. Following decompression of either the roots of the neural foramina or the canal, the en bloc resection can be fixed with the aid of translaminar screws. Fusion can be added. To preserve height, bone graft may be added in the facet joints.

Monoblock Transverse Arthropediculotomy

Monoblock tranverse arthropediculotomy may be unilateral or bilateral. The ligamentum flavum is excised inferior and superior to the desired level to be excised. The dural sac and nerve root as they exit towards the foramen are protected. Three osteotomies are done using fine osteotomes or a fine oscillating saw. The first cut is through the pars interarticularis superior to the superior articular facet to be excised. The osteotomy enters the intervertebral foramina. Similar osteotomies are created through the distal pars interarticularis and directed slightly upward. Similar osteotomies are created through the distal pars interarticularis and directed slightly upward. This provides a wedge effect for subsequent replacement of the bone fragment. The third osteotomy is performed in the frontal plane at the base of the pedicle. If unilateral resection is to be done, an additional osteotomy in the sagittal plane is done through the spinous process. Following further decompression, the arch is then replaced. The oblique cuts through the pars interar-

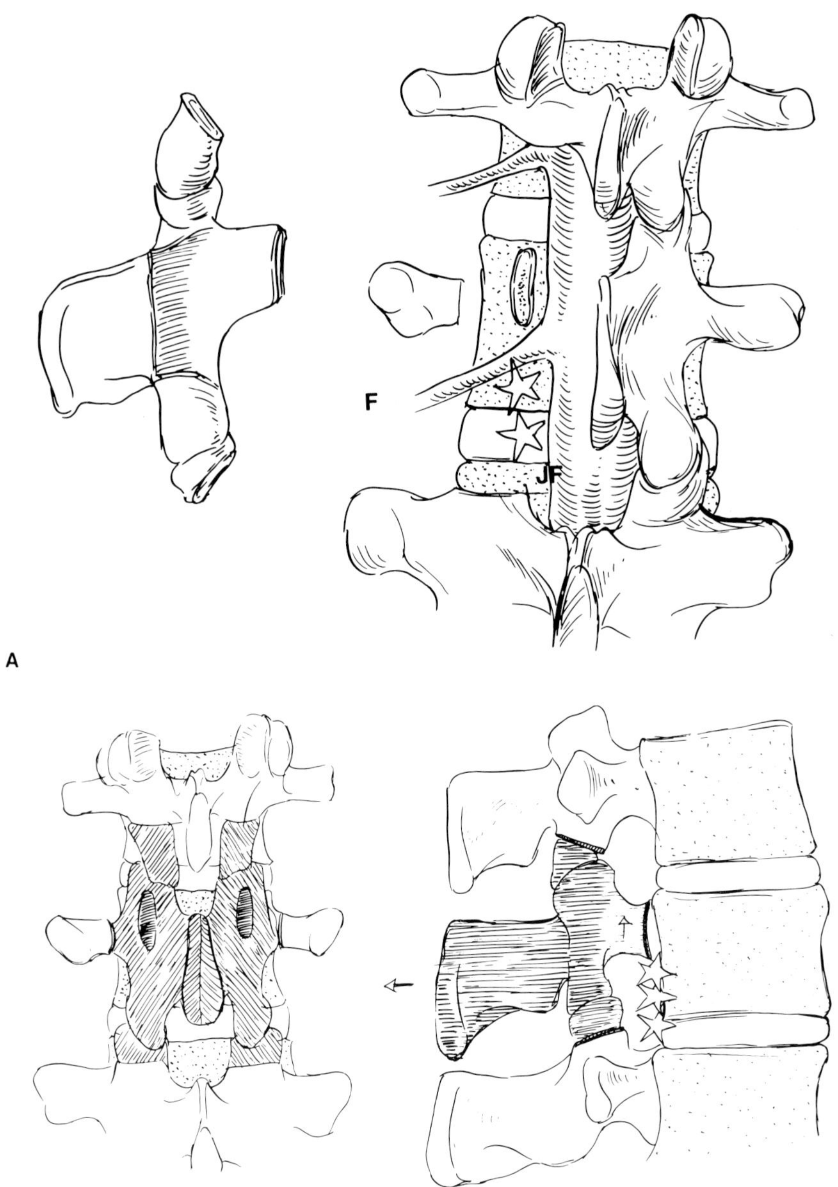

Figure 16. Unilateral **(A)** and bilateral **(B)** mono-block transverse arthropediculotomy.

ticularis allow some degree of stability, and internal fixation may be used for direct fixation through the pars (Fig. 16).

POSTOPERATIVE MANAGEMENT

Management of the patient following spinal cord decompression of either the thoracic, thoracolumbar, or lumbar spine depends on the pathology, the level of surgery, and the general condition of the patient.

For transpleural approaches an evacuation of the pleural cavity through chest suction of 20 cm of water is necessary. Most tubes are removed approximately 48 hours postoperatively but may be left in significantly longer, depending upon drainage. Once drainage has decreased to less than 50 ml a day, they may be safely removed.

Pain Management

Thoracotomy incisions are best managed with injection of Marcaine on the intercostal nerves at the site of incision. This decreases pain resulting from respiratory movements and morbidity related to atelectasis and other respiratory problems. Epidural morphine is also of value in controlling pain.

The mainstay of postoperative pain management is patient-controlled analgesia. This is maintained until bowel sounds return, at which time early administration of mild narcotics such as acetaminophen with codeine 30 mg is administered.

Infection Control

Antibiotics are administered prophylactically at the beginning of the operation and maintained for a minimum of 24 hours. Patients who are at high risk or debilitated may receive antibiotics for a longer period.

Antiembolism Measures

Pulsatile stockings are placed intraoperatively and maintained while in the hospital. All patients are anticoagulated for approximately 10 days. Patients who have a previous history of thrombophlebitis and/or thromboembolism are anticoagulated for approximately 3 months.

Nutrition

Fluid administration in the immediate postoperative period is usually in the form of a 2/3/1/3 solution. In patients undergoing multiple-stage surgery, parenteral peripheral nutrition is administered. Total parenteral nutrition may be administered to debilitated patients.

Respiratory Toilet

Patients with spinal cord decompression may undergo a prolonged procedure and may require considerable fluid replacement, resulting in a fluid overload. Thus the risk of pulmonary edema and/or respiratory distress syndrome exists. Vigorous chest physiotherapy is mandated, including sitting the patient up early, use of a respirometer, breathing exercises, chest manipulation, good fluid control, and adequate moisture. It may be necessary to dry the patient out by administering a diuretic. Respiratory assistance through continued intubation may be necessary, depending on the patient's age, level of surgery, and degree of pulmonary retraction required during surgery for thoracic procedures.

Positioning in Bed

During the first 12 hours following posterior approaches, patients are allowed to lie on their wound to compress it, which decreases the likelihood of hematoma development. Patients are then rolled off their backs and positioned with pillows to prevent accumulation of perspiration and other fluids that may macerate the wound. The dressing is changed at 48 hours and daily thereafter. Sutures are usually maintained for a minimum of 10 days following surgery, and the wound is kept dry during this time.

Ambulation

Patients are usually kept at bed rest for the first 48 hours following spinal cord decompression. If there is neurological deficit, the patient is log-rolled every 2 hours to prevent skin breakdown. All cases are managed on a normal hospital bed. At approximately 48 hours, patients who have sufficient neurological power begin walking. Those with a residual neurological deficit that precludes ease of standing sit in a chair for continued respiratory toilet. Patients with neurological deficit begin muscular rehabilitation 48 hours after surgery through a combination of passive and active exercises designed in conjunction with physiotherapy. Springs and weights are usually used for resistive exercises. Orthoses may be used to prevent the development of contractures in patients with neurological deficits (e.g., drop foot).

Radiological Control

Radiographs should be taken immediately postoperatively to assess the position of internal fixation implants. They should be taken again approximately 48 hours following surgery and on the day of discharge.

COMPLICATIONS

Skin

If there has been a previous incision, the old skin scar should be excised. A diluted solution of 1:500,000 epinephrine (1:1,000 adrenaline to 500 ml of saline) injected intracuticularly, subcutaneously, and in the muscle planes will decrease soft tissue bleeding for up to 2 hours during surgery. Meticulous coagulation of bleeding points should be carried out as the various layers are dissected. Skin edges should be sutured so that edges are everted. In older people, in prolonged cases, or where there is considerable subcutaneous fat, the skin is sutured with interrupted 2-0 nylon sutures rather than staples, intracuticular sutures, or running sutures because it is felt that this will decrease the risk of postoperative wound healing difficulties. If there is considerable subcutaneous fat, the compartment should be drained as well. The risk of infection is also minimized by pulsatile irrigation periodically during the procedure to wash out the wound. All necrotic tissues should be debrided prior to closure.

Hemorrhage

The degree of blood loss depends on the extent and length of surgery. Most cases requiring spinal cord decompression should have a cell saver available. In addition to the cell saver, the postoperative collection and readministration of blood in the first 6 hours can be of help. If suction of blood greater than 2,000 ml through the cell saver occurs, the patient should receive fresh-frozen plasma as well as platelets to prevent coagulopathy. Most blood loss is secondary to oozing from tissues and may be minimized in bony tissues by the use of bone wax; however, bone wax may interfere with subsequent arthrodesis and should be used judiciously. In anterior decompressions, during corpectomy, large pledgets of Gelfoam that have been gently compressed with patties or gauze can aid in controlling bleeding. Epidural bleeding, which may be extensive in acute burst injuries requiring anterior decompression or in certain tumor types, can be controlled by the use of Gelfoam and/or bipolar coagulation.

The greatest blood loss may be encountered through inadvertent division of large vessels. Blood loss is likely to be greater from large venous vessels and is more difficult to control and repair than blood loss from a large artery. Large blood loss is particularly encountered with lesions in the distal spine, primarily from the iliolumbar veins; similarly, it may be encountered from the azygos veins in a thoracotomy. For this reason, I prefer to use the left-sided approach where possible, since it is felt that the aorta may protect venous structures. A knowledge of anatomy and the judicious tying off of large veins is important in exposure.

Dural Tears

A dural tear occurring during a posterior approach is usually easily repaired with proline on a very small needle, although it may be necessary to remove more bone to gain easy access. Anterior dural tears are much more difficult to repair, and it may not be possible to remove more bone to gain access. These may be controlled by applying Gelfoam and allowing time for the dural tear to close spontaneously. The addition of free soft muscle tissue to the site of the dural tear may also help to control bleeding. Large dural tears may require repair with free dural grafts or fascial grafts sutured or glued in place.

Neurological Injury

Neurological injury is rare following anterior spinal cord decompression regardless of the pathology and is considered to be less than 1% in good hands. Patients with pre-existing neurological problems are probably best given a dose of Decadron preoperatively and maintained over a period of 4 to 5 days, decreasing the doses postoperatively.

The use of somatosensory or motor evoked potentials have greatly aided the surgeon in assessing neurological difficulties. However, there may be a latency period of up to 20 minutes following injury before they can be recorded, particularly somatosensory potentials. These potentials may be obtained through cortical evoked or spinal evoked means.

In the lower lumbar spine, the risk of neurological injury during the application of pedicle fixation may be minimized through the use of direct pedicle hole stimulation and electromyographic (EMG) peripheral recordings. Following development of the pedicle hole and prior to insertion of the pedicle screw, the hole may be stimulated for an EMG response. Following insertion of the screw, restimulation is important. If there is any positive response at a low threshold, a new hole should be developed.

Wound Infection

Wound infection following either anterior or posterior decompressive surgery is extremely rare, generally less than 1%. The incidence increases with the use of arthrodesis and particularly with the use of internal fixation.

If wound infection fails to respond to local dressings and the use of systemic antibiotics after 4 to 5 days, then the wound should be opened and debrided, and a decision should be made to leave the wound open or to close it primarily over suction drainage. Suction drainage may be used to instill regional antibiotics and provide a constant irrigation system as well.

If internal implants have been used for fixation and they are not loose, they should be left in place. If they are loose, they should be removed and an alternate form of fixation used, either external fixation (braces, casts, complete bed rest)

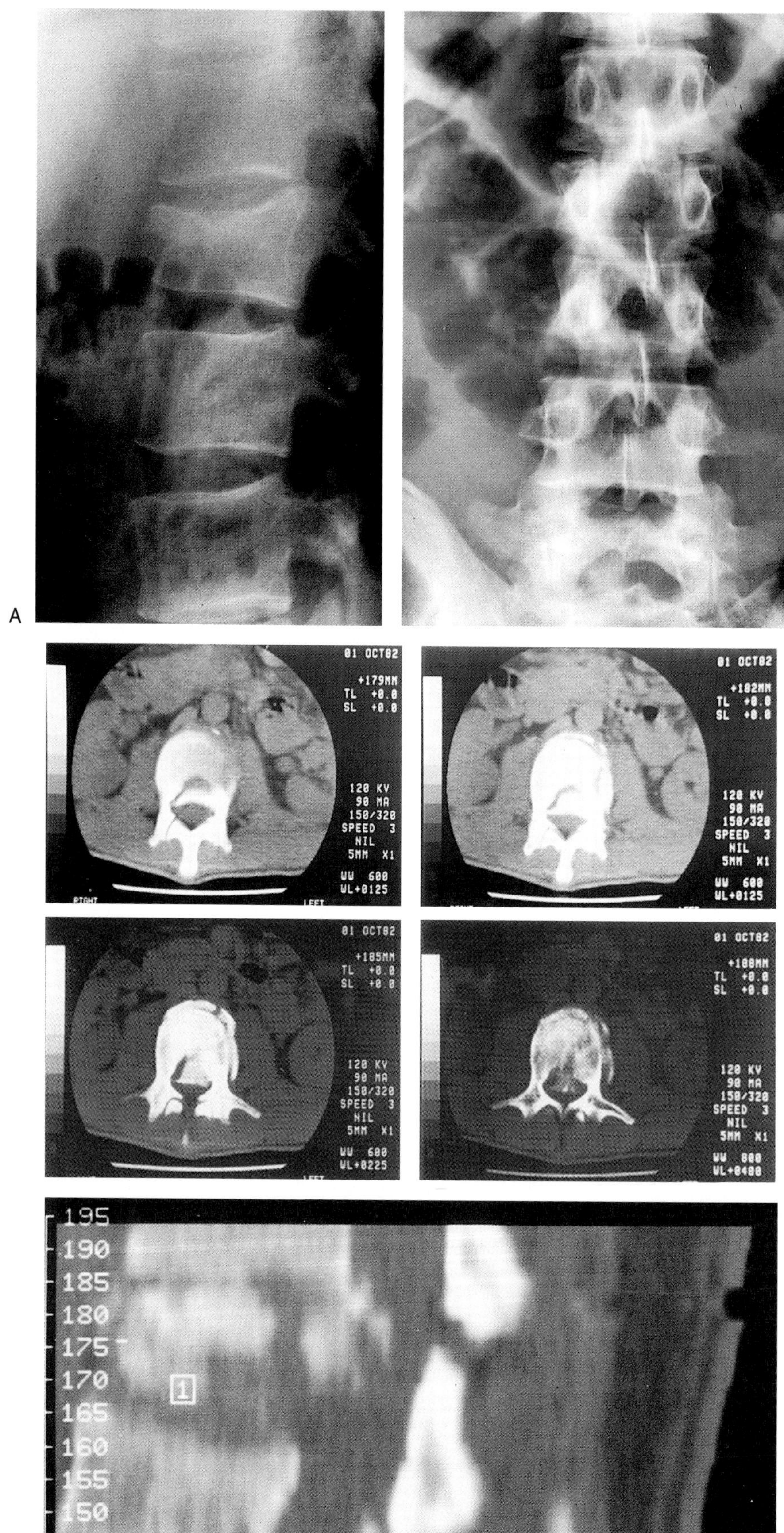

Figure 17. **A:** Lateral views of a burst fracture neurological assessment Frankel grade B. **B:** Preoperative anterior posterior view. Note widening of pedicles of L2. **C:** 1 and 2, CT scans with sagittal reconstruction demonstrates significant canal occlusion. **D:** Postoperative lateral demonstrates fusion at 2 years with good correction of deformity after anterior decompression, grafting, and stabilization. **E:** Postoperative anteroposterior radiograph of another patient demonstrating cross-linkage producing a quadrilateral frame and enhancing rotational control.

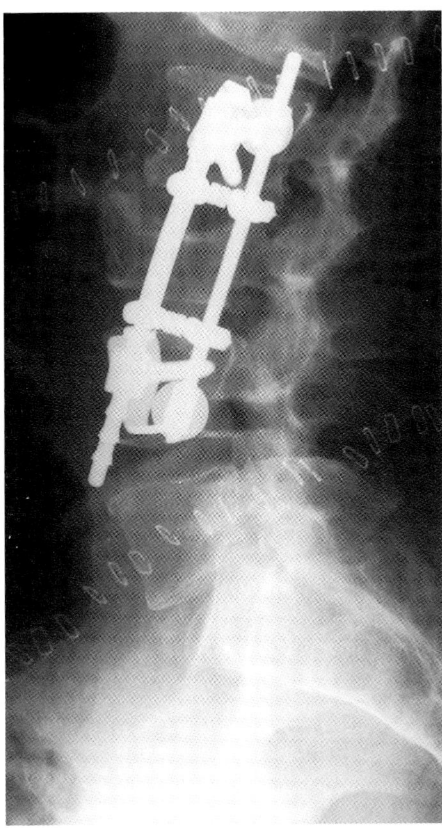

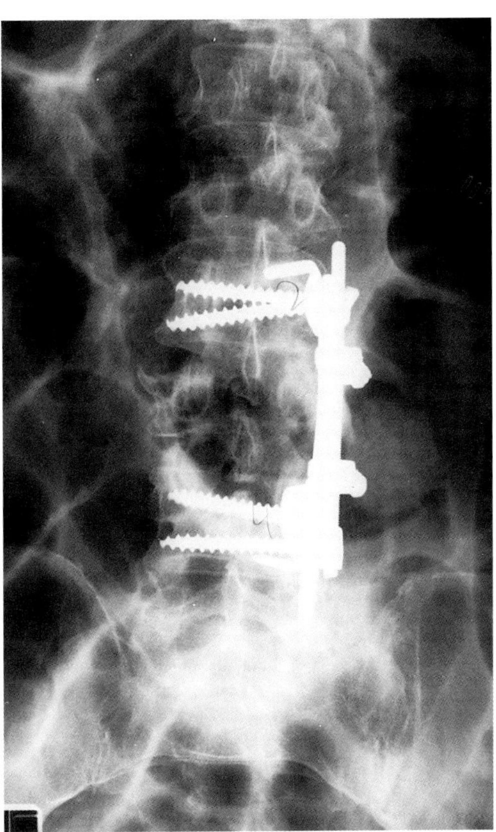

Figure 17. *Continued.*

or fixation from the opposite side of the spine (anterior or posterior depending on the site of infection).

If local opening and packing of the wound or irrigation does not work, the use of implantable antibiotic polymethylmethacrylate beads, depending on the cultures, should be considered. If the implants are loose, they should be removed regardless of the form of antibiotic treatment. If the wound is left open, delayed closure may be obtained. If the tissues are too rigid, a rotation flap may be necessary to close the wound.

ILLUSTRATIVE CASE FOR TECHNIQUE

A 20-year-old male fell 12 m, sustaining a burst injury of L2 (Fig. 17). His neurological status was Frankel grade B. Decompression, correction of deformity, grafting, and stabilization were carried out within 24 hours. At 2 years' follow-up, he was functional Frankel grade D. Postoperative immobilization is usually with a plastic molded orthosis. In less accommodating patients a body cast is utilized. Ambulation was dependent on the degree of neurological damage. Early transfers and walking were permitted.

RECOMMENDED READING

1. Benson, D.: Infectious disease of the spine. In: *The Adult Spine*, Vol. 1, 1st ed., edited by J. Frymoyer, p. 787. Raven Press, New York, 1991.
2. Dick, W.: The fixateur interne as a versatile implant for spine surgery. *Spine*, 12: 882–900, 1987.

3. Hirahayashi, K., Watanabe, K., and Wafano, K.: Expansive open door laminoplasty for cervical spinal sternotic myelopathy. *Spine*, 8: 693–699, 1983.
4. Kostuik, J. P.: Anterior fixation for burst fracturs of the thoracic and lumbar spine with or without neurological involvement. *Spine*, 13: 286–293, 1988.
5. Kostuik, J. P.: Compression fractures and surgery in the osteoporotic patient. In: *The Adult Spine*, Vol. 1: edited by J. Frymoyer, p. 661. Raven Press, New York, 1991.
6. Kostuik, J. P.: Laminoplasty of the thoracic and lumbar spine. In: *The Adult Spine*, Vol. 1 edited by J. Frymoyer, p. 1833. Raven Press, New York, 1991.
7. Kostuik, J. P., and Matsuzaki, H.: Anterior stabilization, instrumentation and decompression for post-traumatic kyphosis. *Spine*, 14: 379–386, 1989.
8. Kostuik, J. P., and Weinstein, J. N.: Differential diagnosis and surgical treatment of metastatic spine tumours, In: *The Adult Spine*, Vol. 1, edited by J. Frymoyer, p. 861. Raven Press, New York, 1991.
9. Kostuik, J. P., and Skubic, J. W.: Thoracic pain syndromes and thoracic disc herniation. In: *The Adult Spine*, Vol. 2, edited by J. Frymoyer, p. 1443. Raven Press, New York, 1991.
10. Kostuik, J. P., Errico, T. J., Gleason, T. F., and Errico, C. C.: Spine stabilization of vertebral column tumours. *Spine*, 13: 250–256, 1988.
11. Lozes, G., Fawaz, A., Herlan, M., and Jomin, M. Des segments anterieurs et lateraux des rachis dorso-lombaire par transverso-orthro-pediculotomie. *Conser. Neurochir.*, 33: 497–499, 1987.
12. Malcolm, B. W., Bradford, D. S., Winter, R. B., and Chou, S. M. Post traumatic kyphosis. *J. Bone Jont Surg, [Am.]*, 63A: 891, 1981.
13. Roy-Camille, R., and Benazet, J. P.: Extradural tumours of the spine. In: *Atlas of Orthopedic Surgery*, Vol. 1, edited by C. Lourin, R. Roy-Camille, and L. Riley Jr., p. 273. Masson, Paris, 1989.
14. Tsuzuki, N., Tanoka, H., and Seichi, A.: Laminopediculoplasty, a new method of reconstructing the posterior elements of the thoracic spine. *Inter. Orthop. (SICOT)*, 13: 39–45, 1989.
15. Weinstein, J. N.: Surgical approach to spine tumours. *Orthopedics*, 12: 897–905, 1989.
16. Weinstein, J. N.: Differential diagnosis and surgical treatment of primary benign and malignant neoplasms. In: *The Adult Spine*, Vol. 1, edited by J. Frymoyer, p. 829. Raven Press, New York, 1991.

Master Techniques in Orthopaedic Surgery,
THE SPINE, edited by D. S. Bradford,
Lippincott-Raven Publishers, Philadelphia, © 1997.

19

Cotrel-Dubousset Instrumentation

Harry L. Shufflebarger

INDICATIONS/CONTRAINDICATIONS

Cotrel-Dubousset (CD) posterior spinal instrumentation was introduced in France in 1982, the result of a joint effort between Yves Cotrel and Jean Dubousset. Cotrel developed the hardware and Dubousset the software, or theory. Subsequently, collaboration of the two resulted in the basic implants and instruments of CD, as initially reported (2). Use of this system spread subsequently throughout Europe, then to North America, and then throughout the world. The theory associated with the development of the instrumentation, which represents as important a contribution as do the implants, was developed by Dubousset and reported by Graf et al. (4). Initially developed for scoliosis, the use of CD has extended to any pathology requiring posterior instrumentation.

CD is indicated whenever posterior spinal instrumentation is indicated. This includes deformity of any etiology, degenerative conditions, spinal trauma, and situations requiring spinal reconstruction. The variety of both implants and constructs possible with CD affords a versatility not previously available, and, to a degree, yet not available with similar systems (1,2,3,7).

The only absolute contraindication to placement of CD is active infection in the area to receive the implants. An exception is acute hematogenous disc space infection. In this event, posterior CD may be placed in conjunction with anterior debridement. Relative contraindications are the same as for placement of any posterior spinal instrumentation and include inadequate bony stock to support the instrumentation, very small size of patient, and past history of spinal infection.

H. L. Shufflebarger, M.D.: 1150 Campo Sano Avenue, Coral Gables, Florida 33146.

PREOPERATIVE PLANNING

Planning for CD instrumentation placement is as important as the actual surgical procedure and requires careful examination of the patient. Most comments here are directed toward the patient with spinal deformity but are appropriate for patients with other spinal pathologies. For the deformity patient, pay careful attention to the shape of the torso. Look for an elevated left shoulder, which indicates a structural left high thoracic curve. Look at the relative prominence of the thoracic and lumbar rotary prominence. A significant lumbar prominence usually indicates a significant lumbar structural curve, which should be included in the fusion level. Be cognizant of the sagittal plane alignment. Note the flexibility of both the coronal and sagittal plane deformities. It is particularly valuable to examine the patient in the *prone* position. An excellent approximation of the correction obtainable with surgery can be gained from the prone examination.

Complete radiographic evaluation is necessary for planning of the procedure. Erect 36-inch anteroposterior (AP) and lateral and supine right and left AP bending radiographs are required (Fig. 1). With a significant kyphotic deformity (either thoracic, thoracolumbar, or lumbar), sagittal bending films are necessary. Three-dimensional analysis of radiographs, in conjunction with information gained from examination of the individual patient, permits formulation of a plan for placement of the various CD implants, to be discussed.

The strategic decisions are several and include the following: (a) proximal and distal fusion levels, (b) hook sites and patterns (6), and (c) effect of forces on sagittal contours. Confusion regarding the levels of instrumentation and the direction of forces has resulted in a complication peculiar to this type of posterior system, namely, imbalance. Lonstein (5) reported several causes of this complication: inadequate evaluation of structural curves; improper hook placement patterns; and failure to consider the crankshaft phenomenon. Only via a complete

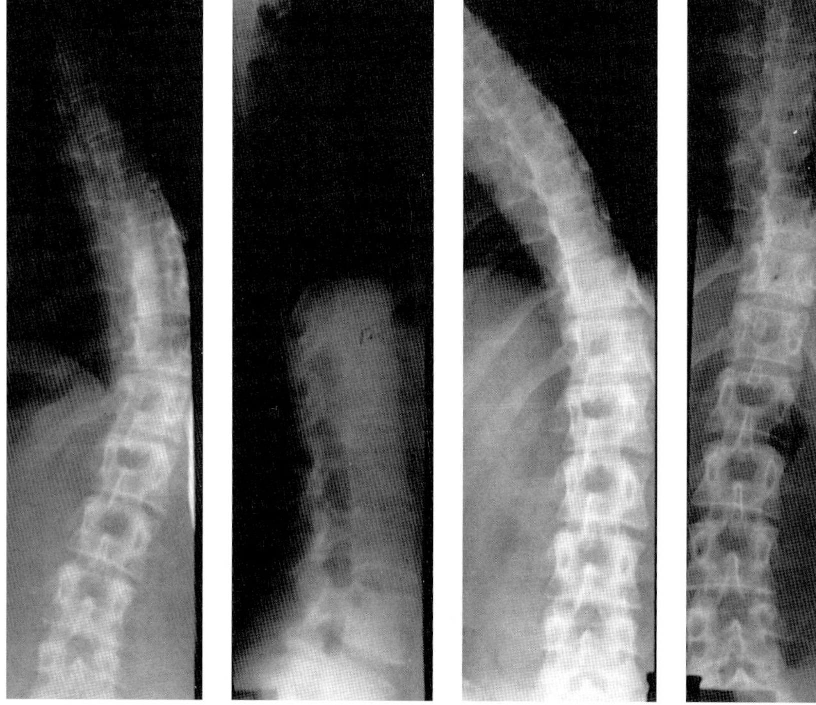

Figure 1. The four required radiographs for strategic planning in the use of CD are the erect AP and lateral films and the right and left supine bending films.

understanding and evaluation of the three-dimensional nature of the spinal pathology can an adequate instrumentation plan be developed. The strategy is no different for any spinal pathology. Reconstruction of the sagittal plane is the primary consideration and goal of spinal instrumentation with CD.

Fusion levels depend upon several parameters: (a) all sagittal abnormal levels must be included in the fusion at the proximal and distal end (avoiding the complication of junctional kyphosis); (b) the disc space distal to the distal end vertebrae must have mobility in right and left bending, in flexion and extension, and in rotation or axial movement; (c) the proximal and distal end vertebrae must fall within the stable zone of Harrington or the center sacral line on the appropriate bending film (this usually requires construction of this line on the two bending in conjunction with the erect AP film); and (d) the inferior end vertebra end plate should be parallel with the horizontal floor reference on the appropriate bending film. Satisfaction of the above criteria will permit a balanced result in the three dimensions regardless of the presenting pathology, including scoliosis problems.

SURGERY

Organization of the Surgical Suite

The preferred surgical table is the Tower table, which unfortunately is no longer commercially available. It allows a modified knee-chest position in which the pelvis is free to move in all directions. Also the lumbar spine can be placed in adequate lordosis by variation of position of the knee rest (Fig. 2). If the Tower table is not available, a regular surgical table with chest rolls placed in the transverse rather than the longitudinal position is preferred. Addition of the Mayfield horseshoe headrest permits access to the upper thoracic spine and lower cervical spine if required.

The Mayfield overbed instrument table is employed, allowing the instrument nurse to distribute all necessary instruments on a single table. Two electro-cauteries are useful, allowing the first assistant to be of maximum value. Paper drapes consist of two U-sheets, placed from the bottom and the top. Bilateral wing sheets complete the isolation of ancillary equipment. The Mayfield overbed table drape joins this with the patient field. Cell saver and somatosensory evoked potential (SSEP) measuring equipment are routinely present (Fig. 3).

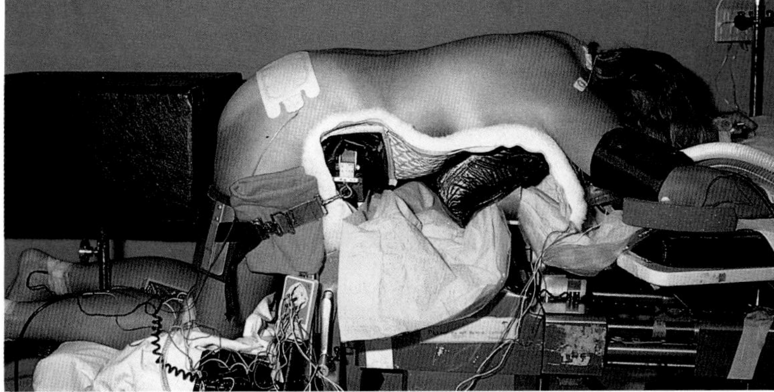

Figure 2. The patient is in a modified knee-chest position on the Tower table.

Positioning and Anesthesia

The position of the patient is of course prone. Trunk support is achieved by the components of the Tower table or the chest rolls. The head is supported either on the support incorporated in the Tower table or on the Mayfield ring headrest if a regular surgical table is employed. Potential pressure areas should be protected and include the knees, ankles, and elbows. Care must also be taken to protect the eyes.

Anesthesia is general endotracheal, with nitrous oxide and narcotic as the primary agents. Intentional hypotension is not employed, but systolic pressure is maintained at approximately 80 to 90 systolic. Foley catheter is routine. Arterial lines and central venous lines are not routine, except in high-risk patients. All

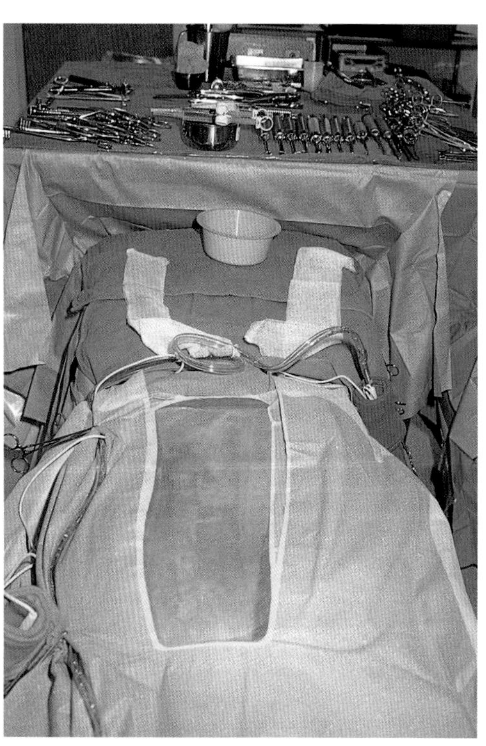

Figure 3. The draped patient and the Mayfield table constitute the main surgical setup.

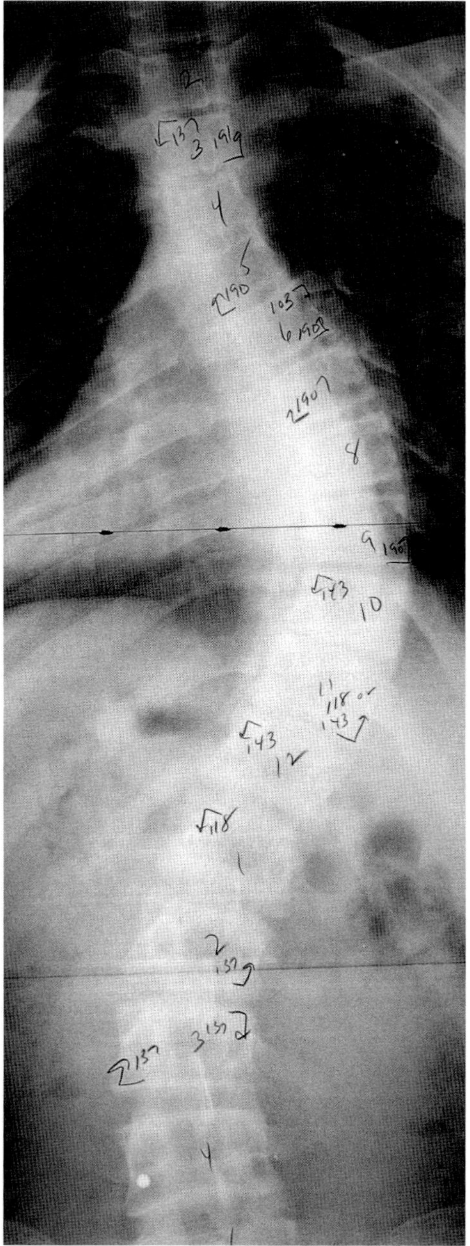

Figure 4. The plan for CD is written on the radiograph, denoting type and direction of implants.

normal patients have predonated autogenous blood, usually 2 units. Designated donor blood is available for those unable to donate. Calculation of allowable blood loss to reach a hematocrit of 30% is done. Transfusion is withheld until the allowable blood loss is exceeded.

Surgical Approach and Exposure

The surgeon and first assistant accomplish simultaneous exposure of the required spinal segments. Exposure is from tips of both transverse processes in the thoracic and lumbar spine. Levels are verified by anatomy. The 11th and 12th ribs are exposed, as well as the appropriate lumbar transverse processes. Intraoperative radiology is not necessary to identify levels, as long as the 11th and 12th ribs along with the first lumbar transverse process are identified. All soft tissue is removed from the spine in preparation for instrumentation and fusion.

Implant Selection and Placement

The large variety of hooks available with the CD system may be extremely confusing at initial glance. For scoliosis problems the number of hooks required is relatively few and the selection relatively simple.

Implants are available in either closed or posterior open versions. The posterior open implant requires a hook blocker to convert it to a relatively closed implant. The blocker must be placed on the rod prior to insertion. Since the blocker and the canal in the hook are conical, the blocker must be placed in the correct direction. It will only enter the open implant from one side. Care should be taken to ensure that the blockers are placed on the rod in the proper directional orientation. An experienced surgical technician will be of great assistance here.

The implant placement plan must be marked on the radiograph before beginning the procedure. I prefer to use arrows denoting the direction of the implant. I also prefer to mark the catalogue number of the implant on the film. This assists the technician in pulling implants from the trays. For example, the closed lumbar lamina hook is #84103. This designation is written on the plan, with an arrow noting the direction (Fig. 4). An implant tray containing all the various hooks by catalogue number will facilitate the technician's hook selection. Of course, this requires some effort on the part of the surgeon.

CD hooks can be additionally divided into pedicle and lamina hooks. The possibilities of placement of each are limited and clearly defined.

Pedicle Hooks. Pedicle hooks can only be used in the thoracic spine and are always directed up, or cephalad. Two designs of pedicle hooks are available. The initial hooks, open and closed (#84100 and #84102), have a relatively long distance between body and blade. These hooks are rarely used currently. The hooks designed later have a decreased distance between body and blade (3 mm less) and are the pedicle hooks used at this time (#84190 and #84191; Fig. 5). This decreased distance results in a significantly reduced posterior prominence.

Pedicle hooks can usually be placed from T1 to T10 or T11, depending on the anatomy of the facet joint. The placement begins with identification of the thoracic facet joint. The capsule is removed. The "white" articular cartilage of the superior articular process of the next vertebra distal must be identified. The facet can then be entered with a small blunt modified Cobb elevator, with a stop to prevent canal penetration (Fig. 6). The pedicle finder instrument can then be used to feel the pedicle. Inability to displace the pedicle finder both proximally and laterally will ensure location of the pedicle.

Usually a small portion of the inferior edge of the lamina of the level to receive the pedicle hook must be removed. The twofold purpose is to gain access to the pedicle and to furnish a square seat for the pedicle hook. Impaction of the hook with a mallet is rarely required. With the tightening maneuvers to be described, adequate seating will be ensured (Fig. 7).

The stability of the pedicle hook relies on several anatomic structures. The hook rests on the superior articular process of the next distal vertebra, on the lamina of the instrumented vertebra, and into the pedicle of the instrumented vertebra. The #84190 and #84191 pedicle hooks provide much better bony contact than the earlier version.

Insertion of the pedicle hook requires use of a hook holder and a hook inserter (Fig. 8). The hook inserter should be left to stabilize the hook while the hook holder is removed. Distal to T10 or T11, the facet anatomy precludes placement of a pedicle hook. Lamina hooks must be placed in these locations.

Lamina Hooks. Lamina hooks are available in a large number of designs. The design variations are in blade width, blade style, and the relation of the blade to

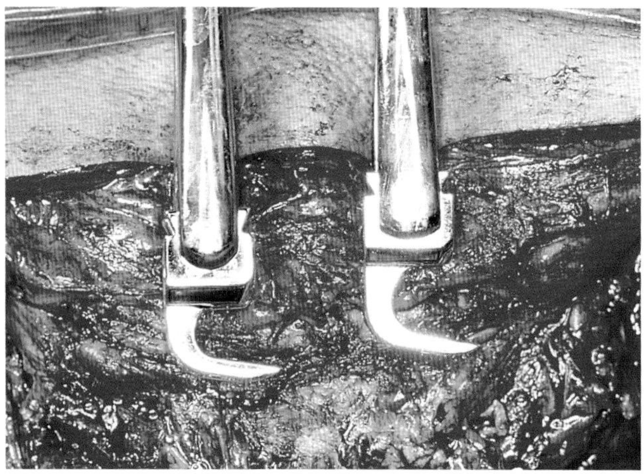

Figure 5. The difference in the body-to-blade distance of the two CD pedicle hooks is demonstrated. The preferred hook (*left*) has the smaller distance.

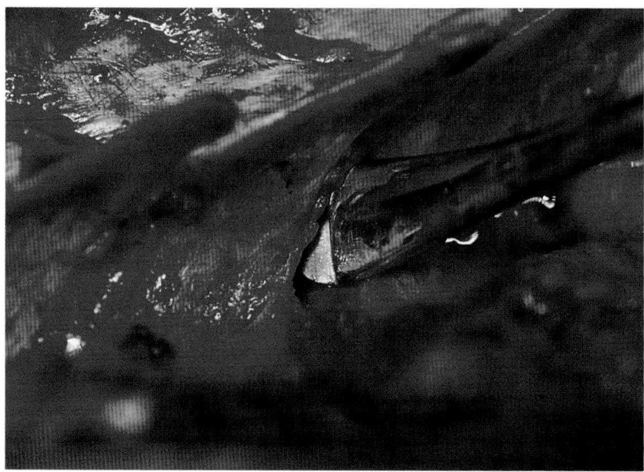

Figure 6. The initial entry into the thoracic facet joint is by a small modified Cobb elevator.

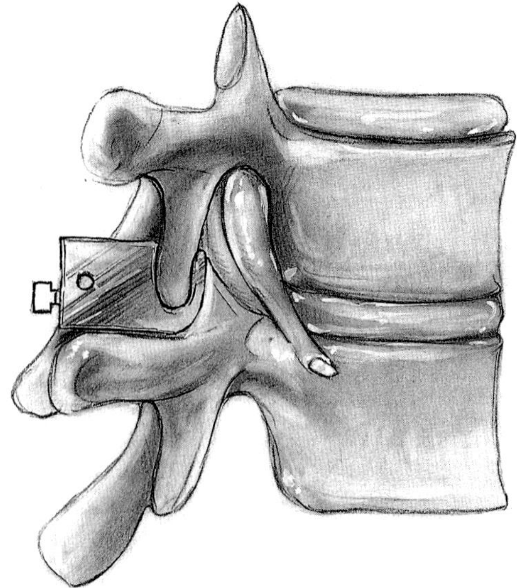

Figure 7. The stability of the pedicle hook is dependent on the lamina of the instrumented vertebra, the superior articular process of the next distal level, and seating into the pedicle. (Courtesy of Dr. Y. Cotrel, Paris, France.)

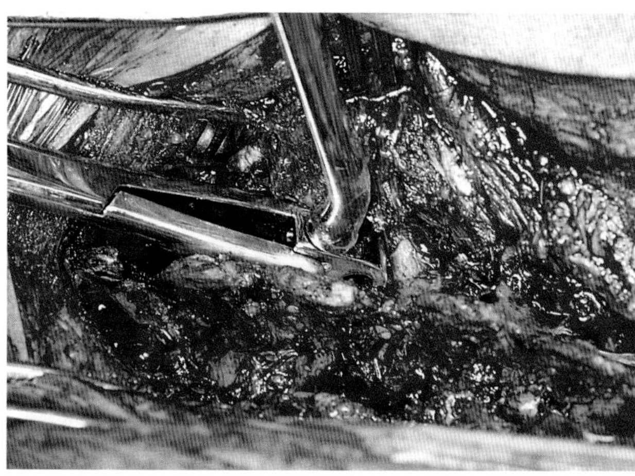

Figure 8. The insertion of the pedicle hook requires control with the hook holder and advancement and seating with the hook inserter.

the body of the hook. Only the most useful designs for CD in scoliosis will be described.

Only three sites of placement exist for lamina hooks. The first is on the superior surface of a transverse process. This will only be in the thoracic spine and will be anatomically possible only between T3 and T10 or T11. The transverse process lamina hook should always be combined with a pedicle hook, producing a pedicle-transverse grip or claw. The claw may be over one or two levels; I prefer the one-level claw (Fig. 9). Above T3, the transverse process becomes more horizontal and will not align with the pedicle hook. If a claw is desired, it should be a pedicle-lamina claw, using a supralamina hook in the canal (preference, #84137 4-mm lumbar lamina hook or #84142 45-degree offset blade; Fig. 10). For placement of the regular transverse process hook, the lamina elevator is used to make the initial path, followed by placement of the regular 7-mm-blade lumbar lamina hook (#84103). The direction of forces provided by the pedicle-transverse claw is either caudal or cephalad, depending on the requirements of the deformity and the sequence of loading.

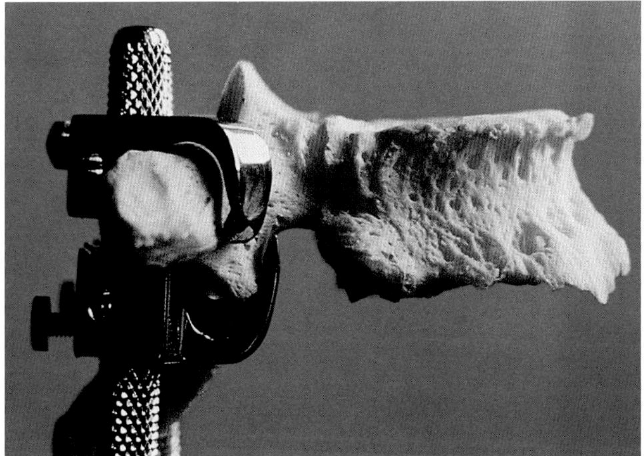

Figure 9. The pedicle-transverse claw or grip is constructed with a lamina hook over the cephalad surface of the transverse process and a pedicle hook at the same level, or one level caudal. (Courtesy of Dr. Y. Cotrel, Paris, France.)

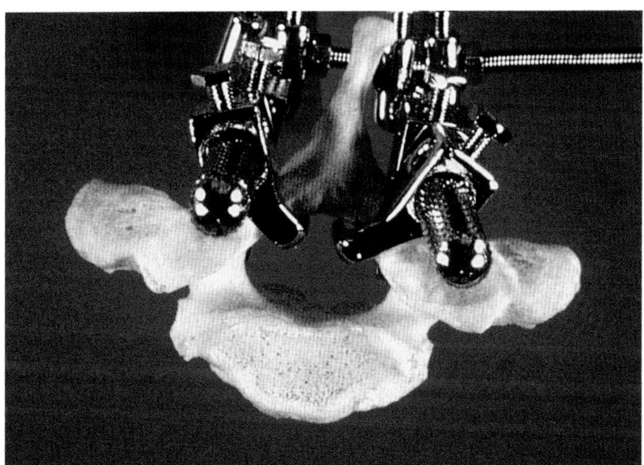

Figure 10. The pedicle-lamina claw is constructed with a supralaminar hook and a pedicle hook. (Courtesy of Dr. Y. Cotrel, Paris, France.)

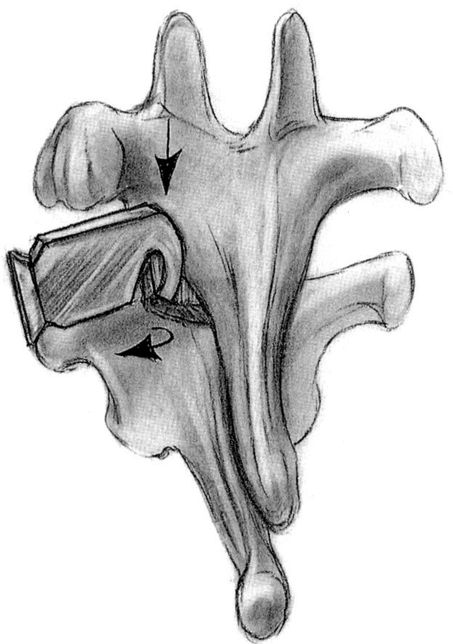

Figure 11. The insertion of the supralamina hook usually requires a twisting and tilting action to ensure placement. (Courtesy of Dr. Y. Cotrel, Paris, France.)

The second placement possibility for lamina hooks is in the supralamina position. This hook will be within the spinal canal. The method of placement involves dividing the ligamentum flavum, removing the flavum, and removing a moderate amount of the inferior edge of the lamina of the vertebra above the level to be instrumented. A Kerrison rongeur accomplishes this. The hook can be easily inserted using only a hook holder (Fig. 11). Usually the lamina of the vertebra cephalad to that to be instrumented will be more posterior than the level at which the hook will seat. Therefore, removal of a portion of this posterior projection will decrease the posterior prominence, allowing easier insertion of the rod into the hook and placement of the blocker (Fig. 12). Direction of the supralaminar hook is caudal.

The choice of hooks for the supralaminar position varies depending on the spinal level and the direction of anterior-posterior forces produced by the rod. In the thoracic spine, the rod is usually bent into kyphosis, producing a posteriorly directed force. This precludes the possibility of pushing the hook into the canal. Lamina hooks #84137 or #84143 (closed or open, lumbar lamina design, 4-mm-diameter blade) are preferred. In the lumbar spine, the lordotic rod bend will produce an anteriorly directed force, with a great possibility of pushing the hook into the canal. Therefore, in T12 through the entire lumbar spine a supralamina hook should be of the thoracic lamina design, #84118 or #84125 (open or closed; Fig. 13), and no danger will exist of pushing the hook into the canal with the lordotic rod.

The third possibility for placement of lamina hooks is in the infralamina position. The direction is cephalad. Rarely is the placement of infralamina hooks necessary in the thoracic spine. Pedicle hooks supply the proximally directed forces. The placement of the infralamina hook is quite simple. The lamina elevator is introduced under the inferior edge of the lamina of the vertebra to be instrumented, dissecting the ligamentum flavum from its origin without actually incising the flavum or entering the spinal canal (Fig. 14). The selection of hook design is also relatively simple. As the infralamina surface is usually significantly more posterior and thicker than the supralaminar surface (particularly in the lumbar spine), a lumbar lamina hook can be placed without danger of intracanal displacement. The reduced or 4-mm-blade hook is preferred (#84137 or #84143, closed or open). Use of CD for the posterior approach to scoliosis requires a small selection of implants, tailoring the spinal anatomy for the implant, and preventing displacement of the implant into the canal.

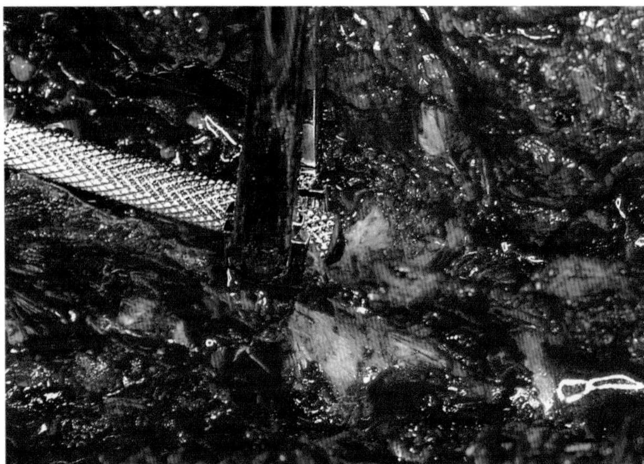

Figure 12. Removal of the posterior portion of the lamina of the next cephalad vertebra is frequently required to allow clearance of the rod into the supralamina hook.

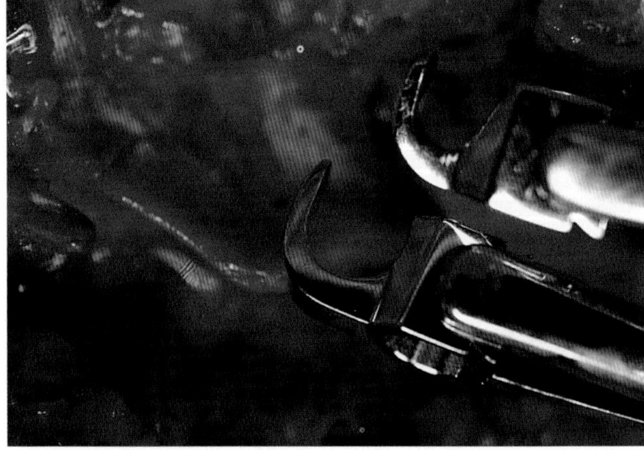

Figure 13. The original two types of lamina hooks, thoracic (*left*) and lumbar (*right*).

Derotation Maneuver (Double Idiopathic Scoliosis)

Figure 15 demonstrates the classic plan for a double thoracic idiopathic scoliosis. This deformity will be used for description of the derotation maneuver technique. Hooks have been placed at the indicated positions.

Rod Bending. A rod of the appropriate length must first be selected. A #10-gauge solid copper electrical wire (stripped of insulation) is used as a template, bent to normal sagittal contours (Fig. 16). The flexible electro-cautery cord can

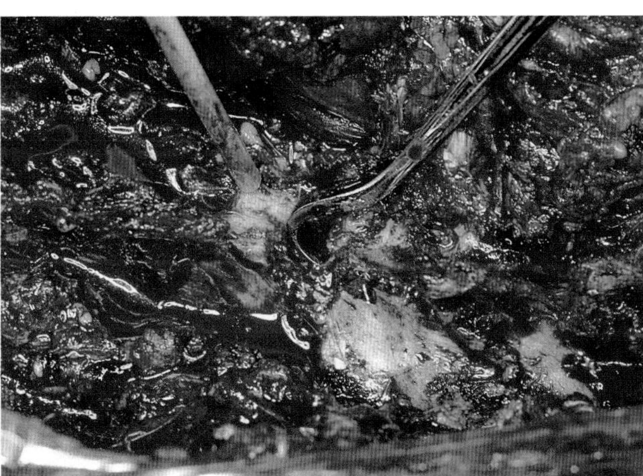

Figure 14. The lamina elevator is used to dissect the ligamentum flavum from its origin to secure placement of the infralamina hook.

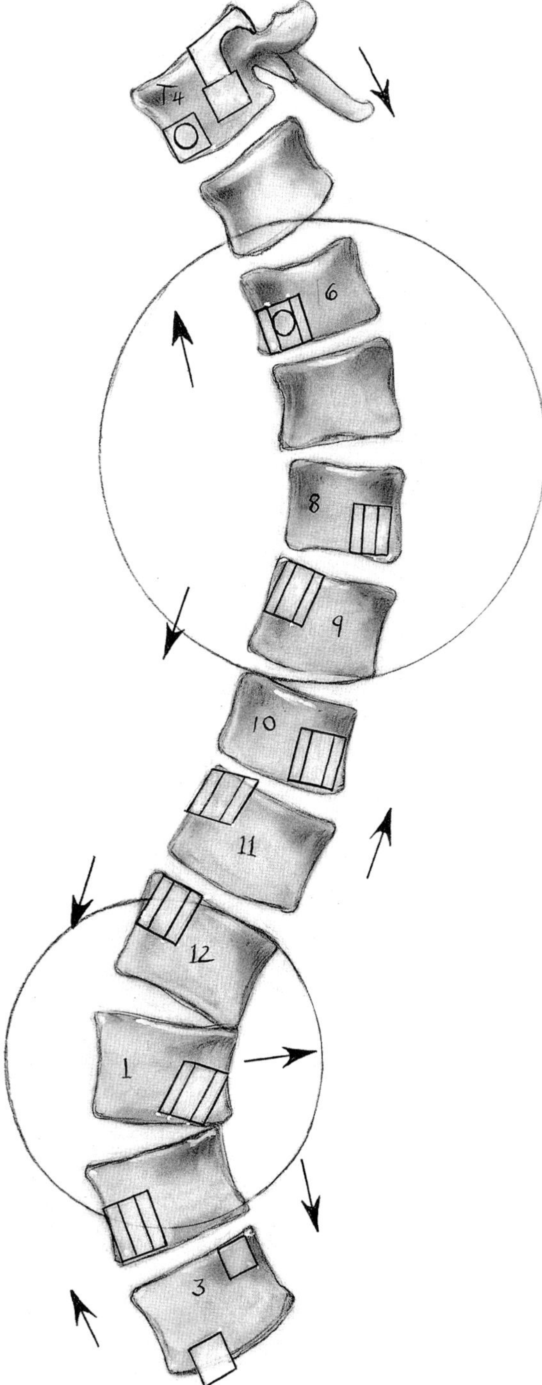

Figure 15. The plan for double structural idiopathic scoliosis (see text).

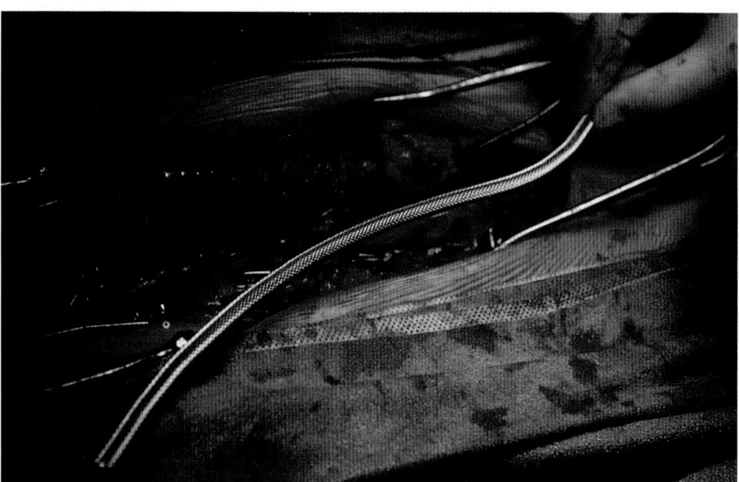

Figure 16. The necessary contours for reconstruction or preservation of the sagittal plane are bent into the CD rod.

then be used to determine the length of rod required. A 5-mm protrusion of the rod through the closed end hooks is necessary. In selecting rod length, remember that length will be lost in the thoracic section (of a lordotic curve with distraction direction forces) and gained in the lumbar segment (with compression direction forces). It is difficult to cut a rod after placement without significantly more dissection.

With the proper length rod selected, place the CD blocker on the rod. Use the French bender to bend the rod. Align the set screw of the blocker on the rod with the groove on the top of the French bender. This will permit the rod to be bent in only one plane. The bend should be smooth and harmonious. Acute bends may induce a stress riser and premature breakage.

A knowledge of normal segmental sagittal anatomy is required to bend the rod properly. In relatively flexible deformities, the bend should approximate normal segmental sagittal anatomy. A thoracic kyphosis of about 30 degrees and a lumbar lordosis of about 45 degrees should be placed in the rod. The apex of the thoracic kyphosis should be at T7 or T8 and the apex of the lumbar lordosis at the L2–L3 interspace. The change from kyphosis to lordosis should be at the T12–L1 interspace.

Arthrodesis. After hook placement and rod bending, the preliminary steps of arthrodesis are accomplished. Thoracic facet joints are destroyed by an electric bur, although any method preferred by the surgeon may be used. Lumbar facet joints are also excised with a rongeur. Autogenous bone graft is then obtained, either iliac or rib (if thoracoplasty is indicated).

The next step is decortication of the thoracic and lumbar transverse processes and lamina on the side to be instrumented first. The spinous processes should be left intact to minimize prominence of the instrumentation. These can be decorticated after placement of both rods. The autogenous graft is placed, packing the facet joints. The second side will be decorticated prior to placement of the second rod.

Rod Placement, First or Left. The following points are important to remember:

1. The more mobile the hooks are, the easier it will be to place the rod in the hooks. Adequate bony resection during hook placement will ensure this.
2. The more mobile the spine is, the easier it will be to insert the rod into the hooks. Adequate facet resection will ensure this.
3. Lack of tension forces on rod and implants will facilitate insertion and rotation. *Don't* distract anything.
4. Ensure that the blockers are in the proper direction on the rod, and in the approximate proper position.

The rod has been bent to approximate normal sagittal contours, as described above. In this instance, the rod bend will approximate the curves. Enter the rod into the T4 closed pedicle hook, with a hook holder on the hook. It is easiest to do this holding the rod in your hand. Advance the rod far enough proximally to clear the distal closed lamina hook at L3. Any of the several rod-holding instruments can be used as preferred. These include the large and small rod holder or the vise grip clamp (supplied with the CD set). I prefer a Schlein clamp (Zimmer Company; Fig. 17) for rod manipulation. For this step, the rod will be in the unrotated position, 90 degrees to the final position.

Next the rod is advanced distally to enter the L3 hook. A hook holder must be placed on the L3 hook to prevent dislodgment. This hook holder should remain in place until the tightening sequence is complete. An assistant should always control the hook holder on the inferior convex hook.

Then, remove the T4 hook holder, as it is no longer required. Place hook holders on the several intermediate hooks, particularly at T6, T9, T11, and T12. The hook holders should straddle the rod. This action will ensure that the rod is aligned with the posterior open body of the hooks. Also be sure that the blockers are in proper position and direction relative to their respective hooks (Fig. 18). At this

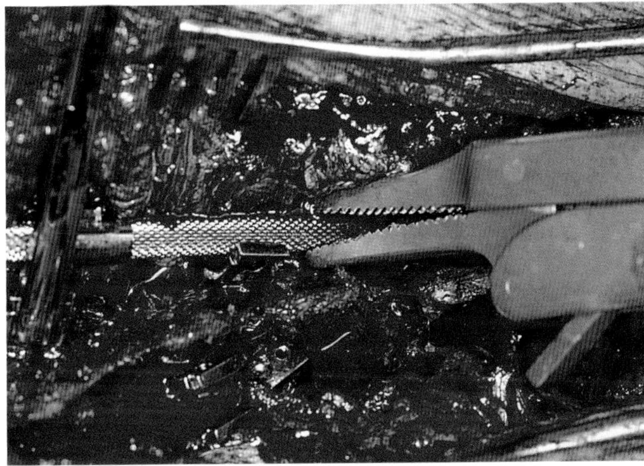

Figure 17. The Schlein clamp is the most useful available vise-grip instrument to provide a fixed point for mechanical action on the rod. Either distraction or compression, as needed, may be applied.

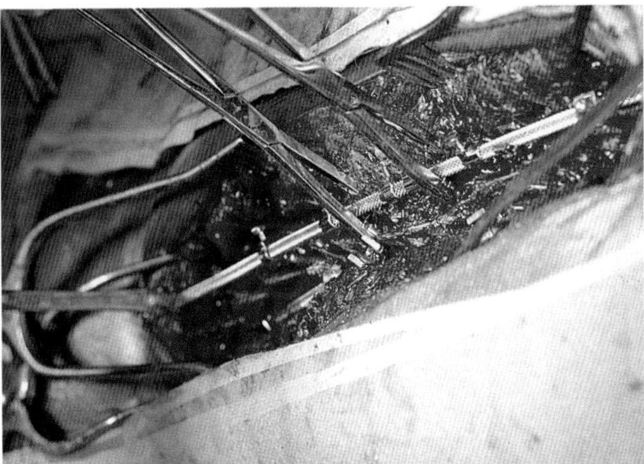

Figure 18. After insertion of the rod into the proximal and distal hooks, hook holders, straddling the rod, ensure alignment of the rod with the posterior open hooks.

point, the T9 and T11 hooks will be farthest from the rod. Entry of the rod into the several open hooks and insertion of the blockers can be accomplished in several ways. The rod should be entered into the T6 hook, and the blocker can be easily inserted. The CD rod introducer (attached to the bulb hook holder) may be applied to the T9 hook. Using the screw device brings the rod to the hook (Fig. 19). The blocker driver #1 can then initiate insertion of the blocker (Fig. 20), maintaining axial rotation control. Blocker driver #2 will complete blocker insertion. Using the rod inserter on this single hook will usually bring all the other hooks to the rod. If not, the same maneuver can be repeated. On occasion, two rod introducers are required, usually on the T6 and T9 hooks. The hex tube will be required for loosening and tightening the set screw in the blocker as it is moved. An alternative is to leave the set screws out of the blocker and move the blocker with a tonsil hemostat in the screw hole. In addition, set screws should not be placed in the closed hooks until rod rotation is complete. Manipulations and vibrations may cause displacement of the set screws either into the hook or outside the hook, resulting in obvious technical problems.

At this point, the rod has been entered into all hooks and blockers have been placed. All hook holders, except the one on L3, can be removed. It is necessary to maintain the hook holder on L3, with an assistant holding it, to prevent displacement during rod rotation.

Rod rotation is the next step. All tension must be released. Don't distract anything. Note that as the rod is rotated, the distance between the T6 and T9 hooks will increase, tending to displace the blockers toward each other and to unload the hooks, permitting potential displacement (Fig. 21). The "rotation protector" (Fig. 22) will maintain constant minimal tension on these hooks, preventing blocker displacement. The earlier C-rings are no longer necessary. Any of the previously mentioned rod-holding instruments can be used for the rotation maneuver. Observe all hooks during the slow rotation procedure. There is some tendency for pedicle hooks to rotate medially due to the friction of the knurled rod on the hooks. Placing a hook holder on the hook during rotation will prevent this. The rod must be fully rotated for optimal results. Less than full rotation is unstable and may result in loss of correction in the postsurgery period. When full rotation is achieved, the rod must be held in this position with one of the rod-holding devices until tightening is begun. The L3 hook must continue to be stabilized and held in position with a hook holder and an assistant.

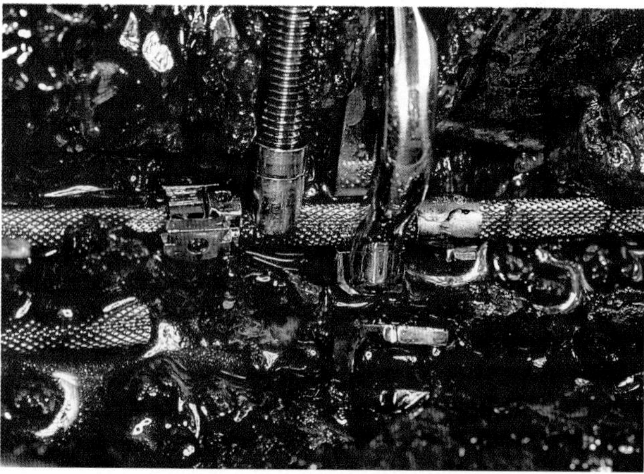

Figure 19. The rod introducer brings the hook (and the spine) into open hooks at some distance from the rod. Firm control of the introducer is necessary.

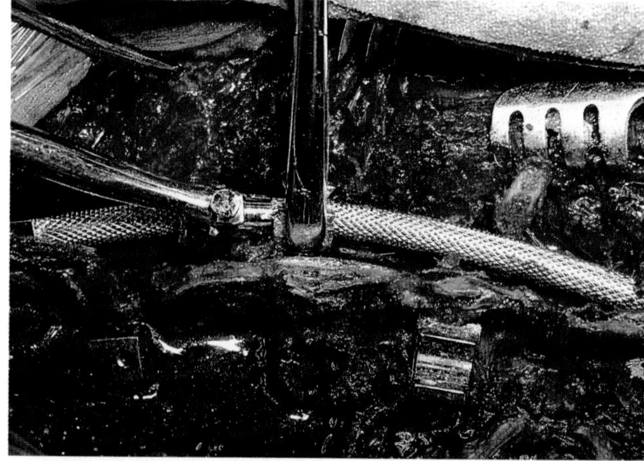

Figure 20. Blocker driver #1 initiates insertion of the hook blocker. Driver #1 maintains axial rotatory control of the blocker, and #2 permits final seating.

Tightening Sequences. Two tightening sequences are possible on this first rod. Either the thoracic segment from T4 to T11 can be tightened first, or the distal lumbar segment first. I prefer the distal lumbar segment, primarily to minimize the length of rod protruding distally. The rod should have been advanced to about a 5-mm protrusion from the L3 hook. Remove the hook holder from the L3 hook and place a set screw. If a significant posterior force exists on the L3 hook, use the rod pusher and an assistant to provide an anterior force (Fig. 23). Tighten the set screw with the hex tube. Provide a fixed point on the rod proximal to the T11 hook (Schlein clamp preferred). Use the CD distractor to distract above the T11 hook, thereby compressing between this hook and the L3 hook. Figure 24 illustrates the method of distraction against a fixed point on the CD rod. This will provide lumbar lordosis and secure the L3 hook placement. Repeat the distraction process proximal to the T12 hook. Repeat it again above the T11 hook. Remember, tightening a hook will loosen any hook in the same direction. Tighten back and forth between T11 and T12 until neither moves.

Next place a fixed point on the rod proximal to the L3 hook. Use the CD compressor to tighten the L3 hook. This step is essential to ensure adequate seating

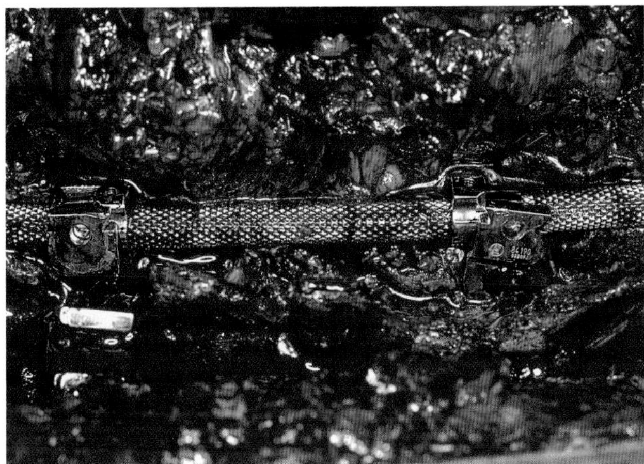

Figure 21. The tendency for the apical concave blockers to displace open hooks with rod rotation due to lengthening of this segment is demonstrated.

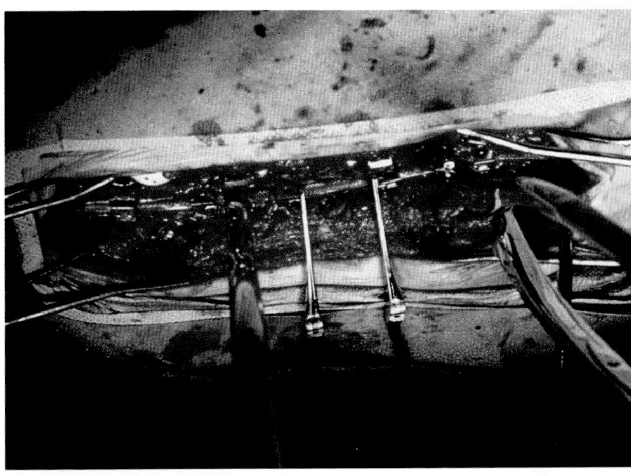

Figure 22. The hook protector, like a self-retaining retractor, prevents displacement of the blockers by application of a constant minimal pressure.

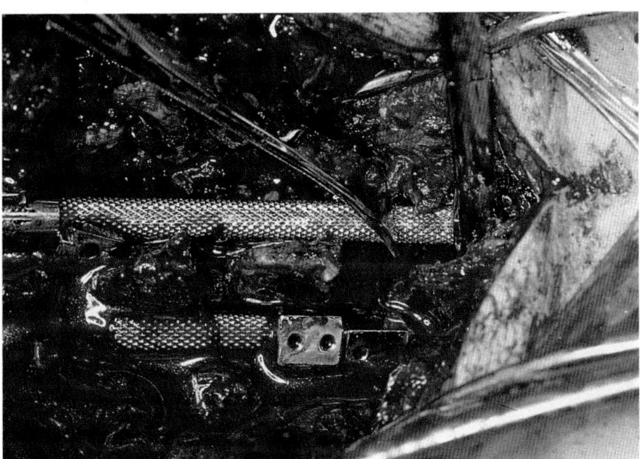

Figure 23. Control of the inferior convex hook is essential. Control is established with a hook holder and the rod pusher.

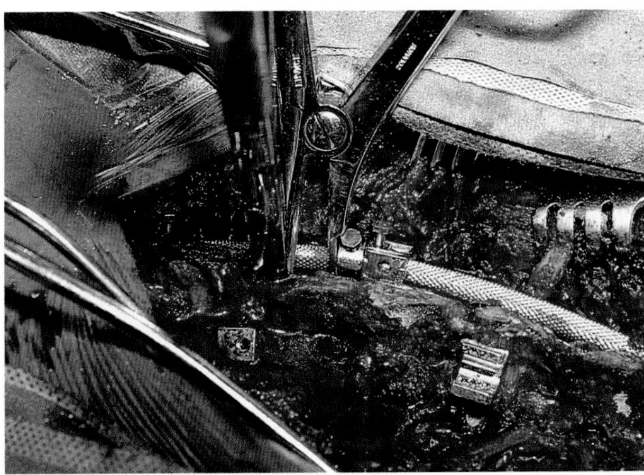

Figure 24. Distraction against a fixed point on the rod (Schlein clamp) provides seating of hooks.

of this inferior convex hook (Fig. 25). Repeat the process with the L2 hook. Retighten the L3 hook. At this point the lumbar segment is secure.

The thoracic segment can now be tightened. With a fixed point on the rod (as previously depicted), tighten the T6 and T9 hooks, using the CD distractor. Check that the T11 and T12 hooks remain tight. Finally, using the distractor against a fixed point on the rod, tighten the T4 hook. Retighten the T6 hook.

Rod Placement, Second or Right. With the first rod in place, the second rod can now be inserted. This should be bent to less kyphosis and lordosis than the initial rod, thereby providing the detorsion forces. Blockers must be placed in the proper position and orientation. The rod is then advanced through the T4 pedicle transverse claw. The less tension on the hooks, the easier the passage. The rod is placed in the final position relative to axial rotation. At this point, the rod should be protruding a significant amount posteriorly (Fig. 26). Place a hook holder on the L3 hook. Place a fixed point on the rod just distal to the T4 pedicle hook. Tilt the L3 hook distally. Using the rod pusher, exert an anterior directed force on the rod just proximal to the L3 hook. The position of the rod regarding length must be perfect relative to the canal in the L3 hook (Fig. 27). Several adjustments may be required in the length of the rod relative to the position of the terminal hook. With optimal rod length, push the rod in an anterior direction with the rod pusher, engage the L3 hook, and tilt the L3 hook cephalad. The rod is now secure in the L3 hook. Using the previously placed fixed point distal to T4, use the CD distractor to advance the rod distally, until it emerges from the distal end of the L3 hook. Usually the slope of the L3 lamina will not permit more than a few millimeters of protrusion, which is adequate.

At this point, the rod will have entered the T8 and T10 hooks, and the blockers can be easily inserted. The L1 hook may require the rod introducer for blocker placement. A useful maneuver for placement of this blocker, and others on the right side, can be termed *capture*, due to the conical design of the blocker. Tilt the hook away from the blocker. Using blocker driver #1, exert an anterior directed force on the blocker just as it engages the hook. With a hook holder on the hook, keeping the anterior and proximal directed force on the blocker, tilt the hook back toward the blocker. Usually this will engage the blocker into the hook. Final seating of the blocker is accomplished with blocker driver #2.

Tightening Sequences. The tightening sequences are relatively simple for this second rod. Begin by tightening the T4 pedicle transverse claw. The set screw on the transverse process hook is tightened, followed by distraction from a fixed point on the rod distal to the pedicle hook. The T8 and T10 hooks are then tightened from a fixed point on the rod distal to the hooks by distraction. This should be

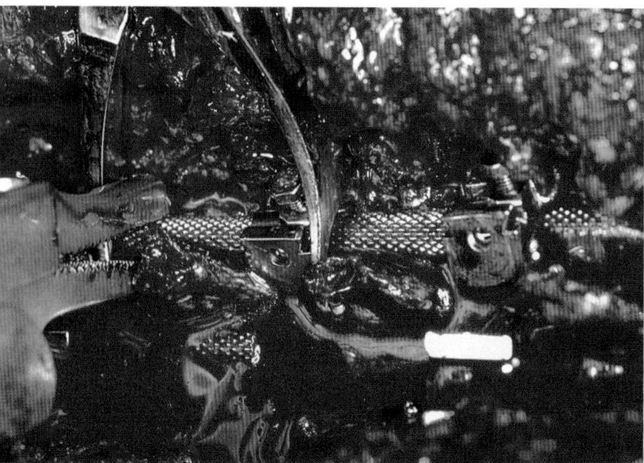

Figure 25. Compression against a fixed point on the rod (Schlein clamp) is a second method of hook seating.

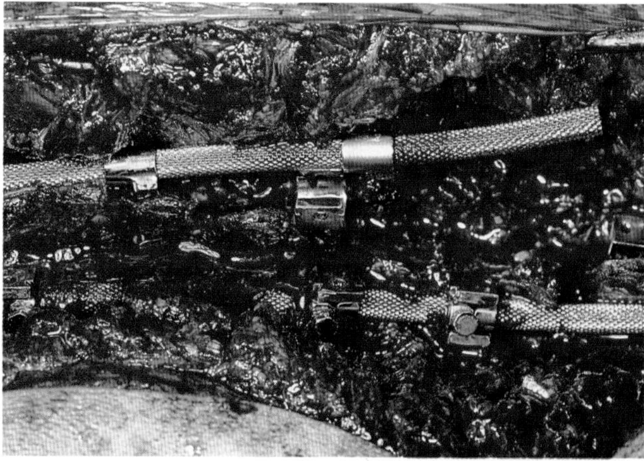

Figure 26. Posterior protrusion of the second or convex rod. The anterior directed force required for placement of this rod provides the final element of the detorque force.

repeated on the two hooks until both are tight, and neither moves. The L1 hook is then tightened in a like manner. This particular hook has a tendency to tilt and to be inadequately loaded. Placement of a security bolt on the side away from the entrance of the blocker will prevent further unloading in the postsurgery period. Finally, the L3 hook is tightened using a fixed point on the rod and the distractor.

Following completion of tightening of the right rod, the left rod should be tightened again, following the order of the initial tightening sequence.

Transverse Connecting Devices. The device for transverse traction (DTT) has been an integral portion of the CD rectangle since its inception. The author has never observed failure of the DTT. The DTT is available in the United States in two versions, the regular (original) and the low profile. The low profile decreases the posterior prominence of the instrumentation by 4 mm. This, combined with the low-profile pedicle hook, decreases the posterior prominence by 7 mm. This is quite significant in the adolescent patient and has resulted in significantly less use of the 5-mm rod system.

A third DTT is available in the rest of the world; Food and Drug Administration approval is pending (Fig. 28). The first two DTTs consist of a small threaded rod

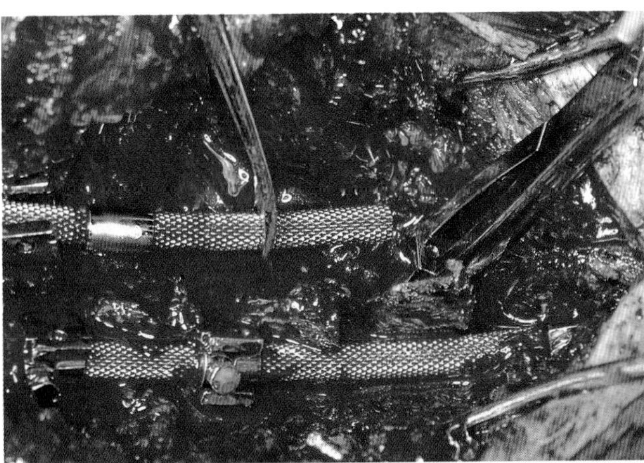

Figure 27. The position of the rod prior to introduction into the inferior right rod is critical. The rod must be at the appropriate point to permit entry into the hook by the maneuver of tilting the hook to the upright position.

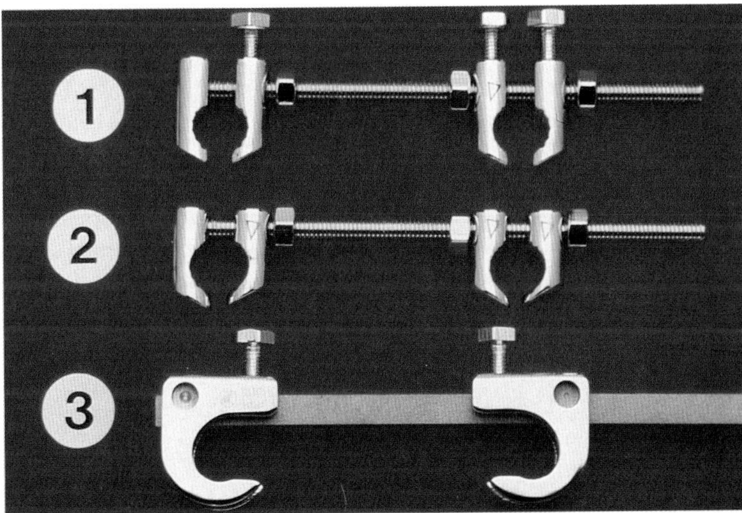

Figure 28. The three varieties of DTTs are depicted. As of this writing, only #1 and #2 are available in the United States. (Courtesy of Dr. Y. Cotrel, Paris, France.)

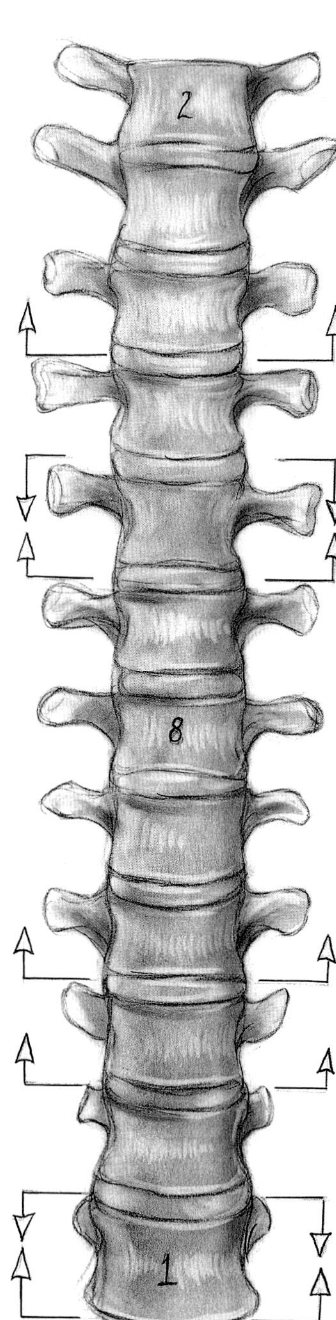

Figure 29. The strategic plan for surgical treatment of Scheuermann's kyphosis (see text).

with two small opposing hooks at each end. Fixation to the rod is obtained by tightening nuts on the threaded rod. With DTT #3, the rod is rectangular, and fixation to the CD rod is obtained by hooks with set screws. Placement of #3 is much easier than #1 and #2. The strength of the transverse rod becomes an issue as the distance between CD rods increases.

In the example in Figure 15, a low-profile DTT (#2) is placed at the proximal end, as close to the T4 hooks as possible. This should be tightened in a compression direction. A second DTT is placed as close to the L3 hooks as possible. This distal DTT can be the original DTT #1, as the lumbar musculature covers it very well. It also should be tightened in compression. Frequently, because of the relatively medial placement of lamina hooks at the distal end, space for the DTT with both central nuts present will not exist. DTT #1 has a significant advantage in this situation. One of the central nuts can be removed. The end of the DTT with the fixed hook can then be tightened. The position of the medial hook of the two can then be fixed with a set screw in the top of the hook. The nut can then be used to tighten the other side. This is not possible with DTT #2, since no position exists in these hooks for set screws.

In instrumentations more than 30 cm in length, a third DTT should be placed, in the approximate center. The third DTT increases the torsional rigidity significantly. It should be placed in a distraction direction.

Completion of Procedure. Subsequent to completion of the instrumentation, the remaining bone graft is placed. If evoked potentials have not changed (or if a wake-up test has been passed), termination of the procedure begins. All set screw heads are broken off, by simply continuing to turn the set screw until it breaks. The screw head is discarded. Care is necessary to ensure that all screw heads are removed from the wound.

Closure is then accomplished. The deep fascia is closed with a running #0 Vicryl suture, or with another method, as the surgeon prefers. A subcutaneous Jackson-Pratt drain is inserted through a separate stab wound. The subcuticular layer is closed with a running 2–0 Vicryl suture, and the skin is closed with staples. Sterile dressings are applied and patient turned onto the bed and awakened. Voluntary motion of the lower extremities is demonstrated prior to transfer to the recovery room.

Cantilever-Compression use of CD (Kyphosis)

Although CD is best recognized for the derotation method of correction, the use of cantilever action and compression forces between segments is employed quite frequently. Figure 29 presents the plan of hook placement for a Scheuermann's kyphosis. To shed light on the various techniques, CD repair of this condition is discussed before repair of thoracolumbar scoliosis and other spinal pathologies.

Implant Selection and Placement. Note on the plan that no implants are present in the periapical area, the apex being T8. It is dangerous to place hooks in the apical areas of a kyphosis, since the significant anterior directed forces can displace a hook into the spinal canal. The implant placement will be divided above and below the apex (Fig. 29).

Above the Apex. Above the apex, a minimum of two, and preferably three, pedicle transverse claws or grips are necessary. These must be placed at alternating levels. The claws are preferred over supralaminar intracanal hooks. Violation of the canal is avoided, and the claw provides a sagittal plane rotation action that a single supralamina hook cannot. I prefer a symmetrical bilateral instrumentation. Staggered instrumentation has been suggested to distribute the load over the entire segment proximal to the apex. The latter instance has not been found to be necessary.

The hooks are all closed. It is relatively easy to pass the CD rod through a series of closed hooks in the absence of coronal plane deformity. The preferred pedicle hook is the low-profile one (#84191). The transverse process hook is the regular lumbar lamina hook (#84103). If malalignment between pedicle and lamina hook exists, an extended body lamina hook may be substituted (#84142). At T2, alignment of the transverse process hook with the pedicle hook usually will not be possible, because of the horizontal orientation of the T2 transverse process. Here a pedicle-lamina claw should be created. A supralamina hook is placed in the canal. The thin-blade lumbar lamina hook can be used (#84137). An option is #84142, a hook with a 45-degree oblique blade, furnished in left or right versions. One or the other will align with the pedicle hook. Placement of these hooks is as previously described.

Below the Apex. Three sets of hooks are preferred below the apex. The proximal two sets of hooks are either pedicle or lamina, depending on the thoracic spine facet anatomy. These should be open. The pedicle is a low-profile one, #84190. The lamina hook should be either thoracic, #84118, or thin-blade, #84143. The terminal implants, here at L1, should be a lamina-lamina claw (Fig. 30). An open hook should be used in the supralamina position, the thin-blade #84143. A closed hook should be used in the infralamina position, thin-blade #84137.

An alternative for the distal L1 implant is the posterior open sacral screw. Placed bilaterally, easier introduction of the rod into the posterior open terminal implants is possible. The screws can be protected with infralamina hooks at the same level. The lamina hook with offset body, #84172 right and left, is suggested.

Rod Bending. The bend of the rod is as described previously. Judgment of length is critical to prevent difficulty of placement.

Arthrodesis. Arthrodesis and posterior shortening as necessary are accomplished during hook placement. Decortication is done prior to rod placement.

Rod Placement and Tightening Sequences. In the absence of coronal deformity, it makes no difference which rod is placed first. With coronal deformity, the convex rod should be placed first. The bent rod is passed through the series

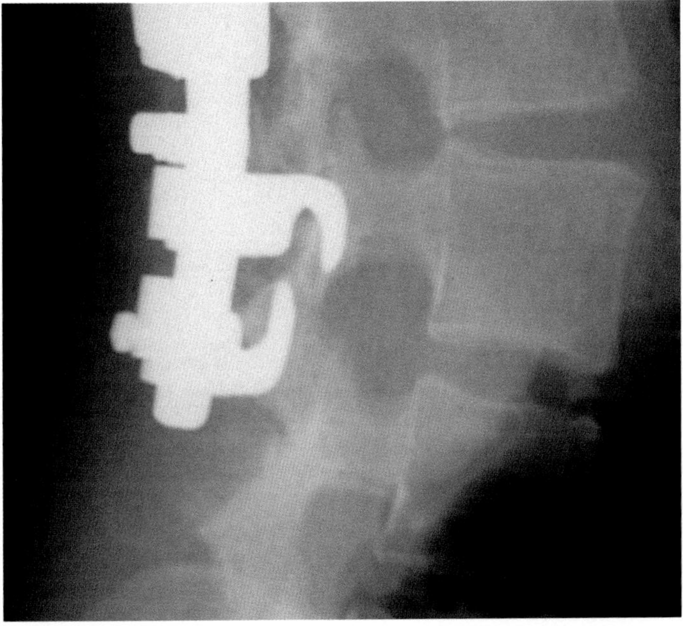

Figure 30. A lamina-lamina claw is demonstrated. The extended body lamina hook is in the supralamina position.

of proximal implants closed, the tip just emerging from the proximal hook (Fig. 31). Tighten the T2 claw, as previously stated. Distraction is then applied distal to the T4 hook, using the distractor against a fixed point on the rod (Schlein clamp). Tighten the set screw. This action compresses the area between T2 and T4. Repeat the distraction step distal to the T6 pedicle hook, accomplishing the same maneuver. Retighten the T4 hook and then the T6 hook. Repeat these maneuvers until neither hook moves. Compression mechanics have been used to correct the kyphosis in this segment above the apex (Fig. 32).

The next step in kyphosis correction is cantilever mechanics. With the proximal segment secure, anterior force is placed on the distal end of the rod, using the rod pusher. The two posterior open hooks are entered and the blockers placed. Distraction distal to each hook via the distractor against a fixed point on the rod is supplied. Alternate between hooks until neither moves. While cantilever corrects the apical kyphosis, the distraction forces distal to the hooks affords additional correction via compression forces between the intervening segments.

At this point, the distal end of the rod will still protrude from the wound. Remove the distal closed lamina hook. Place it on the rod. Divide the paraspinal fascia and musculature to gain a clear view of the L1 infralamina position. Again, push the rod and the hook on the rod, in an anterior direction, a sufficient distance to introduce the blade of the hook just distal to the inferior edge of the lamina. With the good position of the hook relative to the lamina, proximal advancement of the hook can be accomplished. I prefer to place the blocker driver #2 (no tines) against the inferior edge of the hook, and use a mallet to seat the hook (Fig. 33). After the hook is seated, the compressor is used against a fixed point on the rod proximal to the distal hook. Retighten every hook on this side.

When doing the cantilever maneuver, it may be helpful to place a short rod on the other side distally. This can then be used as a handle to pull the spine posterior during the application of the anteriorly directed cantilever forces.

The second rod can then be placed like the first. The tightening sequences are the same. The first rod should then be retightened. DTTs should be placed as previously described. The final events are also as previously described.

Cantilever-Compression (Thoracolumbar Scoliosis)

Use of CD in thoracolumbar deformities requires use of the cantilever-compression action described in the treatment of kyphosis. The resulting mechanics repli-

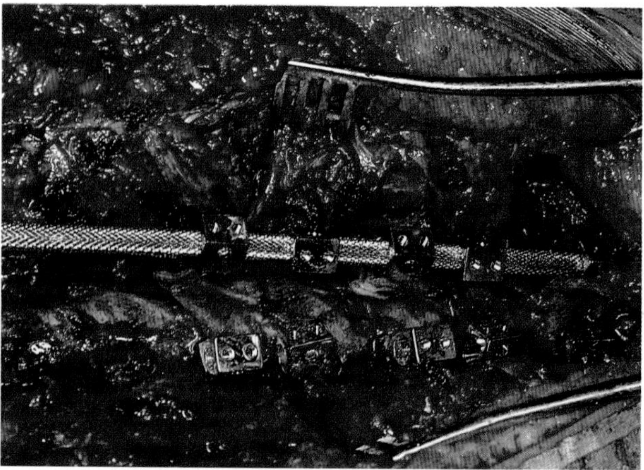

Figure 31. The proximal segment of the rod for kyphosis correction has been placed, and tightening will follow (see text).

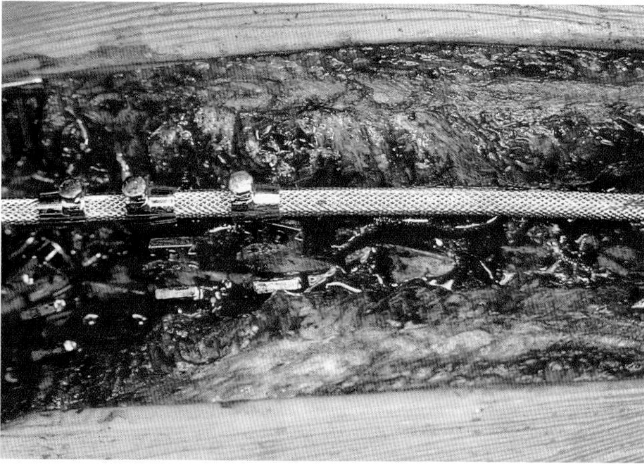

Figure 32. Completion of the "above-the-apex" instrumentation sequence leaves the rod with a significant posterior position.

cate the derotation maneuver of the double structural curve. Figure 34 presents the plan for a thoracolumbar scoliosis. The convex left side should be instrumented first.

Implant Selection and Placement. The convex implants include a closed supralamina hook at T11, thoracic design (#84125). At T12, the open version of the same hook is placed (#84118). Below the apex (L1), as in the kyphosis problem, hooks are placed toward the apex. The L2 infralamina hook is open and usually thin-blade (#84143). The terminal L3 hook is closed and infralamina, usually thin-blade (#84137). The convex hooks include a closed infralamina hook (or pedicle hook, depending on facet anatomy) at T11, either a thin-blade lamina hook (#84137) or a low-profile pedicle hook (#84191). L1 receives an open thin-blade lumbar lamina hook, #84143. L3 receives a closed supralamina hook, thin-blade, #84137. The technique of implant placement is as previously described.

An alternative method of instrumentation for the lumbar segment of this deformity is use of pedicle screws. These can be placed bilaterally at levels L1 through L3. Because of the more lateral placement, a more effective lever arm for derotation is present. Posterior open sacral screws are the preferred implant. A domino connector will usually be required to join the distal screws to the proximal hooks.

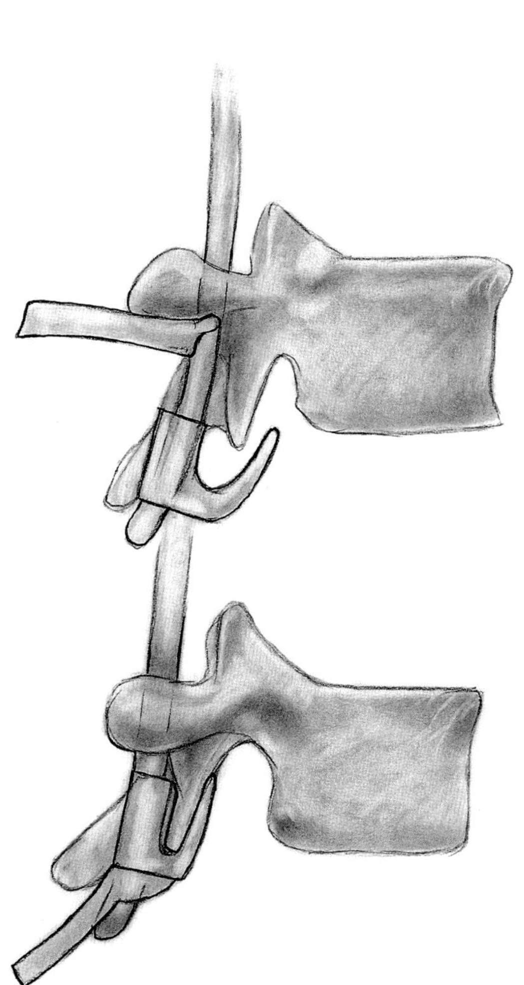

Figure 33. The method of seating the caudal hook in correction of kyphosis requires placement of the hook on the rod and anterior and cephalad directed forces to seat the hook. (Courtesy of Dr. Y. Cotrel.)

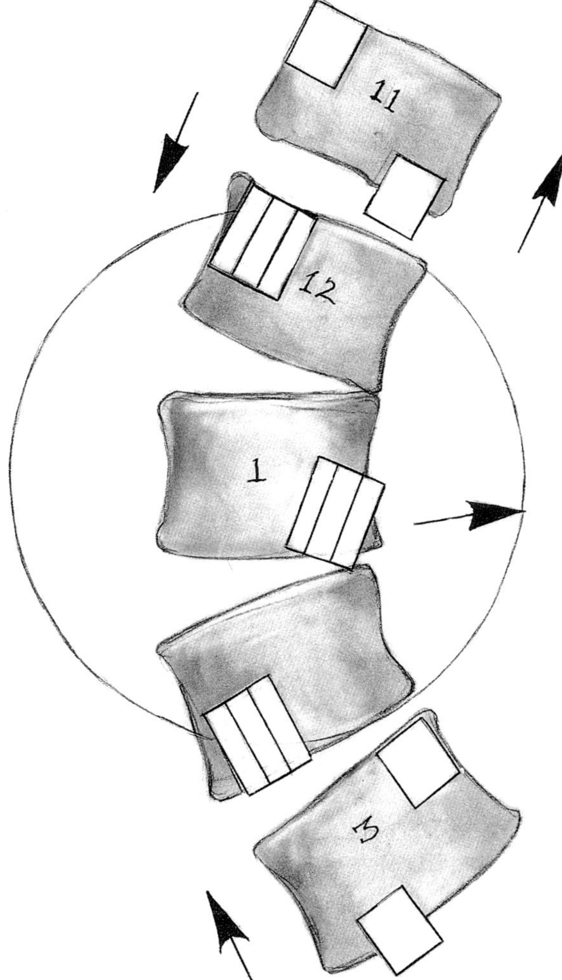

Figure 34. A simplistic but actual diagram of a strategic plan for use of CD in a thoracolumbar idiopathic deformity.

Rod Bending. The bend of the rod will resemble the bend for the double curve. The conversion from thoracic kyphosis to lumbar lordosis should occur at the T12–L1 interspace. In this instance, a single coronal curve is present in two sagittal segments. (Thoracic kyphosis and lumbar lordosis constitute the two sagittal segments.) Due to the required S-shaped bend in the rod, and the single coronal deformity, the derotation maneuver cannot be accomplished.

Arthrodesis. Facet excision and decortication is accomplished before rod placement as previously described.

Rod Placement and Tightening Sequences. *First or Left Placement.* With the rod bent as described, it is inserted in the final position in terms of axial rotation. The rod is placed into the T11 closed hook. Using a cantilever maneuver with the rod pusher, as described for the kyphosis correction, anterior force is supplied. Be sure to allow the rod to enter the T12 open hook, and then the L2 open hook. It is assumed that the blockers have been placed in the correct position and direction. Continuing the anterior force, tilt the L3 hook caudally with the hook holder, as with the inferior convex hook in the double-curve example. The position of the rod is critical. It must be in the exact position to be engaged when the L3 hook is tilted to the upright position. In the kyphosis correction, it was impossible to advance the rod or change its distal position because of the application of compression forces and set screw fixation of the proximal hooks to the rod. In this situation, release of the anterior tension on the rod permits easy reposition of the rod. With good position of the distal end of the rod, the L3 hook is tilted to the upright position, engaging the rod. Keeping anterior pressure on the rod, it is then advanced through the hook. Control of the L3 hook must be maintained with the hook holder until the convex side is completely tight.

After insertion of blockers into the open hooks, tightening begins with tightening the set screw on the L3 hook. Distraction is then done proximal to the T12 hook (as in the double-curve example), using the distractor against a fixed point on the rod (Schlein clamp). This action compresses across the intervening segments (T12 and L3). Lordosis is provided by rod bending and compression. This is exactly the situation with kyphosis correction, and with establishment of lumbar lordosis in the previously discussed double thoracic and lumbar curve. Next, the hook at L2 is tightened, either by distraction distal (distractor against a fixed point on the rod) or compression proximal (compressor against a fixed point on the rod). Then the T11 hook is tightened, best accomplished with the compressor against a fixed point on the rod distal to the hook. Finally, the L3 hook should be tightened. This is best accomplished with the compressor, using a fixed point on the rod proximal to the hook.

Second or Right Placement. The second or concave rod should be bent to less lordosis than the first. This will supply a posterior force on the L1 hook. Insertion of the second rod is accomplished by placing the rod into the T11 closed hook and advancing it into the L3 closed hook. The rod will be somewhat posterior to the apical L1 hook. Insertion of the blocker is accomplished either with the rod introducer or by the capture method. The sequence of tightening is not important. Each hook can be tightened by distraction against a fixed point on the rod. The first rod should then be retightened.

The mechanics of correction are similar to that for kyphosis correction, cantilever and compression. But the effect is derotation, as for the double curve. Consider that the anteriorly directed force on the convex side provides two points of a torque moment. A posteriorly directed force on the concave rod produces the other portion of the torque moment. Therefore, derotation or detorsion is achieved. The thoracolumbar (or lumbar) idiopathic curve requires use of cantilever and compression mechanics of kyphosis correction.

Transverse Connecting Devices. Two DDTs are applied, as near to the ends as possible. A low-profile device should be used at the proximal end (DTT #2) and

DTT #1 placed distally. The placement is as previously described. Termination of the procedure is as previously described.

Removal of CD Instrumentation

Insertion of spinal instrumentation requires the ability to remove it. Removal of CD is destructive of the instrumentation. A portion of the instrumentation can be removed and extension accomplished from the intact instrumentation using the domino connector. The following discussion of removal is systematic for removal of the entire instrumentation. Portions, for example the distal end, can be removed as described for the entire instrumentation. Metal-cutting instruments, such as the Midas Rex drill, are not required; only a bolt cutter and the CD instruments are necessary.

After exposure of the instrumentation, the DTTs should be removed first. Cut the threaded rod. Next, cut between the opposing hooks on each rod. A small end-cutting bolt cutter accomplishes this task. Berry sternal needle holders are then useful to remove the DTT hooks.

The next step is to remove the blockers from the open hooks (Fig. 15). The easiest method to remove the blockers uses the closed hook inserter. For the T6 hook, the closed hook inserter is positioned proximally, contacting the portion of the blocker into which the set screw was placed. Use a mallet to hit the hook inserter. This will drive the blocker distally, out of the open hook (Fig. 35). Repeat this maneuver on each open hook. After all the blockers are driven out of the open hooks, the rod can be elevated posteriorly into the wound. Cut the rod adjacent to the closed hooks at the ends. Remove the rod.

Next remove the open hooks. Remove any bone that may prevent tilting the hook. Use the large rod holder to grip the open hook securely (Fig. 36). Tilt the hook in the direction necessary to permit it to rotate out of its site. Next remove the rod from the closed hooks. This is easily accomplished by breaking the grip of the set screws on the rod. Place a hook holder on the closed hook. Place a Schlein clamp on the rod. Use the Schlein clamp to rotate the rod, keeping the hook position secure with the hook holder. After adequate mobility in rod rotation is attained, use the distractor against the Schlein clamp to advance the rod out of the hook. Rotation of the rod should continue during the application of the distraction force. Here the knurled surface of the rod acts as a file on the set screw. With the rod out of the closed hook, the closed hook can then be removed with the closed hook inserter or with the hook holder.

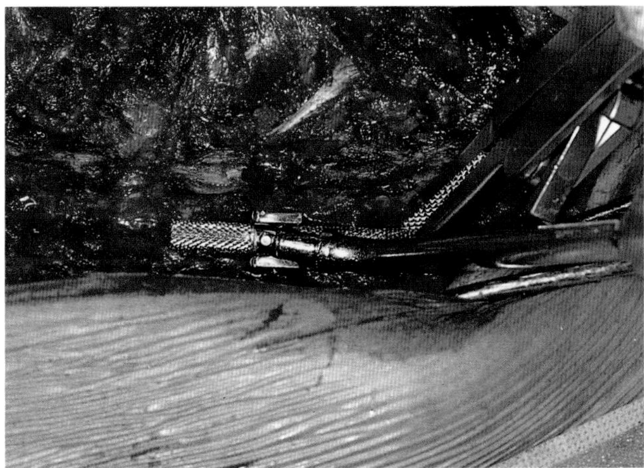

Figure 35. The closed hook inserter is used, with a mallet, to remove the blocker from an open hook.

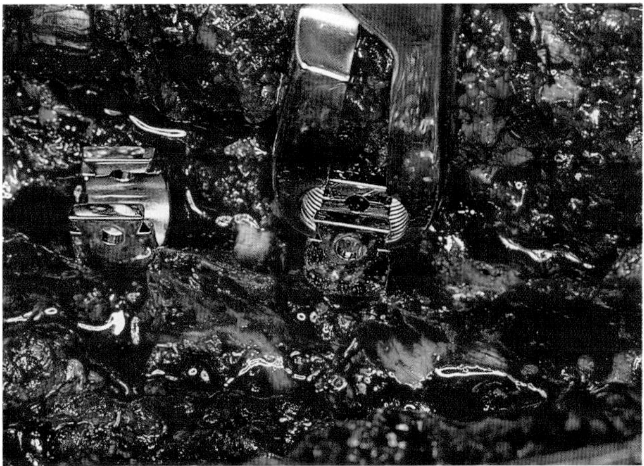

Figure 36. The large rod holder provides an excellent grip for removal of open hooks, after removal of rod and blockers.

If only a portion of the instrumentation is to be removed (e.g., for extension), the same steps are employed. Only the end hooks need be removed. A domino connector may then be placed for extension of the construct.

POSTOPERATIVE MANAGEMENT

Postoperative care of the patient undergoing spinal fusion with CD is relatively uncomplicated compared with postoperative care before CD was developed. No external support (brace or cast) is employed, except for certain patients with myelodysplasia or cerebral palsy. In patients otherwise normal except for the spinal problem, immobilization has not been used since the CD system was first employed in 1985.

A subcutaneous Jackson-Pratt drain is used and is removed on the first postoperative day. The patient is ambulated on the first day. Usually by the third day, intravenous and Foley catheters are removed and the patient is permitted to shower. Hospital discharge is usually on the 6th or 7th postoperative day, with skin staples removed the day of discharge.

After discharge, the patient is permitted to be up and about as wished. Lifting more than 8 to 10 pounds and bending from the waist are discouraged for the first 3 months. Driving is permitted when narcotics are no longer required. After 3 weeks, the patient may use a swimming pool. Follow-up examination and radiology are done at 1, 3, 6, 12, and 24 months in the uncomplicated patient.

At 1 month, the adolescent can usually return to school. For the adult, return to sedentary work is usually possible at 6 to 8 weeks. Activities are liberalized at 3 months. Lifting to 15 to 20 pounds, swimming with any stroke, nonviolent dancing, and bicycle riding are permitted. At 6 months, most activities are permitted, including team sports (noncontact), running, skating, weight-lifting up to 30 pounds, and other low-impact activities. At 1 year, any activity or sport is permitted. A formal rehabilitation program is usually not required, except in the occasional degenerative condition. The nondegenerative patient usually resumes all presurgery activities at the above time intervals.

The amount of correction obtained radiographically is variable. In general, adolescents can expect approximately 60% to 70% improvement in the coronal deformity and adults somewhat less. The sagittal plane can usually be restored to or maintained at relatively normal values in both the adolescent and adult. A minimal amount of loss of correction may be expected, usually no greater than 5 degrees.

COMPLICATIONS

Strategic Complications

Strategic complications are the primary cause of the imbalance problems (5,6,8).

Failure to Include all Structural Curves in the Instrumentation. An imbalance may be in the coronal, sagittal, or axial plane. Imbalance is most frequently produced in the double structural left high thoracic-right thoracic curve pattern, with failure to appreciate the left curve. The false double major curve is also a frequent source of imbalance. In this instance, the cause is inability of the lumbar segment to balance. Several contributing factors are present, including: (a) large and structural lumbar curve; (b) poor hook patterns, particularly with distraction direction forces across the thoracolumbar junction (6,8); and (c) failure to appreciate the presence of a thoracolumbar junctional kyphosis.

Failure to Recognize the Potential for the Crankshaft Phenomenon to Develop. This is associated with large residual coronal and axial deformities after surgery in relatively immature patients. It can be prevented by a preliminary anterior growth arrest and fusion.

Ending the Fusion on an Apical Vertebra. The apex may be in the coronal plane, producing imbalance in this plane, or in the sagittal plane, producing sagittal imbalance.

If imbalance is produced, treatment may be observation, bracing, or surgical extension of the instrumentation. The decision depends on the severity of the imbalance and is a judgment issue for the surgeon.

Technical Complications

Technical complications include all implant placement problems. These may occur at any point in the multiple steps necessary for placement of CD instrumentation. Careful attention to detail at every step is required to minimize possible technical errors. Prominence of the instrumentation is in this category. Prior to the development of the lower-profile pedicle hook and DTT, this was relatively frequent. Removal of the instrumentation was required on occasion. With current instrumentation, prominence is no longer a problem.

Failure to apply two DTT devices results in torsional instability of the construct and may lead to failure. Accurate placement of hooks is essential to successful use of CD. Inaccurate placement may result in hook displacement.

Neurologic Complications

Neurologic complications may arise either within the spinal canal (cord, conus, or cauda equina injury) or outside the spinal canal (nerve root injury, usually due to pedicle or sacral screws). The frequency of this complication has decreased significantly over the past several years.

Neurologic injury within the spinal canal may arise during any portion of the procedure. Careful attention to detail and avoidance of distraction forces should minimize neurologic injuries. The cord is more vulnerable to the combination of derotation and distraction than are either of these alone. Distraction should not be a significant part of the procedure. The use of SSEP and the wake-up test when indicated should minimize this complication. Neurologic complications outside the spinal canal are usually due to impingement of either pedicle or sacral screws on a nerve root or plexus.

If a potential neurologic injury is indicated by a change in SSEP amplitude or latency, forces on the spine should be adjusted and a wake-up test performed. Depending on the subsequent SSEP and wake-up test results, the procedure may either be continued or abandoned. If a neurologic injury is indicated after completion of the procedure, investigation by myelography and/or computed tomography scan should ensue. Prompt removal or revision of the instrumentation may be required, which usually results in recovery.

Infectious Complications

Infections may occur either acutely or later. The treatment of acute infections requires wound debridement and either closure over closed irrigation systems or delayed secondary closure. Appropriate antibiotic administration should accompany the surgical portion of the treatment. Removal of the hardware is not desirable. Late removal due to persistent infection may be required. Hopefully, the arthrodesis will be secure by this point. If early removal is required, external support is usually indicated.

Late infection, usually over 2 years after placement of the instrumentation, appears to be unique to CD (9). The patient usually presents with either swelling over the instrumentation or a draining sinus. Usually no signs of systemic infection are present. Culture is generally negative. Removal of the instrumentation is required. At removal, an extensive granulomatous material is present over the entire instrumentation. Cultures are usually negative and pathology is nonspecific. The cause may be corrosion due to slight motion between the blocker and the open hooks. The incidence in my practice is approximately 6 in 1,000.

Miscellaneous Complications

Pseudarthrosis has not been a major problem in patients undergoing CD for spinal deformity (9). If the instrumentation remains intact for 3 months, this problem is not usually encountered. If pseudarthrosis evolves, repair and revision of the instrumentation is usually required. In conditions other than deformity, pseudarthrosis is more common. Use of autograft bone exclusively may decrease

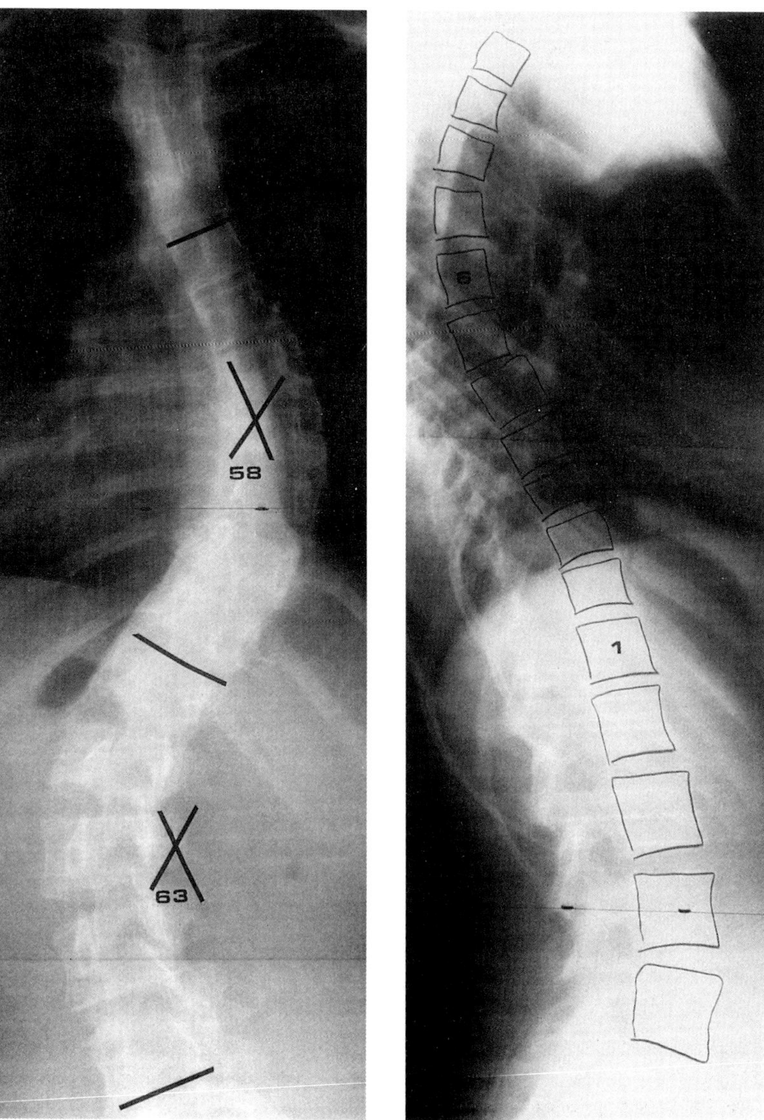

Figure 37. This figure demonstrates the strategy and techniques for double structural idiopathic scoliosis.

the incidence in these areas. It goes without saying that meticulous technique is a routine part of the CD procedure.

Implant displacement may occur in the postoperative period. The most frequent site is the inferior convex hook in the lumbar spine in deformity (9). Replacement is usually required and is relatively easily accomplished.

Bursitis or irritation may occur over the proximal thoracic DTT in deformity patients. Symptoms will usually resolve with use of a nonsteroidal antiinflammatory medication. With time, the frequency and severity of symptoms usually diminishes.

ILLUSTRATIVE CASES FOR TECHNIQUE

Double Structural Idiopathic Scoliosis

Figure 37 presents the radiographs of a patient with adolescent idiopathic scoliosis treated with posterior spinal fusion and CD instrumentation. On the coronal

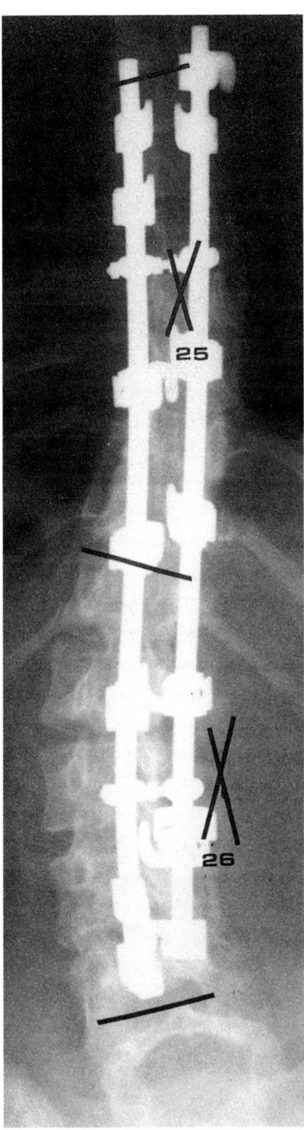

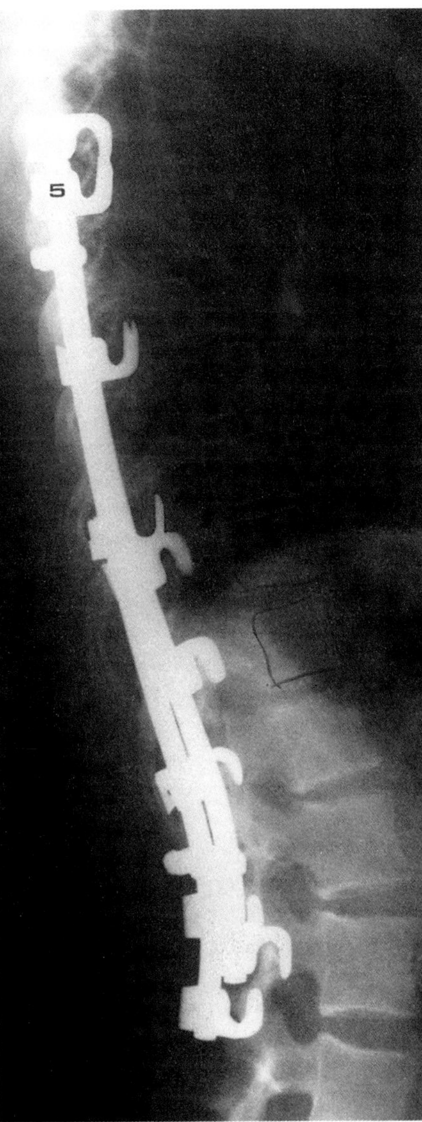

Figure 37. *Continued.*

view, note the implant pattern, which is similar to the technique described. On the sagittal view, note the bending of the rod to approximate normal sagittal contours.

Cantilever-Compression (Kyphosis)

Figure 38 presents the radiographs of a patient with Scheuermann's kyphosis. Note an implant pattern similar to that described. Also note that no implants have been placed in the apical segments. Normal sagittal contours have been produced.

Cantilever-Compression (Thoracolumbar Scoliosis)

Figure 39 shows the radiographs of a patient with thoracolumbar idiopathic scoliosis. The cantilever-compression biomechanical action has been employed.

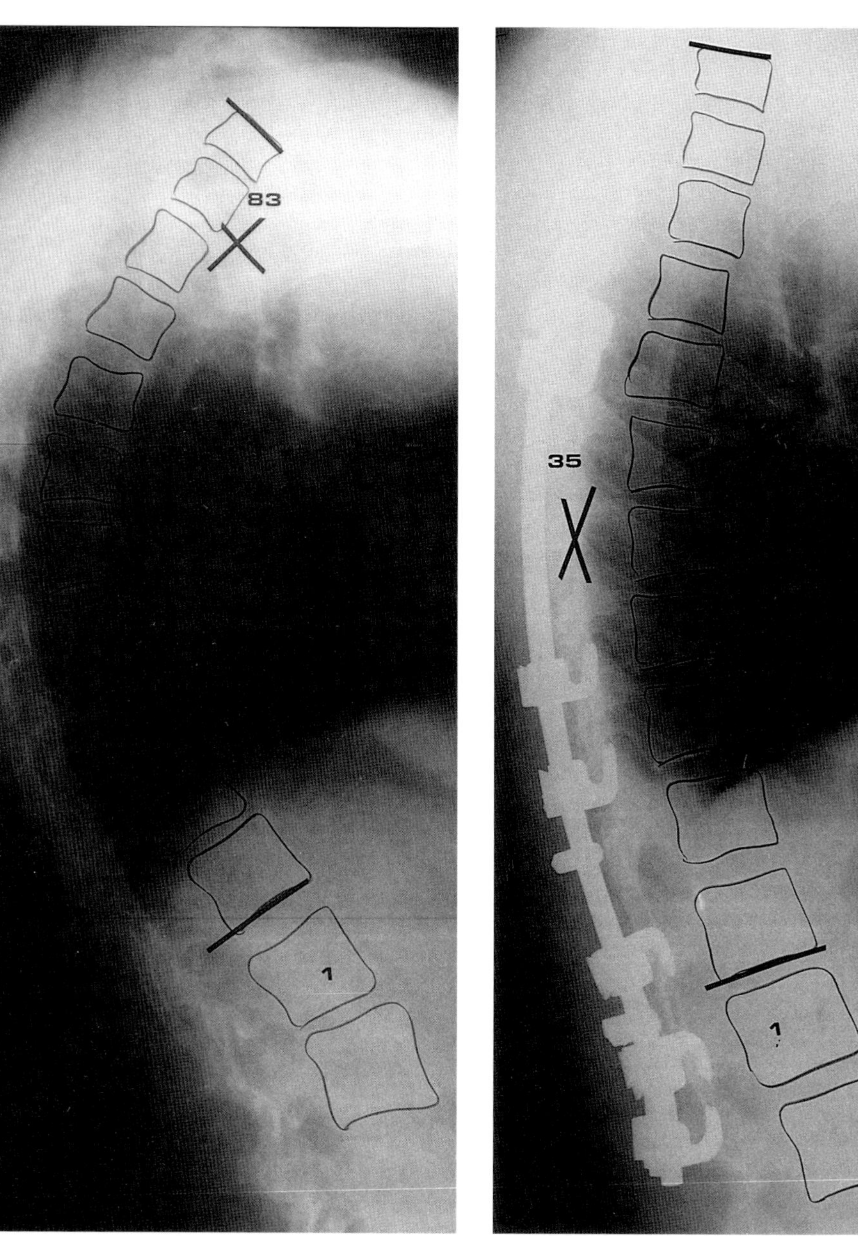

Figure 38. The excellent results possible in the treatment of Scheuermann's kyphosis.

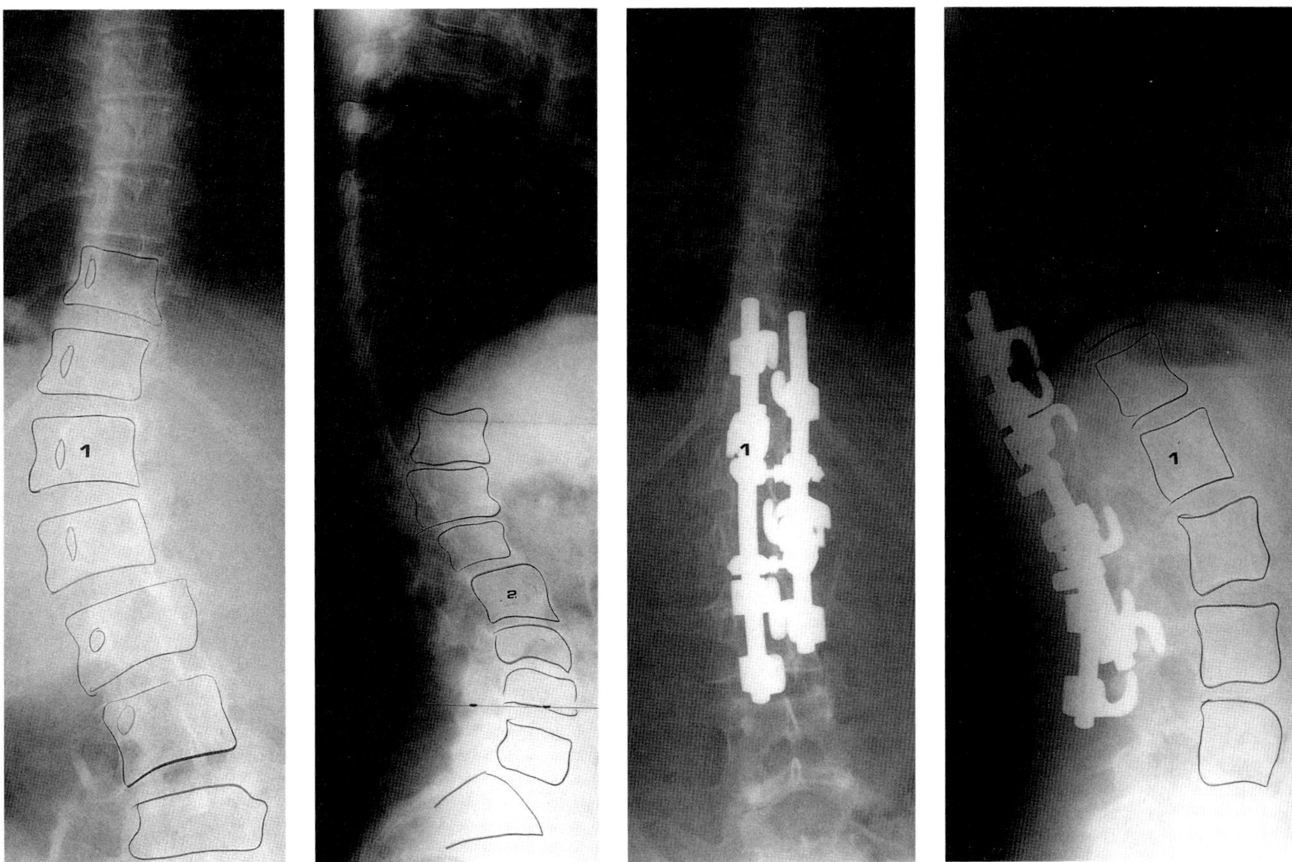

Figure 39. CD instrumentation in the treatment of an idiopathic deformity is a combination of the strategy used for the double structural curve and for Scheuermann's kyphosis.

Note an implant pattern similar to that described. Note that a single coronal deformity exists in the two separate sagittal segments. In the sagittal plane, note the conversion from thoracic kyphosis to lumbar lordosis at the thoracolumbar junction.

RECOMMENDED READING

1. Chopin, D.: Cotrel-Dubousset instrumentation for adolescent idiopathic scoliosis. In: *The Textbook of Spinal Surgery*, pp. 183–217. J. P. Lippincott, Philadelphia, 1991.
2. Cotrel, Y., Dubousset, J., and Guillaumat, M.: New universal instrumentation in spinal surgery. *Clin. Orthop.*, 227: 10, 1988.
3. Dubousset, J., and Cotrel, Y.: Application technique of Cotrel-Dubousset instrumentation for scoliosis deformities. *Clin. Orthop.*, 264: 103, 1991.
4. Graf, H., Hecquet, J., and Dubousset, J.: 3-Dimensional approaches to spinal deformities. *Rev. Chir. Orthop.*, 69: 407, 1983.
5. Lonstein, J.: Decompensation with Cotrel-Dubousset instrumentation. Presented at the Annual Meeting of the Scoliosis Research Society, Minneapolis, Minnesota, 1991.
6. Shufflebarger, H.: Theories and mechanisms of posterior spinal derotation systems. In: *The Pediatric Spine*. Raven Press, New York, 1994.
7. Shufflebarger, H.: Cotrel-Dubousset instrumentation. In: *The Pediatric Spine*. Raven Press, New York, 1994.
8. Shufflebarger, H., and Clark, C.: Fusion levels and hook patterns in thoracic scoliosis with Cotrel-Dubousset instrumentation. *Spine*, 15: 916, 1990.
9. Shufflebarger, H., Thomson, J., and Clark, C.: Complications of CD in idiopathic scoliosis. Presented at the Annual Meeting of the Scoliosis Research Society, Minneapolis, Minnesota, 1991.

Master Techniques in Orthopaedic Surgery,
THE SPINE, edited by D. S. Bradford,
Lippincott-Raven Publishers, Philadelphia, © 1997.

20

Anterior TSRH Instrumentation

John A. Herring

INDICATIONS/CONTRAINDICATIONS

Anterior instrumentation for lumbar and thoracolumbar scoliosis, pioneered by Dwyer (3) and improved by Zielke (6), has proved to be a remarkably effective method for correction of spinal deformity. The Texas Scottish Rite Hospital (TSRH) system is simpler to apply than either the Zielke or Dwyer systems and is considerably more effective in derotating the vertebrae while maintaining lordosis. Anterior instrumentation and fusion usually involves only four or five vertebrae, allowing the surgeon to avoid fusing one or more lumbar levels that would have been included in a posterior instrumentation construct. We have obtained much better derotation of lumbar and thoracolumbar curves with anterior TSRH instrumentation than with posterior constructs and have therefore expanded our indications to include some curves previously not considered amenable to anterior surgery alone.

Thoracolumbar scoliosis with an apex at the 12th thoracic or first lumbar vertebra is usually best managed with an anterior instrumentation and fusion. This is especially true when the patient has not reached Risser stage 1 and may have considerable anterior spinal growth remaining. Patients with thoracolumbar curves often have a compensatory thoracic scoliosis, with the apex toward the contralateral side. The magnitude of this secondary curve is the major determinant of the need for posterior rather than anterior fusion. When the secondary curve is mild, an anterior fusion of the primary curve is appropriate, and the secondary curve will spontaneously stabilize. If the secondary curve is associated with a significant

J. A. Herring, M.D.: Department of Orthopaedic Surgery, University of Texas Southwestern Medical Center at Dallas and Texas Scottish Rite Hospital for Children, Dallas, Texas 75219–3993.

rotational deformity and is greater than 30 to 35 degrees, a posterior fusion that includes the thoracic curve may be the treatment of choice instead of the anterior procedure.

Primary lumbar curves are also very well corrected by anterior instrumentation and fusion. When a secondary thoracic scoliosis exists, as in the King and Moe type 1 pattern, the magnitude and flexibility of the thoracic curve determines the feasibility of anterior correction. When the thoracic deformity is clearly evident on examination and the curve exceeds 35 degrees, an anterior instrumentation of the lumbar curve may leave the patient with significant residual thoracic deformity. On the other hand, when the lumbar curve is large, a purely compensatory thoracic curve may reach 50 degrees or more but may not be accompanied by clinical rib hump deformity. These patients may be well corrected with anterior fusion of the lumbar curve alone.

PREOPERATIVE PLANNING

The preoperative assessment should include a thorough general evaluation to detect any renal, cardiorespiratory, hematologic, or metabolic problems that would adversely affect the patient's recovery. We routinely obtain 2 units of autologous blood preoperatively, an amount that is usually more than adequate to replace operative blood loss. If we plan to use a postoperative orthosis, measurements can be made preoperatively to facilitate fitting.

The choice of levels for instrumentation is based on the standing anteroposterior (AP) radiograph, standing right and left bending films, and occasionally supine forced bending radiographs. The upper vertebra to be instrumented is almost always the upper level of the measured curve. The lower level is chosen based on the degree of flexibility of the spine below the curve. The first example (Fig. 1) is a lumbar curve with an apex between L1 and L2, with L3 as the lower vertebra in the measured curve. On the right bending film the L3 vertebra reaches the horizontal, and on the left bending film the L3–L4 interspace opens to the right. Thus sufficient flexibility exists below the curve to allow compensation after correction, and the instrumentation may stop at L3.

SURGERY

Exposure

The spine is exposed through a thoracoabdominal approach with peripheral detachment of the diaphragm. The incision begins posteriorly just proximal to the angle of the rib and extends around to the costal cartilage and then down the lateral abdominal wall (Fig. 2). The rib level chosen should be one or two levels above the upper vertebra to be instrumented. Thus a ninth-rib approach will be chosen for instrumentation beginning at the tenth thoracic level. The ninth rib is an excellent utility level for a thoracoabdominal approach to lumbar vertebral instrumentation. After subperiosteal removal of the rib, the subdiaphragmatic space is located by splitting the costal cartilage (Fig. 3).

The diaphragm is detached peripherally, and it is helpful to use distinct marking sutures to repair the diaphragm accurately later (Fig. 4). At each vertebral level the surgeon must isolate and double ligate the transverse vessels that cross the vertebral bodies (Fig. 5). Tenuous ligatures may be easily pulled off, resulting in rapid bleeding. To prevent this it is necessary to clear the vessels over a 1-cm area to have secure ligation on either side. The psoas muscle should be dissected

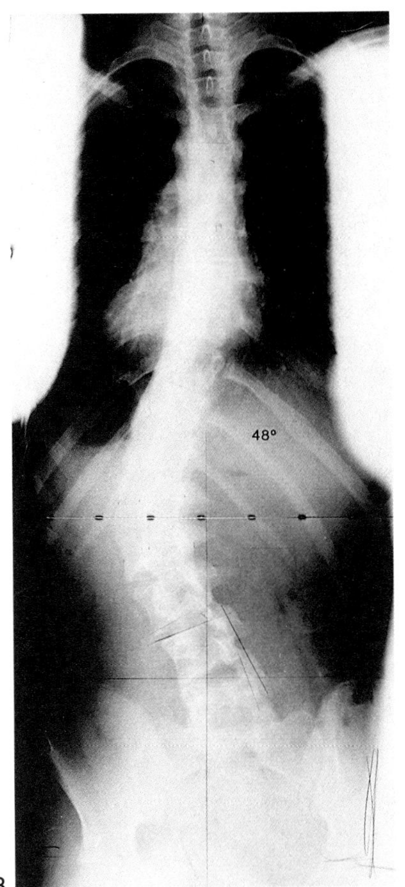

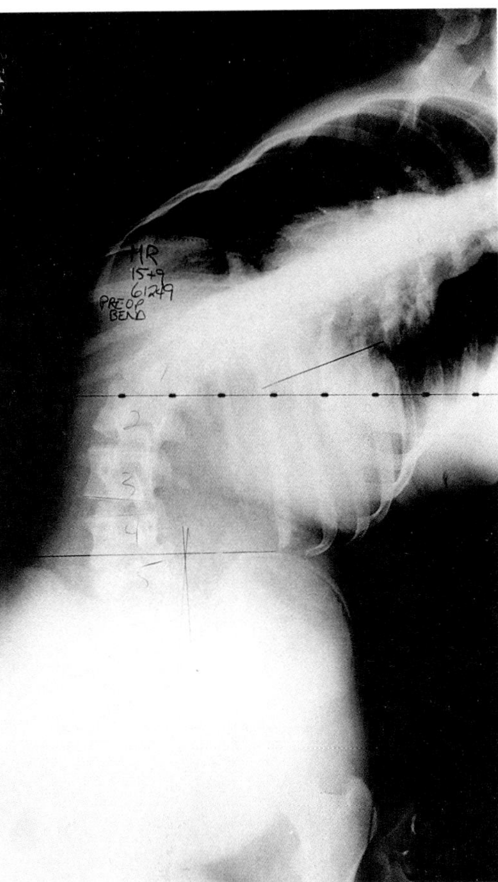

A,B

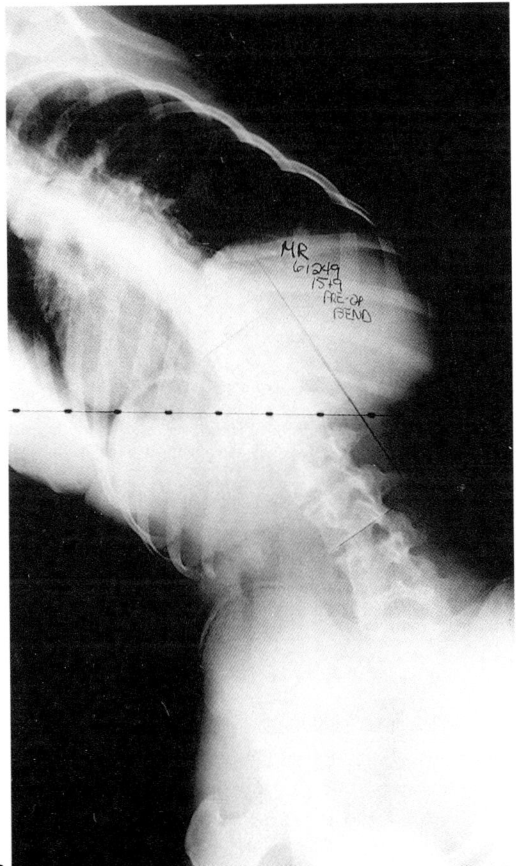

C

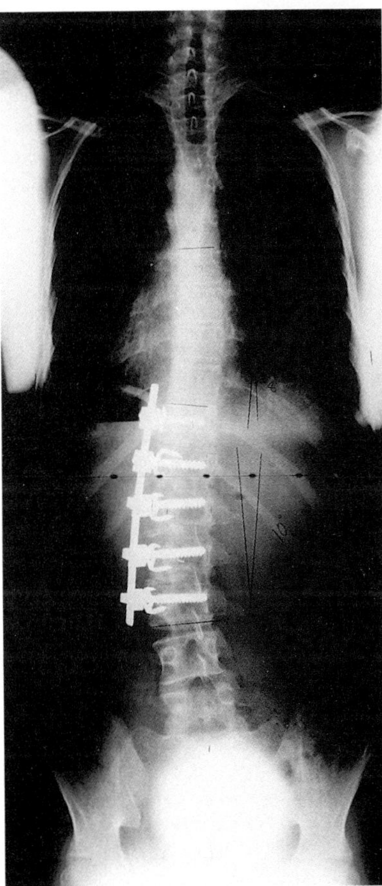
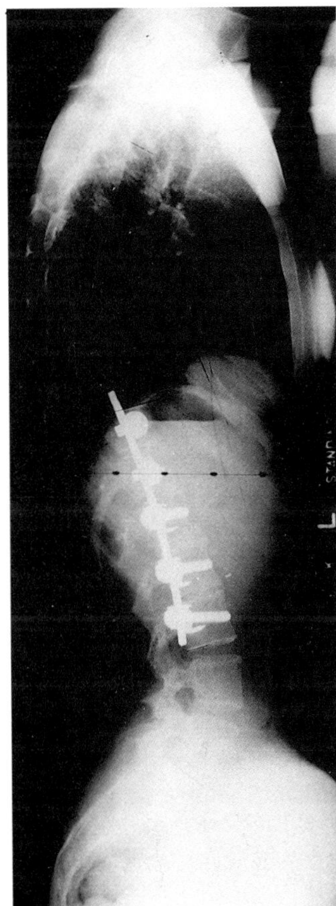

D,E

Figure 1. Case 1, a patient with a primary lumbar idiopathic curve with the apex at the L1–L2 interspace. **A:** Anteroposterior radiograph showing a 48-degree left thoracolumbar scoliosis. **B:** Right bending radiograph showing that the second and third lumbar vertebrae become horizontal with bending to the right. **C:** Left bending radiograph showing complete correction of the primary curve. The interspace between the second and third lumbar vertebrae opens on the right. These bending films indicate that fusion to the second lumbar vertebra will produce a balanced spine. **D:** Postoperative radiograph showing correction of the scoliosis to 10 degrees. **E:** Lateral radiograph showing maintenance of lordosis in the instrumented segment.

free from the lumbar vertebrae over as wide an area as possible (Fig. 6). Cautery should be used with care, since the lumbar nerve roots course through the substance of the psoas muscle and may be injured during exposure.

Discectomy

The discectomy begins with a sharp incision into the disc space (Fig. 7) through which the nucleus pulposus is removed with rongeurs. Rongeurs are also used to remove the anulus fibrosus peripherally over the entire disc space (Fig. 8). A small portion of the anulus may be left in place just over the neural canal as a safety measure. After removal of the anulus, a marked increase in intervertebral mobility should be seen. If the spine remains stiff, usually more anulus is present, which requires removal. After the anulus is removed, the cartilaginous vertebral end plate is removed with ring curettes (Fig. 9). A Cobb elevator may be used to open

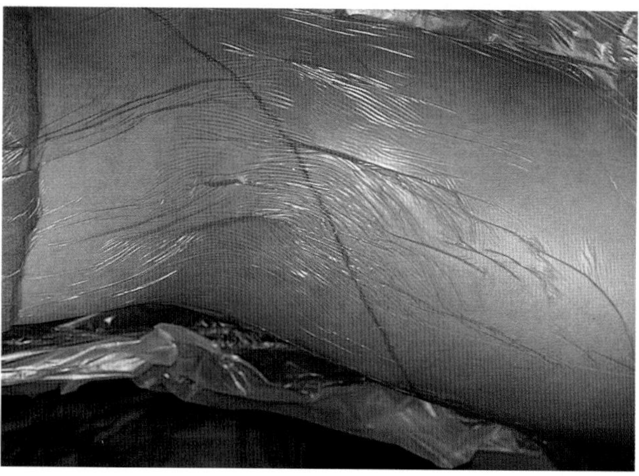

Figure 2. The incision extends over the tenth rib, across the costochondral junction, and obliquely down the abdominal wall.

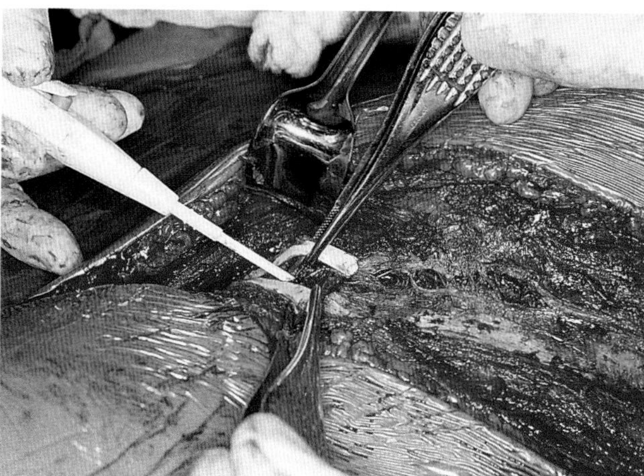

Figure 3. The costal cartilage is split, giving access to the subdiaphragmatic space.

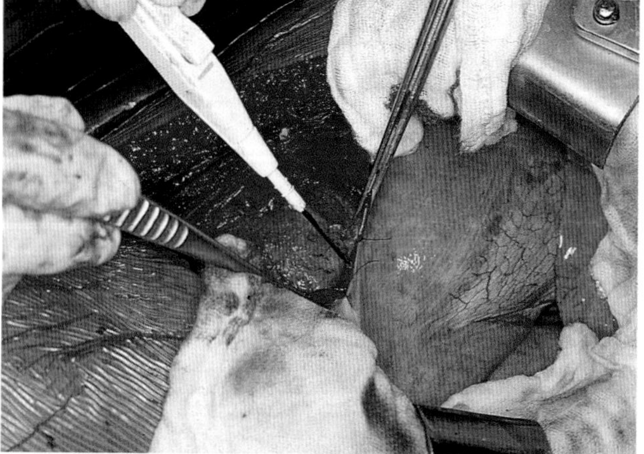

Figure 4. The diaphragm is divided with the cutting cautery 1 to 2 cm from the peripheral attachment to the thorax. Marking sutures are placed at intervals to make accurate closure less difficult.

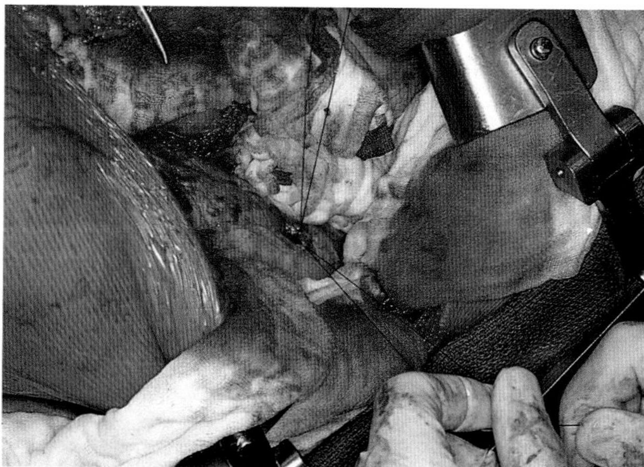

Figure 5. The transverse vessels are isolated as they cross the vertebral bodies. The vessels should be elevated over a 1-cm distance and ligatures tied as far apart as possible. Metal clips are not recommended, as they may be pulled off during the instrumentation procedure.

the interspace for the ring curette. All the cartilage on both sides of the interspace should be removed. It is preferable to "soften up" the bony end plate but not fully remove it, in order to maintain vertebral strength.

Screw Placement

Each screw is placed in the same anatomic location in each vertebra. The starting point is just anterior to the base of the pedicle, right in the center of the vertebral body. The entry hole is aimed so that the screw will bisect the vertebral body.

The screws must also be aligned with one another in a gentle curve that corresponds to the vertebral rotation within the deformity (Fig. 10). I prefer to mark the entry site on each vertebra and check to see that the holes will form a smooth

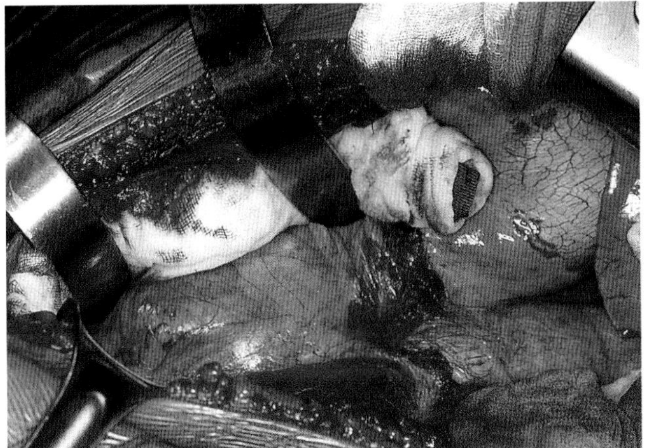

Figure 6. The psoas muscle is dissected from the vertebral bodies to allow access to the base of the pedicle portion of the vertebra.

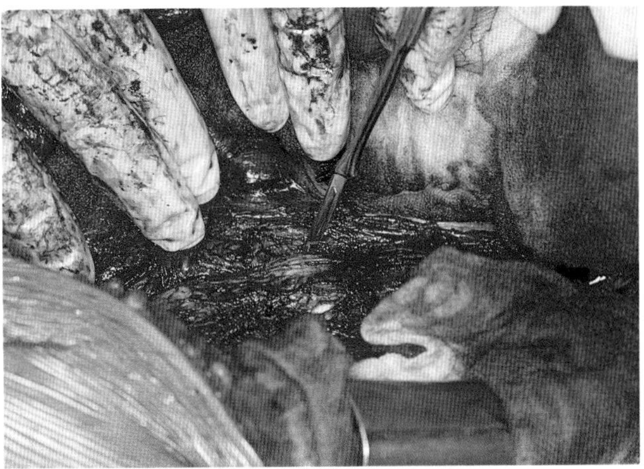

Figure 7. An elliptical incision is made in the intervertebral disc.

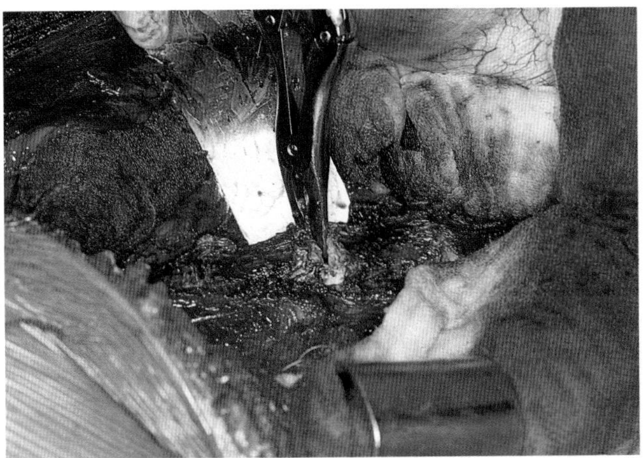

Figure 8. The nucleus pulposus and the anulus fibrosus is removed with a rongeur. The surgeon's finger protects the far side of the interspace from protrusion by the instrument. When the anulus is adequately removed, the intervertebral mobility will be noticeably increased.

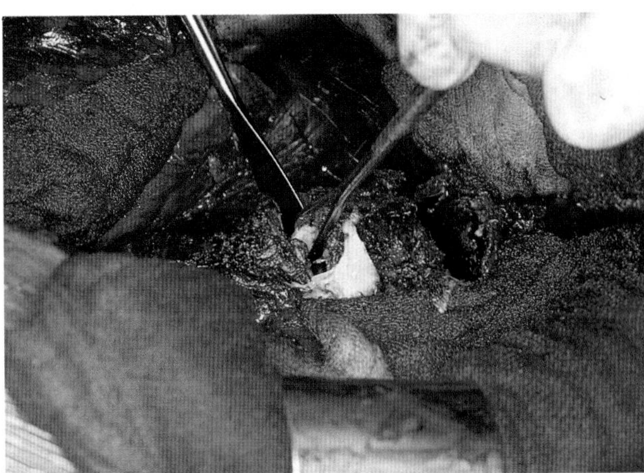

Figure 9. Ring curettes are used to remove the cartilaginous end plate on both sides of the interspace. A Cobb elevator inserted into the interspace and twisted on its side serves to open the interspace for better visualization.

line before placing the first screw. Because the apical vertebra is the most rotated into the deformity, the apical screw will be the most posterior in the construct, even though the anatomic entry site is the same on each vertebra. The appropriate width staple is chosen for each vertebra so that the tines enter the vertebral body close to the end plates (Fig. 11). The staples are inserted with an awl, which also makes the starting hole for the vertebral screws. If the bone is hard, a small osteotome may be used to help start the staples.

The length of the screw is estimated using a caliper over the vertebral body (Fig. 12). The screw is then inserted and directed toward the surgeon's finger, which is placed on the opposite side of the vertebral body. The tip of the screw must be palpated as it exits the vertebra (Fig. 13). It is very important that the screw grip the second cortex and equally important that it not protrude more than a few millimeters beyond the cortex. The screw should be parallel to the disc spaces and perpendicular to the cortex of the body. The groove in the screw should face posteriorly, since the rod will always be placed behind the screw. This is necessary because the nuts of the I-bolts must face forward in order to be accessible for tightening.

Rod Contouring

The rod is contoured to match an ideal lordosis. Thus the lower thoracic segment of the rod should be straight, whereas the lumbar segment should approximate a 40-degree lordosis. The corrected spine will usually reflect slightly less lordosis than the actual rod contour; thus a slight exaggeration of the lordotic curve should be contoured into the rod. This contour almost always matches the scoliotic contour of the vertebrae. The rod should be placed against the screws, and it should be relatively easy to displace the vertebrae enough to bring the screw up against the rod. If the vertebrae cannot be brought against the rod, either the screw placement or the rod contour is incorrect. The rod is cut to length with a minimum of overhang beyond the end screws. The hex end of the rod should be at the end with the best exposure for applying the rotation wrench.

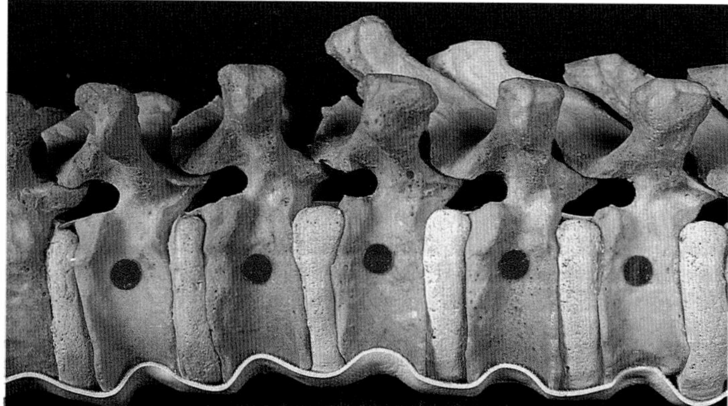

Figure 10. The screws enter each vertebra at a point just anterior to the junction of the pedicle with the body. The apical vertebra is the most severely rotated vertebra, and the screw in that vertebra will lie most posterior in the field. The screws must be aligned with one another without abrupt changes in angulation.

Assembly of the Construct

One I-bolt is placed on the rod for each screw in the construct. The nuts should be backed off until resistance is felt so that they may be easily placed over the screws. The vertebrae may need to be manually displaced laterally to reach the rod. Once the nuts are placed in each screw, the nuts are tightened until the rod is secured in the groove of the screw (Fig. 14).

Rod Rotation

The rotation wrench is applied to the rod, and the central portion of the rod is gripped with vise pliers. The rod is gradually rotated until the contour of the rod

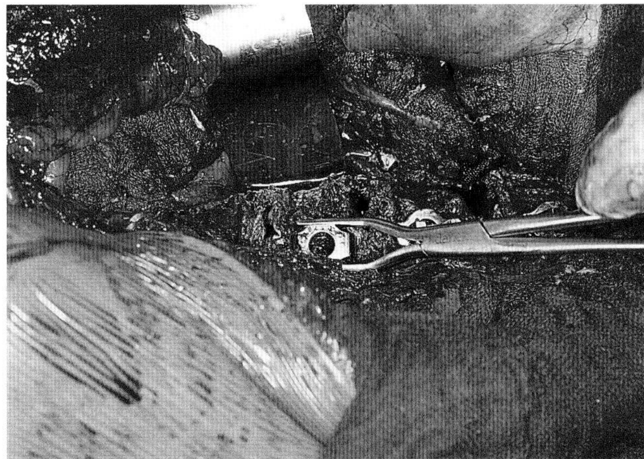

Figure 11. The staples are inserted into the vertebrae with the tines as close as possible to the end plates. They are held in place with a staple holder and inserted with an awl-driver tool.

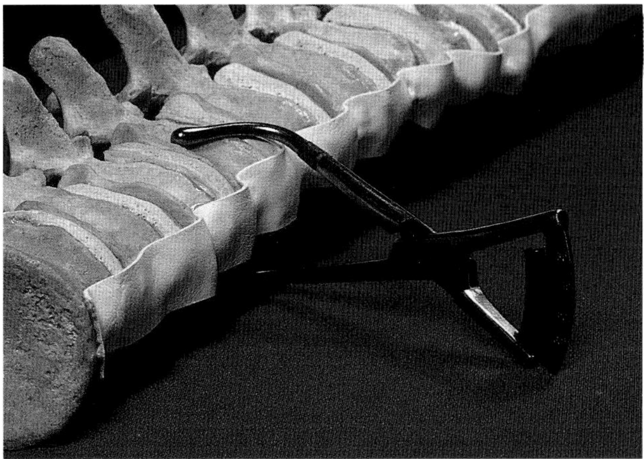

Figure 12. A caliper is used to estimate the appropriate length of the screw.

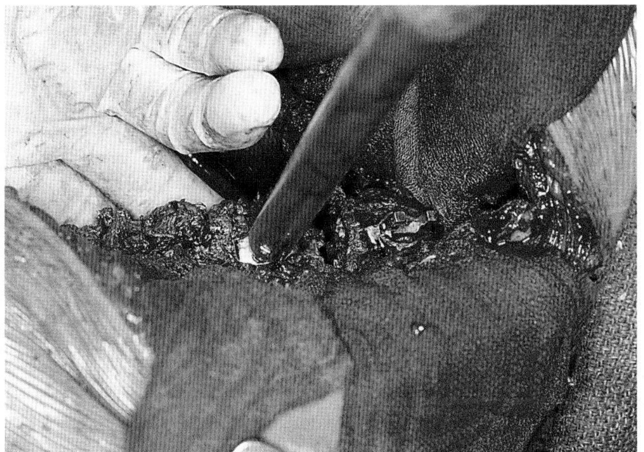

Figure 13. The screw is directed obliquely across the vertebral body toward the surgeon's finger. The tip of the screw should be just palpable as it exits the opposite cortex of the vertebra. A screw that does not grip this cortex may have inadequate purchase, and a screw that is too long may cause vascular injury.

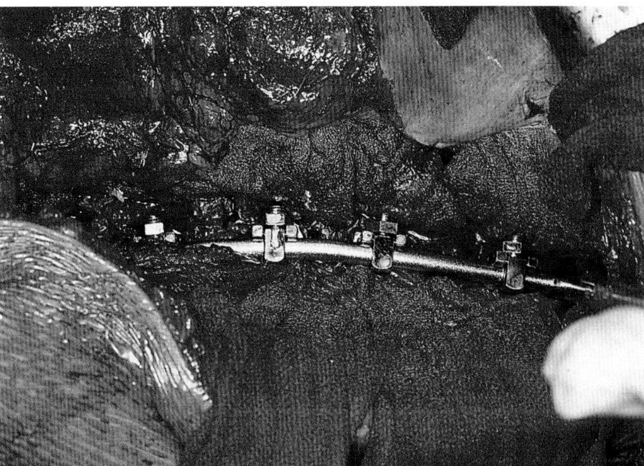

Figure 14. The rod is contoured into a gentle lordotic curve. The curve of the rod should slightly exceed the desired final lumbar lordosis, since some of the contour is not translated to the vertebrae. The I-bolts are placed into the heads of the screws with the nuts facing anteriorly. The groove of the screw head must abut the rod. The nuts are tightened enough to hold the rod in place.

lies in the AP plane (Fig. 15). In the final position the rod should mirror the normal spinal lordosis. Manual pressure on the flank may facilitate rotation in more rigid deformities.

Compression

The apical vertebra is fixed to the rod by firmly tightening the nut at that level. Bone graft is placed into the disc spaces. The adjacent vertebrae are compressed to the apical vertebra using a compression device. Intermittent pressure with a rod pusher enables the vertebrae to be more easily approximated. After the compression maneuver, the nuts are tightened firmly. Finally the end vertebrae are compressed toward the apex, and again the nuts are tightened. The surgeon should watch the screw-vertebral interface during these maneuvers to avoid loosening the screws. Final nut tightening is performed against a screw stabilizer so that maximum torque may be applied between the nut and the screw (Fig. 16). The periosteum of the vertebral body is elevated to expose more bone surface for fusion, and residual bone graft (usually strips of rib) is then laid over the adjacent vertebral bodies.

Closure

The pleura and psoas muscle are closed over the instrumentation using an absorbable running suture (Fig. 17). The diaphragm is closed with both running and interrupted sutures using the marker sutures for realignment. A chest tube is

A
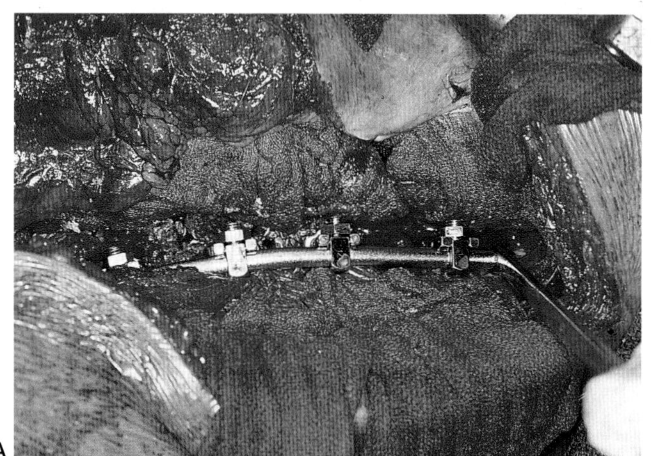

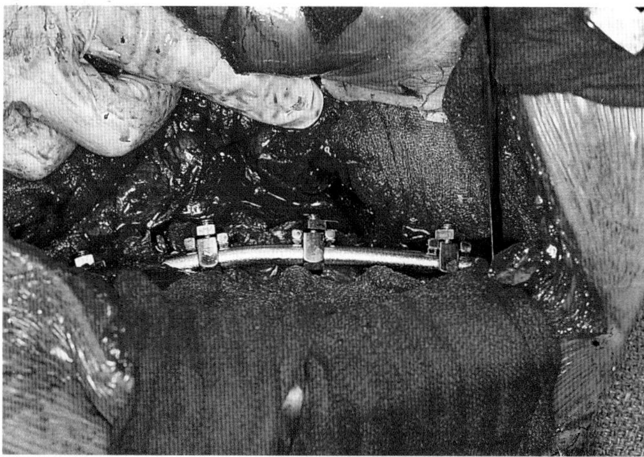
B

C
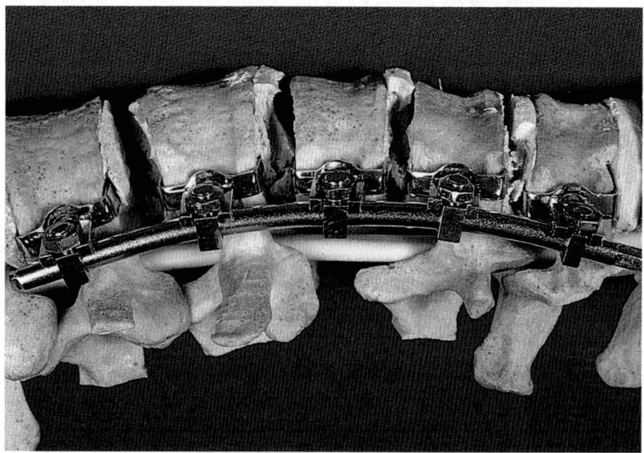

Figure 15. The rod is rotated with the rotation wrench until the lordotic contour of the rod is fully rotated into the sagittal plane. The apical nut is tightened to maintain the rotation. **A:** Rod in place before rotation **B:** Rod in place after rotation **C:** Model of spine with the rod rotated into the lordotic position.

placed in a lateral position so that it will not be occluded when the patient lies supine. The intercostal space is closed with interrupted pericostal sutures and running intercostal sutures.

POSTOPERATIVE MANAGEMENT

The chest tube is removed on about the third postoperative day providing no pneumothorax or hemothorax are present. Hospital discharge is usually on the sixth or seventh postoperative day. In cooperative patients with normal bone strength, no postoperative immobilization is required. These patients should refrain from lifting and bending activities for 4 months, and no sports are allowed for at least 6 months. If any question exists on the adequacy of vertebral fixation, relative either to screw placement or vertebral strength, a prefabricated brace such as the Boston overlap type is used for 3 to 4 months postoperatively. A similar brace or cast immobilization is used for uncooperative patients. Follow-up radiographs are taken at 2, 4, 6, and 12 months and are evaluated for intervertebral fusion and integrity of the construct.

COMPLICATIONS

Immediate postoperative complications include respiratory difficulties, which are uncommon in healthy patients. Pneumothorax, hemothorax, chylothorax, and delayed splenic rupture have been reported after anterior exposures. Lower lumbar exposures in male patients may be complicated by retrograde ejaculation if the superior hypogastric plexus is injured. This sympathetic ganglion is usually found at the third or fourth lumbar vertebral level, and care should be taken to avoid injury to this structure. Later complications include screw loosening in the vertebra and loosening of the nuts with loss of fixation to the rod. The later complications may be prevented by careful intraoperative screw placement and nut tightening. We have seen progression of the thoracic curve above the instrumented curve. This problem is more likely when the thoracic curve exceeds 40 degrees and the patient is immature.

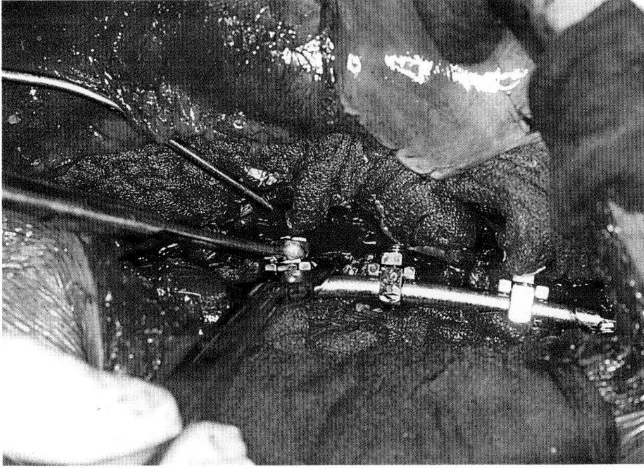

Figure 16. The bone graft is placed into the intervertebral spaces and the adjacent vertebrae are compressed to the apical vertebra. Ideally the spaces are fully closed by the compression maneuver. After compression the nuts are tightened against a screw stabilizer. The rod should be well seated into the groove of the screw, and the cork-screw device may be used to accomplish this. The nuts should be made as tight as possible.

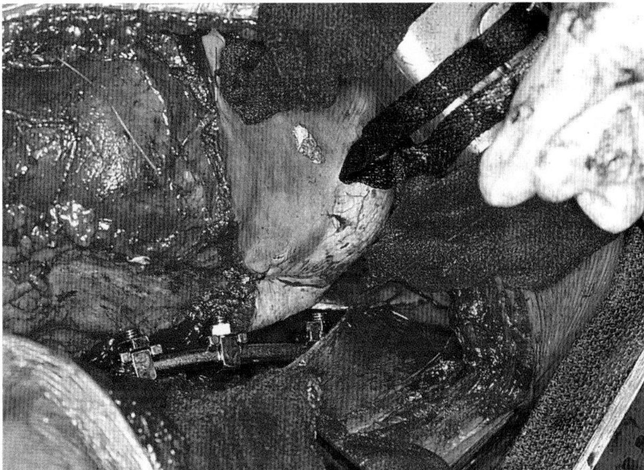

Figure 17. Bone graft is placed over the vertebral bodies after elevating the periosteum. The pleura and psoas muscle are closed over the instrumentation.

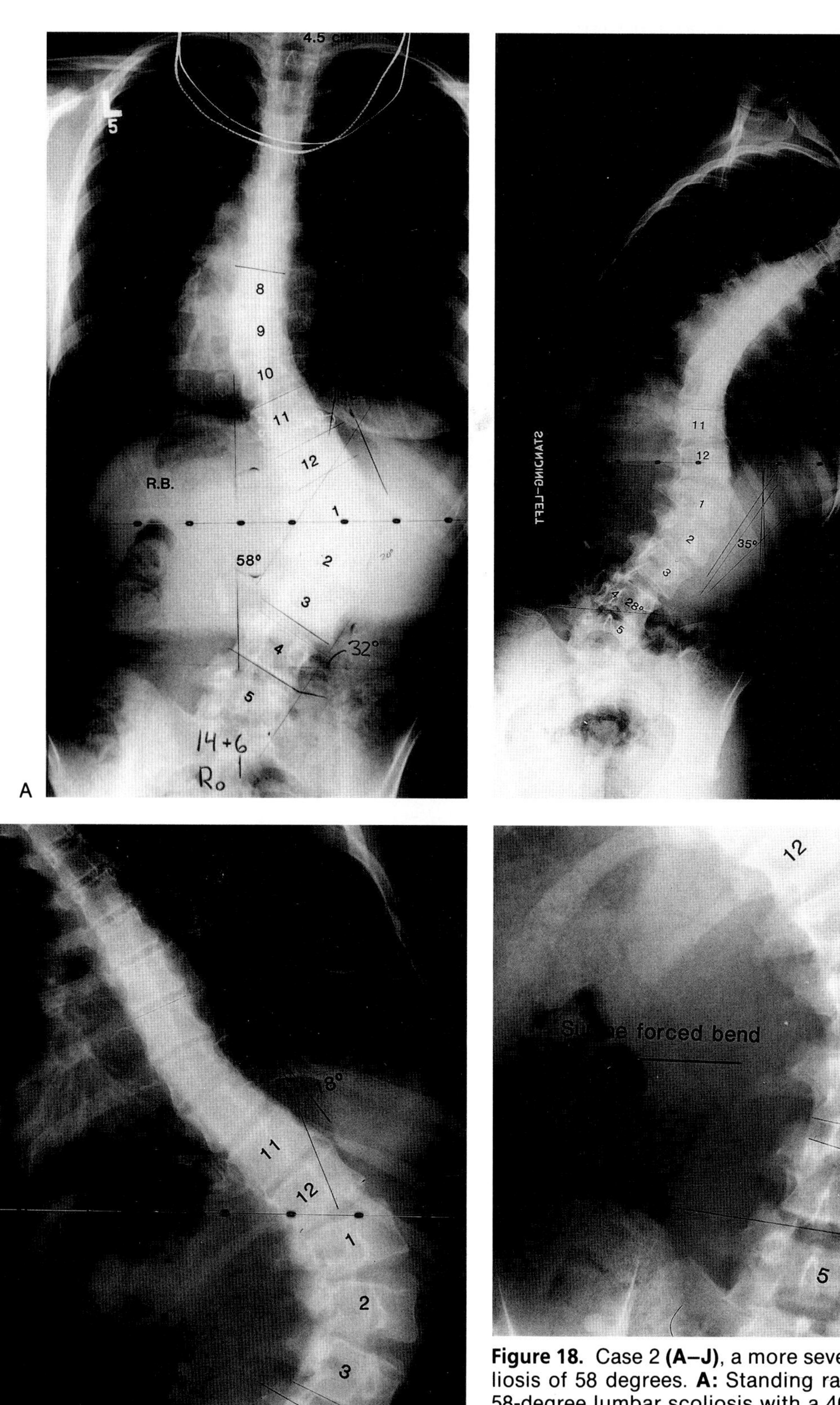

Figure 18. Case 2 **(A–J)**, a more severe right lumbar scoliosis of 58 degrees. **A:** Standing radiograph showing a 58-degree lumbar scoliosis with a 40-degree compensatory thoracic curve. **B:** A standing right bending radiograph that shows correction of the primary curve to 35 degrees. **C:** The standing left bending radiograph shows almost no correction of the tilt of L3 and L4. Based on this film, surgery was postponed. **D:** A supine forced bending radiograph done the next day shows good flexibility of the lumbar segment with the L3–L4 space opening on the right. Based on this information an instrumentation to L3 was performed.

ILLUSTRATIVE CASE FOR TECHNIQUE

In the second example (Fig. 18), a more severe right lumbar curve of 58 degrees, the standing bending films fail to show realignment of the L3 vertebrae, indicating a possibly rigid lower lumbar segment. However, the forced supine bending radiograph demonstrates sufficient flexibility of these lower vertebrae. An instrumentation to L3 provided excellent correction of the rotational deformity and trunk shift. The persistence of an open disc space at the L3–L4 level is noted; the significance of this finding is conjectural.

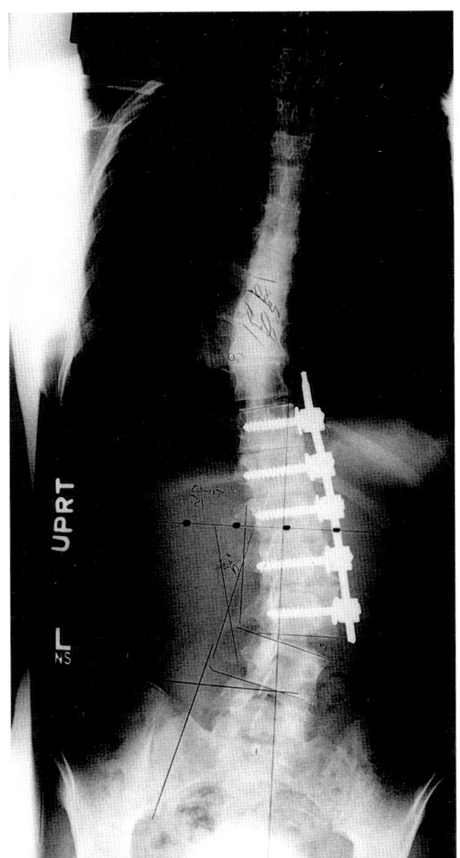

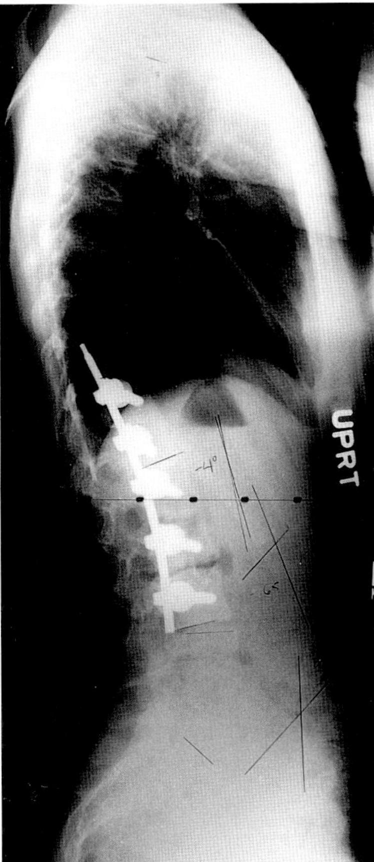

E,F

Figure 18. (*Continued.*) **E:** A postoperative standing radiograph showing correction of the primary curve to 28 degrees. The trunk is well balanced. The L3–L4 interspace is open, a finding of uncertain significance. **F:** A standing lateral postoperative radiograph showing excellent maintenance of lordosis.

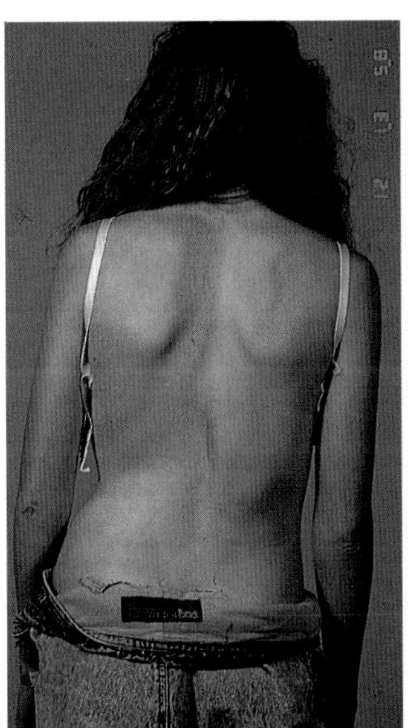
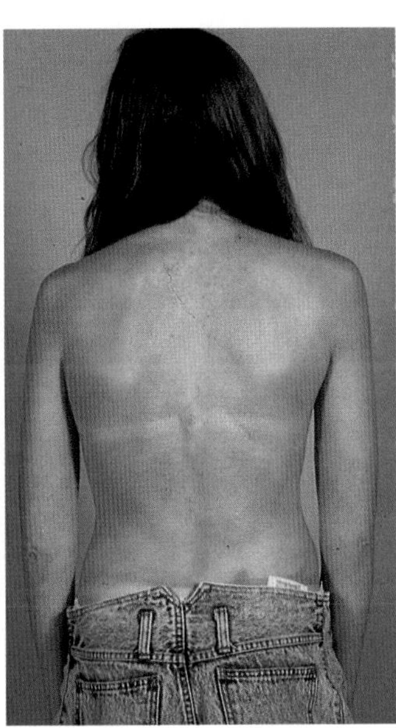
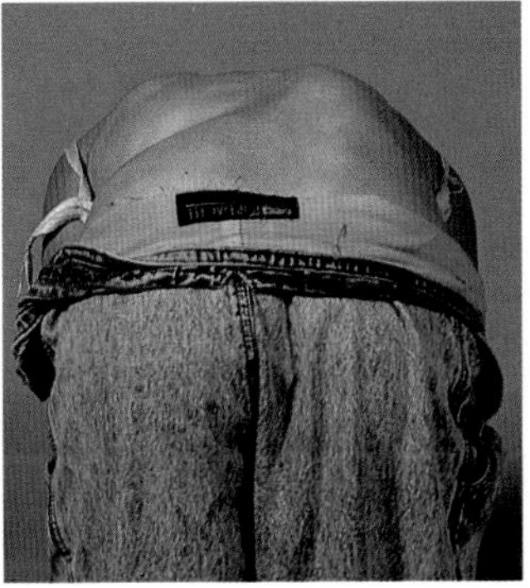
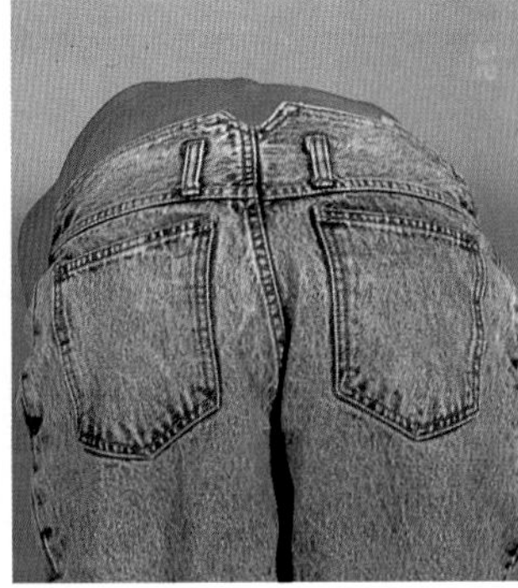

G,H

Figure 18. (*Continued.*) **G:** A preoperative photograph showing trunk shift to the right. **H:** A postoperative photograph showing correction of the trunk shift. **I:** A preoperative photograph in the forward bend position demonstrating elevation of the right flank due to lumbar rotation. **J:** A postoperative photograph showing complete correction of the lumbar rotation.

RECOMMENDED READING

1. Anderson, P. R., Puno, M. R., and Lovell, S. L.: Postoperative respiratory complications in non-idiopathic scoliosis. *Acta Anaesthesiol. Scand.*, 29: 186–192, 1985.
2. Colletta, A. J., and Mayer, P. J.: Chylothorax: an unusual complication of anterior thoracic interbody spinal fusion. *Spine*, 7: 46–49, 1982.
3. Dwyer, A. F.: Experience of anterior correction of scoliosis. *Clin. Orthop.*, 93: 191–214, 1973.
4. Flynn, J. D., and Price, C. T.: Sexual complications of anterior fusion of the lumbar spine. *Spine*, 9: 489–492, 1984.
5. Hodge, W. A., and Dewald, R. L.: Splenic injury complicating the anterior thoracoabdominal surgical approach for scoliosis. *J. Bone Joint Surg.*, 65: 396–397, 1983.
6. Zielke, K., Hack, H. P., and Harms J.: Spinal instrumentation. In: *The Paediatric Spine*, edited by D. S. Bradford and R. M. Hensinger, p. 491–517. Thieme, New York, 1985.

Master Techniques in Orthopaedic Surgery,
THE SPINE, edited by D. S. Bradford,
Lippincott-Raven Publishers, Philadelphia, © 1997.

21

Posterior TSRH Instrumentation

John A. Herring

INDICATIONS/CONTRAINDICATIONS

The Texas Scottish Rite Hospital (TSRH) instrumentation system is a versatile system that enables the surgeon to tailor the surgical construct to the best correction of many different deformities. The principal corrective manuever is rod rotation with hooks placed in distraction to correct a thoracic scoliosis or compression to correct a lumbar curve. When the nuts are lightly tensioned, distraction is maintained, and the rod may be rotated without loss of hook position. The open hook design allows the rod to be used as a cantilever to correct the lateral curvature of a thoracolumbar scoliosis. In addition, the rod may be used as an anteroposterior (AP) cantilever in the correction of kyphotic deformities. The open hooks also allow for a single rod to be used in a double thoracic deformity, with the upper hooks seated after rod rotation.

Another major versatility is the ability to use the same instrumentation system anteriorly and posteriorly. This is especially helpful when doing sequential or simultaneous anterior and posterior procedures. A final advantage of this system is the ease of revision or removal of instruments. Months or years after a primary procedure, the I-bolt connecting nuts can be loosened for rod removal or for additional instrumentation. Existing hooks within the fusion mass may be reused with a new construct. Hooks designed to fit beneath a thick fusion are also available.

The well-established indications for an instrumentation and fusion in idiopathic scoliosis include the following:

A progressive curve in a skeletally immature patient that is too severe for brace management

J. A. Herring, M.D.: Department of Orthopaedic Surgery, University of Texas Southwestern Medical Center at Dallas; Texas Scottish Rite Hospital for Children, Dallas, Texas 75219–3993.

A deformity that is cosmetically unacceptable in a skeletally mature patient.
A deformity that is likely to progress in adulthood.

The contraindications to this procedure include pulmonary function inadequate to undergo a major surgical procedure, an active infection in any organ, anemia, and any other major medical conditions that have not been carefully evaluated. With the use of blood salvage techniques, refusal to receive transfusion is not a contraindication in the ordinary case.

PREOPERATIVE PLANNING

A thorough general physical evaluation is essential in preparing for a major surgical operation. Any history of excessive hemorrhage should be evaluated with appropriate hematologic studies. A careful neurologic evaluation including evaluation of abdominal reflexes is necessary to detect the occasional case of tethered spinal cord or syringomyelia. A magnetic resonance imaging (MRI) scan of the spinal cord should be performed if any question exists of a neurogenic etiology. The presence of a left thoracic primary scoliosis requires a neurologic evaluation, usually including an MRI scan, because of the frequent association between this curve pattern and underlying spinal cord disorders. Autologous blood collection should be used whenever feasible.

Specific preoperative studies should include standing AP and lateral radiographs, along with standing right and left bending radiographs. A spot lateral radiograph of the lumbosacral spine is helpful to rule out spondylolisthesis. The

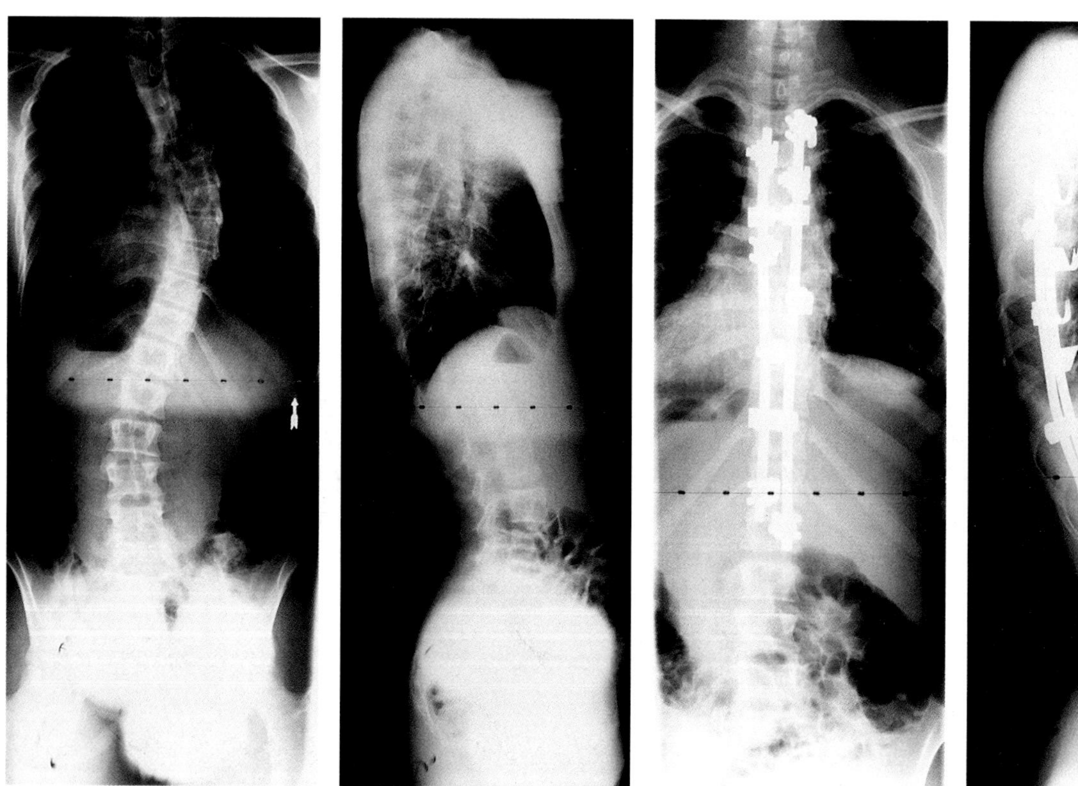

A,B C,D

Figure 1. King-Moe type III curve. The hook placement pattern is known as the standard right thoracic pattern. **A:** Anteroposterior radiograph showing a 40-degree right thoracic scoliosis. **B:** Lateral radiograph showing a normal contour. **C:** Anteroposterior radiograph showing postoperative correction to 14 degrees. *Right,* two upgoing pedicle hooks and two downgoing laminar hooks; *left,* a proximal claw of a transverse process hook and a pedicle hook, a central pedicle hook, and a lower upgoing laminar hook. **D:** A postoperative lateral radiograph showing a physiologic kyphosis.

hook insertion plan is drawn on the radiograph preoperatively and referred to intraoperatively.

In the King-Moe curve pattern III, which is usually a right thoracic deformity, the "right thoracic pattern" for hook placement is used (Fig. 1). First the end vertebrae of the curve are determined by marking the maximally inclined vertebral end plates at the top and bottom of the curve. These vertebrae may usually be used as the end vertebrae instrumented, but the lateral radiograph must also be evaluated. If the lower vertebra chosen lies at or above a junctional kyphosis, instrumentation will need to be carried one or two levels lower so that the lower hook lies below the kyphosis.

The right side of the right thoracic pattern consists of a pedicle hook proximally, a laminar hook distally, and at the apex of the curve a pedicle and laminar hook facing opposite directions with two or three vertebrae between them. On the left side is a transverse process-pedicle claw hook configuration at the top. These hooks may be on a single vertebrae, or preferably two adjacent vertebrae. At the apex of the curve is a pedicle hook, and at the caudal end an upgoing laminar hook.

In the King-Moe type IV curve, the lower vertebrae of the curve extend into the lumbar spine (Fig. 2). In these cases it is necessary to use a reverse hook

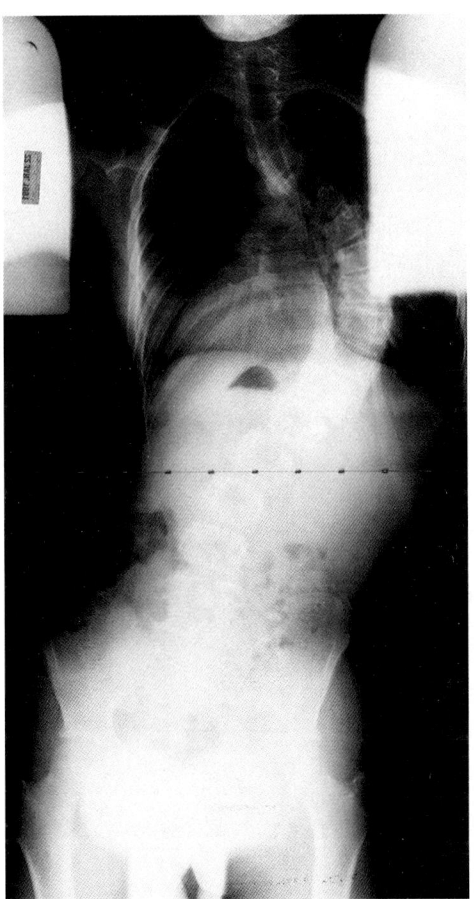

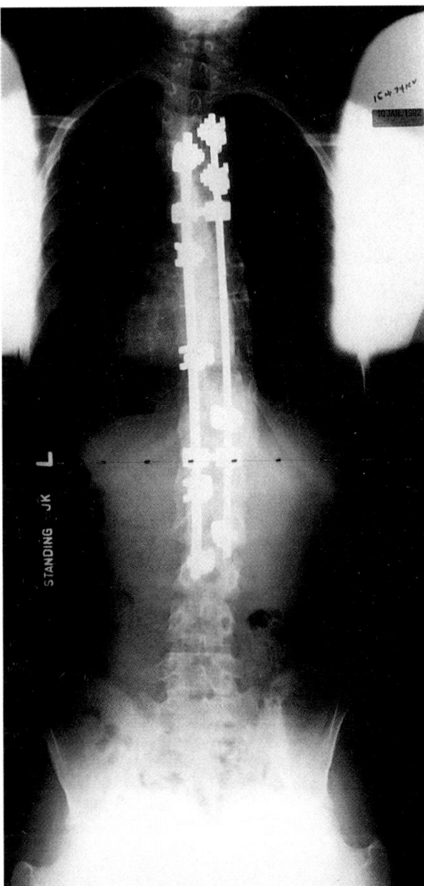

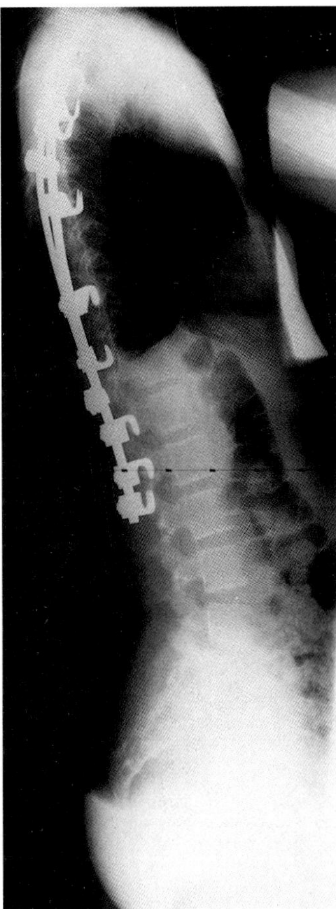

A,B C

Figure 2. A King-Moe type IV curve. The hook placement used here is known as the hook reversal pattern. **A:** Anteroposterior radiograph showing an 86-degree right thoracic scoliosis. **B:** Anteroposterior radiograph following instrumentation with correction of the scoliosis to 18 degrees. Compared with the right thoracic pattern in case 1, an additional upgoing hook is seen at L2 on the left. On the right the lowest hook is now downfacing. The purpose of this pattern is to induce lordosis into the lumbar portion of the construct. **C:** A postoperative lateral radiograph showing a neutral thoracolumbar junction.

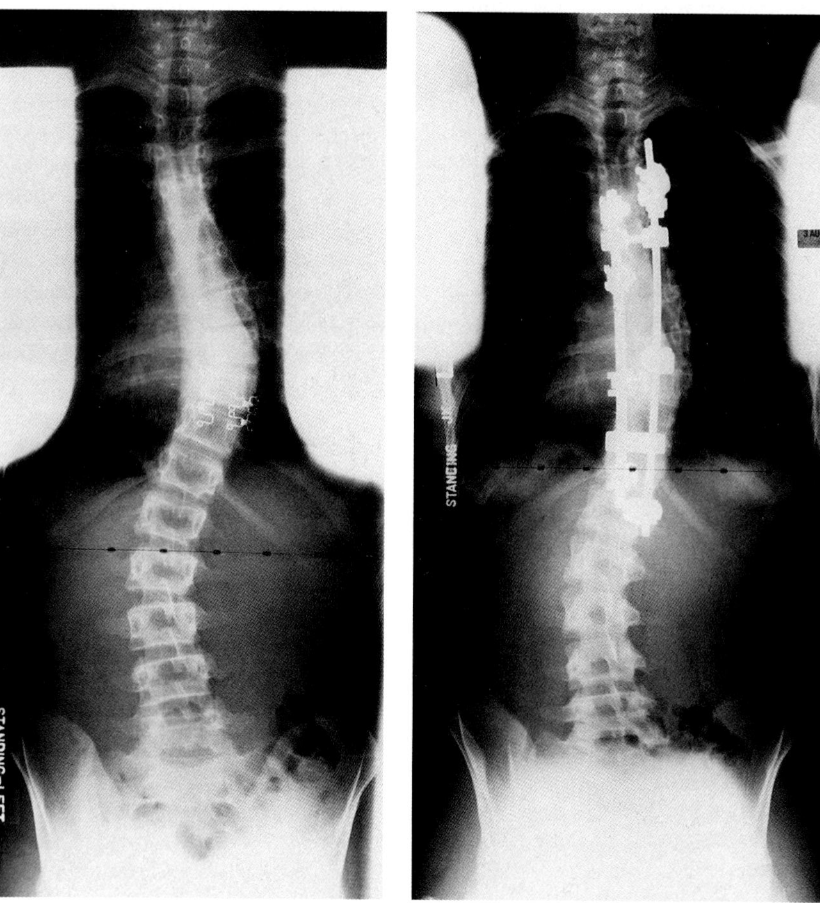

A,B

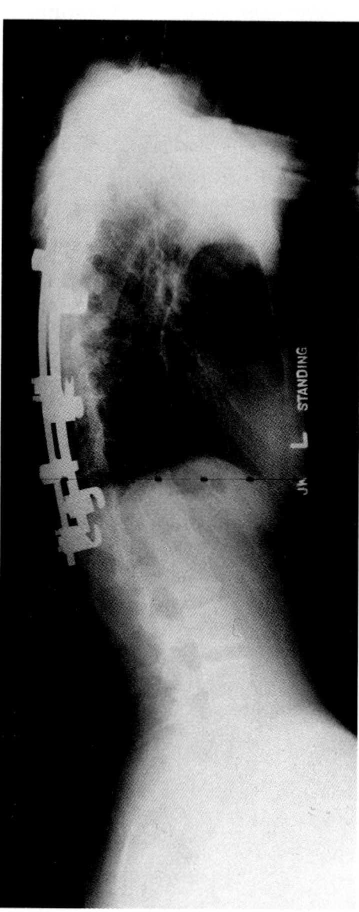

C

Figure 3. A King-Moe type II curve. The lumbar component of this deformity is mild, and the right thoracic pattern of hook placement is appropriate. **A:** Anteroposterior radiograph showing a 40-degree right thoracic and a 30-degree left lumbar scoliosis. **B:** Postoperative radiograph showing correction of the curve to 32 degrees. Greater degrees of correction of the thoracic portion of the King II curve may result in decompensation to the left. **C:** Lateral radiograph showing a normal kyphosis.

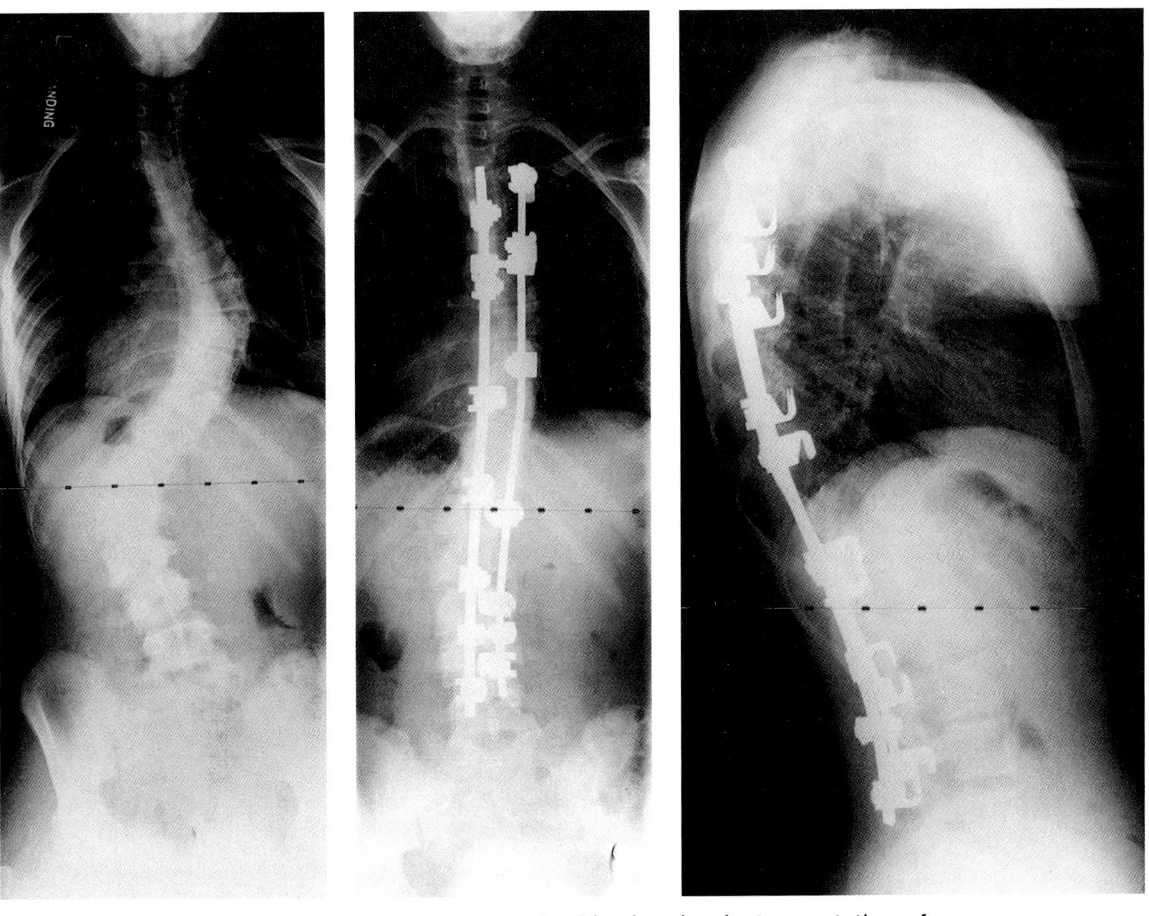

Figure 4. A more severe King-Moe type II curve. In this situation instrumentation of both the thoracic and lumbar curves is necessary. **A:** Anteroposterior radiograph showing a right thoracic curve of 60 degrees and a left lumbar curve of 55 degrees. **B:** Postoperative radiograph showing correction of the thoracic curve to 21 degrees and the lumbar curve to 25 degrees. The spine is well compensated. The hooks on the left, from top to bottom, are two upward pedicle hooks, three downward laminar hooks, and two upward laminar hooks. *Right*, a transverse-pedicle claw, a central pedicle hook, two upward laminar hooks, and a downward laminar hook. **C:** Postoperative lateral radiograph showing kyphosis of the thoracic spine and lordosis of the lumbar spine. The compression instrumentation of the lumbar segment is essential to produce the lordosis.

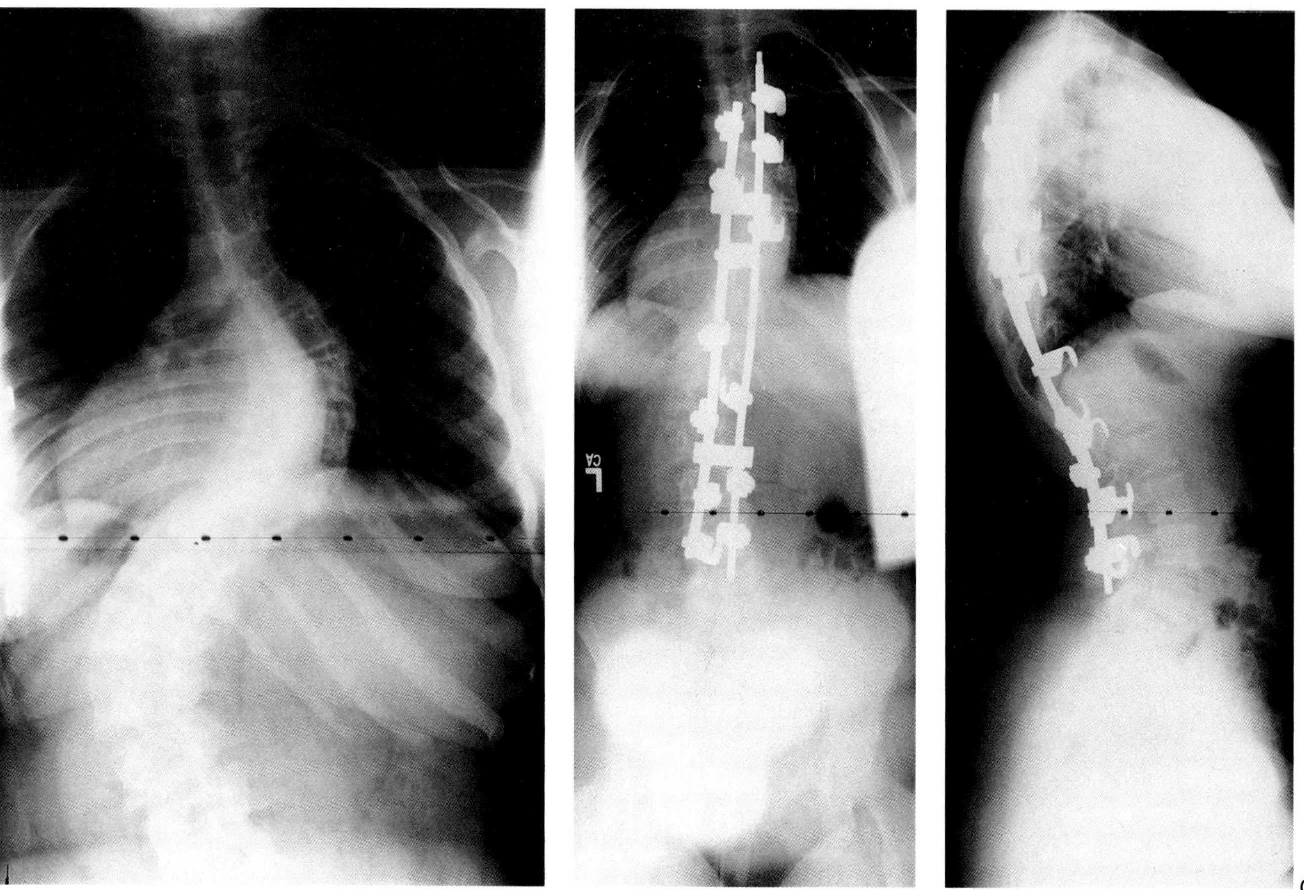

Figure 5. A more severe King-Moe type II curve, which requires instrumentation of both the thoracic and lumbar curves. **A:** Anteroposterior radiograph showing 74-degree curves. **B:** Postoperative radiograph showing correction of the curves to 34 and 28 degrees. The spine remains balanced. **C:** Postoperative lateral radiograph showing normal sagittal contours.

pattern on the concave side of the curve to restore lumbar lordosis in the appropriate segment of the curve. This can be easily added to the lower end of the right thoracic pattern by having an upgoing hook on the lower vertebra and a downgoing hook at the end of the thoracic segment. At the same time the lower hook of the convex side is now placed in a downgoing direction on the same lower vertebra. In the King-Moe type II curve, decision making is more difficult. In less severe curves with a lumbar component of less than 40 degrees, often a selective fusion of the thoracic component is appropriate (Fig. 3). This is done with the usual "right thoracic" pattern. If the lumbar curve is more severe and significantly rotated, a double curve instrumentation pattern is required (Figs. 4 and 5). With small variations this resembles a right thoracic pattern on top of a left thoracic pattern. Thus a distraction pattern is present on the left side of the right thoracic curve, and a compression pattern on the left side of the left lumbar curve. It is important to apply compression forces to the lumbar component of any curve in order to restore lumbar lordosis.

SURGERY

Positioning

The patient is positioned prone on a scoliosis operating frame, which allows the abdomen to fall forward without compression. The surgeon should take care that no pressure is placed on the arms by the frame. The lower supports of the frame should be distal to the anterior iliac spines. The spine is exposed subperiosteally out to the tips of the transverse processes over the levels to be instrumented. It is helpful to expose one extra level proximally to facilitate upper hook insertion.

Hook Placement

The first step in placing a pedicle hook is to make a transverse osteotomy in the inferior articular process of the chosen vertebra (Fig. 6). The placement of this osteotomy is such that the tips of the pedicle hook will engage the pedicle as the shoulder of the hook touches the inferior articular process (the location if the pedicle corresponds to the midpoint of the base of the transverse process). The full thickness of the inferior articular process should be removed, exposing the

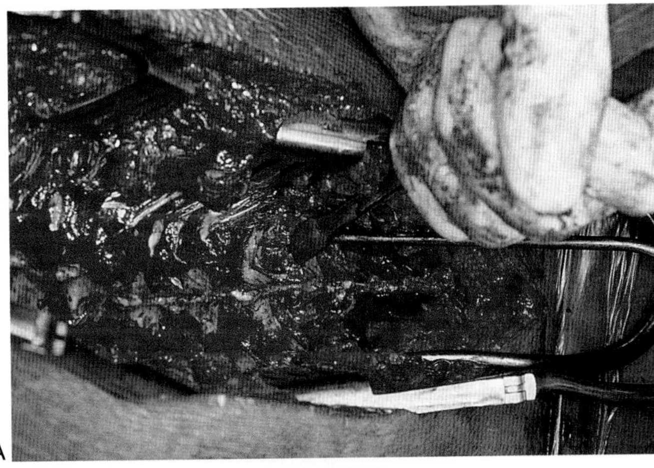

A

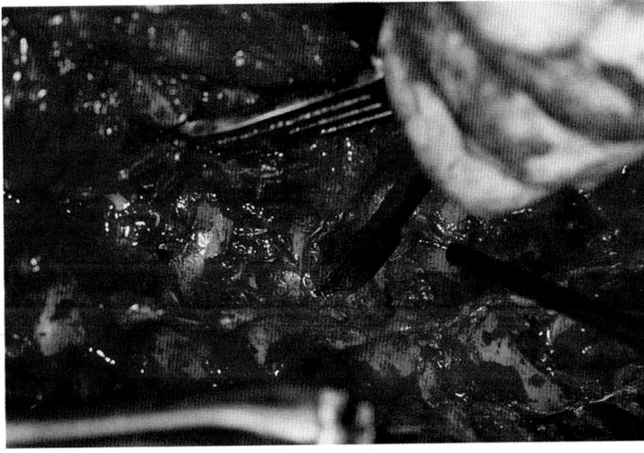

B

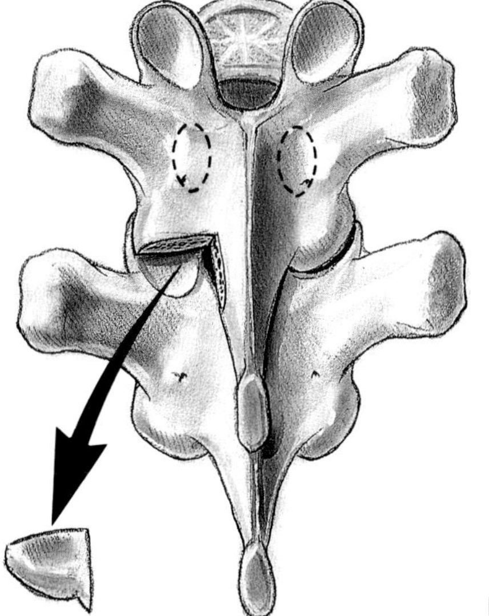

B′

Figure 6. Pedicle hook placement. **A:** A transverse cut is made with an osteotome through the inferior articular process. This cut is placed about 5 mm inferior to the junction of the transverse process with the lamina. **B:** A vertical cut is made in the inferior articular process. After this cut, the segment of bone over the facet is removed **(B′)** and the articular cartilage of the facet is seen.

Figure continues.

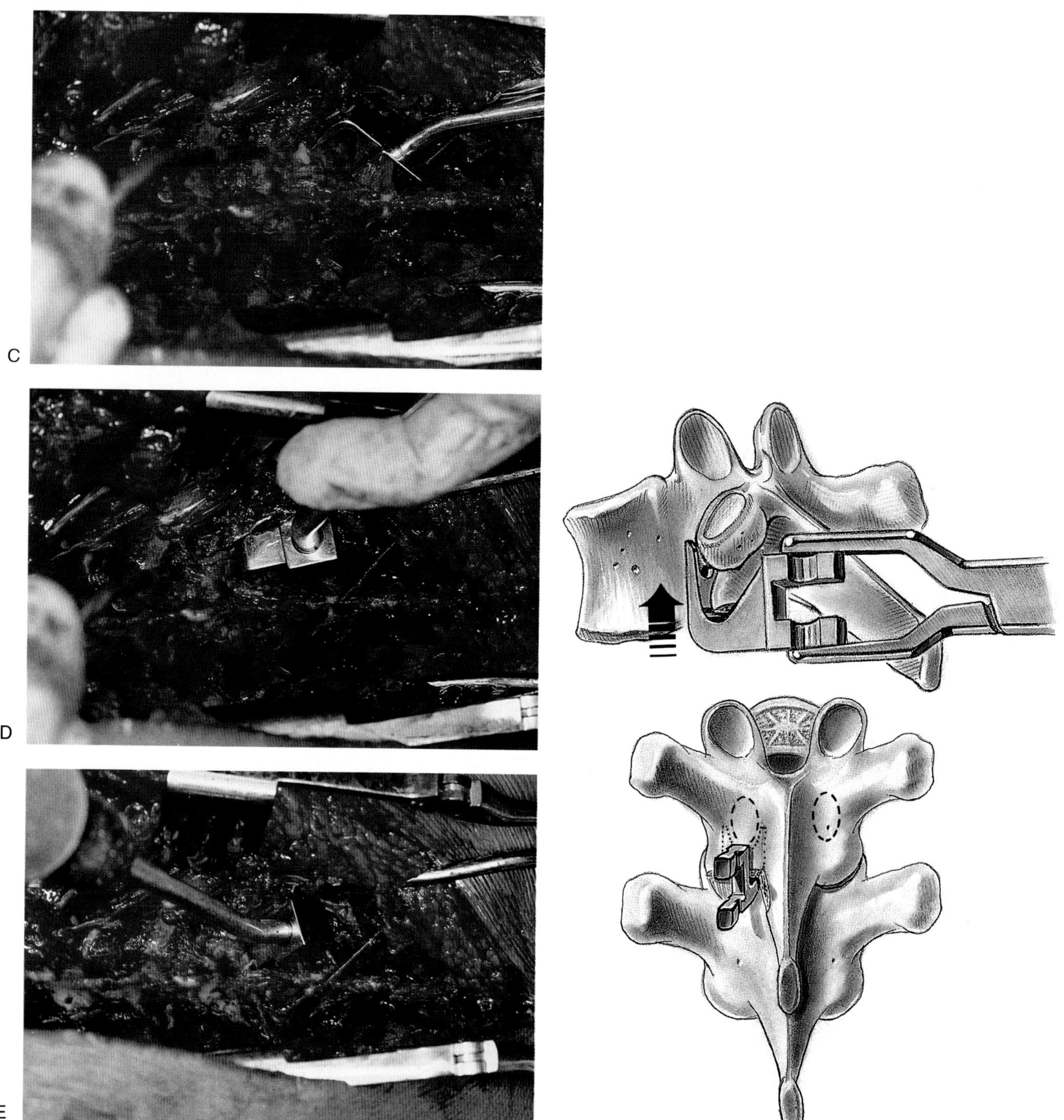

Figure 6. (*Continued.*) **C–E**. A trial pedicle hook is inserted into the facet. The trial hook is gently impacted with a mallet to seat it.

cartilage surface of the superior articular process of the next lower vertebra. The trial pedicle hook is inserted into the prepared site, and a gentle tap with a mallet will firmly seat it.

A caudal-facing laminar hook requires some carpentry to be correctly placed. First the facet is excised with a gouge, removing the inferior articular process of the next cephalad vertebra (Figs. 7 and 8). Then the spinous process of the cephalad vertebra is removed. The ligamentum flavum is then incised sharply and half the ligament removed with a Kerrison rongeur. The caudal edge of the lamina of the cephalad vertebra will usually need to be removed with the rongeur to allow space for placement of the hook. When the space is prepared, the red-handled trial hook is inserted. If the hook will not readily seat, it is often necessary to remove even more bone from the cephalad lamina.

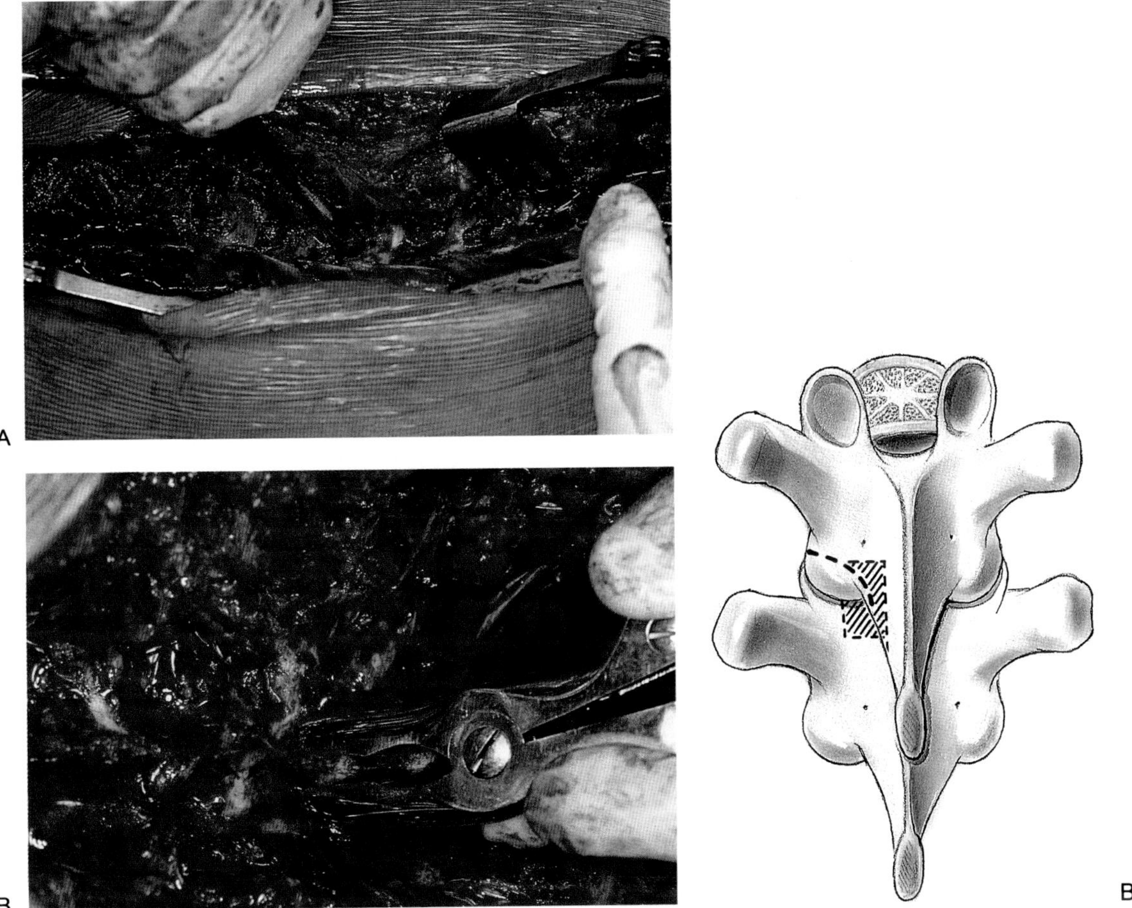

Figure 7. Laminar hook placement, facing in the caudal direction. **A:** A facetectomy is performed at the cephalad facet joint. **B, B′:** The spinous process that overlies the interspace is removed.

Figure continues.

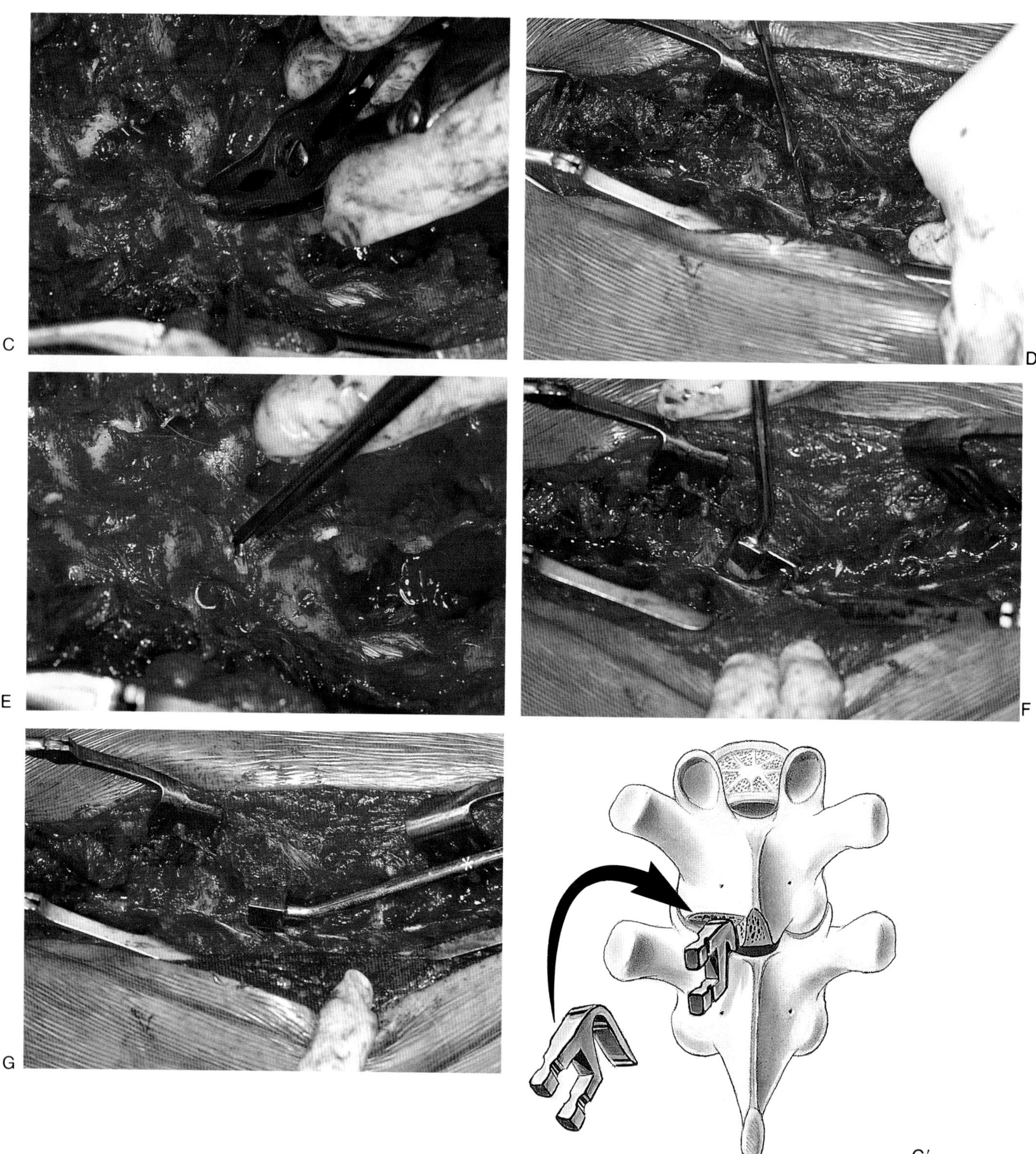

Figure 7. (*Continued.*) **C:** The interspinous ligament is removed. **D:** The ligamentum flavum is sharply incised. **E:** The ligamentum flavum is removed with a Kerrison rongeur. **F,G:** A trial hook (*) is placed into the interspace **(G′)**.

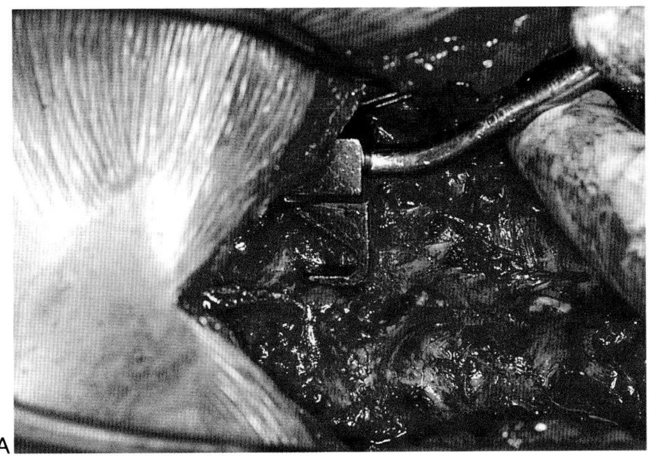

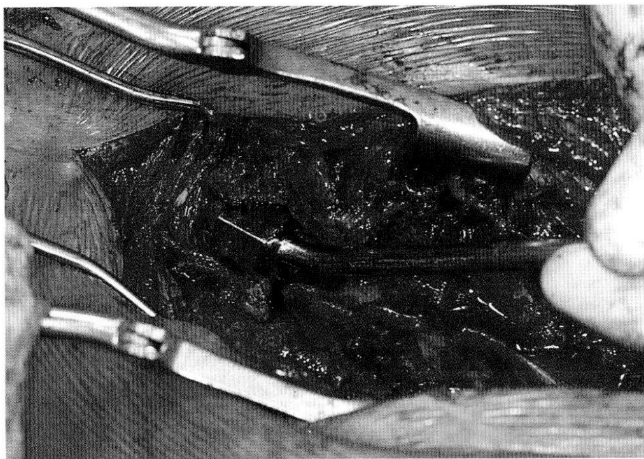

Figure 8. Lower laminar hook placement, caudal facing. **A:** The interspace is prepared as in Fig. 3. **B:** A trial hook is placed into the interspace.

An "upfacing" laminar hook may usually be placed with minimal laminar preparation (Fig. 9). The laminar elevator is inserted through the ligamentum flavum and the blue-handled trial hook inserted beneath the caudal edge of the lamina. When this hook is placed in the caudal-most vertebra to be instrumented, the interspinous ligament is exposed but preferably not excised. The final position of this lowest hook must be carefully monitored because it is easily dislodged. For a claw hook placement, the upper transverse process is exposed and a laminar elevator is then passed over the process (Fig. 10). The black-handled trial hook is then placed in the same location. A pedicle hook is then placed either on the same vertebra or preferably on the next lower vertebra.

Facetectomy and Decortication

After placing and removing the trial hooks at each level, a facetectomy is performed bilaterally (Fig. 11). The surgeon must keep track of the eventual hook

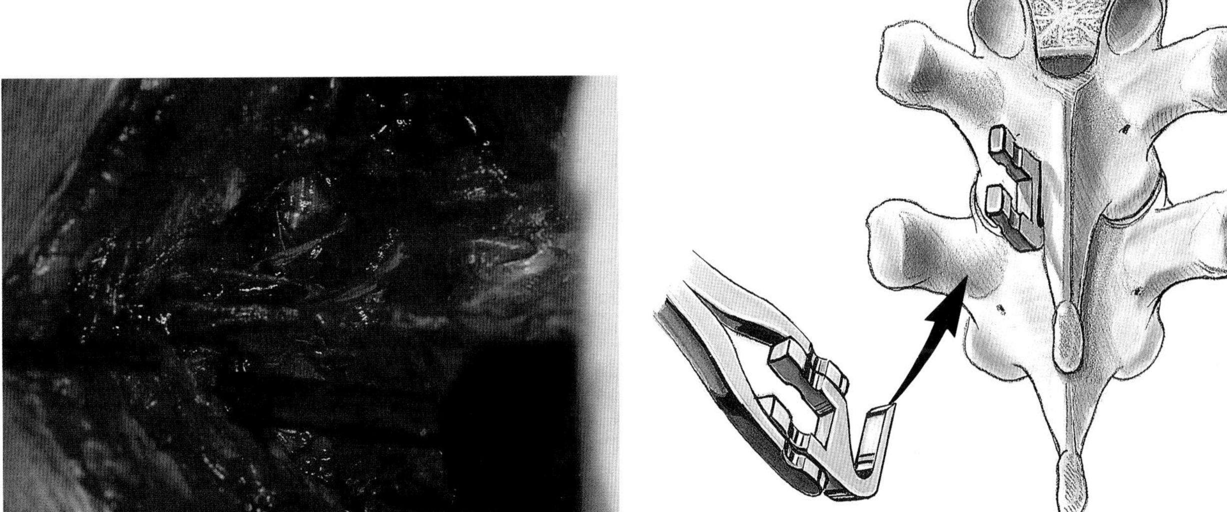

Figure 9. A&B: Placement of a cephalad-facing lower laminar hook. An elevator is used to pierce the ligamentum flavum over the caudal surface of the lamina. The trial hook is placed into the interspace (*black handle*).

A

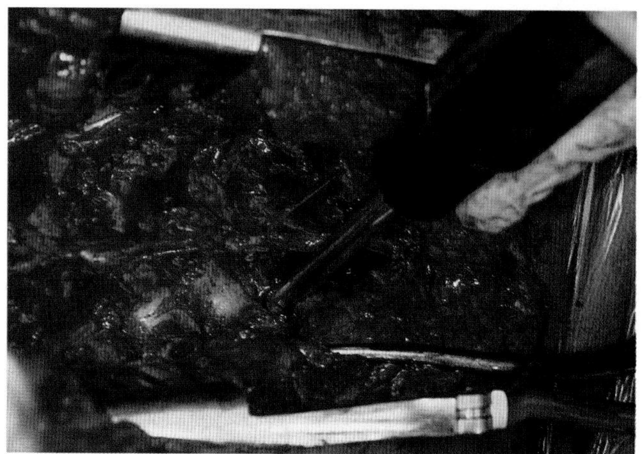

B

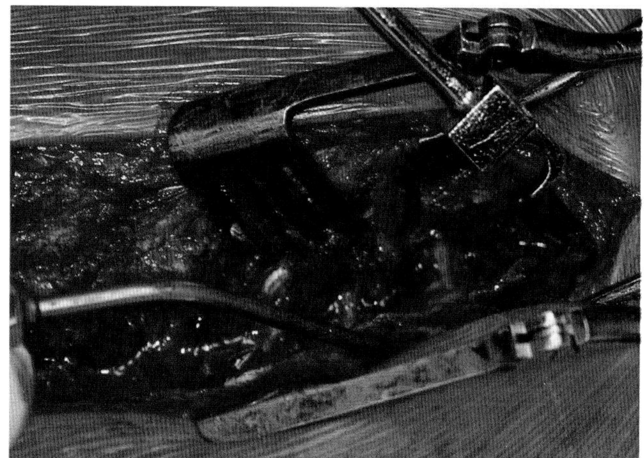

C

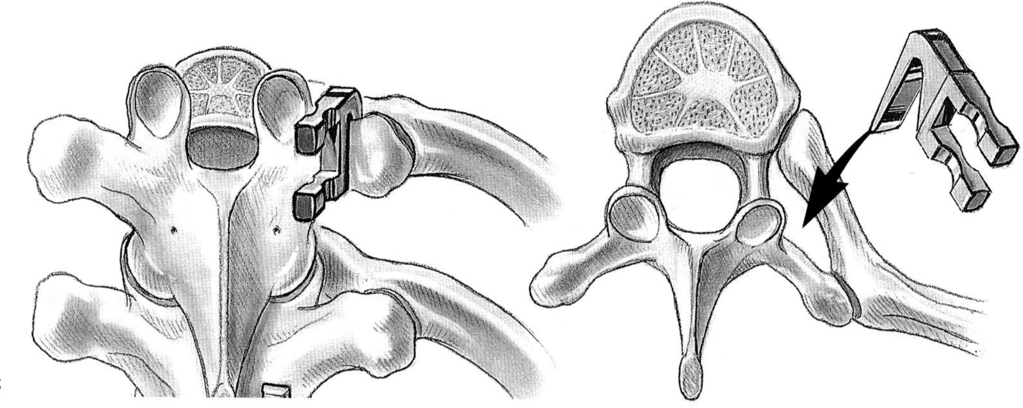

Figure 10. Transverse process hook placement. **A:** An elevator is passed beneath the periosteum of the transverse process. **B:** The trial hook is placed over the transverse process. **C:** Placement of the transverse process hook. The hook fits over the transverse process, between the process and the rib.

placement and avoid facetectomy of a pedicle hook site. Next the laminae and transverse processes are decorticated on the side of the spine to be instrumented first, usually the concave side.

Hook Insertion

The final hooks are then placed appropriately on the concave side and firmly seated. In most instances it is helpful to remove the hook holders. Bone graft taken from the iliac crest is then placed over the exposed bony surfaces.

Rod Contouring

Next the rod is contoured to match an ideal kyphosis. This contour also usually matches the existing scoliotic deformity (Fig. 12). The contoured rod is placed in the hooks to be certain the rod contour fits the spinal deformity. Some space between the apical hooks and the rod may be later closed by pulling the apical

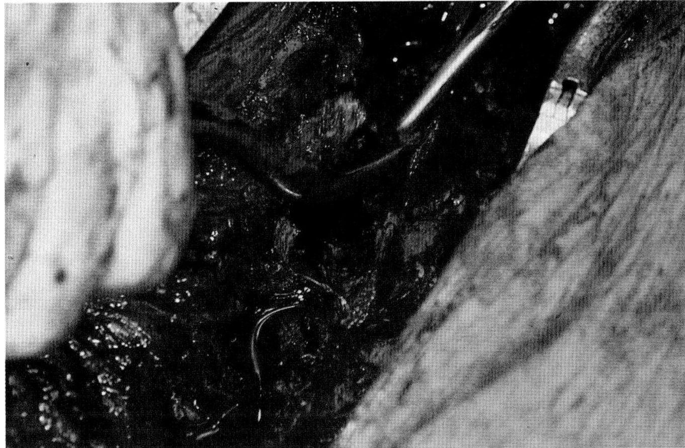

Figure 11. After all trial hooks have been placed, the facet joints are excised bilaterally. The laminae are decorticated on the concavity of the deformity and bone graft is placed over the laminae and transverse processes. Hooks are then inserted on the concavity.

A

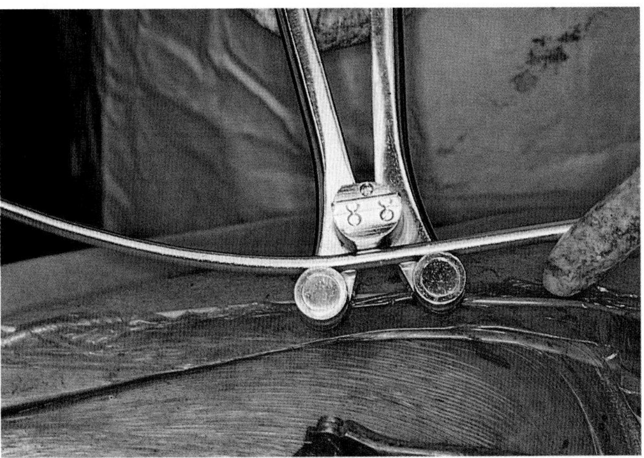

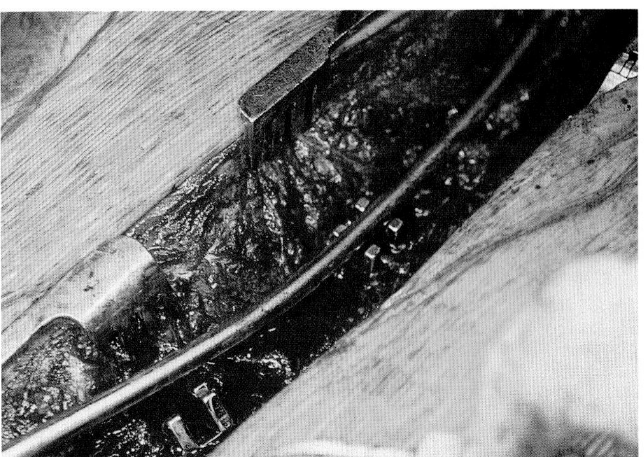

B

Figure 12. The rod (usually the ¼-inch flex rod) is contoured to an ideal kyphosis. **A:** The French benders are used to contour the rod. **B:** The rod is placed into the hooks to evaluate the contour.

vertebra to the rod. In a rigid deformity, this may not be possible, and further contouring of the rod will be required. The rod is cut to appropriate length, allowing for some distraction.

Assembly of the Construct

The rod is now inserted into the hooks with one I-bolt for each hook. An additional crosslink I-bolt must be placed on the rod in the appropriate position for each crosslink prior to insertion into the hooks (Fig. 13). The crosslinks should be placed as close to the ends of the construct as possible. Once the I-bolts are in the hooks, the nuts are tightened enough to hold the rod in the hook. If the hook will not reach the rod, the "corkscrew" is used to bring the hook over to the rod. Again, tightening the nut will keep the rod in the hook. Teamwork during the assembly process is important. The assistant should make sure that all the I-bolts are in position before locking the individual I-bolts in place. If this is overlooked, the I-bolts may end up fixed between the hooks, and the rod will have to be removed from the hooks to move the bolts.

Distraction and Compression

Next the hooks are seated by distraction between the two apical hooks using a rod holder and a distraction device (Fig. 14). Distraction will be maintained if the

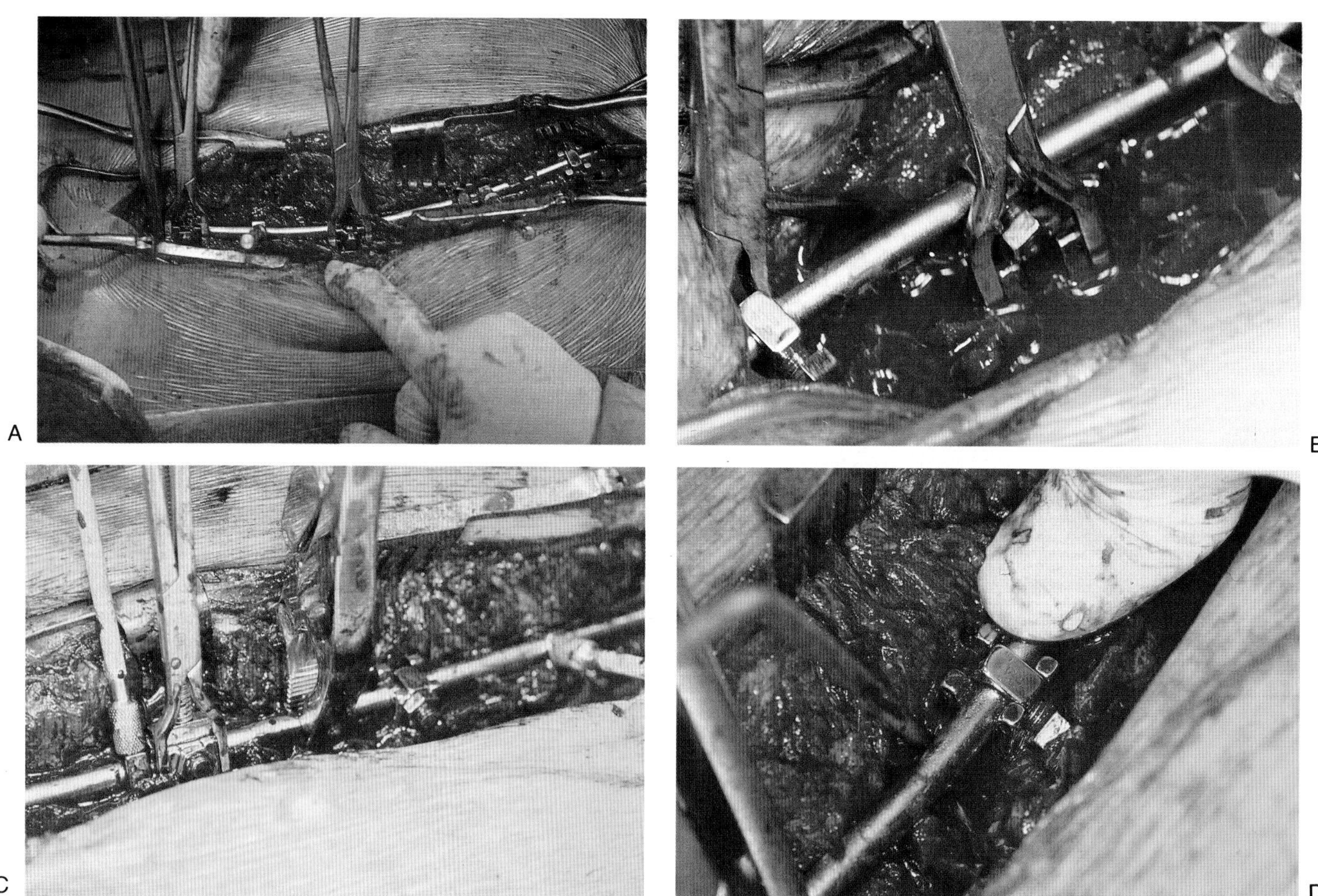

Figure 13. Assembly of the rod and I-bolts. **A:** I-bolts are lined up next to appropriate hooks and manually inserted into the hooks. Extra I-bolts are in place for crosslink placement. **B:** The nuts may exit either side of a double upright hook. **C:** The nuts are definitively seated with the corkscrew. **D:** A properly placed I-bolt will keep the rod deeply seated within the uprights of the hook.

nuts are tightened down moderately, and rotation of the rod will still be possible. Following this, the end hooks are seated with distraction. Again the nuts are moderately tightened to maintain the distraction. If a compression hook is used at the bottom, compression is applied to that hook and maintained by moderate nut tightening.

Rod Rotation

The rod is rotated by applying the rotation wrench to one end of the rod and a holding wrench to a lower portion of the rod (Fig. 15). The rod is gradually

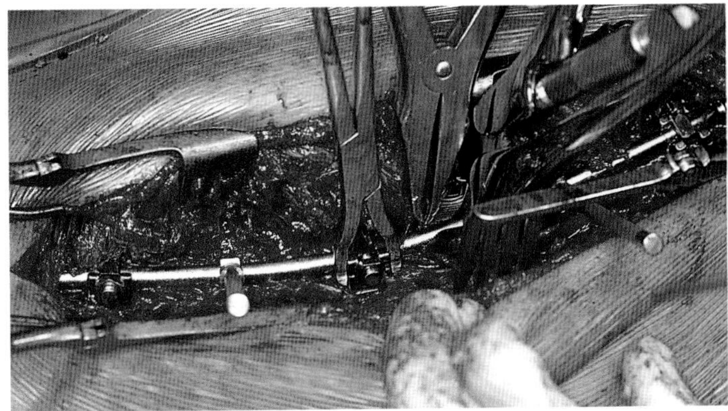

Figure 14. The apical hooks are distracted apart and stabilized by lightly tightening the nuts. The end hooks are also distracted moderately to seat them.

A

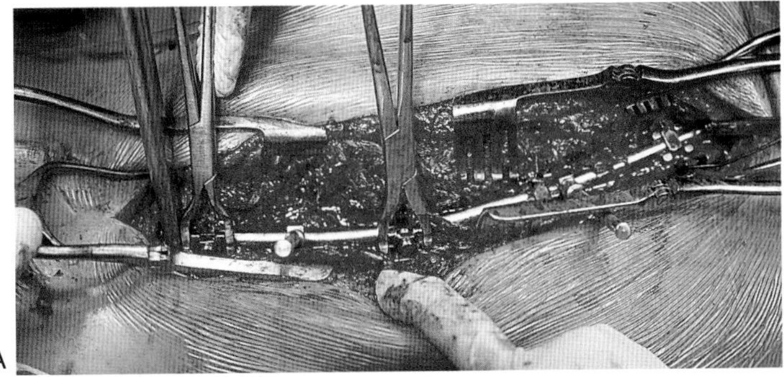

B

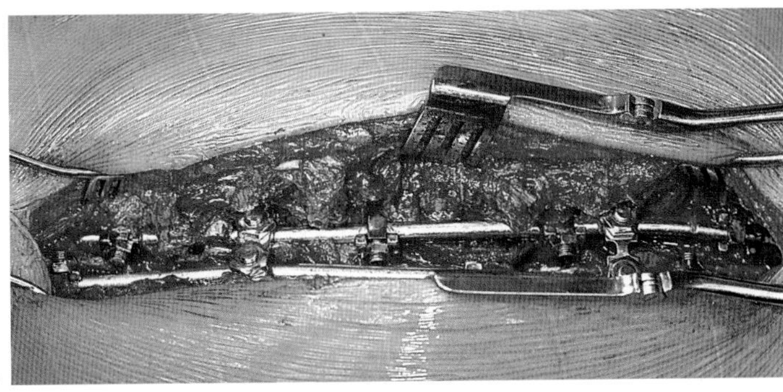

Figure 15. Rotational correction maneuver. **A:** The concave rod is in place and the nuts tightened just enough to maintain distraction and hook seating. The rod is then rotated so that the curvature lies in the sagittal plane. **B:** The rods are in place after rotation. The curvature of the rod is now in the sagittal plane and the scoliosis has been corrected. The convex rod has also been inserted.

rotated in a direction to convert the scoliotic contour to a kyphotic contour. If rotation is difficult, or if a hook is noted to be rotating with the rod, the appropriate nuts should be loosened slightly. As the rod is rotated, pressure over the rib prominence may facilitate rotation. Once the rotation is complete, with the rod now in a fully kyphotic position, the apical nuts are tightened firmly. Seating of the apical hooks should be checked, and a bit more distraction may be applied even after rotation if necessary. Likewise a small amount of additional distraction may be applied to the end hooks prior to final tightening. Excessive distraction, however, is unnecessary and increases the risk of neurologic complications.

Convex Instrument Placement

The laminae are decorticated on the convexity of the deformity, and the hooks are placed as planned. Bone graft is laid over the laminae and facets. The rod with extra I-bolts for the crosslinks is inserted. The upper claw is compressed with a compression device and the nuts tightened. The apical pedicle hook is compressed and the nut tightened, and the lower hook is compressed and also tightened.

Final Tightening

At this point all nuts are tightened against the hook-stabilization device. The nuts should be as tight as possible, and when feasible a closed wrench should be used. Next extra bone graft is placed over any exposed bony surfaces (Fig. 16).

Crosslink Placement

The crosslink plates are chosen so that the groove in the plate fits over the rod (Fig. 17). If the rods are nonparallel, the plates should be contoured with plate benders to match the alignment of the rods. The I-bolts are stabilized with a Kelly clamp while the nuts are placed. The nuts are tightened maximally with a torque wrench (Fig. 18).

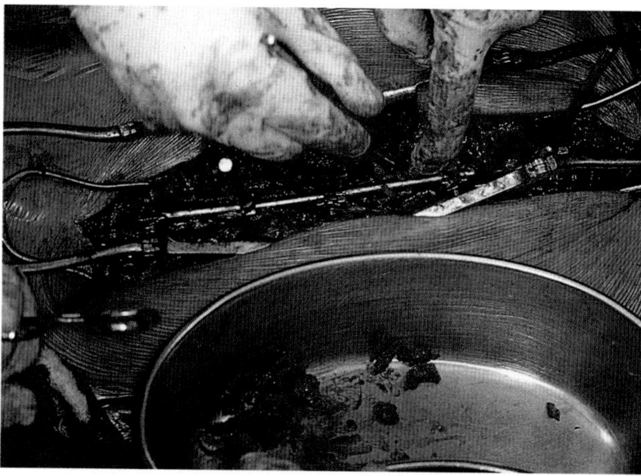

Figure 16. All remaining bone graft is placed over exposed bony surfaces.

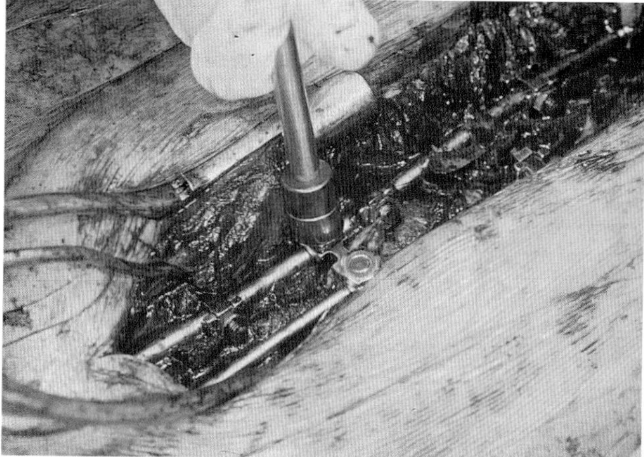

Figure 17. The crosslinks are placed and tightened with the T-handled wrench.

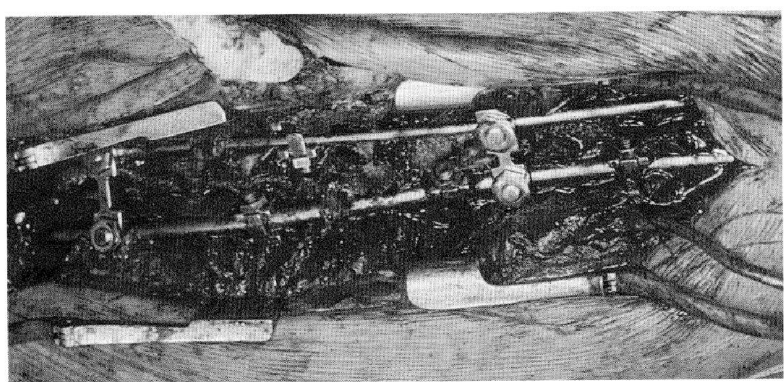

Figure 18. The final appearance of the implant.

Closure

The apophyses are closed with interrupted mattress sutures, following which a routine closure is performed.

POSTOPERATIVE MANAGEMENT

The patient is allowed up the following day. No postoperative immobilization is necessary except in the juvenile patient in whom bone strength is lacking. The patient is seen for wound evaluation 2 weeks postoperatively. Subsequent follow-up is usually at 3-month intervals for the first year. No sports are allowed in the first 6 months, and contact sports are excluded for 1 year. Bicycling and swimming are allowed after 4 weeks. The fused segments of the spine are permanently stiff, but the patient may resume normal activities; they usually notice no functional disability from the loss of motion unless the fusion extends below L4.

COMPLICATIONS

Five possible surgical complications are noted. Hook dislodgment can occur, most likely with an upfacing hook on the lowest vertebra instrumented. This may be due to incorrect contouring of the rod in the sagittal plane with considerable posteriorly directed force at the lower vertebral level. This hook is sometimes placed with inadequate exposure to be certain it is beneath the lamina. The treatment of this problem is usually replacement of the hook at a second operative procedure.

Laminar fracture during rod rotation is caused by too great a force applied to a stiff deformity or one in which there is osteopenia of the vertebrae. The usual treatment is to replace the hook at another level.

Pseudarthrosis is a potential complication, and with rigid instrumentation may not be manifest for many years. One should avoid placing up- and down-going hooks at the same level on both sides of the spine, since this pattern is associated with pseudarthrosis development. The patient may present with back pain and curve progression. Eventual loosening or rod fracture will occur if the pseudarthrosis remains unhealed. It is difficult to confirm the diagnosis preoperatively, but computed tomography and technetium bone scanning may suggest the diagnosis. The treatment is removal of the instrumentation, exploration of the fusion mass, and reinstrumentation with a compression construct across the pseudarthrosis.

Wound infection is a potential complication of any surgical procedure. Cases of low-grade infection presenting several years after the initial surgery have been seen with this and other types of instrumentation. The patient may complain of intermittent swelling over the incision area, back pain, and occasionally fever. The erythrocyte sedimentation rate will be elevated. Treatment is removal of the hardware and primary closure of the wound over drains. Appropriate antibiotic treatment is also recommended.

Decompensation of the spine in a patient with a King-Moe type II curve has been noted. This is most likely with more severe deformities, especially if only the thoracic curve is instrumented. The usual presentation is a left shift of the shoulders over the pelvis in a patient who was shifted to the right preoperatively. Most patients need no treatment, but an occasional severely shifted patient may require instrumentation farther into the lumbar spine.

General complications include postoperative atelectasis, urinary tract infection, anemia, and ileus.

22

L-Rod Instrumentation

Ben L. Allen, Jr.

INDICATIONS/CONTRAINDICATIONS

L-rod instrumentation (LRI) of the scoliotic spine has been available since the mid-1970s and is now a mature technique (6,7). Although the alloys used in the instrumentation have been improved, LRI techniques have not undergone substantive modification since the early 1980s (1,2,4,5). Many of the desirable features of LRI such as provision of secondary spinal contours, secure pelvic fixation, and no need for a postoperative cast or brace, which were not available with classic Harrington instrumentation, are now available in a variety of other spinal instrumentation systems. It is therefore reasonable to ask what advantages (if any) LRI continues to offer versus newer implant systems. For the third world and wherever cost is a major factor, an LRI implant is relatively inexpensive, and extremely inexpensive compared with new systems. The instrumentation required for LRI is minimal, and some needs can be met by adaptive use of available tools, whereas new systems require a large inventory of system-specific instruments. The LRI technique is readily applied to severe and unusual spinal contours and does not depend on nearly normal facet geometry, as do hook-based systems.

The goals of the LRI surgical procedure are: (a): to achieve maximum "safe" correction of the deformed spine, (b) to provide a means of holding the correction, and (c) to stimulate a massive spinal arthrodesis. Upon completion of LRI, the instrumented portion of the spine is secured by sublaminar wires at each vertebral level to rods that lie at the base of the spinous processes on either side of the spine. Thus there are two sites of attachment to each vertebral arch; if 10 vertebrae were instrumented, 20 sublaminar wires would secure the spine to the rods.

The paramount disadvantages of LRI are the large number of judgments the surgeon must make during an LRI procedure and the medicolegal threat of a lawsuit should the surgeon inflict a neurologic injury while passing a sublaminar wire (3).

B. L. Allen, Jr., M.D.: Shriners Hospitals for Crippled Children, Greenville, South Carolina 29605.

The author presently uses LRI for most neuromuscular scoliosis cases, for severe scoliosis of any etiology (a Cobb angle of more than 100 degrees), and in cases associated with fragile bone. In experienced hands, LRI is reasonable to use as a general purpose technique for correction and fixation of the spine in scoliosis, other spinal deformities, and some spinal fracture cases that can be managed by a transverse loading system not providing a load bypass for the instrumented spinal segment. The surgeon should especially consider LRI for the patient with unusually fragile bone and for the patient in whom (for whatever reason) a hook-based system would be difficult to apply.

The paramount contraindication to LRI, when posterior spinal instrumentation is indicated, is lack of experience in the technique. Although many surgeons use LRI safely, the neurologic injury rate has been high in some centers, especially early in their experience, and has been higher than Harrington instrumentation in Scoliosis Research Society morbidity/mortality surveys. Whenever the surgeon contemplates posterior spinal instrumentation and is considering laminar fixation into a surgically opened neural canal, the question of whether some less-invasive technique would have equal efficacy should arise; if so, such a technique should be carefully weighed against the risks associated with laminar fixation.

PREOPERATIVE PLANNING

Proper selection of the length of spine to be instrumented and arthrodesed, while of paramount importance, lies outside the scope of this discussion. In general, instrumentation and fusion should extend at least from neutral vertebra to neutral vertebra in compensated deformities (S-curves) and from the upper thoracic spine to the pelvis in uncompensated deformities (C-curves). Principles that are helpful in deciding the best levels for Harrington instrumentation also apply to segmental instrumentation. The etiology of the spine deformity must be considered in each case, since it too has an important bearing on the selection of levels. One should be attentive to sagittal as well as coronal plane deformities and should avoid ending a fusion below an adjacent-to-the-coronal-plane-deformity kyphosis. If not controlled in such a circumstance, the kyphosis will likely progress.

We routinely take a series of bend or stretch films that define the correctability of each structural deformity of the patient's spine. When a scoliosis cannot be passively corrected to a Cobb angle of less than 50 degrees, then anterior spinal release and fusion to enhance correctability should be performed because residual deformity of 50 degrees is about the threshold at which the LRI implant construct becomes mechanically inadequate and at risk for early fatigue failure.

Since spinal balance is critically important to a good result from surgery, a deformity correction plan that ensures balance should be thought through before the actual surgery is performed. For clear definition of balance problems, stretch films are of much greater planning benefit than bend films and should be obtained. Three balance situations are commonly encountered. The most frequent relates to postsurgical pelvic obliquity in patients with neuromuscular conditions undergoing a long instrumentation and fusion to the pelvis. To achieve a level pelvis, it may be necessary to plan anterior surgery so that the degree of correction of the spinal deformity is sufficiently improved that leveling the pelvis is possible. A second circumstance is that of a double-curve pattern for which fusion to the pelvis is planned; the degree of correction of each curve must be adjusted so that compensation is maintained. This may translate into planning less-than-possible correction of the more flexible curve, to balance the lesser correction possible in the more rigid curve. The third spinal balance factor to be planned is sagittal plane balance: thoracic kyphosis and lumbar lordosis must be in proper proportion for acceptable sitting and standing posture. Whenever a long fusion is to be done, careful attention should be paid to planning the postsurgical sagittal curves, since imbalance in this plane will thrust the trunk forward or backward relative to the pelvis.

Equipment

For scoliosis cases, rods of $\frac{3}{16}$ inch in diameter and 60 cm in length are preferable to larger-diameter rods because of their lesser stiffness and because it is easier to cut the rod to appropriate length than to cover all the possible needed lengths in inventory. Use of the more-flexible rods gives a degree of forgiveness in fitting the rods to the spine and has been shown to have clinical efficacy in most scoliosis applications (8). Rods of $\frac{1}{4}$ inch in diameter, not discussed in this chapter, are necessary for spinal fracture, some revision, and most kyphosis applications of L-rods.

Fully annealed wires of either 1.0 or 1.2 mm in diameter are used to secure the rods to the vertebral laminae. When the larger-diameter wire is used, a single strand passing about a lamina is sufficient for fastening the rod at all intercalary levels; double strands are required for the end wires because of the greater loads at those sites. With the smaller-diameter wires, double strands should be used at all levels. The author's preference is for the 1.2-mm wires, even though the double strands of smaller wire are mechanically stronger when fastened by twisting, because only one wire passing is needed for all intercalary levels compared with two wire passings when the 1.0-mm wires are used, and because no clinical deficiency has been seen in performance of the 1.2-mm diameter wires.

Rods and wires suitable for LRI are available in 316 L or 22-13-5 stainless steel and in MP-35-N; 22-13-5 stainless steel and MP-35-N have very similar mechanical properties. Compared with 316-L stainless steel, they are more fatigue-resistant, less notch-sensitive, and much more easily work-hardened. In the fully annealed state 22-13-5 stainless steel and MP-35-N wires are stiffer than 316-L stainless steel wires of the same diameter. The author presently uses 22-13-5 stainless steel rods and end wires along with 316-L stainless steel intercalary wires; this is felt to be a good blend of easy workability of the wires with adequate fatigue strength of the spinal implant.

Special tools designed for specific steps in LRI make the operation easier. Those mentioned in this chapter, available from the Smith-Nephew Richards Company, are shown in Figure 1. Their use is described in the appropriate technique discussions.

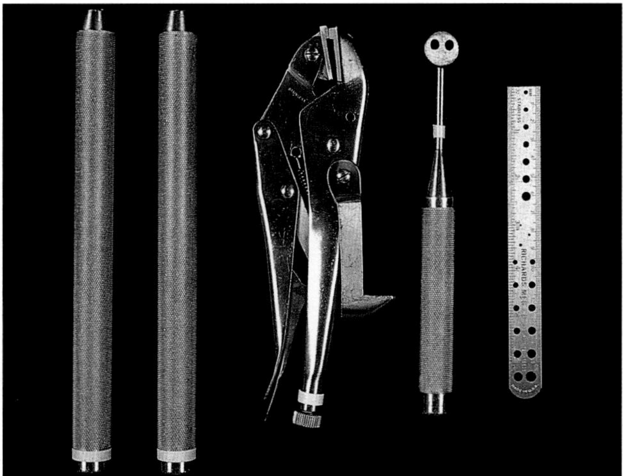

Figure 1. Instrumentation for LRI: from left to right are sleeve benders, pelvic rod clamp, pelvic rod guide, and ruler.

SURGERY

As for any spinal deformity surgery, it is helpful to have the patient positioned on a table or frame such that the abdomen hangs free; relief of any abdominal compression greatly reduces the risk of excessive blood loss during the operation. Beyond this basic need, a number of additional options may be helpful. For LRI a table that allows intraoperative flexion and extension of the lumbar spine is especially helpful; in flexion the interlaminar spaces are widely open, which facilitates passing wires beneath the laminae. The lumbar region should usually be fixed in some extension, or lordosis, so if the table does the necessary positioning, the procedure is facilitated.

During surgery the patient's neck must be protected from torsional injury and the eyes from pressure injury. The anesthesiologist must have free access to the endotracheal tube. We prefer to avoid turning the patient's head to one side because the risks just listed are not sufficiently controlled. Although a horseshoe-style headrest can be safely used to support the head, we prefer to suspend the head with Mayfield tongs attached to the operating table, particularly in Oriental patients, whose eyes are less protected by the orbit than are the eyes of patients of other races.

Our prepping and draping routine provides wide exposure of the patient's back and posterior thorax; the undraped area is covered with an adhesive plastic film. The options for posterior thoracoplasty, insertion of a chest tube if needed, and iliac crest bone grafting are all open.

Technique

As for any scoliosis surgery, the initial step is adequate exposure of that portion of the spine to be instrumented and fused. For the most part this is done in a routine manner, but a few points are worthy of mention. For cases in which a posterior thoracoplasty is planned, it is helpful to make a skin incision that is curved toward the convexity of the scoliosis rather than a straight midline incision. Once the thoracoplasty has been completed, the skin wound will shift toward the concave side, making the curved incision straight. Skin and subcutaneous bleeding quickly come under control when the surgical wound is stretched open with Wheatlander retractors: with this technique any sort of cutaneous and subcutaneous injection for hemostasis is unnecessary. In reflection of soft tissues to expose the posterior spine, one should be careful to remove facet joint capsules since in our fusion technique the facets are not excised.

Description of the surgical technique conveniently divides into five parts once the spine has been exposed: (a) excision of the ligamentum flavum, (b) wire preparation and handling, (c) rod shaping and correction technique, (d) pelvic fixation, and (e) fusion technique and postoperative management.

Excision of Ligamentum Flavum. Excision of the ligamentum flavum is a three-step process to be done at all interlaminar spaces along the length of the spine to be instrumented. In the first step the ligamentum flavum, which is a paired structure, is exposed and thinned until its midline cleavage plane can be seen (Fig. 2). The surgical technique in the thoracic region is slightly different from that in the lumbar region.

Because the caudally slanting spinous processes overlie the interlaminar spaces in the thoracic spine, the obstructing bone must be cut away to access the interlaminar space. A rongeur is placed vertically on the spinous process over the interlaminar space, and the bone is cut, thereby exposing the ligamentum flavum. One should preserve as much of the base of the spinous process as possible because later the rods will be fixed against this bone. The rongeur is used to cut away the superficial portion of the ligamentum flavum. When the midline cleavage is clearly

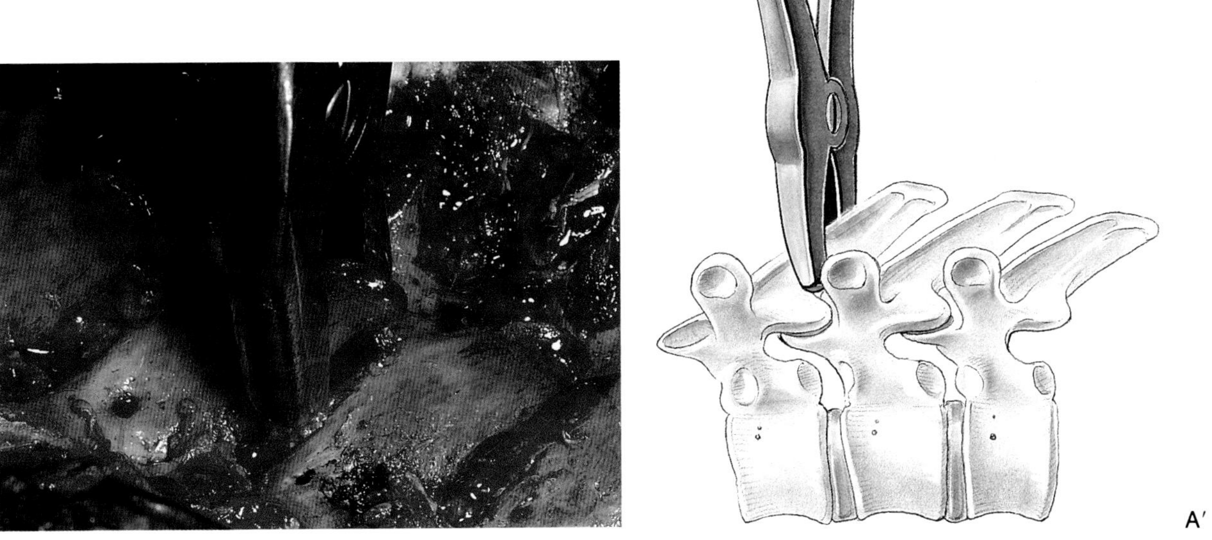

Figure 2. A,A′: The patient's head is to the left. A thoracic spinous process is being cut to expose the ligamentum flavum.

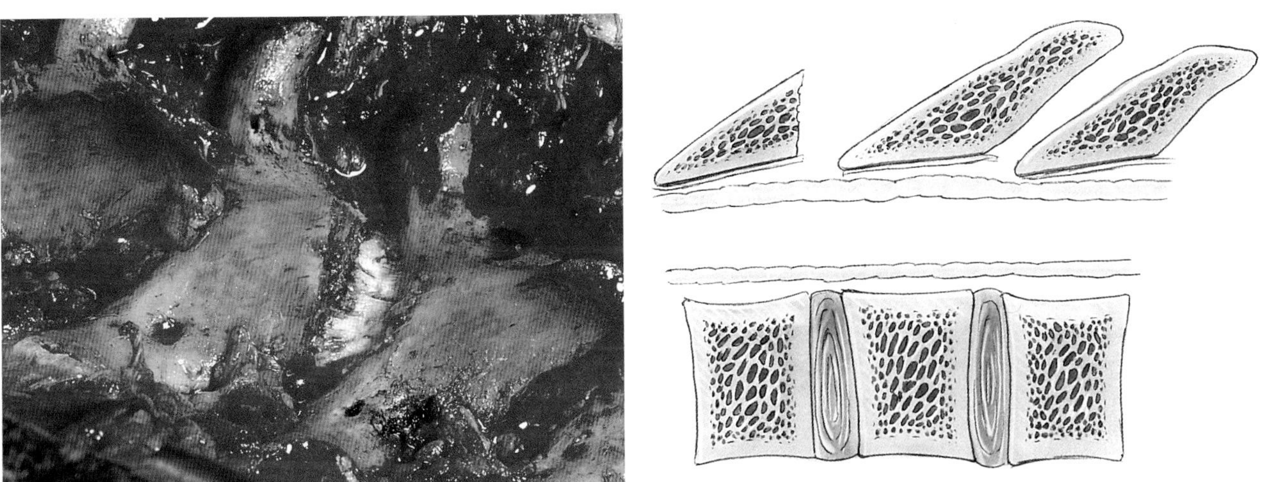

Figure 2. B,B′: The "yellow ligament" can be seen once the spinous process has been removed.

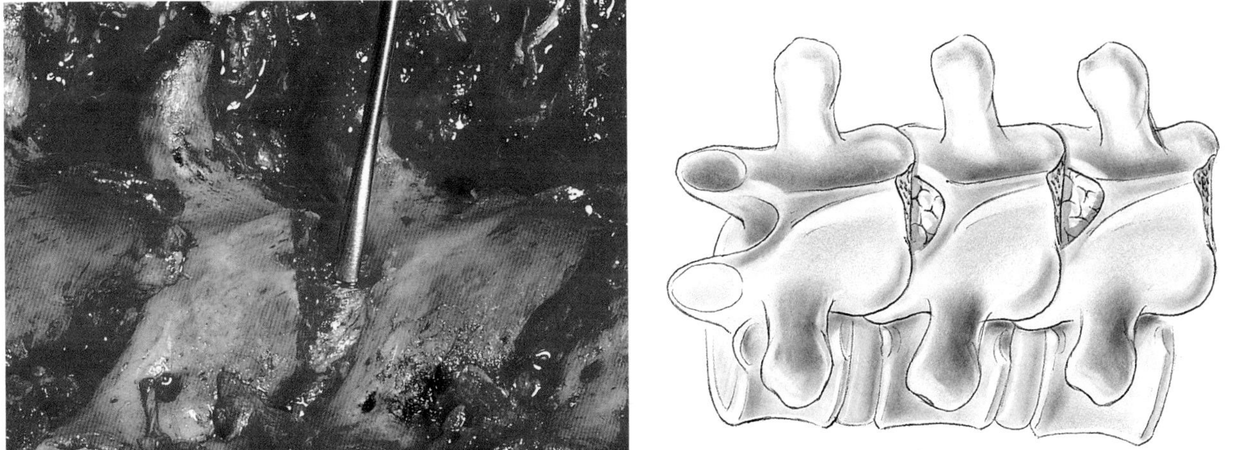

Figure 2. C,C′: The paired ligaments are being separated with a Penfield dissector.

visualized, the initial step has been completed. The first step in lumbar spine surgery is similar to the thoracic technique except that it is unnecessary to remove any bone. The next step is to separate the paired ligamenta flava fully at each interlaminar space. Gently working a Penfield #4 dissector through the midline plane of the ligaments establishes the separation and develops a working plane for the final step, in which Kerrison punches (the largest sizes that can be inserted into each particular space) are used to excise the ligaments.

Wire Preparation and Handling. Either commercially prebent wires, wire from a spool, or straight wires may be used in the operation. If the prebent wires are not available, each wire must be bent into shape for passing beneath a vertebral lamina. To do this, approximately 50-cm lengths of wire are cut from stock and folded into halves. The bends at the tips are left open so that the tip can be easily grasped by passing the tooth of a clamp or a nerve hook through it. Each wire is shaped to the configuration shown in Figure 3. The diameter of the primary bend should be slightly larger than the lamina around which it is to be passed and should have an arc of 180 to 210 degrees. Because the wire must enter the neural canal almost vertically, a second bend is necessary. This second bend should be a smooth curve with an arc of about 90 degrees. An angular secondary bend should be avoided because when the wire is pulled under the lamina, the secondary bend must be reversed; a smooth contour reverses easily, while an angular one requires much greater force for the pull-through. Once a wire has been properly shaped, the strands are slightly separated so that sublaminar twists and rotation can be avoided.

Passing a wire is a four-step process: (a) introduction, (b) advancement, (c) roll-through, and (d) pull-through (Fig. 4). Although not critical, it is usually more expedient to begin at the upper thoracic level and progress to the lower lumbar level.

For introduction, the wire tip is gently placed into the neural canal at the inferior laminar edge in the midline. The initial direction is more or less vertical. The wire is rotated to point the tip cephalad, and, without further rotation, the wire is advanced 5 to 6 mm; this enables the wire tip to clear the sublaminar origin of the ligamentum flavum, which is a soft area. Roll-through follows advancement. The surgeon gently pushes the wire around the lamina, taking care to keep it snugly in contact with the bone. Successful roll-through presents the wire tip from emerging above the lamina.

The wire tip is hooked with a nerve hook or grasped with a clamp, and pulled through until about half its length protrudes above and half below the lamina. Each individual wire must be secured so that, if inadvertently bumped, it will not

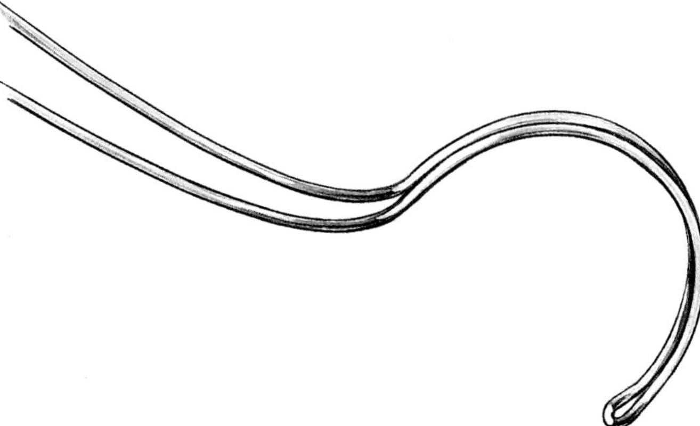

Figure 3. This is the best shape for a wire to be passed under a vertebral lamina.

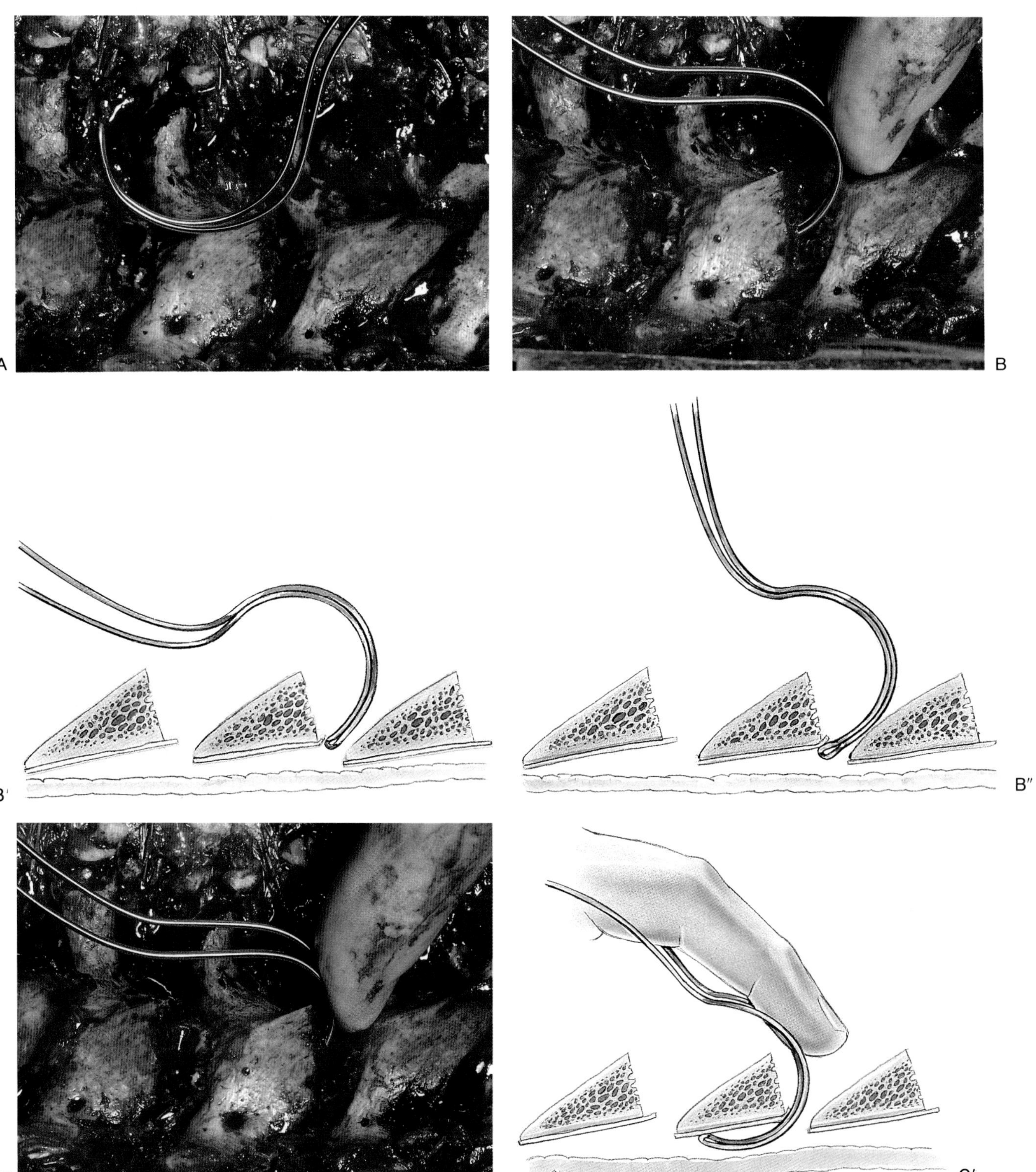

Figure 4. A: The primary bend in the wire should be a bit larger in diameter than the width of the vertebral lamina about which the wire is to be passed. **B,B′,B″:** Introduction of the wire into the neural canal. **C,C′:** Advancement of the wire.

Figure continues.

displace into the neural canal. If the surgeon is using 1.2-mm-diameter wire, the tip is cut from the wire, one length is placed to the right side, and the other is placed to the left side of the particular lamina. Each single wire is crimped about the lamina. The superior half of the wire is kept at the midline and the inferior half laterally at all intercalary levels and at the caudal end. At the cephalad end the inferior wire end is placed medially and the superior end laterally (Fig. 5).

Rod Preparation and Correction Techniques. Two rods are implanted in all straightforward operations for scoliosis. The initial rod is used to effect most correction and the second rod to boost the strength of the instrumentation. When the initial rod is placed on the convex side of the scoliosis, the deformity is said to be corrected by a convex rod technique. This is the most efficient method for thoracic curves in which room exists for the free end of a rod to protrude from the wound. The initial rod is fastened to the upper region of the scoliotic curve with its short limb positioned transversely across the lamina of the second vertebra above the curve, since fixation with wire does not control tilt of the end vertebra as effectively as does a facet hook. The rod is levered to the spine (Fig. 6) and sequential wires are secured as the rod contacts the successive laminae. After all wires except the end ones to the initial rod have been secured, the second rod is placed, and at least the wires about the caudal segment of its long limb are tightened. The areas of decussation are aligned, with the short limb of one rod passing

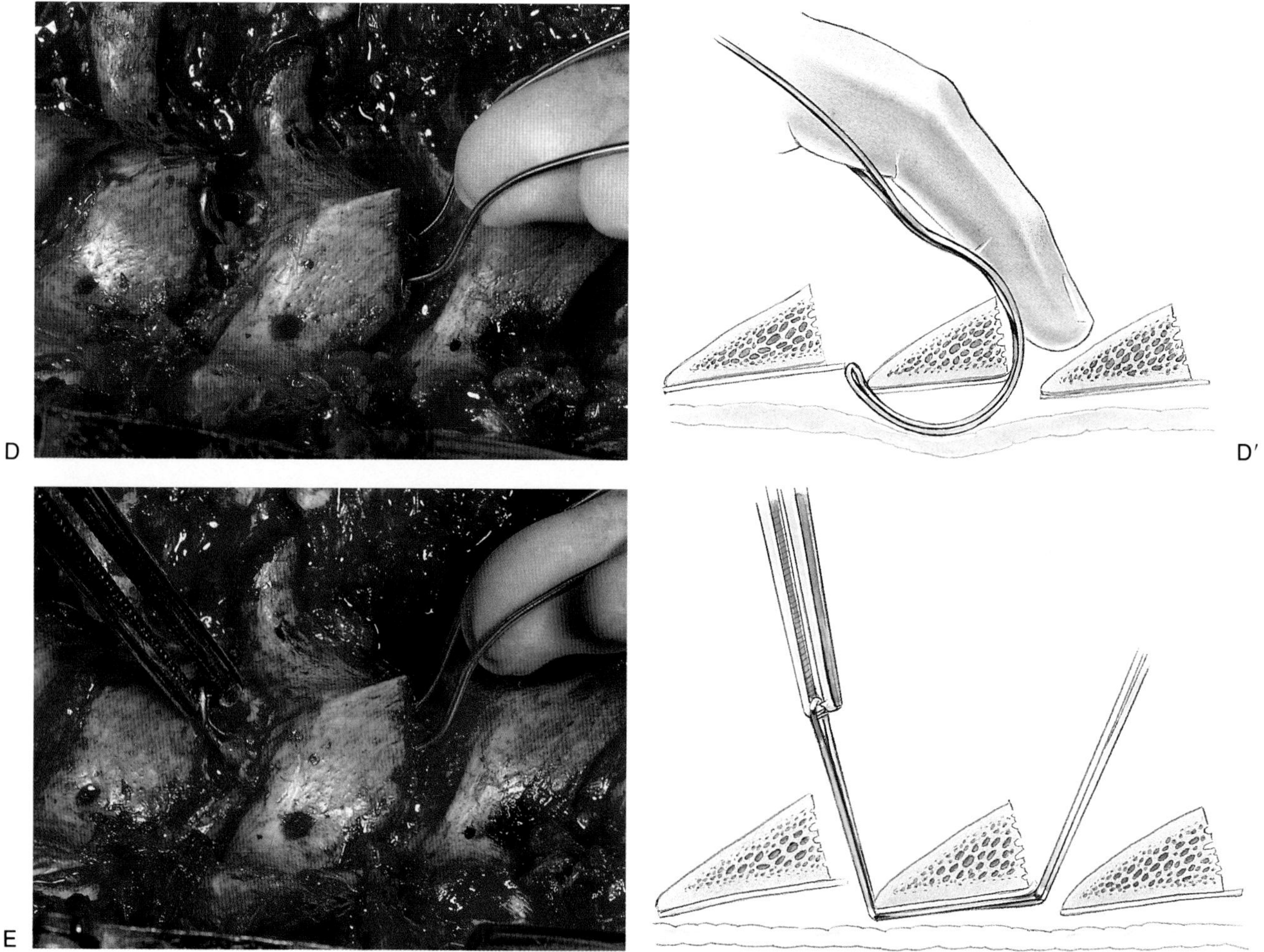

Figure 4. D,D′: Roll-through of the wire. Note the wire tip appearing in the cephalad interlaminar space. **E,E′:** Pull-through of the wire.

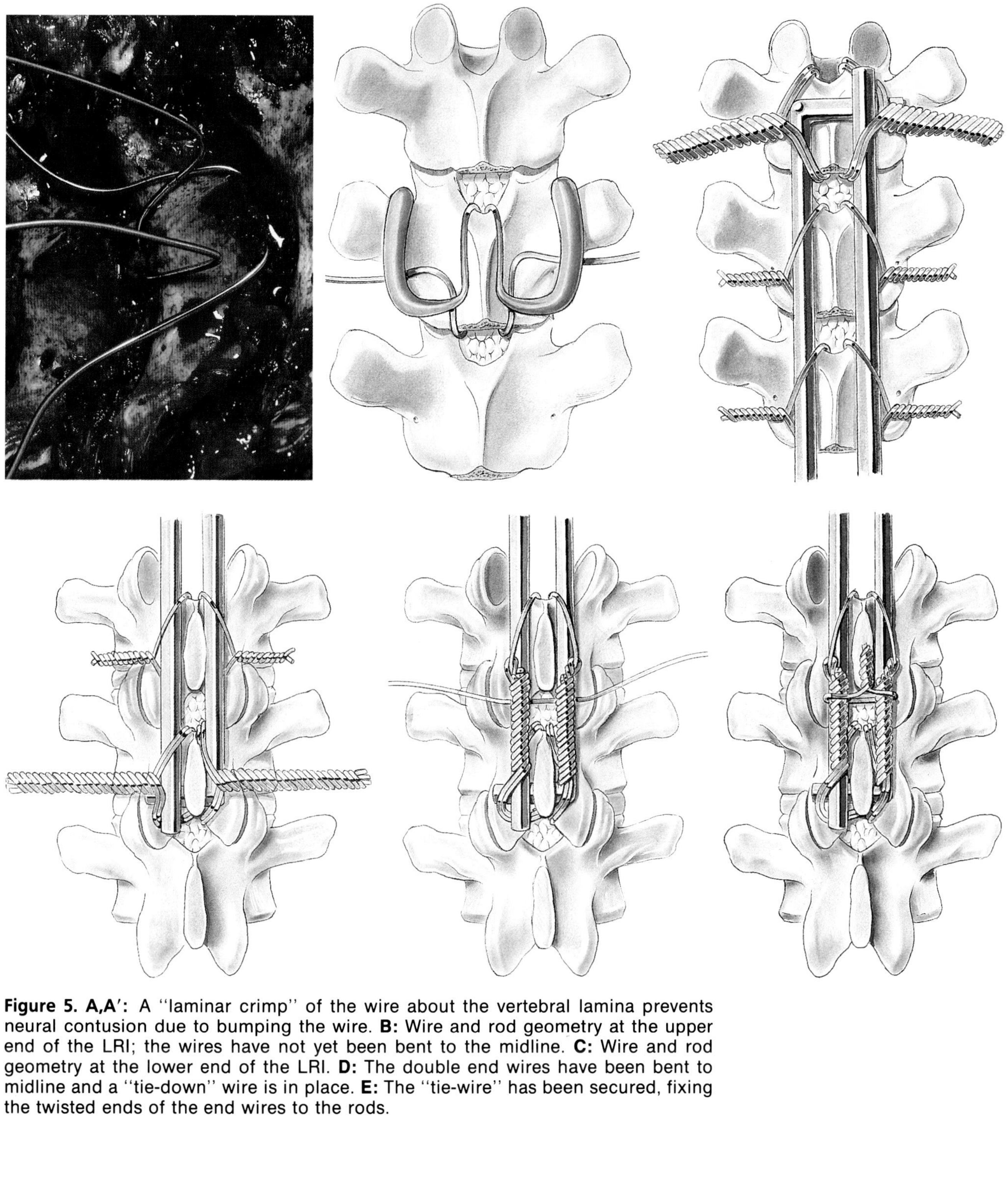

A,A′ B

C,D E

Figure 5. A,A′: A "laminar crimp" of the wire about the vertebral lamina prevents neural contusion due to bumping the wire. **B:** Wire and rod geometry at the upper end of the LRI; the wires have not yet been bent to the midline. **C:** Wire and rod geometry at the lower end of the LRI. **D:** The double end wires have been bent to midline and a "tie-down" wire is in place. **E:** The "tie-wire" has been secured, fixing the twisted ends of the end wires to the rods.

deep to the long limb of the opposite rod, and the double end wires are fastened by twisting. Note the relationships of wires and rods, shown in Fig. 6.

In contrast to the usual deformity in the thoracic spine, lordotic thoracic and lumbar scoliosis are more easily corrected by a concave rod technique (Fig. 7). The initial rod is placed with its short limb passing transversely across the lamina of the lowermost vertebra selected for instrumentation; it should pass through a hole at the base of the spinous process or through a notch cut vertically into the spinous process. The inferior double-end wire on the concave side and the wires to the laminae of the vertebra above the curve with which the rod is in contact are twisted. When lumbar lordosis has been prebent into the rod, the end of the short limb must be held down on the convex side of the deformity. Two forces are used to bring the spine to the rod; an assistant effects manual correction by appropriate pressure on the trunk, and the surgeon pulls the wires that pass beneath the lamina of the apical vertebra toward the rod. When maximum correction has been obtained by these maneuvers, twist the wires immediately above and below the apical wires. The other forces can now be released, and other wires in the area of deformity can be secured.

A
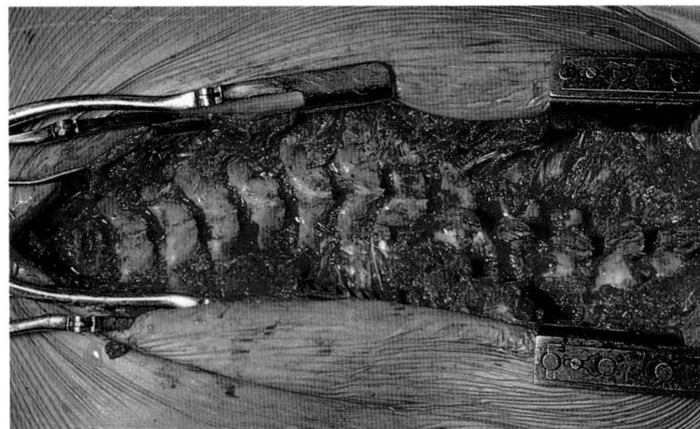

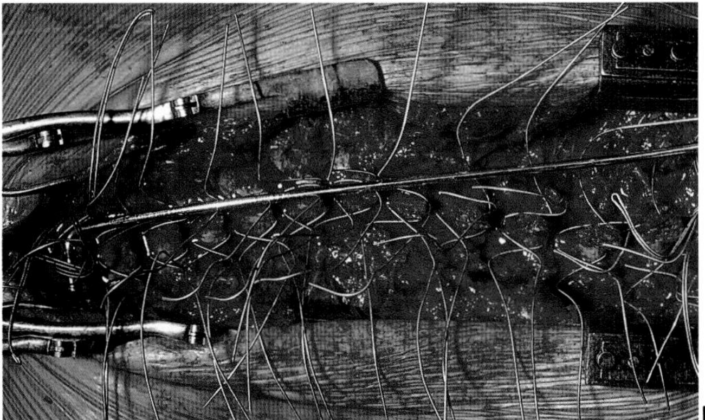
B

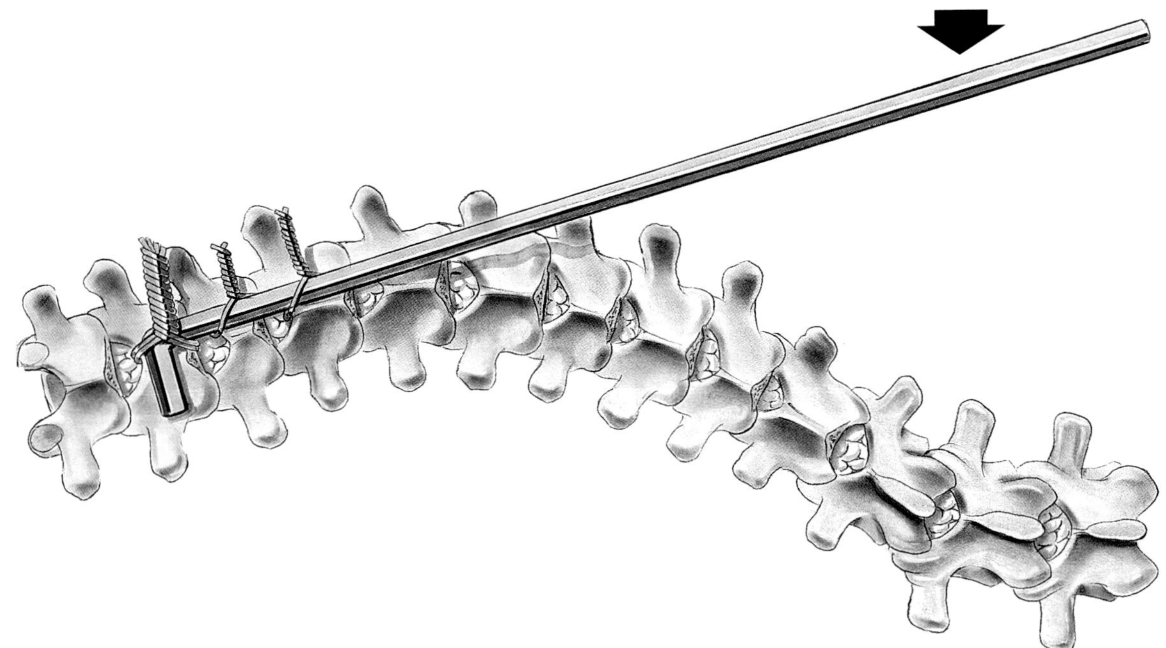
B′

Figure 6. A: The patient's head is to the left; her spine has been exposed and the interlaminar spaces opened. Her right thoracic scoliosis is evident. **B,B′:** Sublaminar wires have been passed and the initial rod has been secured on the upper, convex side of the curve for a "convex correction."

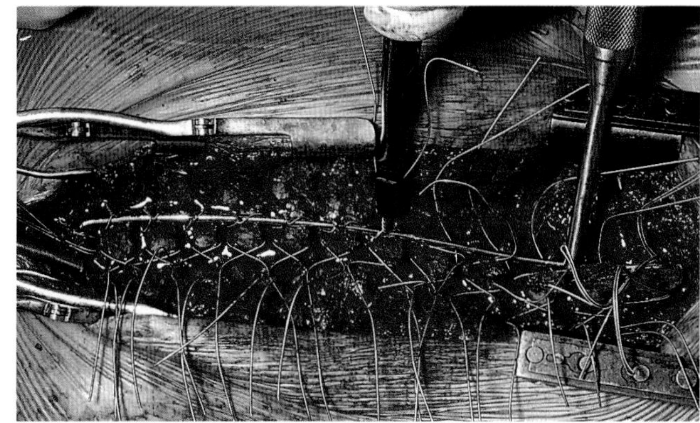

Figure 6. C,C′: Correction is obtained mainly by levering the rod to the spine and sequentially fastening the wires.

C

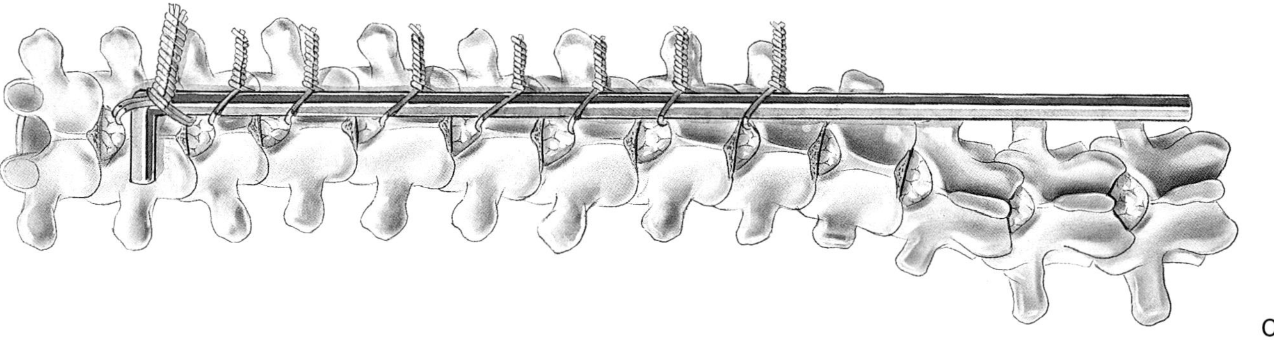

C′

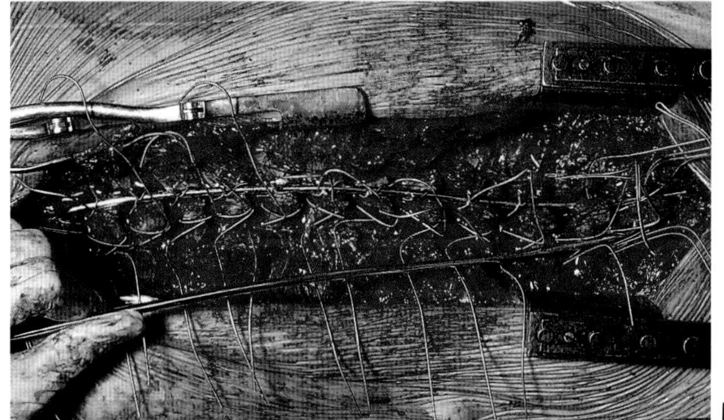

Figure 6. D,D′: The second rod is added before the initial rod has been completely secured.

D

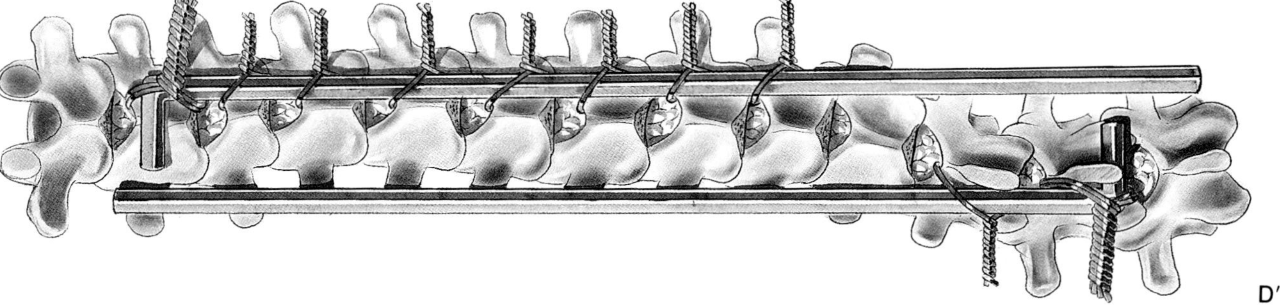

D′

Figure continues.

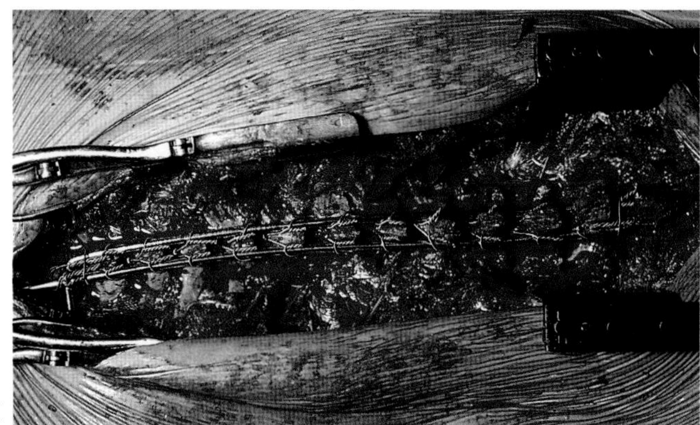
E

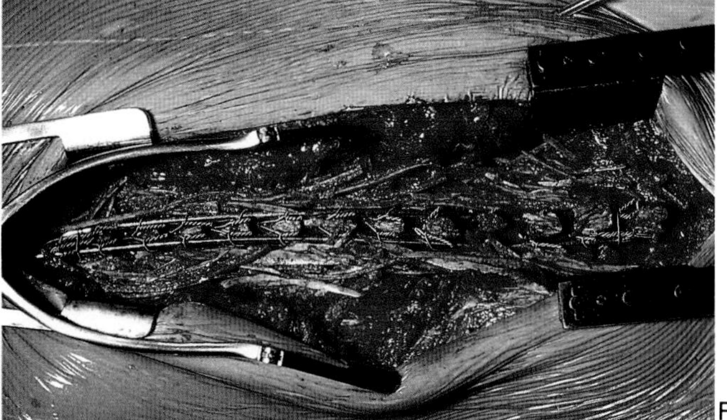
F

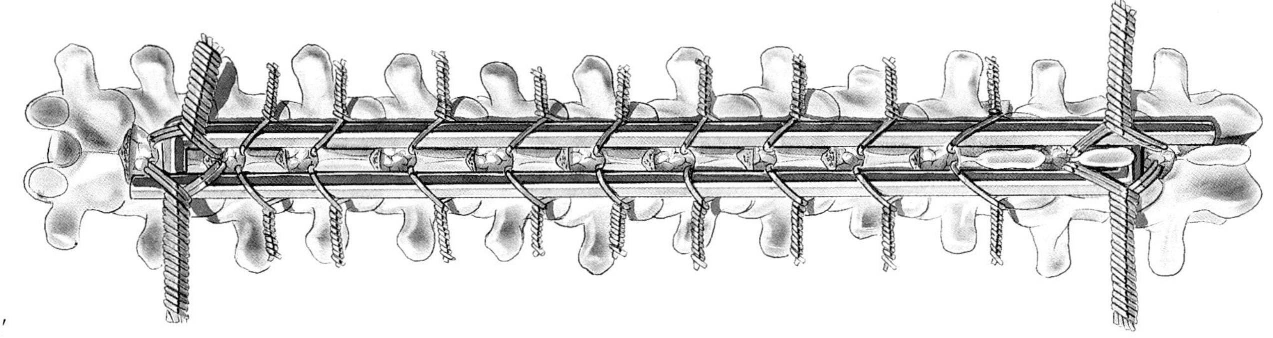
E′

Figure 6. E,E′: The instrumentation has been completed; wires are bent to the midline in the photograph. **F:** Bone graft has been placed lateral to the implant on both convex and concave sides of the spine.

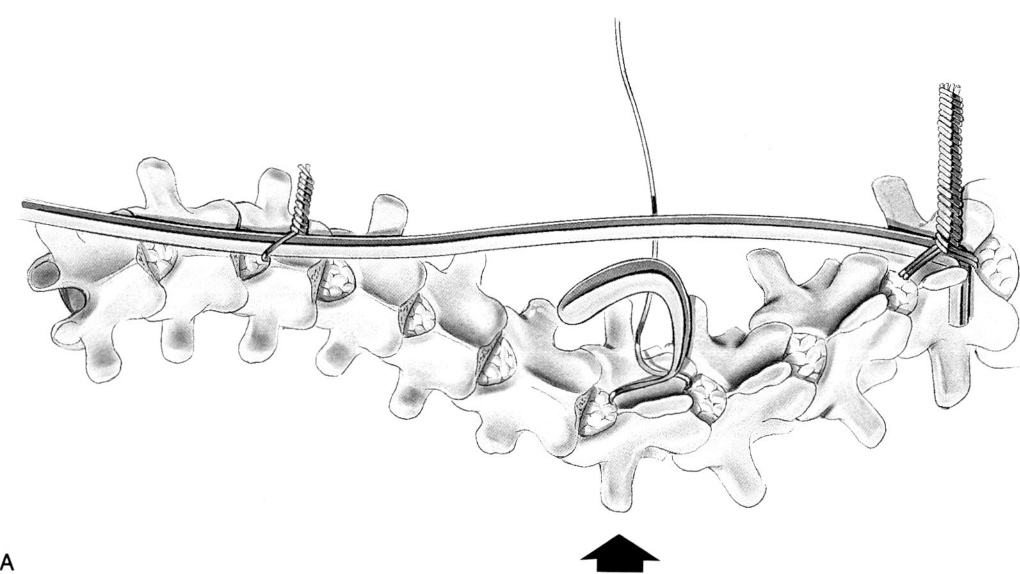
A

Figure 7. A: For a "concave correction" the initial rod spans the concavity of the scoliosis. **B:** The spine is pushed to the rod and apical wires are fastened in a partially corrected position. **C:** A second rod is added to assist in completion of the correction. **D:** Squeezing the rods together provides final correction.

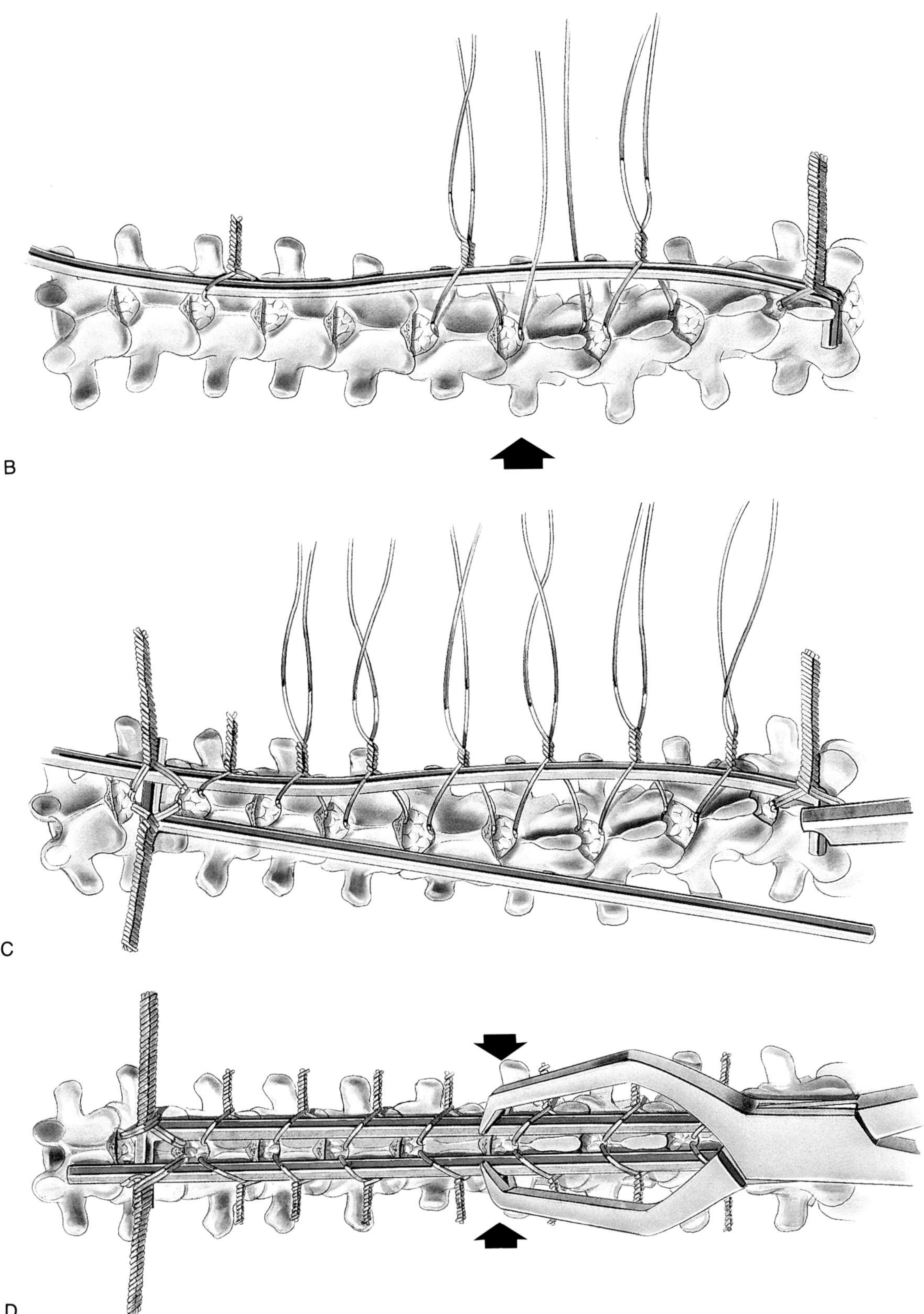

Figure 7. *Continued.*

If the rod is not seated snugly against the lamina upon completion of the first pass, do not waste time attempting to achieve firm contact at this point in the procedure. Place the second rod and secure its long limb from cephalad to caudad. Once it is in position, both rods can be brought into firm contact with the lamina by squeezing them toward the midline with a rod approximator. It may be helpful to lever a rod down to a lamina using the opposite rod as a fixed point; a rod lever or a rod pusher serves this purpose. Using these techniques, it is usually necessary to tighten the concave wires twice and the convex wires once, although all wires should be checked for tightness upon completion of the instrumentation. The rod decussations should be set with the respective short limbs beneath the long limbs when this technique is used for a lumbar curve.

Pure convex and pure concave techniques are applicable only to single curves; double curves are best handled by a combination concave and convex rod technique. Usually this involves beginning with a convex rod placement for the thoracic scoliosis and using the same rod for a concave rod technique for the lumbar scoliosis.

The provision of secondary spinal contours improves the cosmetic result of spinal instrumentation. When the area of instrumentation extends below the third lumbar vertebra, it is essential to provide lumbar lordosis if fixing the patient in a "jump position" is to be avoided. If lumbar lordosis is provided, it is essential to provide compensatory thoracic kyphosis when the instrumentation extends to a mid or high thoracic level. For a nonlordotic thoracic curve that does not require instrumentation below the second lumbar vertebra, attempting to provide kyphosis adds little to the cosmetic result. Planning for maximal apical translation in the posteromedial direction with the concave rod supporting most of the displacement is a good strategy for realizing maximal correction of the rotational component of the deformity.

Making bends in the rods to provide the secondary spinal contours introduces a torsion strain into the instrumentation. Two points of consequence arise as a result: (a) firm fixation of the short transverse limb of the rod is the only maneuver that prevents gross rotation of the entire initial rod, and (b) torsion strain is propagated through the entire length of the rod rather than from segment to segment as is true for lateral bending.

If the preferred concave rod technique is used for a lumbar curve or the preferred convex rod technique for a thoracic curve, the effect of the torsion strain is to rotate the short limb of the rod posteriorly, away from the spine. The relative position of the short limb of the initial rod and the long limb of the second rod at the rod decussation becomes important. If the short limb lies above the long limb, only one set of wires prevents rotation of the initial rod—a tenuous situation when 316 L stainless steel wires are used. However, if the short limb of the initial rod lies beneath the long limb of the second rod, rotation of the initial rod is blocked by the long limb of the second rod, which can distribute the load to multiple wires. This preferred relationship often requires the short limb of the initial rod to be pushed down onto the lamina as the second rod is placed. When MP-35-N or 22–13–5 stainless steel wires are used, one set of double wires may be sufficiently strong that placing the short limb above the long limb is acceptable.

Because torsional stress is propagated throughout the entire length of the rod, torsion strain must be taken into account. Consider a lumbar curve corrected by a concave rod technique (Figure 7). When torsional strain occurs, the long limb of the rod tends to rotate into the curve so that less than the desired correction of lateral bending can be achieved. This effect can be avoided by allowing for rotary deformation when bending the secondary spinal contour into the rod; an offset of 20 to 30 degrees out of the sagittal plane away from the concave side of the spine is usually about right if a full posterior correction of the deformity is planned.

When bending a rod to provide both lumbar lordosis and thoracic kyphosis in a full posterior correction case, the surgeon should keep the secondary contours in the same plane. For example, in the bending of a rod for a concave rod technique correction of a left lumbar scoliosis with a structural right thoracic curve of a lesser degree, the short limb of the initial rod is held in the transverse plane and lordosis is bent into the rod with a 20- to 30-degree offset from the sagittal plane toward the patient's right side. Thoracic kyphosis is bent into the rod in the same plane as the lordosis. When the rod is applied to the spine, torsional stress will strain the lordotic bend into the sagittal plane, and the portion affixed to the thoracic curve will also lie in the sagittal plane.

One key to success is awareness that what is needed is an oblique plane bend that has the proper secondary contour and that with torsion strain will give the selected amount of lateral deviation. Attempting to bend secondary contours and lateral deviations in separate steps is futile.

For maximum rigidity of fixation, it is essential that the rods rest on the laminae firmly against the bases of the spinous processes upon completion of the procedure. However, the wires should not be twisted to approximate a rod to a lamina; these must be brought into proper relationship by some other means. Attempting to pull the spine to a rod or the rod to the spine produces a dangerously overstrained twist that breaks easily at its base. The wire should be twisted only to secure the rod in position; ideally the strands in the twist should lie at about 45 degrees to the axis of the twisted portion of the wire.

After fastening by twisting, all intercalary wires are trimmed to about a 1-cm length and bent caudally toward the midline. This pattern reduces the prominence of the twisted ends and places them away from the site of intended arthrodesis. The end wires must be handled differently, for the strain at the ends of the instrumented segment will cause them to assume a position at right angles to the rods. The result is a palpable wire, perhaps an annoying bursa, or a real threat of pressure necrosis of the overlying skin. The end wires are therefore cut longer, about 2.5 to 3 cm in length, and bent to overlie the rods ipsilateral to each set of wires. After both end wires have been properly bent, a single wire is passed around both rods, and end wires are secured by twisting. This fastens the end wires to the rods and avoids the problem of their "standing up."

Pelvic Fixation. Pelvic fixation is best obtained by driving a length of a rod into each ilium (Fig. 8). Optimum placement of the iliac portion of the rod is intraosseously from a bone entry point at the lower level of the posterior superior iliac spine, across the posterior ilium 10 to 15 mm above the sciatic notch, and into the transverse bar above the acetabulum. The tip of the inserted rod should point toward the anterior inferior iliac spine and not the acetabulum, which occurs when the bone entry point is too cephalad. The optimum rod placement allows a maximum length of rod to be inserted, theoretically reduces stress because of the long lever arm, gives good multiplanar fixation strength because of the triangular configuration at the base of the implanted L-rods, and allows bone for grafting to be obtained from the posterior iliac crest in the usual manner.

Exposure. Wide exposure of the pelvis is critically important for accurate rod placement and judgment of compensation. The midline incision over the spine must be extended to a sacral level below the posterior superior iliac spine; the skin incision should drift 1 to 2 cm off the midline over the sacrum so that the sacral spine does not push directly into the skin wound after surgery when the patient lies supine. The fascial and deeper dissection is midline over the sacrum. Both posterior iliac crests are exposed as if to obtain a bone graft through the midline incision. The sciatic notches must be sufficiently visualized to permit a finger to be hooked into them.

The posterior sulcus at the articulation of the sacrum and ilium must be exposed at the level of the posterior superior iliac spine. This is accomplished from the midline by elevating the erector spinae musculature. The surgeon should be alert to the possibility of accessory posterior sacroiliac joints as the medial aspect of the posterior ilium at the level of the lower margin of the posterior superior iliac spine is cleaned of soft tissue to provide a bone entry point for the rod. In most cases midline exposure only for the bone entry point is sufficient, but in patients with a wider-than-usual sacrum a small second fascial incision adjacent to the bone entry site may be helpful to ensure that the entry point is at the proper level and that the intended rod path will be intraosseous.

Rod Path Preparation. The path for the rod in the ilium is established by driving a sharp pin into the ilium (Fig. 9).

A Steinmann pin of the same diameter as the rod to be used in the spinal instrumentation is selected to make the intraosseous iliac path for the rod to be inserted later. The erector spinae muscles are retracted to provide a clear view of the intended bone entry point, which is just posterior to the sacroiliac joint at the

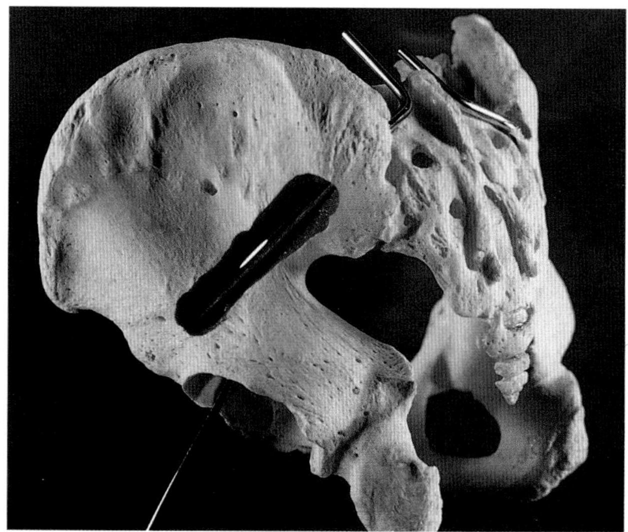

A

Figure 8. A,B,C: The model shows a cutaway view of the pelvic segment of an LRI pelvic fixation by the Galveston method. The drawings show how a Steinmann pin established the path for the rod in the ilium.

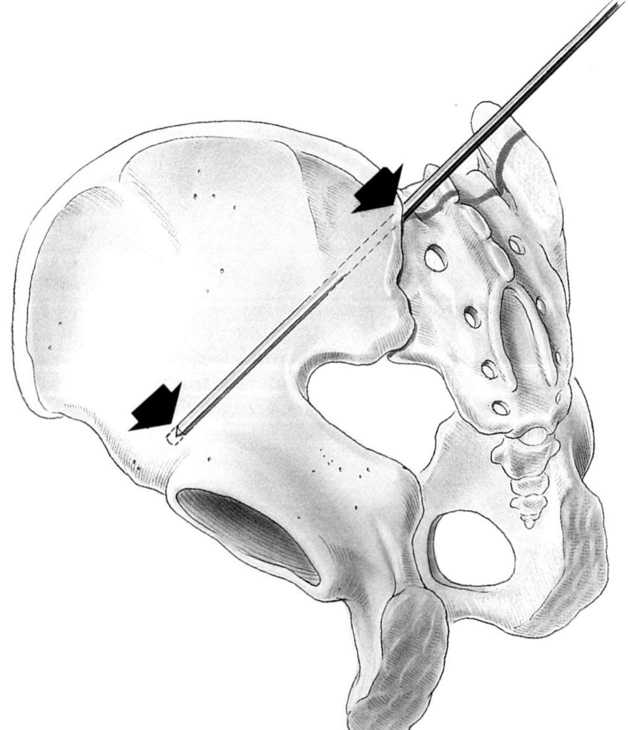

B

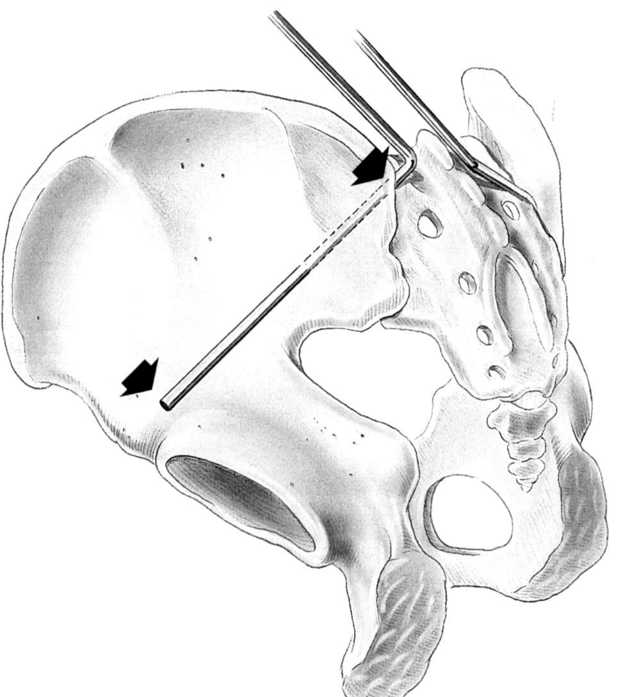

C

level of the lower margin of the posterior superior iliac spine. In cases without accessory posterior sacroiliac joints, the sharp tip of the Steinmann pin may be used to establish the entry point, but when accessory joints are present or when the surgeon is not certain of the anatomy, the bone entry point may be developed with a curette until the surgeon is confident that the entry point provides an intraosseous path for the rod.

The surgeon places a finger in the sciatic notch and with the free hand positions the tip of the pin at the bone entry point. By a combination of feel and sighting down the pin the surgeon aims the pin just above the sciatic notch and just deep to the outer iliac table. An assistant drives the pin with a mallet while the surgeon controls pin direction. Six to 9 cm, depending on the size of the patient, is the desired depth of pin penetration. Pins are placed on both the right and left sides of the pelvis and are left in place to serve as guides for rod shaping.

The length of pin in the ilium and the distance from the pin entrance hole to the ipsilateral, lateral surface of the sacral spinous processes need to be measured and noted for proper dimensioning of the rods later.

Shaping the Pelvic Portion of the Rods. The path that the rod will follow from anterior to posterior is first through the intraosseous path in the ilium for a 6- to 9-cm distance, second from the posterior iliac bone entry point to the base of the

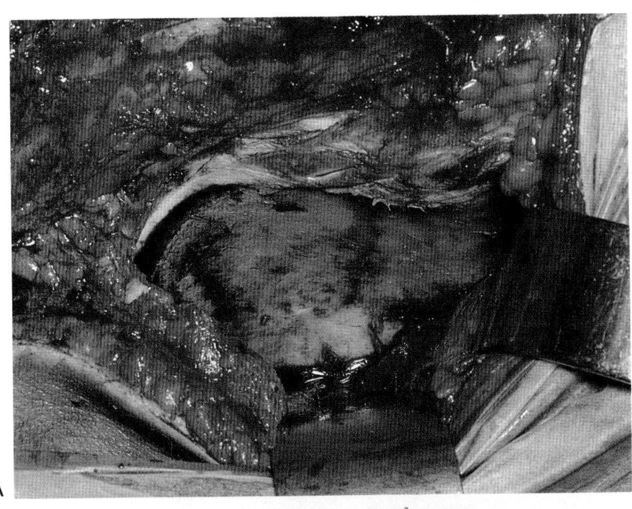
A

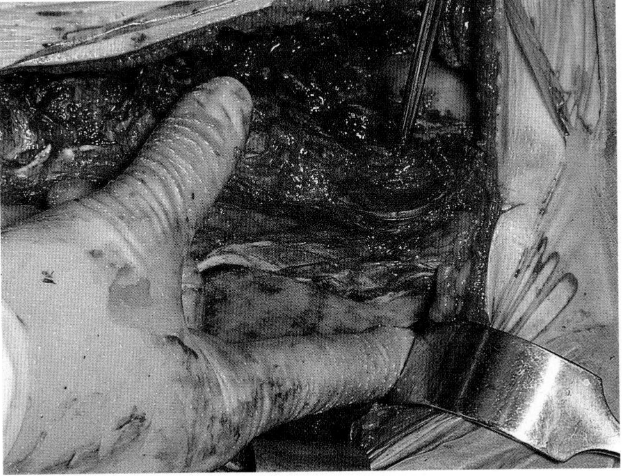
B

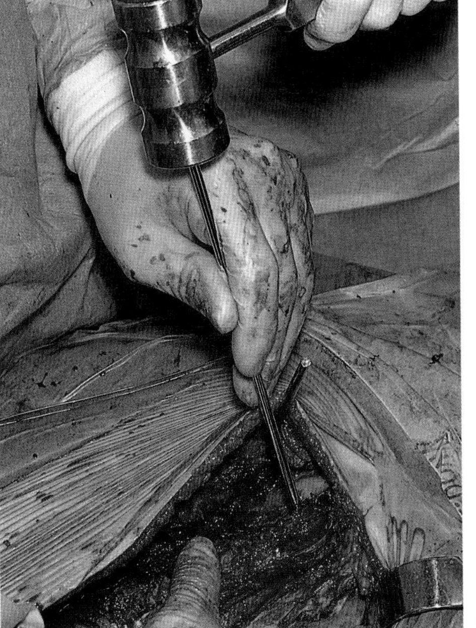
C

Figure 9. A: The patient's head is to the left; each ilium should be adequately exposed in pelvic fixation cases. **B:** The surgeon hooks a finger into the sciatic notch to use as a guide to placement of the pelvic pin. **C:** An assistant drives the pelvic pin while the surgeon maintains the aim.

sacral spinous processes, and third cephalad along the base of the sacral spinous processes extending to the vertebrae to be instrumented. It is necessary to make two bends to accommodate this anatomic placement of each rod, one at the point where the rod will exit the ilium at the bone entry point to place it parallel to the surface of the sacrum and a second at the point at which the rod will reach the sacral spinous processes and turn to extend alongside the spinous processes of the vertebrae. It is convenient to refer to the part of the rod that will lie in the ilium as the iliac portion or segment, the part that runs from the ilium to the midline as the sacral portion or segment, and the part that runs along the bases of the spinous processes as the spinal portion or segment. Right and left rods are prepared in similar manner (Fig. 10).

Sleeve benders are used to make the first bend between the sacral and spinal portions of the rod; the surgeon adds the previously made measurements of the iliac portion and the sacral portion of the rod to calculate the length of rod from its caudal tip to the bend at the junction of the sacral and spinal portions; for this example, consider an iliac depth of 8 cm and a posterior superior iliac spine-spinous process distance of 2 cm, yielding a sum of 10 cm. Ten centimeters are

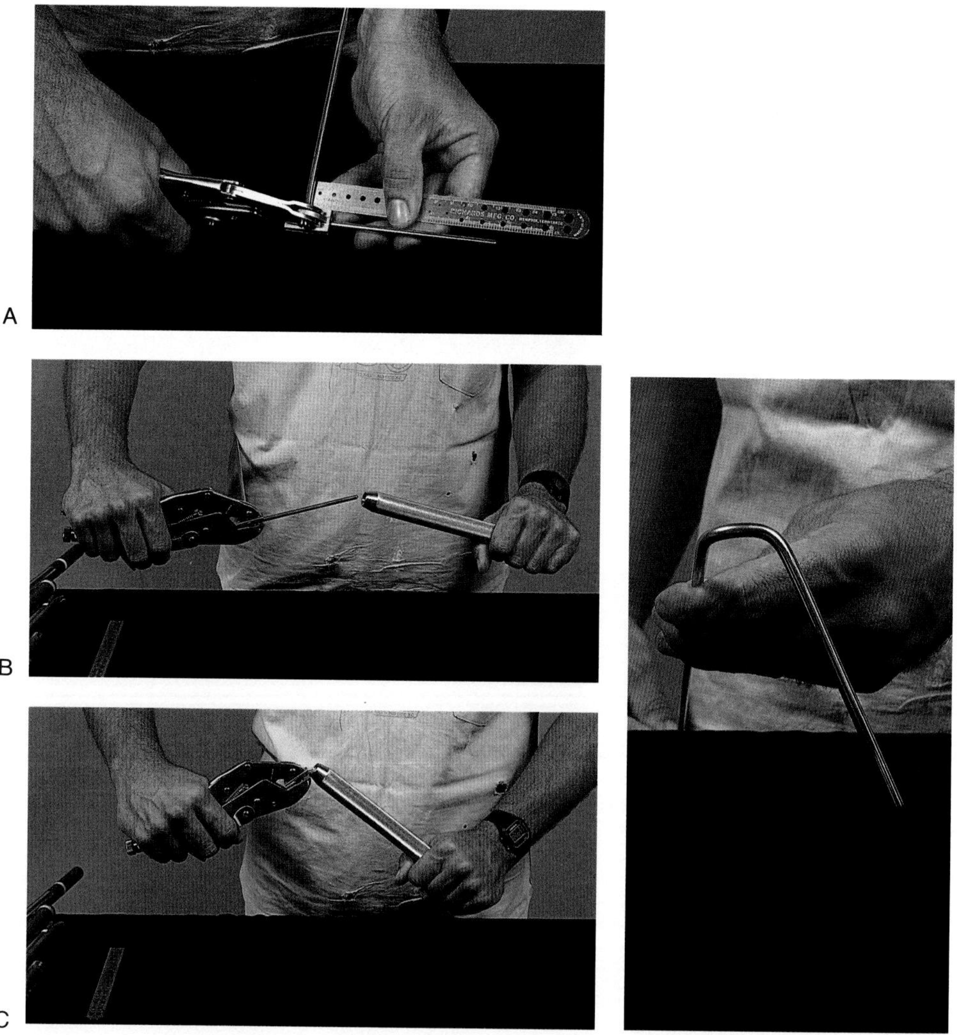

Figure 10. A: The pelvic rod clamp is placed to shape the bend between the sacral and iliac segments of the rod. **B:** A sleeve bender will be placed on the iliac segment. **C:** The bend between the sacral and iliac rod segments has been made. **D:** An "end-on" view of the pelvis-fixing portion of the rod.

measured along the long limb of the rod, sleeve benders are positioned close together at the 10-cm length, and an 80- to 90-degree bend is made.

The second bend between the iliac and sacral portions of the rod will be 2 cm lateral to the bend just completed; it is most easily accomplished with a pelvic rod clamp and a sleeve bender. The pelvic rod clamp is positioned and secured with the tip of its jaws at the 2-cm bend point; the sleeve bender is slipped over the iliac portion of the rod, and the rod is bent to an angle that will direct the spinal segment parallel to the posterior sacral surface and the iliac portion parallel to the previously placed Steinmann pin.

At this point the rod shaping for pelvic fixation is complete except for final small adjustments. While maintaining the iliac rod segment parallel to the Steinmann pin, the surgeon positions the rod such that the spinal portion is perpendicular to a line across the tops of the iliac crests; this represents a zero pelvic obliquity alignment with no provision for residual strain in the rod. The surgeon now shapes the spinal portion of the rod for sagittal contours and desired coronal plane correction (Fig. 11). The bends in the rod should be adjusted until the spinal portion of the rod has the desired coronal plane angle to a line across the tops of the ilia when the iliac portion is parallel to the Steinmann pin. If it is judged desirable to have residual strain in the final implant, this is the time to plan for it. A large surgical T-square is sometimes helpful in rod shaping for a severely decompensated patient. The rod should now be ready for insertion into the pelvis.

Inserting the Rods into the Pelvis. It is important to have the bone entry hole clearly in view and the iliac portion of the rod aimed down the intended path through the bone when insertion of the rod into the ilium is imminent. While the surgeon stands ready with the iliac portion of the rod parallel to the Steinmann pin and the rod tip close to the bone entry hole, an assistant slowly removes the Steinmann pin. As soon as the pin clears the bone entry hole, the surgeon places the tip of the iliac portion of the rod into the hole while maintaining the same angle as the pin. Whereas the first few centimeters of rod insertion can be done by hand, the remainder will require hammering to drive the rod.

Once the rod has been started by hand into the ilium, the surgeon should rotate the spinal segment of the rod to a nearly vertical position and place a pelvic rod clamp on the sacral segment close to the second bend. The surgeon may then either hammer the clamp to drive the rod, or alternatively, place a rod pusher adjacent to the pelvic rod clamp and hammer the pusher. As the rod is being driven home, the spinal portion is rotated to lie in the wound next to the spine.

A

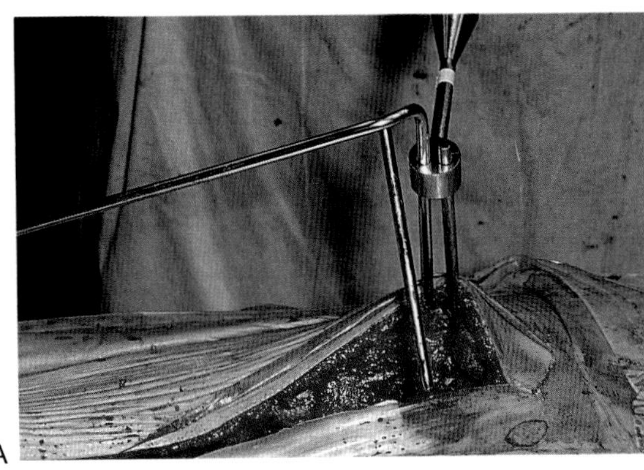

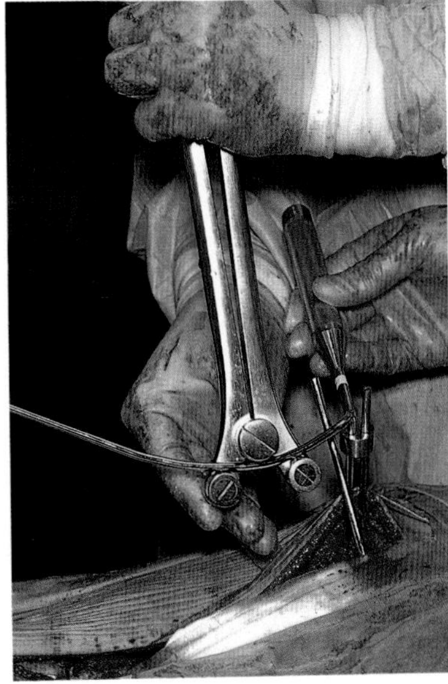

B

Figure 11. A: The patient's head is to the left; the iliac segment of the rod is held parallel to the pelvic pin by a pelvic rod guide while the spinal segment of the rod is shaped. **B:** French benders are useful for bending both lordosis and kyphosis into the spinal segment.

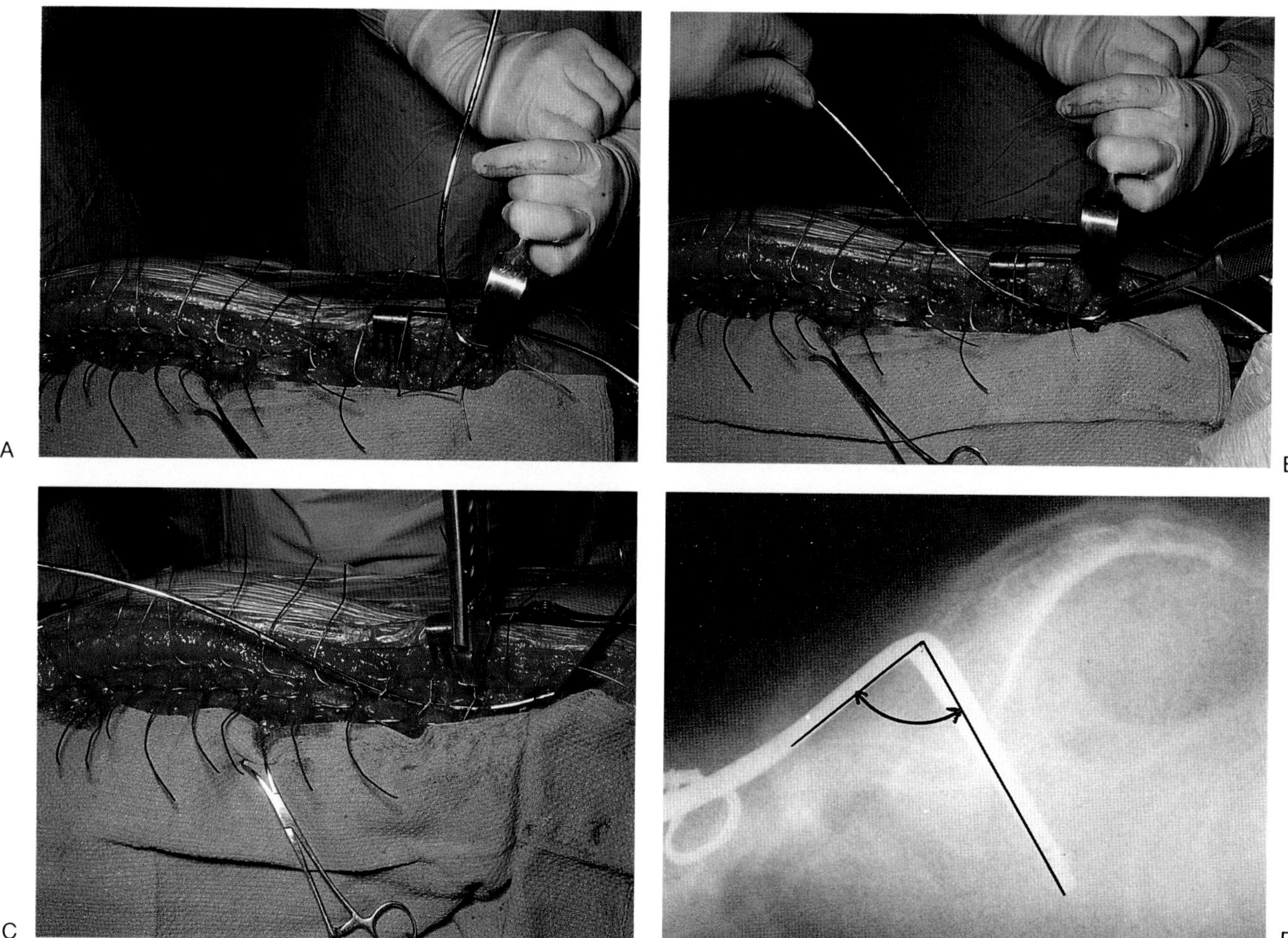

Figure 12. A: The patient's head is to the left. The spinal segment of the rod is vertical for initial driving of the iliac segment into the ilium. **B:** As the rod is driven into place the spinal segment is rotated into position beside the vertebral spinous processes. **C:** Wires at the lumbosacral junction have been fastened. **D:** Radiographically one can see that the iliac rod segment aims above the acetabulum and that the distal portion of the spinal rod segment lies on the posterior sacral surface.

Final seating of the rod into the ilium is done by placing a rod pusher on the extreme caudal end of the spinal segment of the rod and hammering the pusher. Once these steps have been completed for both the right and left rods, the pelvic fixation is complete. (Figure 12).

Fusion Technique. The author favors the addition of a large volume of autogenous bone graft lateral to the LRI to stimulate a spinal arthrodesis; with this method decortication and facet excision are not required. Posterior thoracoplasty, when a significant rib hump is present, provides both an enhanced cosmetic outcome and a voluminous bone graft. The author uses this adjunctive procedure frequently.

POSTOPERATIVE MANAGEMENT

During the first few days postoperatively, medical management appropriate for the patient who has undergone major spine surgery is carried out. The patient is placed in a regular bed and kept flat on the back for 12 to 24 hours unless insensitive skin or other medical problems preclude this position. No orthosis is prescribed and no plaster cast is applied. We do ask patients to restrict their activities to a walking level of intensity for the first postsurgical year. Sitting, climbing stairs, driving a car, riding a bicycle, and light lifting (less than 25 pounds) are permitted as soon as the patient can comfortably do them. Sexually active patients may resume intercourse as soon as they are sufficiently comfortable to do so, with restriction to the missionary position. Standing radiographs of the spine are obtained when the patient is able to stand, at 1 month, 6 months, and 1 year after surgery. Once the fusion is clinically and radiographically solid, further follow-up is a matter of individual judgment. Because prostaglandin E_2 inhibitors interfere with bone formation, we advise patients to avoid aspirin and nonsteroidal antiinflammatory drugs for the first year after surgery. Acetominaphen is an acceptable minor analgesic for use during this time.

We outline our expectations for a patient's first postoperative year in terms of the ranges of activities that reflect our experience with other LRI patients in aggregate. Most individuals will not require narcotic analgesics for more than 2 weeks; acetominaphen with codeine is a reasonable prescription. After 2 weeks most patients take no analgesics, but a small fraction do want a bedtime dose for another week or so. Return to school or to sedentary work is highly variable; the most robust will do so at 3 to 4 weeks, whereas others may not feel capable of returning for 12 to 16 weeks. As long as reasonable individual progress in increasing activity is made, we do not push the individual to do more than desired. For the person whose convalescence seems slower than usual, we encourage walking a certain time or distance several times a day, adding small increments from day to day. Most patients tell us that it took at least 6 months for them to feel completely normal again.

Once the patient feels good, the surgeon's role changes from encouraging activity to guiding appropriate activity. We tell the patient that until the spine fusion has become strong, at about 1 year after surgery, activity puts a load on the spinal implant. Because the implant takes the load, no pain or warning sign shows that it is being overloaded. We explain further that if the implant should break, it would be from fatigue, not catastrophic overloading; the analogy of breaking a paper clip by bending it back and forth helps to convey the concept.

If the fusion is radiographically solid at 1 year after surgery, the patient is advised to resume full activities gradually with the exception of contact sports.

By the end of the first postoperative year, the spinal fusion should be radiographically evident and intact. When rib graft obtained with a posterior thoracoplasty has been used, the graft is visible from day 1; whether it is being resorbed or is stimulating the desired new bone formation can be easily observed each follow-up visit. With a cancellous bone graft, the host response may not be evident for some months, and it is not until no new bone can be seen at 1 year that graft resorption can be considered with confidence. Either way, if a solid fusion is not present, the implant will eventually break from fatigue failure. We recommend doing whatever is required to prove the presence of an intact fusion at 1 year (i.e., oblique x-ray views, tomograms, stress films); if fusion cannot be proved, surgical exploration of the fusion is appropriate, with rebulking and whatever else may be indicated based on surgical findings.

COMPLICATIONS

It seems self-evident that all the medical, anesthetic, and general surgical complications that may occur in spinal operations may be seen when LRI is performed. Their management is well defined and is not discussed here. We focus on the more dire complications of (a) immediate spinal cord injury, (b) delayed onset spinal cord injury, (c) hyperesthetic syndrome, (d) deep infection, and (e) resorption of the bone graft.

The author has no experience with LRI-associated immediate spinal cord injury but nonetheless does have an opinion about intraoperative management in such a case. With open interlaminar spaces, the most dreaded event would be plunging an instrument into the neural canal and striking the spinal cord. Obviously this should not happen; if it did, medical measures, such as steroid administration, should be started and the operation should be completed with a lesser attempt at deformity correction than would have been done otherwise. Evidence shows that splinting an injured spinal cord is beneficial and even though the prospects for recovery from the neurologic injury may not be immediately clear, no justification seems to exist for the spinal deformity to remain as an uncontrolled problem.

From my knowledge and experience, most of the spinal cord injuries associated with LRI have been delayed in onset. Management of these cases is controversial, and available data do not clearly support one approach over another. My preference is to follow these cases expectantly and manage them medically as long as the neurologic deficit is neither dense nor progressive during the observation period; full recovery can be expected when these conditions are met. When a progressive deficit exists, the best course in my opinion is to return the patient to the operating room and bend the implant to a lesser degree of correction, or, if circumstances permit, remove the implant altogether.

The hyperesthetic syndrome is the most frequent neural injury associated with LRI; it probably results from spinal cord contusion, which can occur when sublaminar wires are passed inexpertly. The hyperesthetic, dysesthetic region, because it is so sensitive and painful, may greatly stress the patient. Adequate analgesia and reassurance should be given. In most cases the symptoms resolve in less than a week, but in the rare patient may last for months—the longest duration of symptoms of which I am aware was 6 months. No case of failure to resolve has been documented. Desensitization techniques and mobilization by a physical therapist may be helpful.

In our experience the most effective plan for managing a deep wound infection in the LRI patient is medical suppression coupled with surgical drainage; we avoid reopening the wound, debriding the wound, irrigating the wound, and other invasive measures. The strategy is to control the infection for 1 year until the fusion consolidates; at that time we remove the spinal implant and treat with appropriate antibiotics for about 2 weeks, an empiric time.

Once the problem has been recognized, appropriate antibiotics (determined by culture and sensitivity) should be administered and a small drainage tract established at the caudal extreme of the wound. The usual measures of sepsis (temperature elevation, increased white blood count with left shift, hemoglobin, and serum albumin) are followed. In the usual case the trend to improvement becomes evident within 24 hours. As tolerated, the patient should be mobilized to the degree appropriate for an uncomplicated case. When the threat of severe systemic sepsis has resolved, oral antibiotics, for as long as needed to keep the infection under control, are prescribed. At this point the sedimentation rate may be a useful follow-up measure. Some patients may be taken off antibiotics after several months, whereas others will need continuous suppressive therapy. One should attempt to keep the drainage tract open; from time to time granulation tissue may require debridement. In our experience, the spinal fusion in infected cases proceeds relatively normally, and the infection is fully controlled once the implant has been removed. Although aggressive wound debridement and wide-open drainage would be desirable if a life-threatening, otherwise uncontrollable sepsis were present, we have never encountered such a case.

ILLUSTRATIVE CASE FOR TECHNIQUE

The following case was selected to illustrate both the effectiveness of an LRI-based strategy in correcting a severe deformity and the management of several significant complications. The patient, a 15-year-old boy who had a low thoracic-level myelomeningocele, presented with neglected musculoskeletal problems; he no longer fit into a wheelchair and his recumbent postures were limited. A long, left thoracolumbar scoliosis and fixed contractures of the hips in a windswept position were found. The scoliosis measured 130 degrees (Cobb angle; Fig. 13) and corrected to about 90 degrees on a traction radiograph (Fig. 14). The left hip had a flexion, abduction contracture, and the right hip had a flexion, adduction contracture. Neither hip would fully flex.

Because acceptable correction of the patient's scoliosis was not considered possible (from traction studies), the strategy of a two-stage surgical approach with anterior spinal release and fusion followed by secondary LRI was planned. Bilateral proximal femoral resections were planned for mobilization of his hips. At age 15.6 years he underwent anterior release and fusion (ARF) from T10 to S1 without complication and was placed in tong/gravity traction on a circular bed. Twelve days after the ARF, LRI from T2 to the pelvis and bilateral proximal femoral resections were done, (Fig. 15). His scoliosis had been corrected to about 35 degrees (Cobb angle), and he was well compensated. Uneventful healing from this point, which is the usual course for such a patient, would have yielded an excellent result, but he developed a wound slough at the thoracolumbar junction at the upper end of his myelomeningocele repair.

Over the next several weeks, after his LRI, the wound was locally debrided until it was approximately 2 by 4 cm and extended through the deep fascia. Despite antibiotic coverage, he developed a deep infection with mixed flora. Antibiotics, adjusted from time to time depending on cultures and sensitivities, were administered via a Hickman catheter, and the now clean wound, through which the implant was visible, was managed by frequent dressing changes and further minor debridements. The strategy was to suppress the infection and allow the wound to heal partially by second intention; it was hoped that the strategy of allowing the fusion to heal for 1 year and then removing the hardware could be followed. A concern existed, however, that much of the bone graft in the area of the wound complication had been debrided.

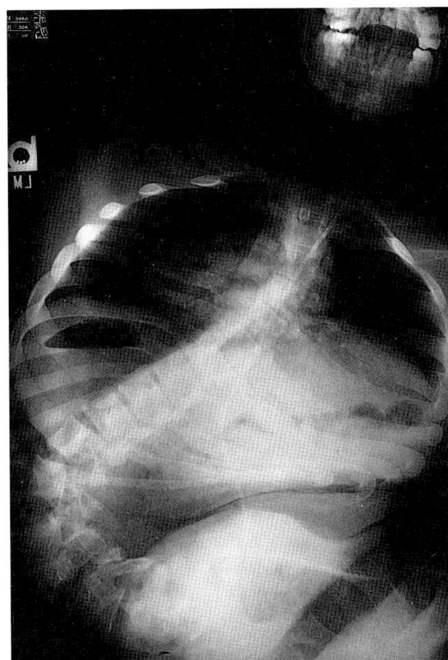

Figure 13. Presurgical, sitting, AP radiograph of the illustrative case.

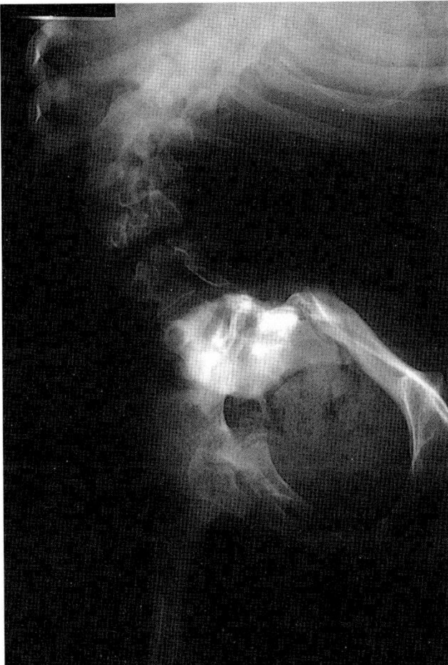

Figure 14. Presurgical traction correction radiograph demonstrating the stiffness of his deformity.

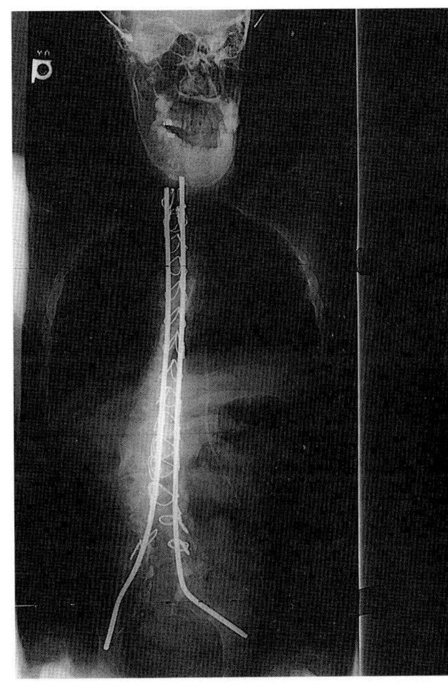

Figure 15. Postoperative two-stage anterior release with fusion and posterior LRI with pelvic fixation, sitting, AP radiograph.

At 2.8 months after surgery he developed a deep venous thrombosis with venogram-demonstrated clots in the superficial femoral vein. Anticoagulation with heparin followed by conversion to Coumadin was begun. Several days into this regimen he hemorrhaged from his back wound to a degree that the hemorrhage appeared to be a more threatening problem than the deep venous thrombosis; anticoagulation was discontinued.

By 111 days after surgery, his wound had almost healed by second intention. He was discharged from the hospital on local dressing changes for the wound and instructed to use a wheelchair at his preoperative activity level, which was limited. Although we would have preferred to keep a sinus tract open, the wound closed fully.

A little over 9 months after surgery his rods fractured, with an acute loss of about 40 degrees (Cobb angle) as well as loss of lumbar lordosis; an obvious pseudarthrosis existed at the level of his previous wound debridement (Fig. 16). Pseudarthrosis repair with reinforcement of his LRI construct was performed (Fig. 17). Despite prophylactic antibiotics he had another episode of wound infection, with positive cultures for methicillin–resistant *Staphylococcus epidermalis* (MRSE). He was treated with intravenous vancomycin and other antibiotics as indicated by culture and sensitivity along with local wound care; his wound once again healed without preservation of a sinus tract.

Since that time, he has remained stable and his fusion appears radiographically solid (at 2.7 years after surgery Fig. 17). He is a candidate for elective removal of his spinal implant.

This case illustrates many of the points made earlier in this chapter. At the outset it was recognized that adequate correction could not be obtained by a simple posterior instrumentation because of the rigidity seen on a traction film. No evidence shows that any implant gives a better result than forced bend or traction films indicate is possible, and LRI is certainly no exception. ARF was appropriate both to enhance correctability and to improve the probability of solid spinal fusion. Although it is true that between-stage traction may not improve correctability, it was used in this case to facilitate respiratory care, which it seemed

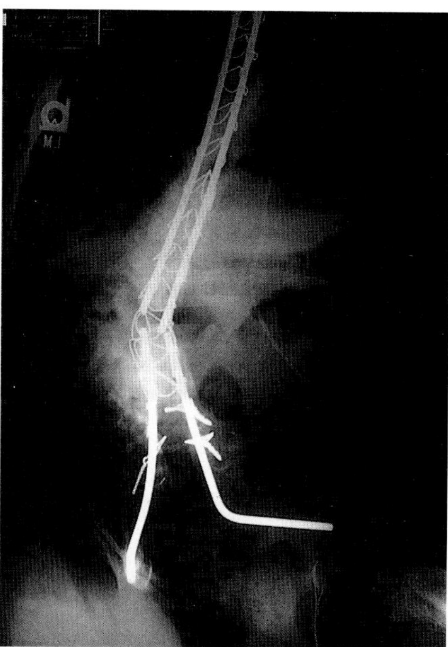

Figure 16. Nine-month postoperative sitting AP radiograph showing the implant failure and the pseudarthrosis site.

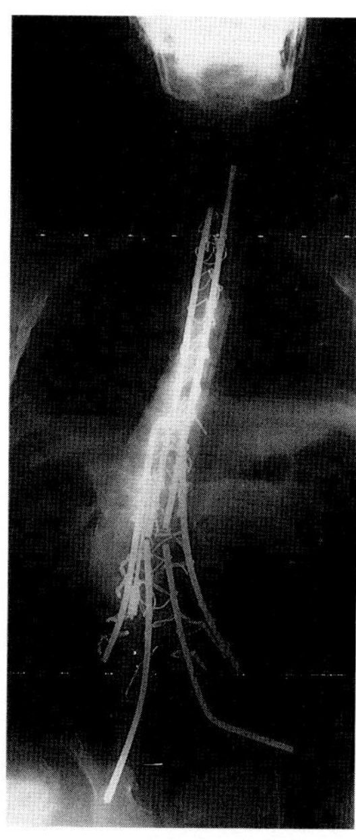

Figure 17. Postrevision surgery with repair of pseudarthrosis, sitting AP radiograph.

to do. Whereas our current practice is to perform same-day two-stage surgery whenever possible, in a severe case such as this one, separate operative times for the stages may be needed to ensure a tolerable surgical injury.

Hip contractures are a major problem in pelvic fixation cases because if the hips are pushed into flexion when hip flexion is limited, the posterior pelvis may be fractured, resulting in loss of pelvic fixation. Although it is not the best of available options for increasing hip motion, proximal femoral resection seemed the best choice for this patient in view of the severity of his loss of hip motion.

The initial goals of adequate correction, compensation, level pelvis, and adequate hip motion were achieved, but then the complication of local wound necrosis arose. Debridement of the wound to a subfascial level was appropriate, but it set the stage for wound infection via an exposed implant and also for pseudarthrosis via removal of bone graft at the depth of the wound. Both of these complications occurred.

Once the wound was open, the use of antibiotics to suppress infection was appropriate; the antibiotics had to be adjusted as the wound flora changed from time to time. Wide wound debridement would have been a mistake because the patient was not uncontrollably toxic and because removal of the bone graft would have compromised the chances for a fusion. He differed from most patients with an infection in that he did not have continuing drainage and his wound healed.

Implant failure at 9 months after surgery was early and unexpected; in most patients with a pseudarthrosis the implant does not break for 3 to 4 years after surgery. The factors in this case are not known, but they include the possibilities of greater than usual stress because the patient walked on his hands and of crack initiation at the site of a scratch on the implant. The degree of acute loss of correction that he sustained after implant failure made revision mandatory; as with his initial surgery, the complication of a deep infection occurred. Once again suppression of the infection controlled the problem, and once again the wound closed. His pseudarthrosis repair healed uneventfully, and a radiographically solid fusion, anteriorly as well as posteriorly, became evident.

This patient is now a candidate for elective implant removal. Even though his path to recovery was difficult and tortuous, he now has an excellent clinical outcome.

RECOMMENDED READING

1. Allen, B. L. Jr., and Ferguson, R. L.: The Galveston technique for L rod instrumentation of the scoliotic spine. *Spine*, 7: 276–284, 1982.
2. Allen, B. L. Jr., and Ferguson, R. L.: The Galveston technique of pelvic fixation with L rod instrumentation of the spine. *Spine*, 9: 388–394, 1984.
3. Allen, B. L. Jr., and Ferguson, R. L.: Neurologic injuries with the Galveston technique of L-rod instrumentation for scoliosis. *Spine*, 11: 14–17, 1986.
4. Ferguson, R. L., and Allen, B. L. Jr.: Staged correction of neuromuscular scoliosis. *J. Pediatr. Orthop.*, 3: 555–562, 1983.
5. Ferguson, R. L., and Allen, B. L. Jr.: The technique of scoliosis revision surgery utilizing L-rod instrumentation. *J. Pediatr. Orthop.*, 3: 563–571, 1983.
6. Luque, E. E.: The anatomic basis and development of segmental spinal instrumentation. *Spine*, 7: 256–259, 1982.
7. Luque, E. R.: Segmental spinal instrumentation for correction of scoliosis. *Clin. Orthop.*, 163: 192–198, 1982.
8. Weiler, P. J., Medley, J. B., and McNeice, G. M.: Numeric analysis of the load capacity of the human spine fitted with L-rod instrumentation. *Spine*, 15: 1285–1293, 1990.

23

Isola Spinal Instrumentation

Marc A. Asher

INDICATIONS AND CONTRAINDICATIONS

Because an idiopathic scoliosis deformity with a Cobb angle of 50 degrees or greater can be expected to progress during a person's lifetime (15), surgical treatment of such curves is universally accepted as appropriate. For a fully mature, middle-aged person with a curve of 50 to 60 degrees that causes no difficulty of any consequence, continued observation is reasonable since cardiopulmonary compromise is not anticipated (10).

A more difficult area of patient selection for surgical treatment involves curvatures between 40 and 50 degrees. Patients with balanced spines and deformities, as well as normal sagittal plane alignment, are usually best managed nonoperatively by brace treatment in the growing child and observation in the adult. Curves from 30 to 40 degrees are virtually always best managed nonoperatively, except when considerable imbalance exists, with both the T1 and inflection vertebrae offset laterally to the same side of the midsacral gravity reference line or when unusually large thoracolumbar junction kyphosis is present in the sagittal plane.

PREOPERATIVE PLANNING

The history and physical examination are used to be certain that no underlying neurologic, congenital, or other explanations exist for the patient's scoliosis. Lack of forward bending flexibility to the point of not being able to touch to the tibial tubercles, left apex thoracic scoliosis, and asymmetrical abdominal cutaneous reflexes are among the important warning signs of possible underlying spinal cord abnormality. The important physical findings for defining the clinical deformity

M. A. Asher, M.D.: Section of Orthopaedic Surgery, University of Kansas Medical Center, Kansas City, Kansas 66160–7387.

are coronal and sagittal plane balance, shoulder height asymmetry, waist and/or trunk asymmetry, and forward bending paravertebral asymmetry.

The principle imaging studies used are standing 36-inch-long, 72-inch tube-film distance, posteroanterior (PA) and lateral radiographs. Recumbent nonstressed right- and left-bending, recumbent anteroposterior (AP), and sometimes cross-table lateral with bolster views may also be helpful.

The goals of surgical treatment of idiopathic scoliosis are as nearly normal spine alignment as possible, maximum motion segment preservation and accommodation of residual deformity in such a manner as to achieve spinal balance. Selection of vertebrae to be fused to achieve these goals has always been controversial but has become more so as understanding of the three-dimensional aspects of scoliosis deformity has increased (13). Rules established for two-dimensional instrumentation systems (5,6,7) no longer seem applicable, at least not fully (8,9,14,16). To achieve our goals, a clear definition of spinal alignment, deformity, and corrective load application is necessary.

Spinal Alignment and Deformity Analysis

Analysis of spine position and scoliosis deformity is based on use of Cartesian coordinate systems. Figure 1 shows a reference system placed in a global manner with the origin centered on top of the S1 body, the vertical gravity reference line through it, and the mediolateral reference line parallel to a line connecting the anterior inferior iliac spine. Angular positions of the various vertebrae in relation to this reference coordinate system are defined using the engineer's right-hand

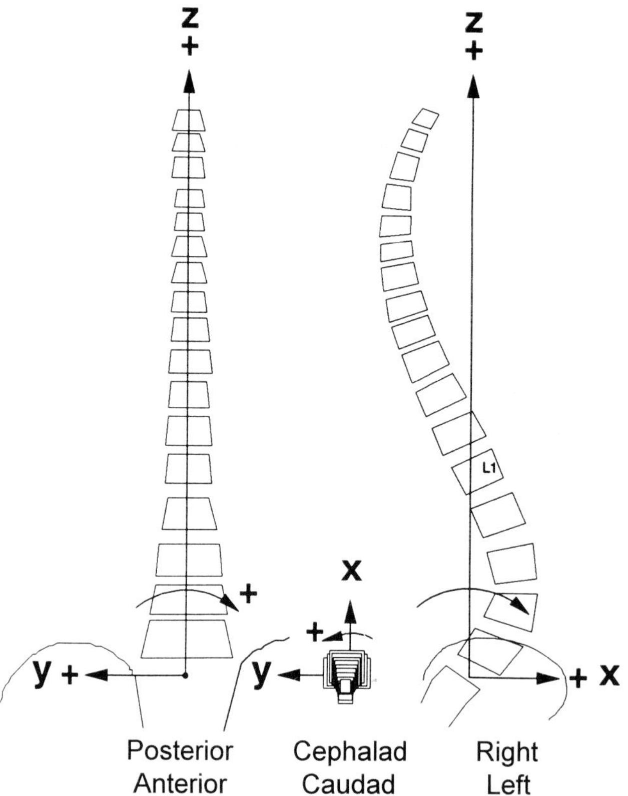

Figure 1. The three planes and 6 degrees of freedom of motion defined by a Cartesian coordinate system. Note that mediolateral translation, coronal plane angulation, and transverse plane angulation are all zero in the normal spine.

rule (Fig. 2). For Cobb measurement, the reference coordinate system is placed on the lower end vertebrae.

In the normal spine 3 degrees of freedom of motion are zero (coronal and transverse plane angulation and medial-lateral translation). Sagittal plane angular position as well as AP and vertical translation vary with each segment (4). Scoliosis deformities are apex (and periapex) vertebra lateral translation, transverse plane angulation, anterior or posterior translation, and vertical translation. The end vertebrae deformities are coronal plane angulation, vertical translation, and sometimes lateral translation, AP translation, sagittal plane angulation, and/or transverse plane angulation.

End Vertebra Selection

The upper vertebral level to be instrumented should have minimal translation laterally in relation to the rib cage, normal sagittal plane alignment, and normal transverse plane angular position (i.e., no rotation). It is usually one level above the upper end vertebrae for short thoracic curves, two levels for long thoracic curves, and the upper end vertebrae for double thoracic curves and compensatory thoracic curves.

The lower vertebrae level to be instrumented in single and double thoracic curves should have minimal translation laterally in relation to the trunk sides as well as normal sagittal and transverse plane alignment. Following instrumentation, it should be transacted by the midsacral gravity reference line. Its selection is dependent on the amount of curve correction that can be achieved. In general it is one below the lower end vertebrae, sometimes at the lower end vertebrae, and very occasionally two below the lower end vertebrae. This is usually one or two above the stable vertebrae.

A compensatory thoracolumbar/lumbar curve cannot be excluded from the instrumentation if, in the coronal plane, the inflexion vertebra is laterally translated toward the convexity of the lumbar curve, or if the lower adjacent motion segment is hyperkyphotic or hyperlordotic. On lateral bends the motion segment below the planned instrumented vertebra should be mobile at least to the point that the end plates become parallel with bending toward the convexity. Following these guidelines, the lower instrumented vertebra is usually one below the apex vertebra/disc of the compensatory curve, one above the lower end vertebra, and one or two vertebrae above the stable vertebra. It is possible to accept up to about 15 degrees of transverse plane angular deformity (rotation) of the lower instrumented vertebra. The lower instrumented vertebra for double curves, thoracolumbar curves, and lumbar curves is usually the same as the lower end vertebra.

Nonstress, recumbent bend films are helpful to decide whether or not supplemental procedures should be utilized to achieve correction. In small curves and in curves in which the bending correction is 50% or more, supplemental procedures are not required for acceptable correction. However, when the curve(s) is greater than approximately 65 degrees with flexibility of approximately 40% or less, supplemental procedures (e.g., thoracoplasty, rib osteotomies, discectomies, or even osteotomies in the extreme cases) should be considered.

Instrumentation Concepts and Sequence

The five broad concepts of application are as follows: foundations, anatomically contoured longitudinal members, variable position connections, force couples, and stable, strong, durable constructs.

The sequence of load application is apex medial and either anterior or posterior translation. If apex anterior translation is needed, convex side instrumentation is required first. If only posterior apex translation is called for, concave side instrumentation is accomplished first. For end vertebral coronal plane alignment, convex compression is done first and concave distraction last.

Component Selection

The Isola components, which have been described in detail in several publications, emphasize minimal internal and external profile, simplicity, and versatility (1, 2). Their application features are the capacity to deliver correction and resist deforming forces and moments in each of 6 degrees of freedom of motion and to allow sequential, fully segmented instrumentation.

Hooks are usually employed at the upper end vertebra, at the convex thoracic apex vertebra, at or near the inflection vertebra, and sometimes on the concavity of the thoracic curve. Screws are routinely employed at the lower end vertebra and the lumbar apex vertebra (Fig. 2). Sublaminar wires are often used on the convex sides of the thoracic and lumbar vertebra.

The patient illustrated in Fig. 3 has a compensatory thoracolumbar curve that cannot be safely excluded when doing three-dimensional instrumentation. This is because the inflection vertebra (T10) is already bisected by the midsacral gravity reference line, and correction of the thoracic curve alone would almost certainly result in coronal plane imbalance to the left. Furthermore, stopping the fusion above L1, or even sometimes above T12, often results in thoracolumbar junctional hyperkyphosis. Following the end vertebra selection guidelines described above, the recommended instrumented levels are T4, one above the upper end vertebra, and L2, one above the end vertebra of the lower curve, one below the apex vertebra of the lower curve, and three above the stable vertebra (Fig. 3).

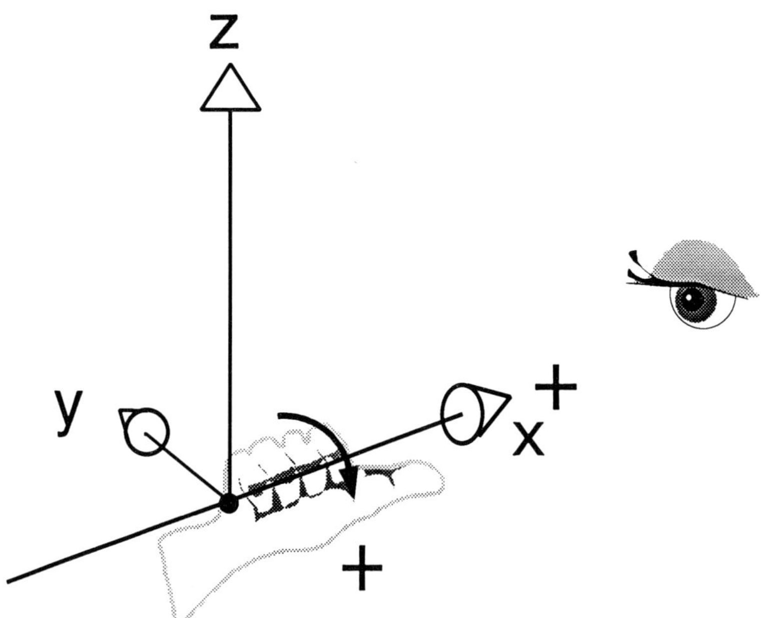

Figure 2. Sense, positive and negative, of angulation around an axis as defined by the engineer's right-hand rule in which the thumb of the right hand points in the positive translational direction along the axis, and the curled fingers define the positive sense of the angular position/motion about the axis (positive being counterclockwise when viewed standing on the positive axis looking down the axis toward the origin.

SURGERY

General anesthesia is used, but with an incomplete pharmacologic paralysis so that two twitches are always present to neural stimulation. This helps warn the surgeon that vital neurologic structures are being approached. Mild hypotension with a mean arterial pressure of around 70 mm Hg is generally utilized, and care is taken to make sure the patient maintains a normal temperature.

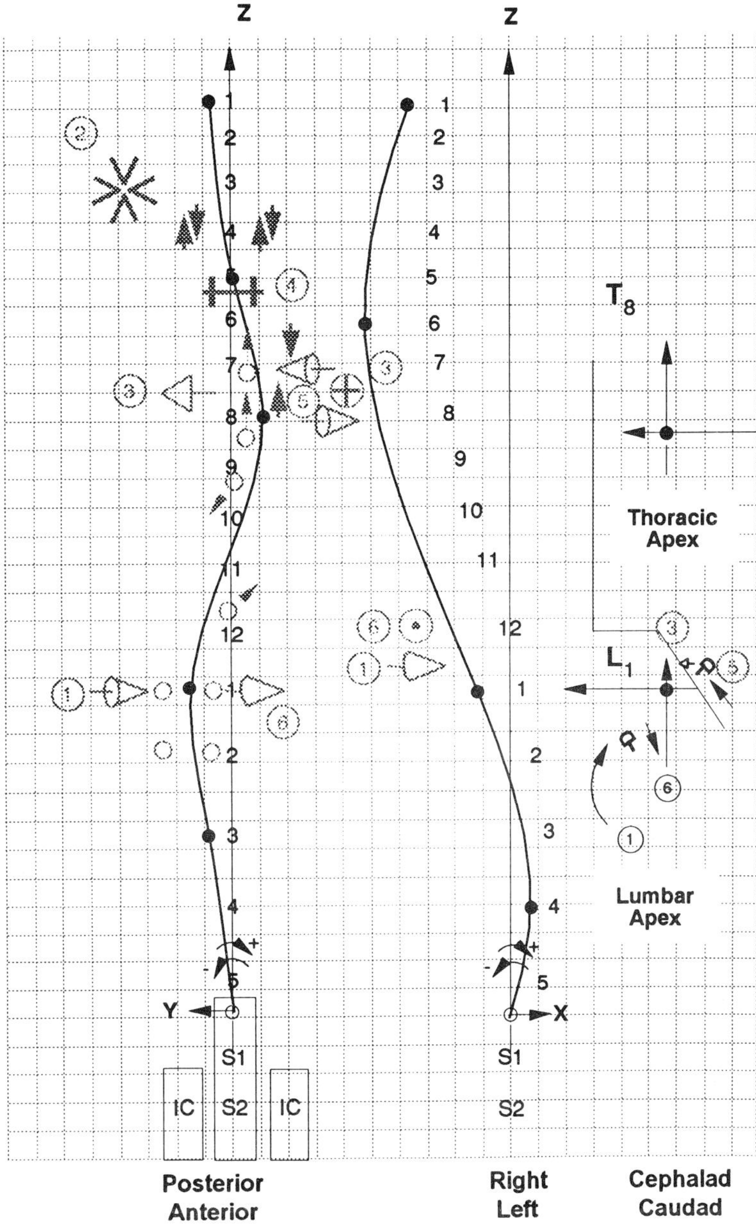

Figure 3. Thoracic and thoracolumbar double curve instrumentation and load application sequence. *1*, thoracolumbar apex medial and anterior translation; *2*, thoracic concave upper end instrumented vertebra foundation; *3*, thoracic apex medial translation; *4*, upper thoracic foundation completion, including transverse connection; *5*, thoracic apex medial translation; and *6*, lumbar apex medial and posterior translation. Loads 1 and 6 provide a transverse plane force couple on the lumbar curve, and loads 3 and 5 do the same for the thoracic curve. Compression on the scoliosis convexities, followed by distraction on the concavities, completes the load applications.

Patients are positioned on a Relton–Hall-style frame, and all bony prominences are well padded. The operative table must have clearance to accommodate cassette placement for PA radiography. Bleeding is minimized at all times utilizing the techniques of electrocautery dissection and coagulation, bone wax, oxycel (cotton-type oxidized cellulose; Desceret Medical Inc., Sandy, Utah), and bipolar coagulations.

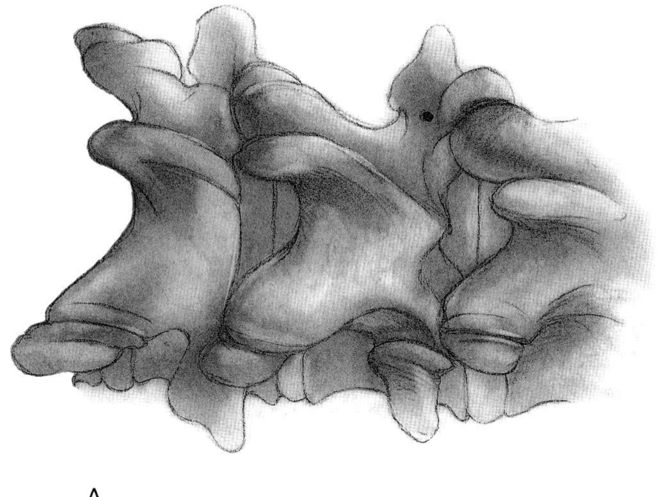
A

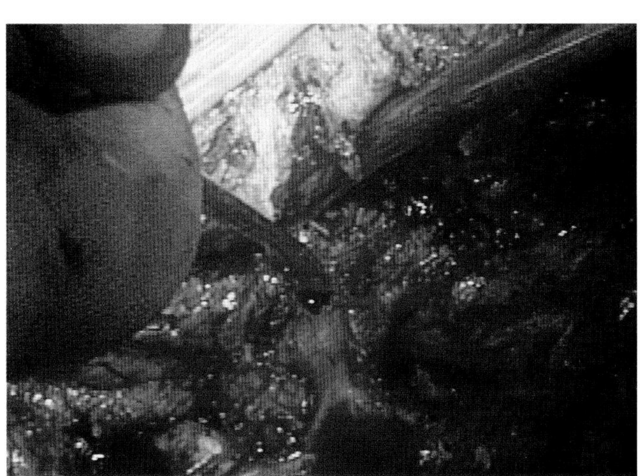
B

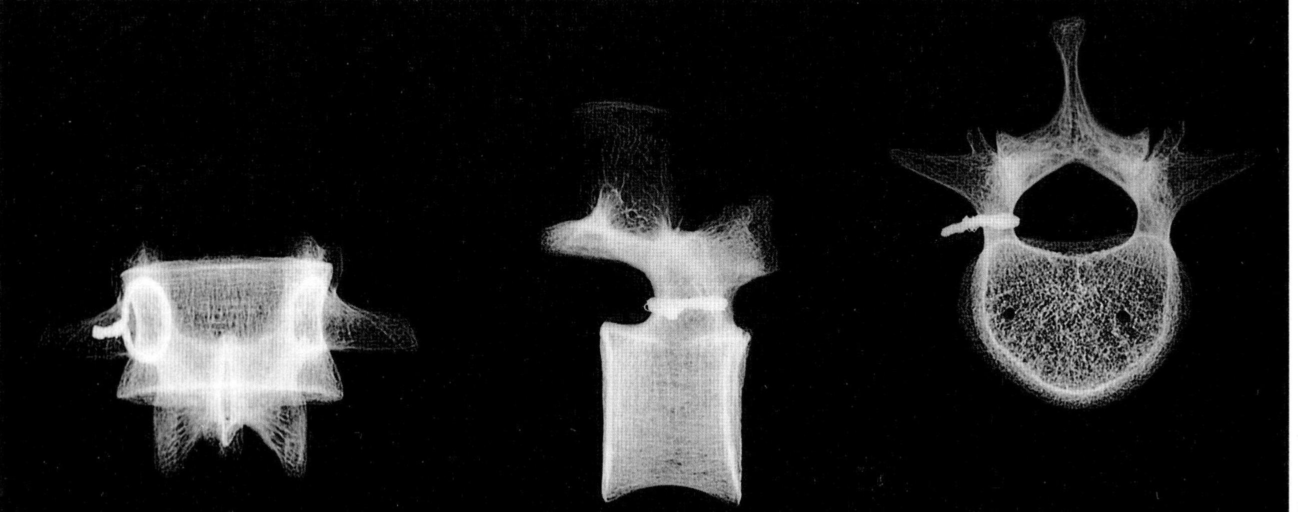
C

Figure 4. In this patient, screws have been placed on both sides of L1 and L2. **A:** Anatomical drawing of T12, L1, and L2 vertebrae in the field visualized. **B:** Curved dural-style VSP probe about to be inserted into the pedicle entry site. **C:** Radiographs in the coronal, sagittal, and transverse planes of lumbar vertebrae with a wire around the pedicle.

Incision

After skin preparation and draping, a longitudinal incision is made from one level above to about one-half level below the planned instrumented levels. An intraoperative PA radiograph is recommended to confirm the levels exposed. Electrocautery dissection is done following the bony contours, trying to avoid disruption of the dorsal primary rami as they pass lateral to the pars interarticularis. The dissection is carried to the tip of the transverse processes in the thoracic spine and to the midpart of the transverse processes in the lumbar spine. Any remaining interspinous ligaments and capsule are removed with curettes or rongeurs. Care is taken to preserve all, or at least most, of the spinous processes since they provide the strut supporting the posterior muscle mass and are the coverage for the implants. Gelpi, extended Gelpi, and long Weitlaner retractors are most helpful in this process.

Pedicle Screw Anchor Placement

Pedicle screw placement is analogous to intramedullary implant placement in a long bone. The point of entry to the pedicle is at the junction of the superior facet process, transverse process, and pars interarticularis for the lumbar spine (12) (Fig. 4A).

The cortical bone overlying the entry point is removed either with a rongeur, gouge, or awl to expose the underlying cancellous bone. The awl should not penetrate to the depth of the spinal canal. The pedicle is probed with the curved dural elevator probe (11, 12) (Fig. 4B). It is important to visualize where the probe is supposed to be and to know what the feel should be. The passage line is perpendicular to a point line joining adjacent laminae in the sagittal plane and coronal plane and directed from lateral to medial to accommodate the transverse plane angular

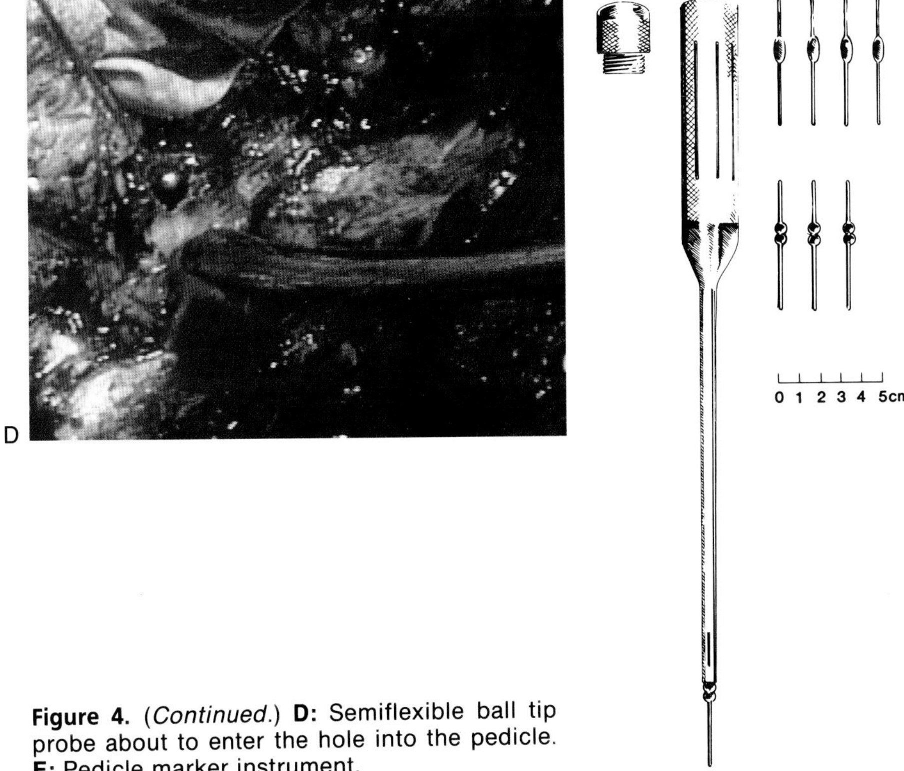

Figure 4. (*Continued.*) **D:** Semiflexible ball tip probe about to enter the hole into the pedicle. **E:** Pedicle marker instrument.

Figure continues.

position of the pedicle. This is typically 0 to 20 degrees. The pedicle is oval, with the larger diameter being cephalocaudal (vertical) (Fig. 4C). This allows for variable angular positioning of the probe in the sagittal plane and is helpful in ensuring proper perpendicular orientation of the screw in relation to the longitudinal member.

The motion used to advance the pedicle probe is a swirl and wiggle to produce a round hole at the opening and an oval hole in the pedicle. If resistance is suddenly lost during insertion, the probe has almost certainly exited the cortical tube leading into the pedicle or the pedicle wall. The probe should be removed and the hole palpated with the semiflexible ball tip probe (Fig. 4D) to determine whether penetration has been medial, lateral, superior, or inferior. After this has been ascertained, the pedicle probe can be properly redirected into the pedicle isthmus. After probing the four walls and floor of the hole with the ball tip probe, pedicle markers may be placed (Fig. 4E). The entry to the hole is plugged with a small piece of bone wax and the 30-mm end of the pedicle marker placed and positioned so that it is perpendicular to the passage line of the longitudinal member. Posteroanterior and lateral radiographs are taken to determine marker position and alignment.

The hole is tapped with an auger tip tap (Fig. 4F). This tap will pull itself into the hole and merely needs to be guided. Only the isthmus needs to be tapped, and the tap used is customarily slightly smaller than the screw to be placed. The VSP screw is inserted with the ⅛-inch (3.2-mm) hex driver until a strong resistance to torque is encountered (Fig. 4G,H). If necessary, for the sake of profile, the acorn connection on the screw may be countersunk into the hole with a large curette prior to screw placement. Variations in AP translation of the acorn junction may be adjusted with the 3- and 5-mm washers.

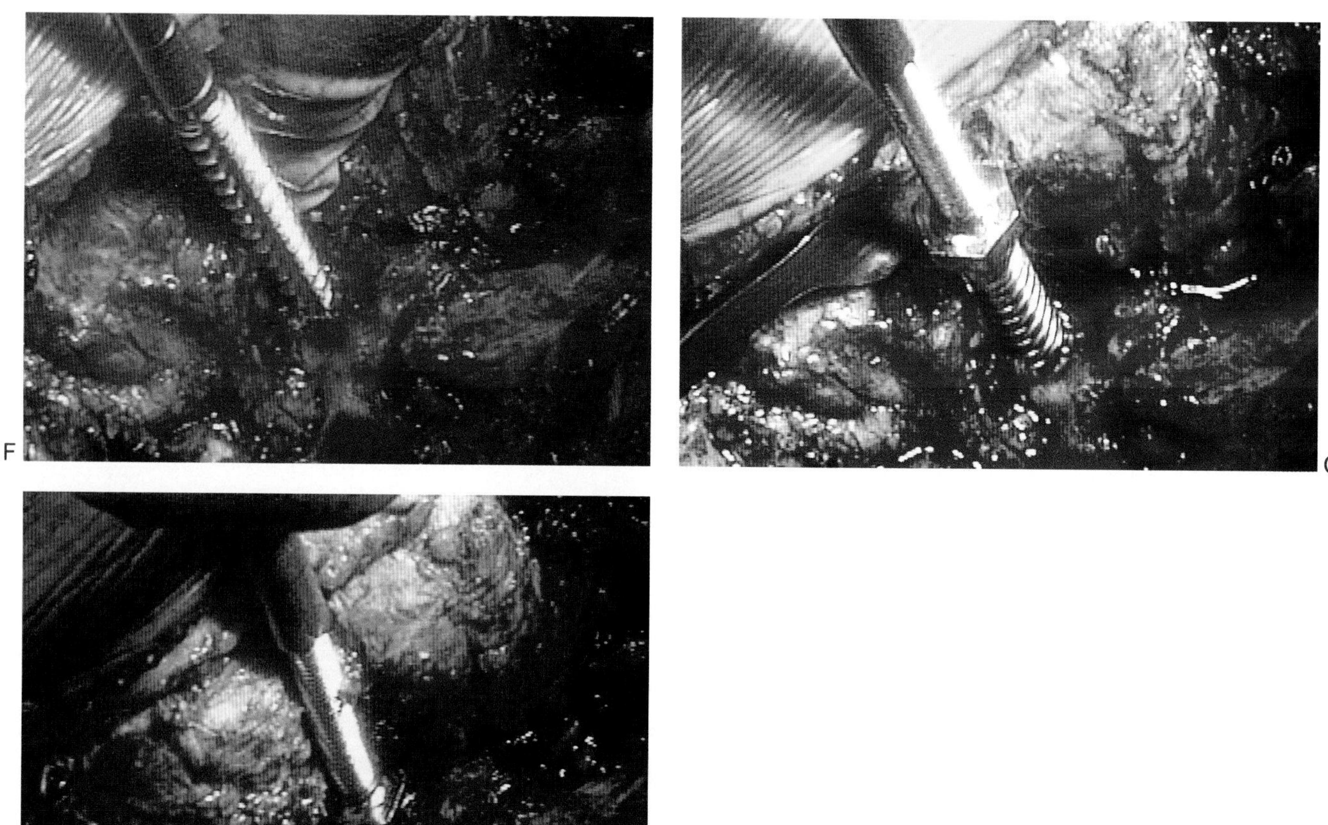

Figure 4. (*Continued.*) **F:** Auger tip tap being partially inserted. **G:** VSP screw partially inserted. **H:** VSP screw completely inserted.

Hook Anchor Placement Intrasegmental Claw

At T4 on the thoracic concave side, a transverse process elevator is passed over the top of the transverse process to prepare it for hook placement (Fig. 5A). A lamina/facet hook starter is utilized to prepare the site under the lamina/facet (Fig. 5B). When preparing for an intrasegmental claw, it is usually not desirable to remove any of the inferior edge of the facet so that enough vertical distance exists to accommodate the claw. The throat height hook selected for passage over the top of the transverse process is typically 9.5 mm. After it has been initially positioned, the holder is removed and the sucker tip inserted into the rod hole to rotate the hook into a perpendicular position in relation to the spine line (Fig. 5C). The lamina/facet hook is inserted with a hook driver (Fig. 5D). The oval shape of the hook hole provides improved hook control by the driver. The throat diameter of the hook is typically two sizes smaller than the transverse process hook throat height.

Thoracic Concave Apex Anchor Placement

To prepare for open hook concave thoracic apex anchors, the sharp inferior edge of the facet is removed with an osteotome and the hook positioned in the

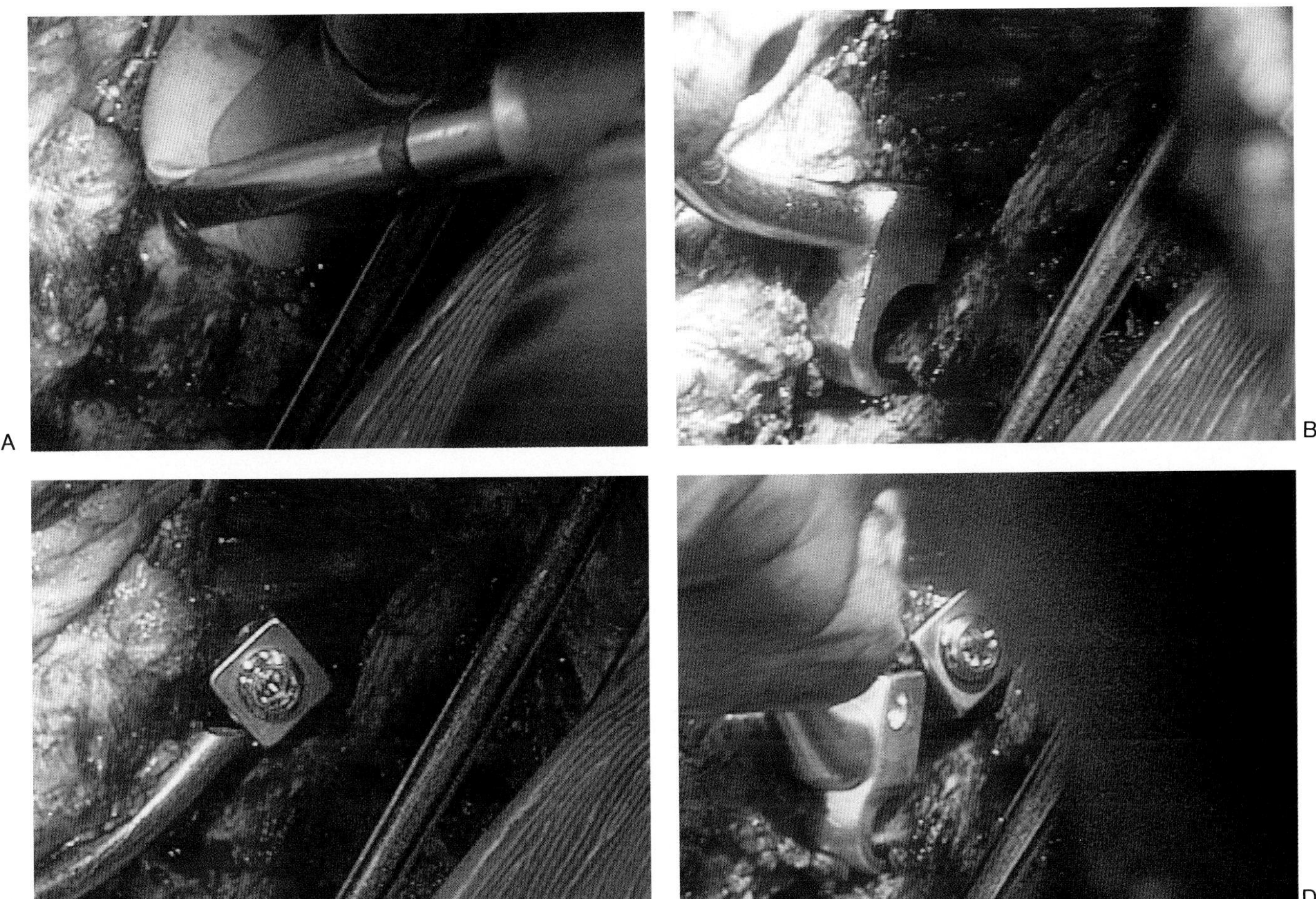

Figure 5. A: Transverse process elevator in place on the left side of T2. **B:** Lamina/facet hook starter in place. **C:** Sucker tip about to engage transverse process hook for rotation perpendicular to the spine. **D:** Lamina/facet hook being inserted to complete formation of upper claw.

facet location (Fig. 6). Sublaminar wires or cables are also useful concave apex anchors and are best utilized in patients with larger and stiffer curvatures in whom a residual mismatch between the longitudinal member and the spine is anticipated.

Inflection Thoracic Concave-Side Anchor Placement

The laminotomy is begun with a curette and/or small gouge to remove enough of the inferior edge of the lamina of the vertebra above the inflection vertebra to expose the ligamentum flavum. A Lempert rongeur is used to nibble through the ligamentum flavum, just exposing epidural fat (Fig. 7A). A Penfield #4 probe and/or Woodson dental instrument are employed to separate the posterior internal venous plexus from the ligamentum flavum (Fig. 7B). Both 1-mm and then 2-mm Kerrison rongeurs are used to sculpt the lamina to accommodate the hook. The laminotomy should be narrow so that the body of the hook will block canal intrusion. The hook throat height should be the smallest possible to just pass around the lamina. The laminotomy site should be prepared as far laterally as possible, which is to the inner wall of the pedicle (Fig. 7C).

A portion of the ridge formed by the spinous process as it joins the lamina on the inflection vertebra should also be removed with a rongeur to accommodate the body of the hook. The hook is rotated into position in the slot (Fig. 7D). It is important to begin with a small throat diameter (e.g., 6.5 mm for the 6.35-mm, $\frac{1}{4}$-inch rods and 5.0 mm for the 4.76-mm, $\frac{3}{16}$-inch rods.)

Rod Preparation

The length of the rod is determined by using two or three hemostats, since is necessary to direct a surgical suture along a line from the facet above the upper instrumented vertebra to the facet below the lower instrumented vertebra. For a short curve, a 0.5-cm length is added to this and for a long curve, 1.0 cm. The rod is cut with the table-top rod cutter (Fig. 8A). Variable radius benders are used to create anatomical sagittal plane curvatures in the rod (Fig. 8B). Templates are not necessary; the goal of rod preparation is to contour the rod to known normal sagittal plane contours. Using the mechanism of variable position connectors, the rod and spine are approximated through the process of capture, manipulation, and stress relaxation until the desired sagittal plane angular position is achieved.

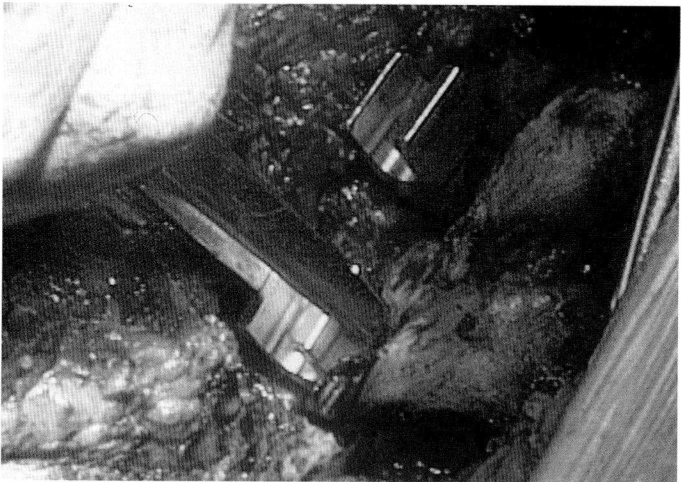

Figure 6. Thoracic concave apex facet hooks positioned.

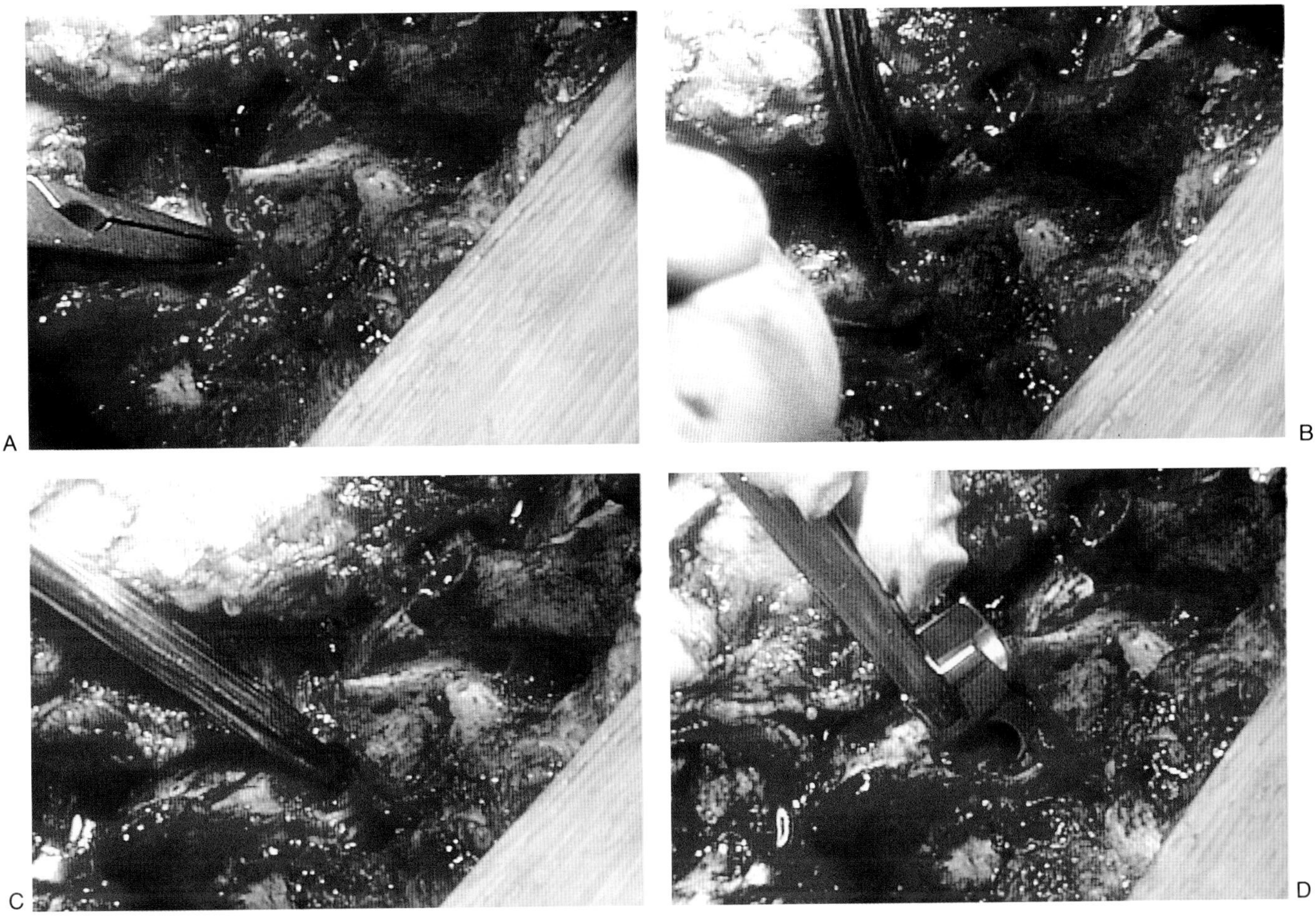

Figure 7. A: Lempert rongeur being used to nibble through the ligamentum flavum. **B:** Penfield #4 probe being used to separate the posterior internal venous plexus from the ligamentum flavum. **C:** A 1-mm Kerrison rongeur being used to create the laminotomy slot. **D:** Rotation of hook into position.

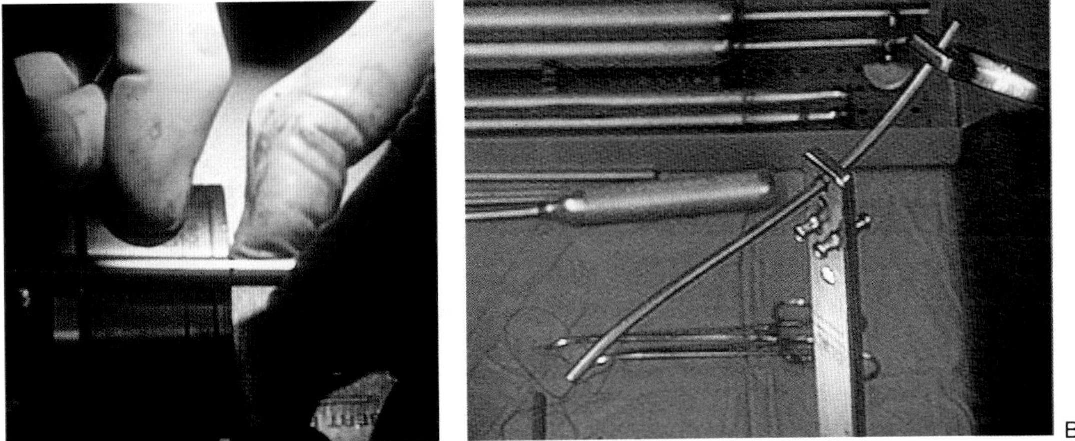

Figure 8. A: Table-top rod cutter head showing addition of 1-cm length to the rod prior to inserting rod into the cutting hole. **B:** Completion of placement of anatomical sagittal plane rod contours with the variable radius benders.

Arthrodesis

Facet and extrafacet decortication and addition of autologous iliac crest bone graft are done prior to longitudinal implant member placement.

Concave Rod Placement

The rod is back-entered through the upper intrasegmental claw (Fig. 9A). To assist with this, it is helpful for this rod to have been prepared so that the upper end of the rod is the machined end. At L1 and L2, the rod connection to the screws with slotted connectors is begun (Fig. 9B). Next the rod and inflection open hook are approximated. The hook holder is replaced with the Camlock approximator (Fig. 9C). Once the hook and rod have been approximated, the sliding cap is inserted (Fig. 9D). The cap set screw is temporarily tightened to allow

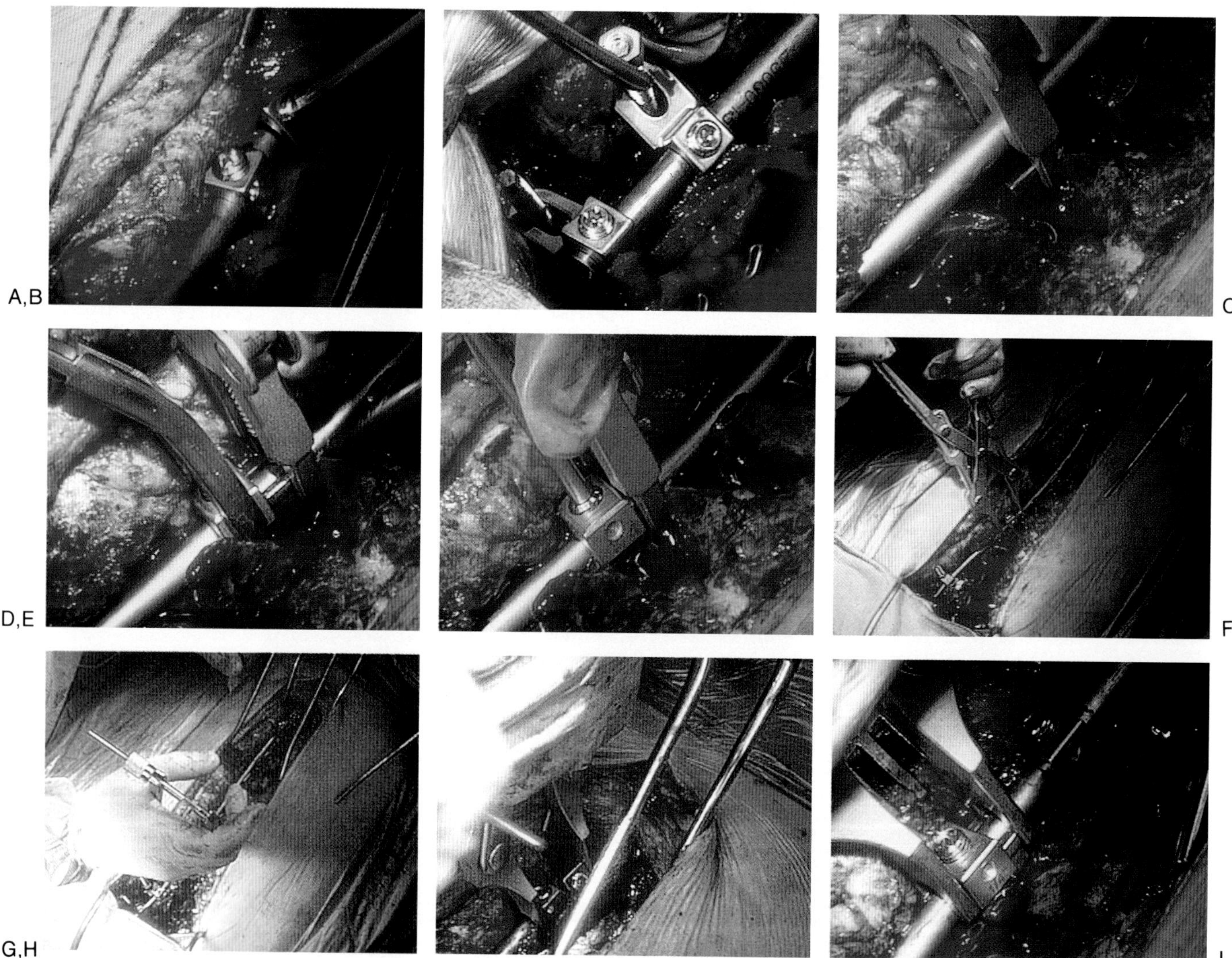

Figure 9. **A:** Back-feeding thoracic concave side rod into the upper claw. **B:** Placement of L1 and L2 slotted connectors. **C–F:** Approximation of inflection hook in rod and closure of open hook. **G:** Rod rotation to translate the lumbar spine anteriorally and medially. Note that the thoracic concave apex open hooks are not engaged with the rod at this point. **H:** Setting of upper end instrumented vertebra claw foundation. **I:** Completion of concave thoracic apex hook to rod translation and capping.

removal of the Camlock approximator (Fig. 9E). A compression instrument applied after the set screw is loosened completes the capping process (Fig. 9F).

Rod repositioning, so that the normal sagittal plane contours are placed in the parasagittal plane, is done with a rod gripper (Fig. 9G). Note that the concave apex thoracic hooks are not engaged. After the rod has been properly positioned, the upper end instrumented vertebra intrasegmental claw is secured, thus controlling rod position (Fig. 9H). The reason that such a thoracic foundation is produced is because the thoracic vertebrae are secure within the rib cage, whereas the lumbar vertebrae are not. The concave apex hooks are approximated to the rod with the Camlock approximator (Fig. 9C–F) and capped (Fig. 9I). Although the set screws are tightened at this point, they will be loosened again when the convex rod is placed.

Convex Rod Placement

Intrasegmental claws are placed at the upper end vertebra and at the apex on the convex side of the thoracic curve. Pedicle screw anchors are placed at the L1 and L2 levels on the concave side of the lumbar curve. Instead of using an inflection hook on this side, the hook is placed distally at the T12 level to help with transverse plane angulation.

The convex rod is prepared with less thoracic kyphosis and lumbar lordosis than the thoracic concave rod (Fig. 10). The exception is at the ends of the curve, where the anticipated proper sagittal plane angulation is placed. The rod is back-entered through the upper claw and, when possible, the apex claw. When this cannot be achieved, the apex hooks are drop-entered after the rod has been placed through the upper claw. Drop entry is made possible by the hook design, which allows for increase of the angle between the hook blade and longitudinal member by 10 degrees for insertion. Note that the rod stands away posteriorly from the lumbar spine.

Transverse Connection and Formation of a Superfoundation

The distance between the outer edges of the two longitudinal members is measured with the caliper (Fig. 11A). If this distance is greater than 25 mm, as it usually is, the nuts of the turnbuckle transverse connector can be placed on the

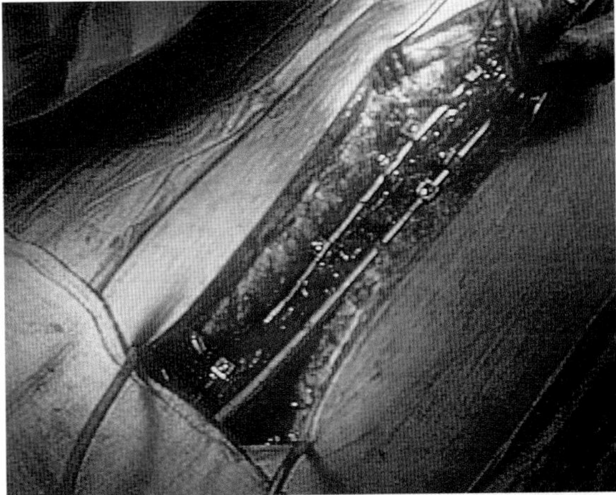

Figure 10. Insertion of thoracic convex rod. Note the rod standing away posteriorly from the lumbar spine lower end.

inside. Starting with the turnbuckle threaded transverse connector in the collapsed position toward the midline, the turnbuckle transverse rod is turned so that the outer jaw tips just clear the calipers (Fig. 11B). Excess transverse connector rod ends are cut off.

When applying the turnbuckle transverse connector, a hook holder is often used on one of the outer jaws, engaging it first and then successively rotating the other three jaws into position. When space constraints are tight because of full segmental placement of vertebral anchors, the profile tolerances may not exist to allow use of the hook holder. In such cases the first hook is caught around the rod and the other three jaws rotated into position (Fig. 11C). Subsequent turnbuckle rod rota-

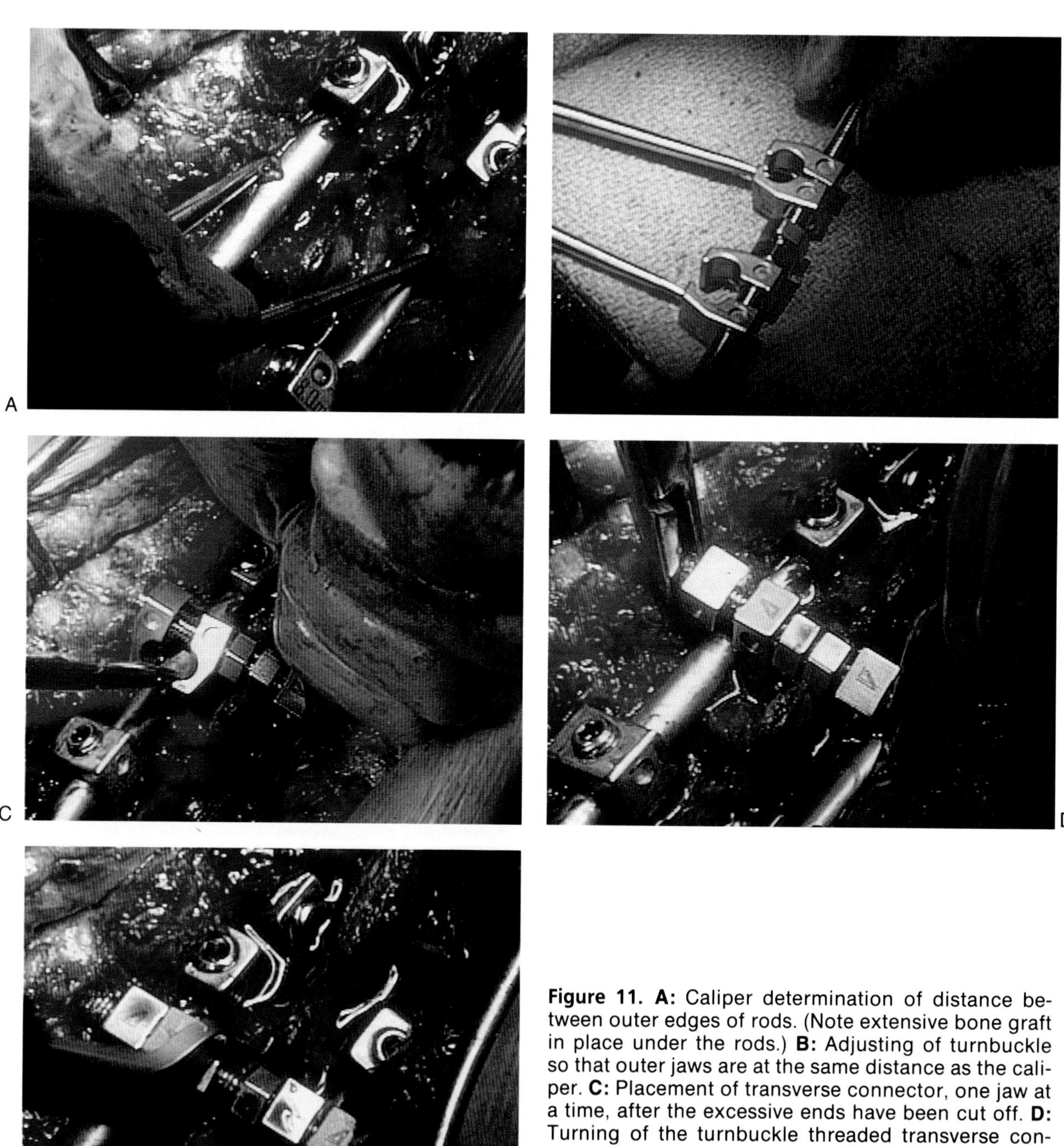

Figure 11. A: Caliper determination of distance between outer edges of rods. (Note extensive bone graft in place under the rods.) **B:** Adjusting of turnbuckle so that outer jaws are at the same distance as the caliper. **C:** Placement of transverse connector, one jaw at a time, after the excessive ends have been cut off. **D:** Turning of the turnbuckle threaded transverse connector rod toward the apex of the *A* symbol on the threaded jaws. **E:** Tightening of nuts by turning in the same direction as the turnbuckle threaded transverse member rod.

tion is somewhat easier if the right-hand thread side is placed on the patient's right side. Using a small needle holder reserved for this purpose, the turnbuckle transverse connector rod is rotated in the direction of the arrow to bring the outer jaws into contact with the rod (Fig. 11D). The same is true when the nuts are placed on the outside and the threaded jaws on the outside, except that the threaded jaws are moved outward to engage the rod.

If mediolateral distraction or compression of the longitudinal member rod is desired, a compression or distraction instrument is used to apply the appropriate force to the longitudinal members.

The nuts are tightened by rotating in the same direction the rod was rotated (Fig. 11E). The tightening torque is about 65 lb/in (7.3 Nm), a feel readily obtained that can be described as just about at the point where the shoulders of the nuts seem ready to round off.

Application of Transverse Plane Force Couples

Using an open laminar hook placed under the lamina of T12 and the Camlock approximator, the rod and spine are approximated (Fig. 12A). This produces anterior, medially directed force on the convex apex of the thoracic curve and a posterior, medially directed force on the apex of the concave side of the lumbar curvature (Fig. 12B). As the rod and lumbar spine are approximated, the nuts on the concave pedicle screws are loosely tightened. It is important to realize that the convex lumbar connections have not yet been tightened.

Completion of Thoracic Curve Instrumentation

At this point, if sublaminar wires have been utilized on the concave side of the thoracic curve, they are further tightened. The convex side of the thoracic curve is compressed (Fig. 13A) by providing some force on the T12 laminar hook. The concave thoracic hooks are checked to be sure they are secured under the lamina and the set screws finally tightened (Fig. 13B). The thoracic convex apex claw is

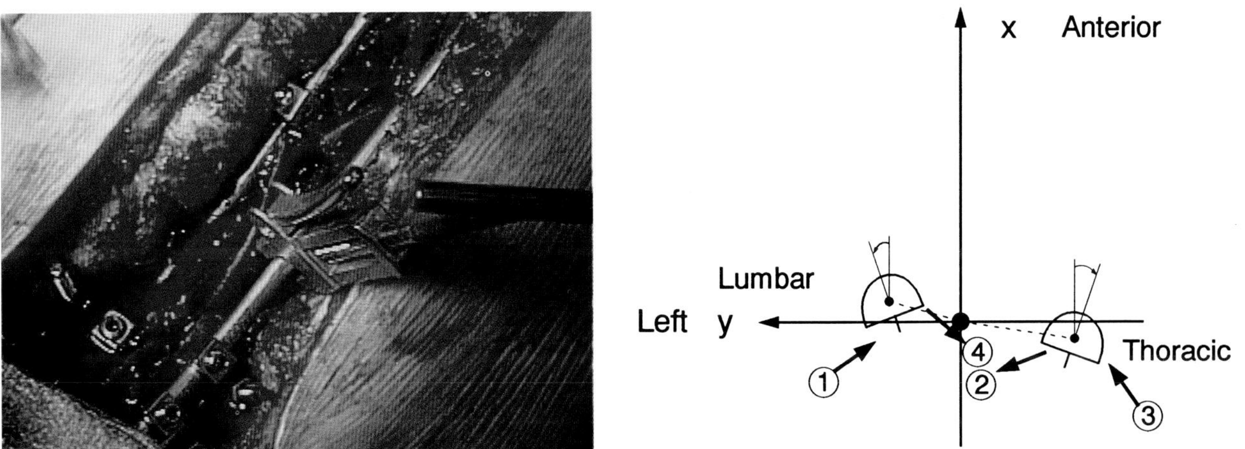

Figure 12. A: Approximation of thoracolumbar curve to lumbar convex rod utilizing the T12 open hook and Camlock approximator. **B:** Diagram of the sequence of load application to the apex and periapex vertebrae as projected onto the transverse plane. *1*, lumbar convex medial and anterior translation; *2*, thoracic concave medial and posterior translation; *3* thoracic apex convex medial and anterior translation; and *4*, lumbar apex medial and posterior translation. Forces 1 and 3 and than 2 and 4 provide transverse plane force couples.

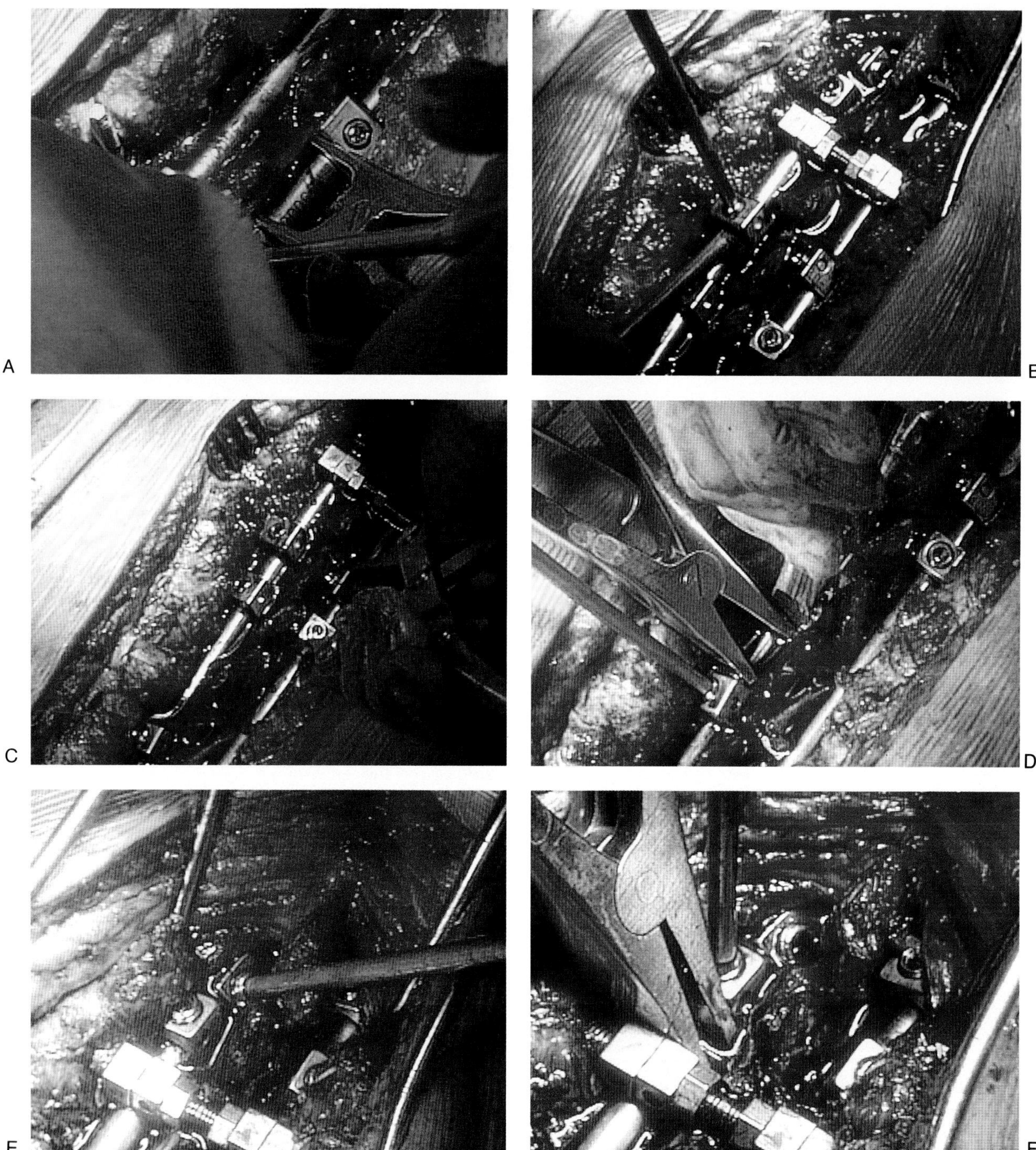

Figure 13. A: Application of compression across the convexity of the thoracic curve at the T12 hook. **B:** Final seating and tightening of the thoracic concave apex hooks. **C:** Completion of the tightening of the thoracic convex apex claw. **D:** Terminal distraction of the thoracic concave inflection hook. **E,F:** Loosening of the thoracic concave side upper end vertebra transverse process hook (E) in preparation for terminal distraction (F), a force seldom used.

tightened because any transverse plane angular correction of the apex vertebra will have already occurred (Fig. 13C).

To complete the thoracic curve instrumentation, concave distraction, the last corrective force, is placed. It is first applied at the inflection hook level (Fig. 13D). Additional distraction on the upper concave hooks is seldom required because of the pronounced tendency to elevate the left shoulder. It is better to leave residual angular deformity of the upper instrumented vertebra and to leave uninstrumented almost all compensatory high thoracic curves in order to preserve motion. If terminal distraction is to be placed on the concave upper foundation, the transverse process hook must be loosened and the VHG connection loosened from the rod by toggling the hook on the rod (Fig. 13E). Distraction may be placed on the lamina/facet hook, again ascertaining that the hook has been loosened by toggling (Fig. 13F).

Completion of Lumbar Curve Instrumentation

The convex side of the lumbar curve is placed in compression and the set screws tightened (Fig. 14A). The anchors closest to the center of the apex are tightened first. It is very important that the set screws be tightened before the nuts on the pedicle screws (Fig. 14B,C). Finally, the distraction necessary to remove any residual coronal plane angular deformity of the lower instrumented vertebra is applied to the concave side of the lumbar curves.

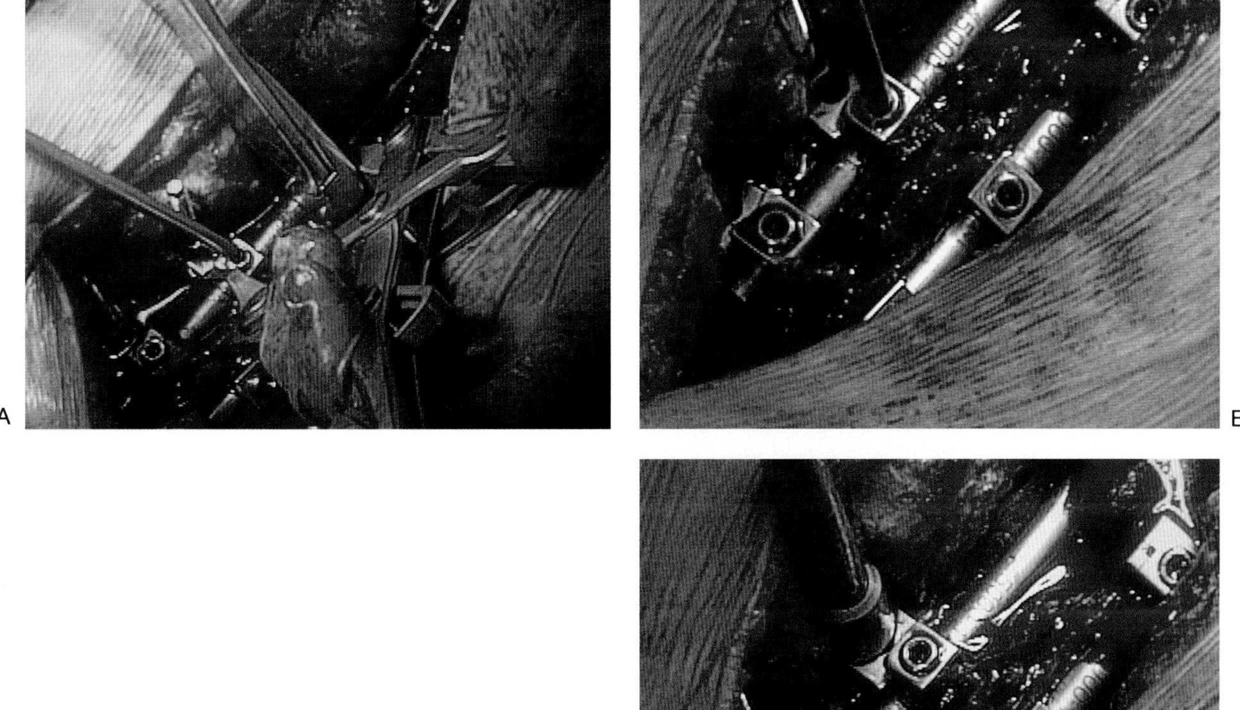

Figure 14. A: Lumbar apex convex compression. **B:** Set screw tightening before pedicle screw nut tightening. **C:** Pedicle screw nut tightening with the cannulated locking wrench.

Instrumentation Completion

All set screws and nuts should be checked for tightness. The recommended torque for the set screws is 60 lb/in (6.8 Nm), 65 lb/in (7.3 Nm) for the transverse connector nuts, and 100 lb/in (11.3 Nm) for the pedicle screw nuts. These torques are readily achieved by feel and are near the maximum torques obtainable with the instruments provided (Fig. 15A). When tightening is completed, excess machined portions of the pedicle screws are cut off (Fig. 15B). (A cannulated screw cutter has now been developed that simplifies this procedure.)

Closure

At this point any additional touch-up decortication is done and bone added; usually the work is minimal, as it has been finished prior to instrumentation. The wound is copiously irrigated using bulb syringes with 1 L of saline followed by 1 L of antibiotic irrigation solution through kidney tapes placed over the operative field to prevent the bone graft from being dislodged. The deep fascia is closed with interrupted permanent sutures that in the lumbar spine are passed through the spinous process (Fig. 16) or under a transverse connector. This layer is supplemented with running locking #0 Dexon hemostatic closure. The deep subcutaneous tissues are closed with running locking #2 Dexon sutures, the shallow subcutaneous tissues with #3 Dexon sutures, either interrupted or running, and the skin with a #3 PDS shallow subcutaneous deep dermis running nonlocking closure. Steristrips and a sterile gauze dressing complete the procedure.

A

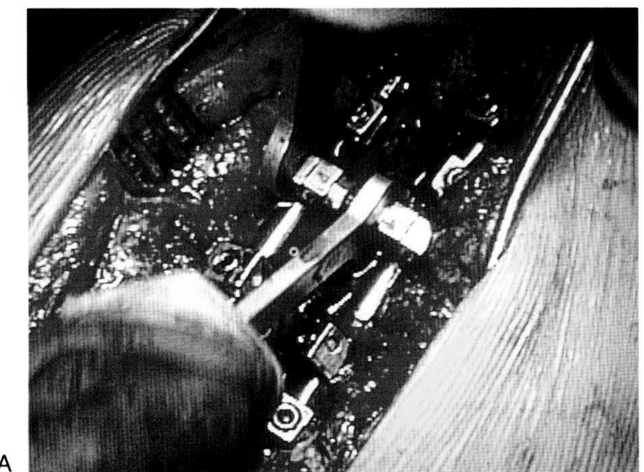

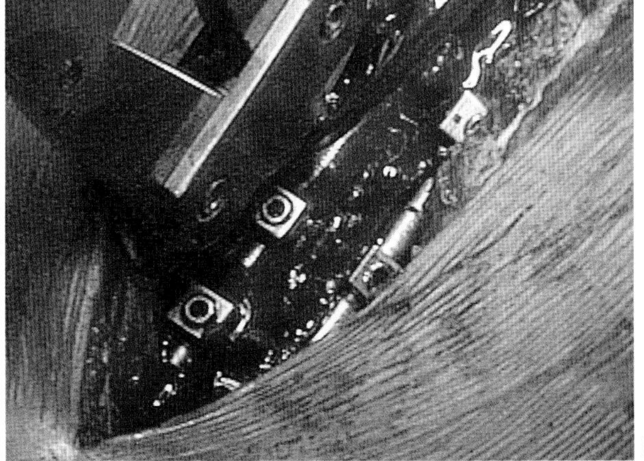

B

Figure 15. A: Checking the transverse connector nuts for tightness. **B:** Cutting off residual screw ends.

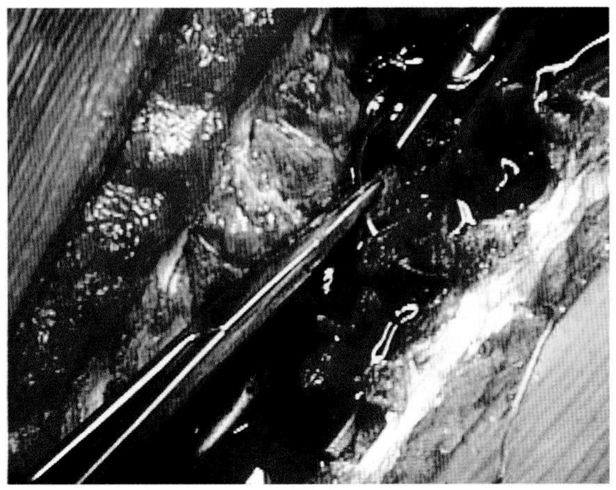

Figure 16. Securing of deep fascia to spinous process in the lumbar spine.

Idiopathic Scoliosis Instrumentation Sequences

Four basic instrumentation sequences are used in the posterior instrumentation of idiopathic scoliosis. Small variations in these four are necessary to accommodate the variety of deformity presentations encountered.

The sequence used in the patient illustrated in Fig. 17 is for a right thoracic major, left lumbar compensatory (minor) curve and is applicable to King-Moe

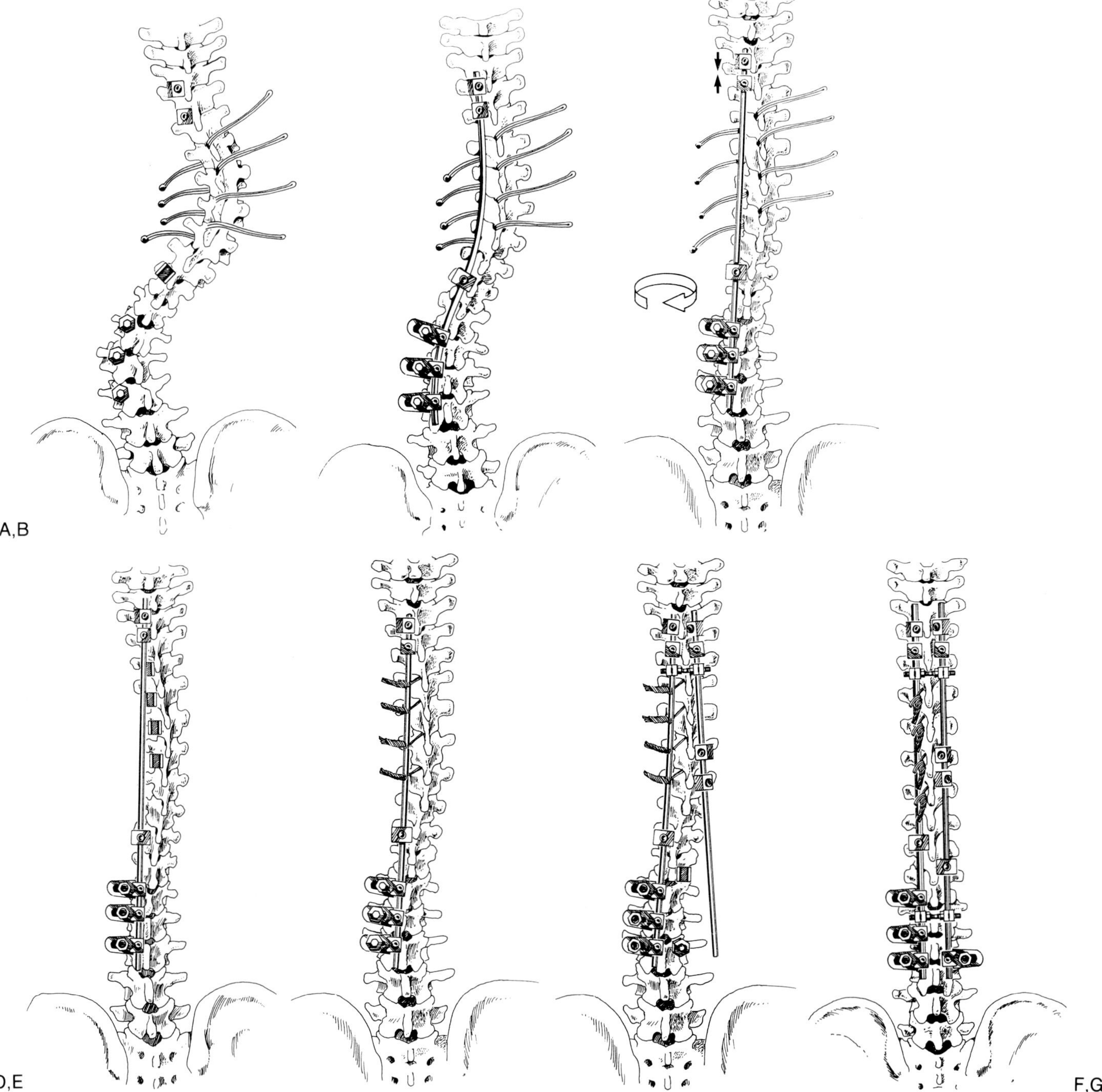

Figure 17. Idiopathic scoliosis right thoracic major, left lumbar compensatory (minor) curve. **A:** Coronal deformity and initial left-side anchor placement. **B:** Following placement of left-side longitudinal member. **C:** Following clockwise longitudinal member rotation. **D:** Substitution of open facet hooks for sublaminar wires in patients with thoracic curves that can eventually be reduced to about 25 degrees or less. **E:** Following thoracic apex medial and posterior translation. **F:** Placement of right-side rod. **G:** Completed construct. (From ref. 13, with permission.)

level II curves with inclusion of part or all of the lumbar compensatory curve and to King-Moe level I curves. Such patients typically have thoracolumbar junction kyphosis, posterior translation of the apex of the lumbar curve, and anterior translation of the apex of the thoracic curve. The left-side implant components are placed first (Fig. 17A). The longitudinal member is prepared with the required sagittal plane alignment built in. The rod is back-entered into the upper transverse process laminar claw and dropped onto the open hook at the inflection site and onto the pedicle screws (Fig. 17B). The nuts on the pedicle screws are taken to finger tightness only, and the set screws in the VHG connection are loosened. Following capping of the supralaminar inflection hook, the rod is rotated in a clockwise manner, and in the process the apex of the lumbar curve is moved anteriorly and the inflection sagittal plane alignment partially restored (Fig. 17C). The rod is held in this position by tightening the upper end thoracic transverse process lamina claw. In thoracic curves that can be reduced to approximately 25 degrees or less, concave facet hooks should be utilized rather than sublaminar wires (Fig. 17D). Also, cables may be used rather than wires or hooks.

The apex of the thoracic curve is translated medially and posteriorly by tightening the sublaminar wires (Fig. 17E). Note that no preliminary distraction is or has been applied. As the apex of the thoracic curve is translated, the spine will lengthen somewhat. It is important to consider the position of the inflection hook and to keep it engaged in its supralaminar position. This may require temporarily tightening and loosening of the facet hook at this level. In some instances, it is necessary to tighten the set screws on the slotted connectors temporarily in order to gain additional rod control while considerable medial and posterior load, which tends to produce a counterclockwise torque, is being applied with wire tightening.

The right convex rod is placed with an upper intrasegmental transverse process lamina claw and an apex transverse process laminar claw with compression applied between the two (Fig. 17F). The amount of compression is dictated by the projected postoperative position of the patient's shoulders. If it is likely that the right shoulder is to be lowered, then very little compression would be applied between these two claws. Transverse connection is applied to complete the upper foundation, and in this manner the set screws can be loosened on the left-side lumbar slotted connectors. As the right rod is delivered to the spine, transverse plane force couples at the apex of the thoracic and lumbar curves are applied (Fig. 12B).

To complete the construct (Fig. 17G), right-side T12 compression is applied, final left concave thoracic wire tightening performed, and left-side T11 supralaminar hook distraction placed. The lower curve correction is completed by placing convex, left-side compression followed by right-side distraction. The lower end instrumented vertebra coronal plane angular position should be reduced to as near zero as possible. The second transverse connector is then added.

The second sequence is for single thoracic curves and is applicable with modification to King-Moe levels III, IV, and II with selective thoracic fusion (Fig. 18). Only the upper portion of the sequence just illustrated is utilized. The hooks at the lower end would be changed to closed hooks with the addition of one or more compression hooks on the convex side at the level of the lower end vertebra and one above. Pedicle screws may be substituted for the lower end vertebra hooks, since they may provide better end vertebra coronal and sagittal plane angular control.

The third sequence is for double thoracic curves (King-Moe level IV) or those with large compensatory high thoracic curves (Fig. 19). As in the sequence for single thoracic curves, rod rotation is not required.

The fourth sequence is for thoracolumbar and lumbar major deformities and basically uses the lower portion of the first sequence. In long curves with the apex at T10 (sometimes T11 or L1) and no compensatory thoracic curve, it is necessary to connect the convex pedicle screws first and rotate (clockwise for left apex

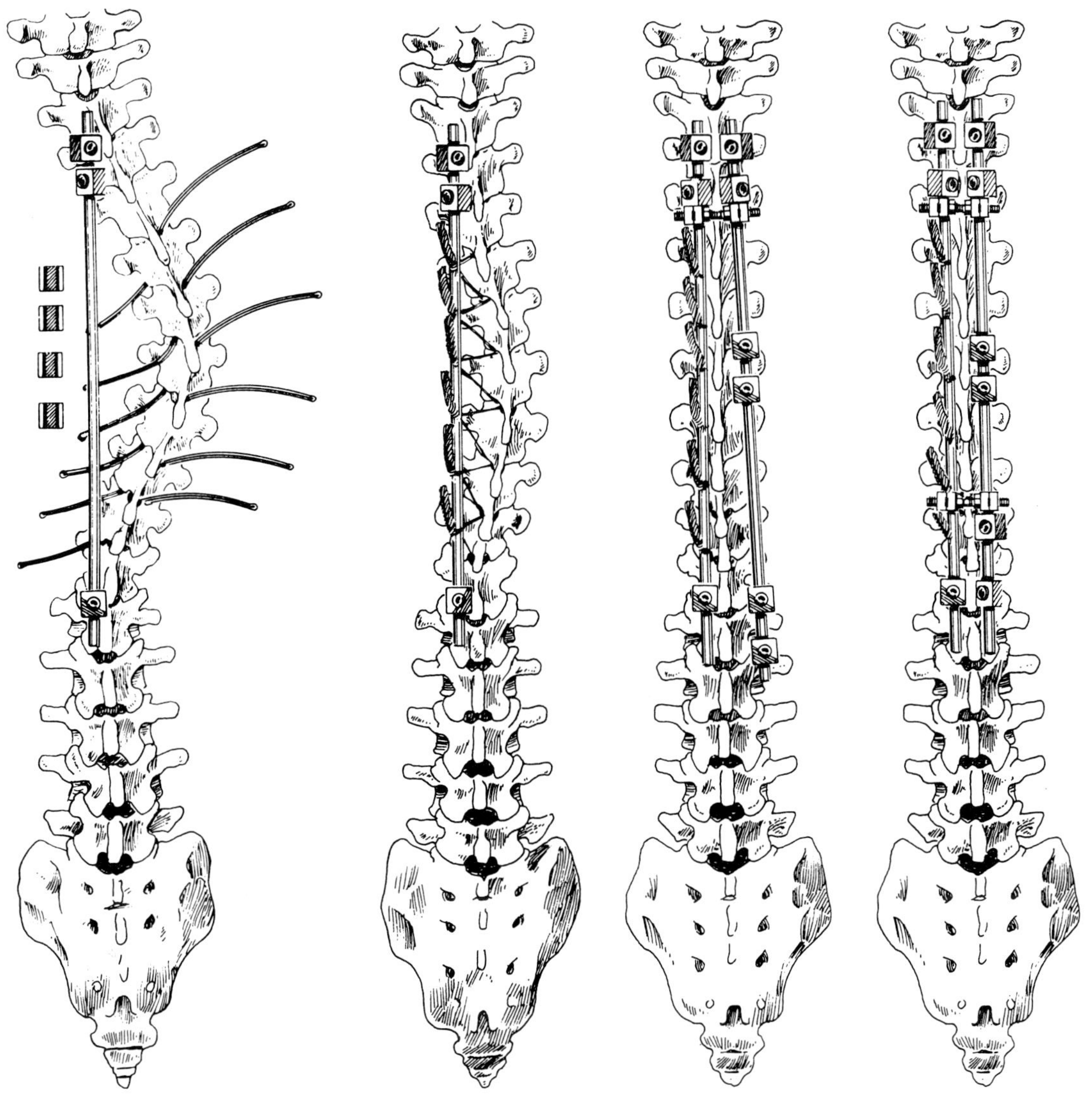

Figure 18. Idiopathic scoliosis right thoracic curve. **A:** Following placement of left (concave) side implants and securing the longitudinal member in the proper sagittal plane position, using the T4 transverse process-facet intrasegmental claw. Open facet hooks may be used instead of wires for curves that will correct to about 25 degrees or less. **B:** Following apex medial and posterior translation. **C:** Following preliminary placement of the convex rod. **D:** Following anterior and medial apex translation (thus completing the apex transverse plane force couple) by reducing the convex rod to the spine. (From ref. 13, with permission.)

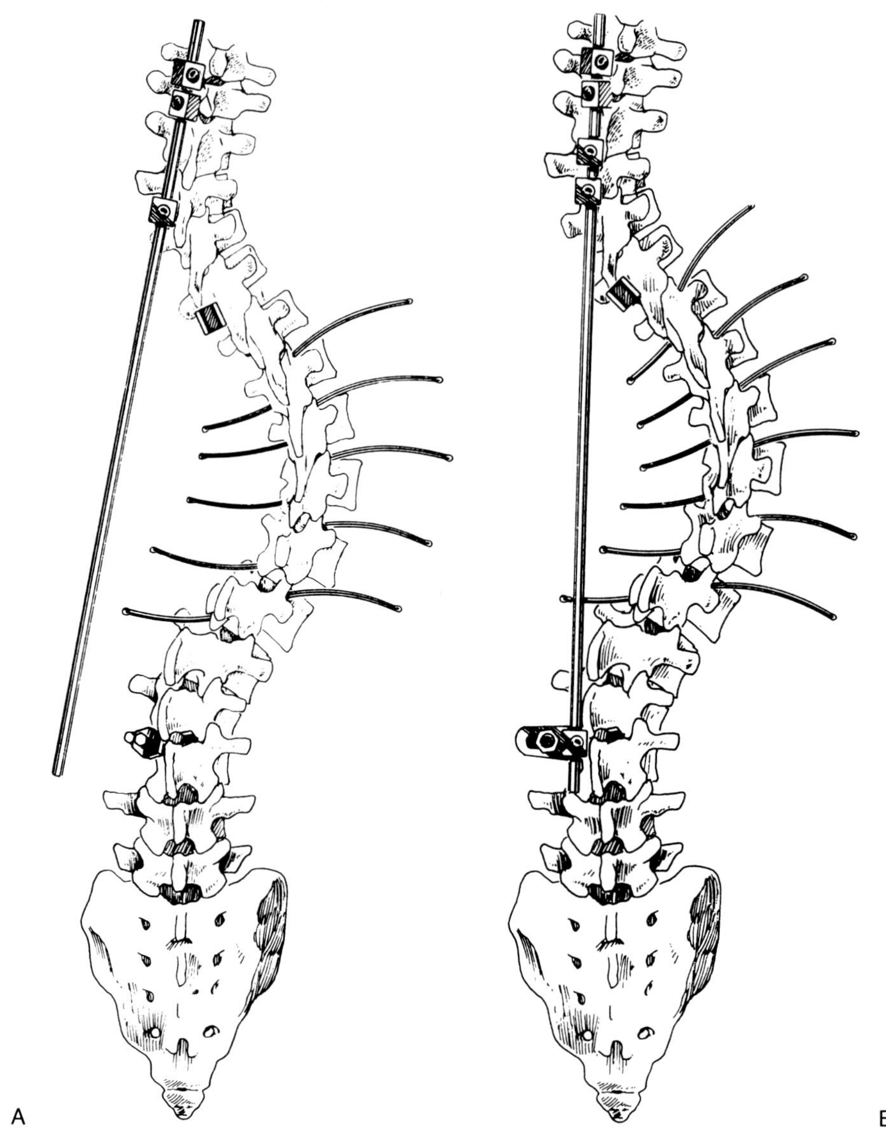

Figure 19. Idiopathic scoliosis left high thoracic, right thoracic curves. **A:** Following placement of the left anchors and initial placement of longitudinal member. **B:** After securing of convex longitudinal member to the lower anchor, resulting in T2 coronal plane angular position correction. **C:** Low thoracic curve apex medial and, if necessary, posterior translation. **D:** Initial placement of right-side rod during which the T2 coronal plane force couple is completed. **E:** Following construct completion. (From ref. 13, with permission.)

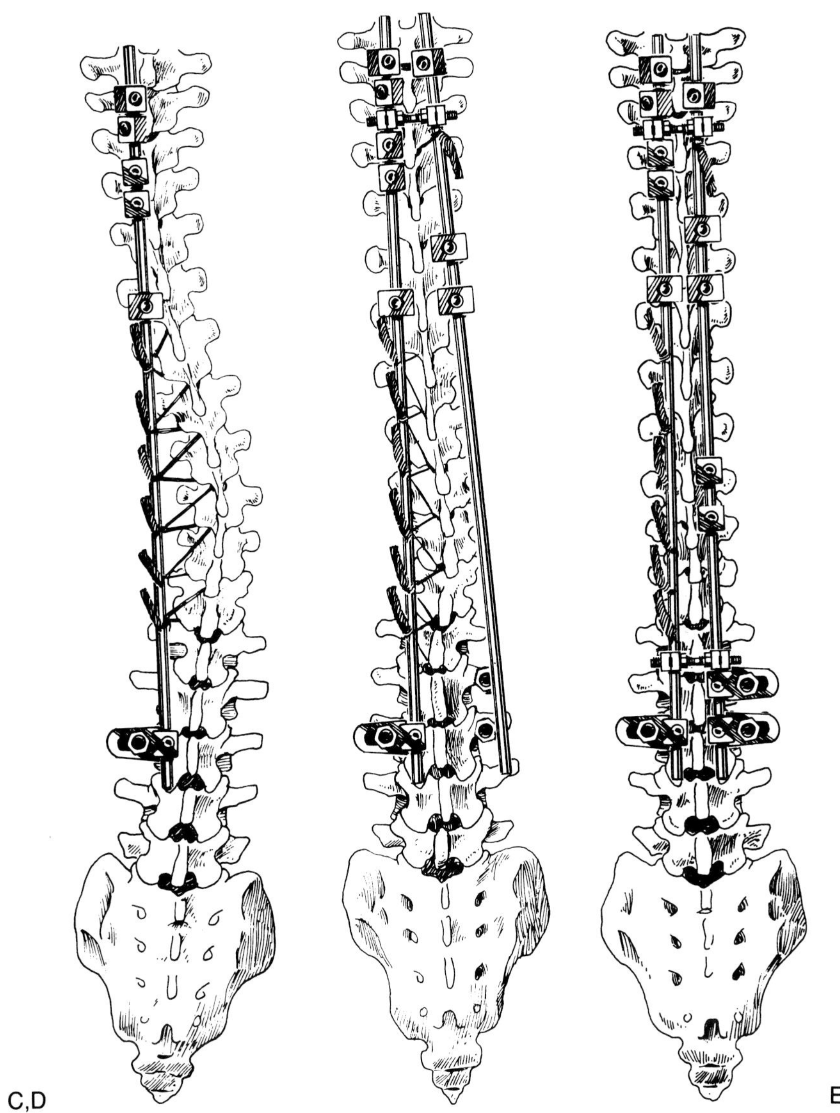
C,D
E

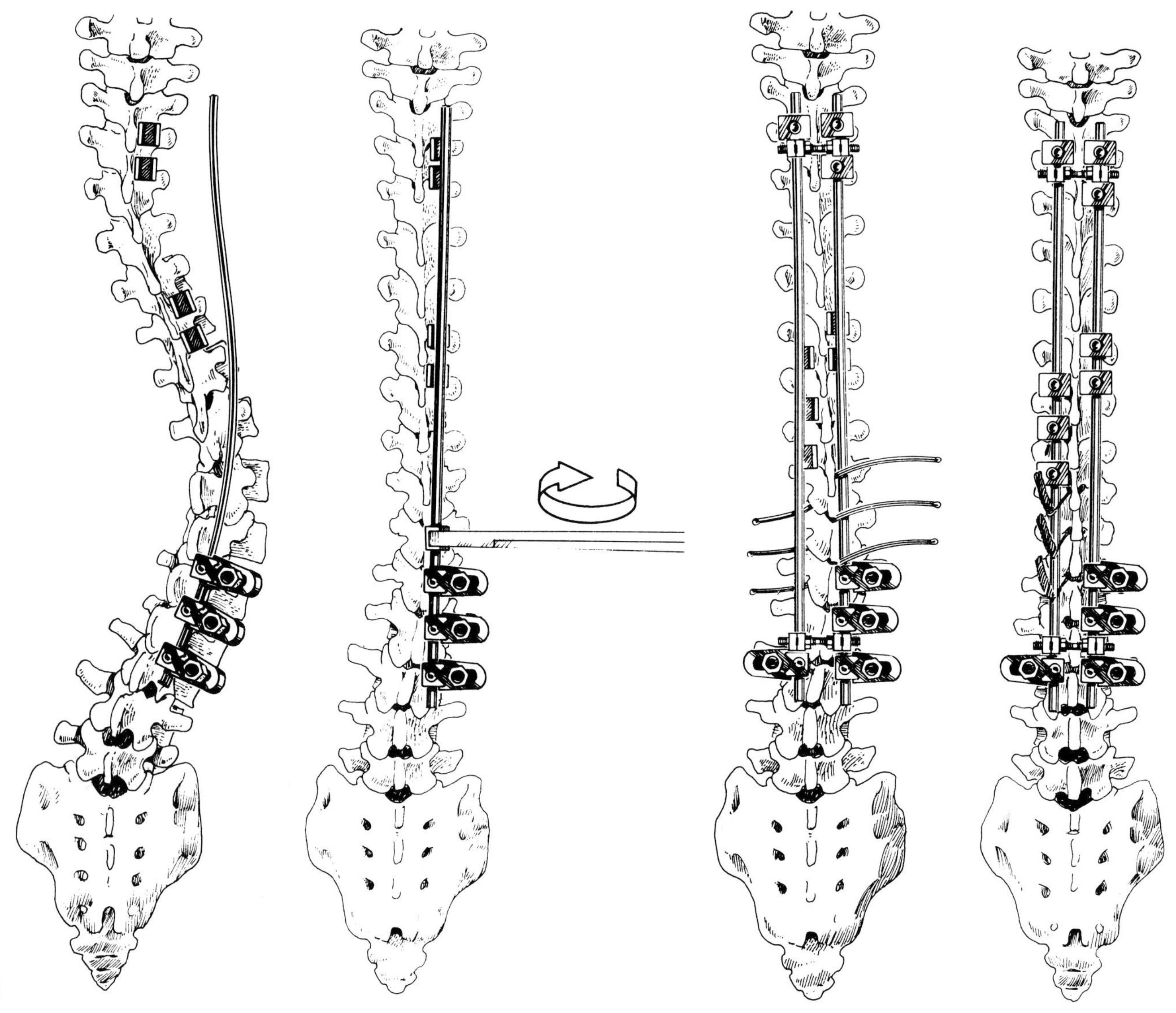

Figure 20. Idiopathic scoliosis thoracolumbar curve. **A:** Following placement of convex side anchors and initial capture of the anatomically contoured longitudinal member to the lumbar anchors. Note that the longitudinal member cannot be captured by the thoracic anchors at this point because the coronal plane deformity is not the same as the anatomic sagittal plane alignment desired. **B:** Following counterclockwise rod rotation and thoracic anchor capture, providing apex medial and anterior translation, making thoracic posterior translation possible in the next phase of instrumentation. **C:** Following placement of left-side implant. **D:** Following apex medial and posterior translation to approximate the spine to the anatomically contoured longitudinal member. (From ref. 13, with permission.)

curves) the rod into the proper sagittal plane position as it is landed into an open intrasegmental claw at the upper end instrumented vertebra (Fig. 20). The concave instrumentation features several apex and periapex translational anchors, either sublaminar wires, open hooks, or (in the lumbar spine) screws.

POSTOPERATIVE MANAGEMENT

Patients are usually in the intensive care unit for one night. Patient-controlled analgesia (PCA) is used for 48 to 60 hours and then replaced with a scheduled intramuscular nonsteroidal agent, and an injectable narcotic medication, as needed. No postoperative immobilization is utilized. Sitting begins within 1 or 2 days and walking within 2 to 3 days after surgery. The Foley catheter can usually be discontinued by the third or fourth postoperative day. Clear liquids are not begun until the patient is hungry, not thirsty. The criteria for discharge are normal food intake, normal bowel movement, and ability to walk stairs. Patients are discharged at about 7 to 8 days postoperatively. Patients usually still require some mild narcotic medication by mouth at this point, although the need generally does not persist beyond 1, or at most, 2 weeks after discharge. Follow-up is done at 3, 6, 12, and 24 months postoperatively with the admonition to remain in touch long term.

The principal rehabilitative tool is walking. Patients are encouraged to achieve 30 minutes of sustained walking for a minimum of three times a week by 1 month following surgery. Patients generally return to school at approximately 4 to 6 postoperative weeks. Older patients who are working usually return to work by about 3 months, depending on deformity and surgery magnitude. At 3 to 4 postoperative months, they are begun on push-ups, prone lying trunk lifts, and sit-ups. They are allowed to return to gym class between 6 and 12 postoperative months, but gymnastics and contact sports are not allowed.

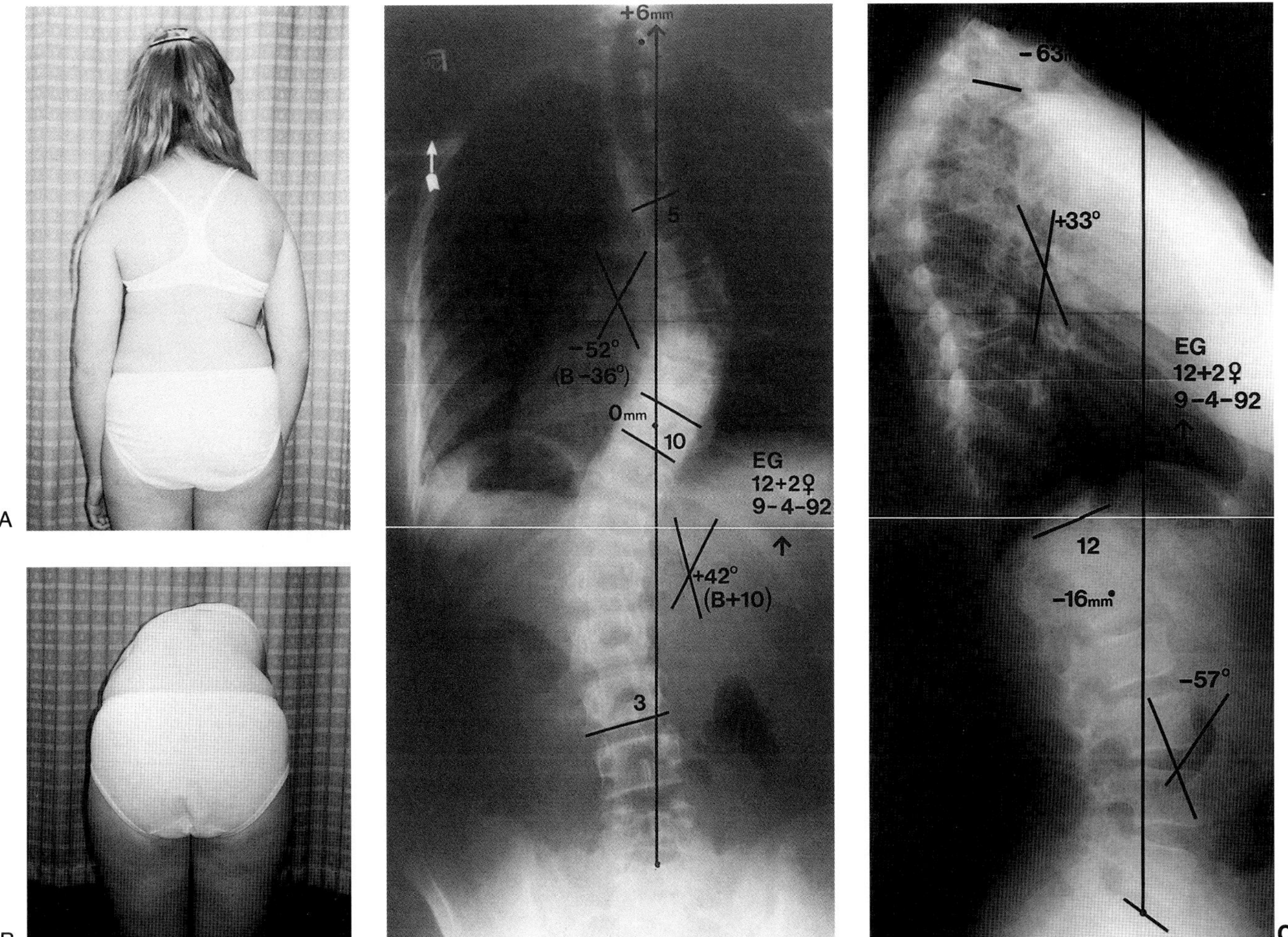

Figure 21. Clinical photographs and preoperative radiographs of a 12-year, 5-month-old girl whose surgery is presented. The upright posterior position **(A)** and the forward bend position **(B)**; standing PA **(C)** and lateral **(D)** 36-inch deformity radiographs.

COMPLICATIONS

The most frequent complication encountered at this time is ileus. In an effort to limit it, the PCA program is stopped at 48 to 60 hours, since it is believed that continuous narcotic medication may be a contributing factor. Oral intake is not begun until the patient is hungry and passing flatus, and bowel tones are audible.

Patients undergoing thoracoplasty often require a chest tube, so one is now placed prophylactically during surgery before the thoracoplasty. Patients undergoing concave rib osteotomies seldom require a chest tube, although observation for hydrothorax is necessary postoperatively. Closed suction drainage in the thoracoplasty or rib osteotomy bed is used to decrease hematoma pressure in an attempt to decrease pleural fusion.

The next most common "complications" are unsightly scars. Every effort is being made to improve cosmetic appearance at closure. The possibility of death, paralysis, and infection is now remote because of improved anesthesia and hemostasis techniques, improved surgical technique (including the elimination of distraction as a primary corrective force), and intraoperative antibiotics coupled with thorough wound lavage prior to closure. Urinary tract infections are identified and treated appropriately.

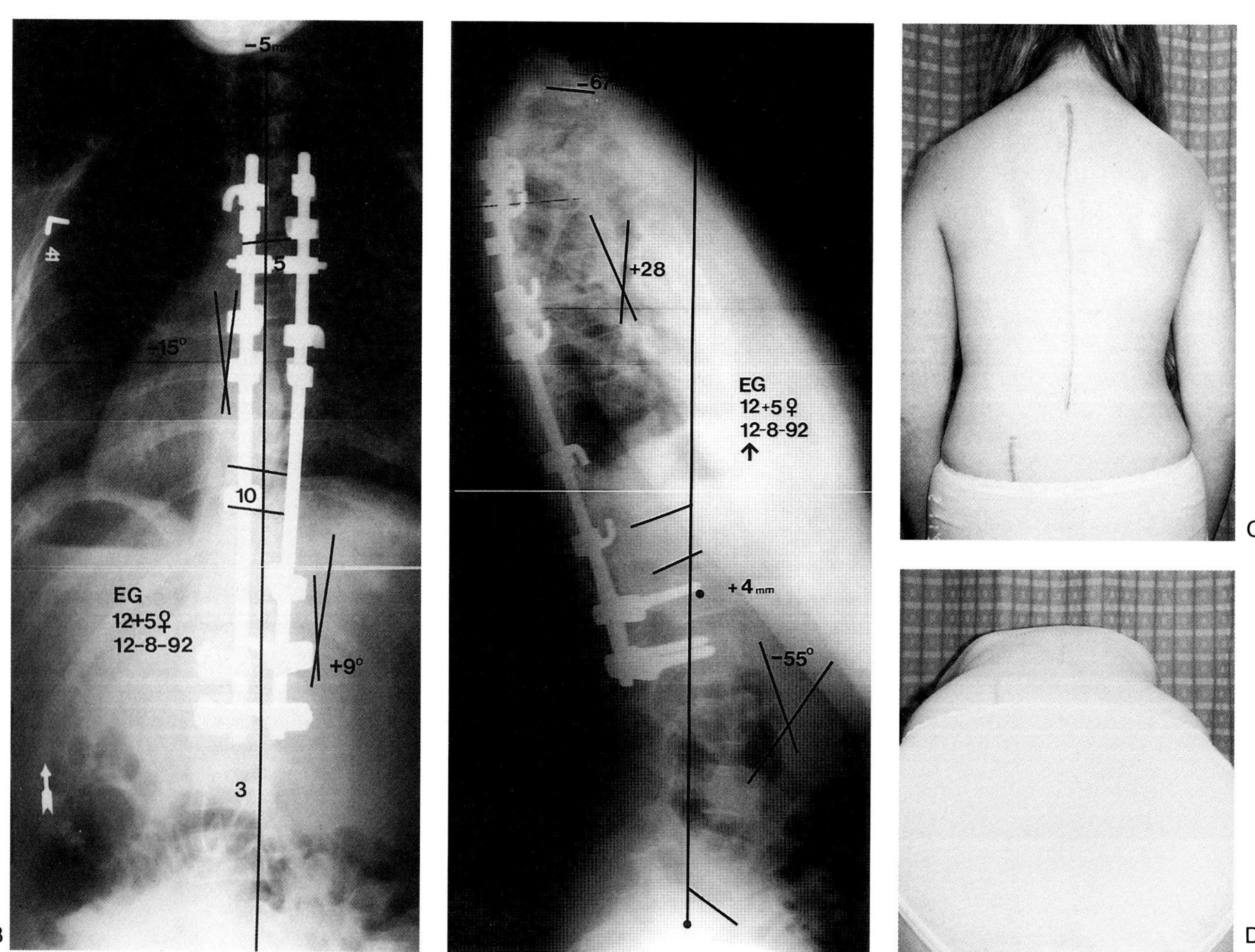

Figure 22. A–F. Postoperative standing posteroanterior **(A)** and lateral **(B)** radiographs, as well as standing 3-month postoperative posteroanterior **(C)** and forward bend **(D)** photographs of the patient.

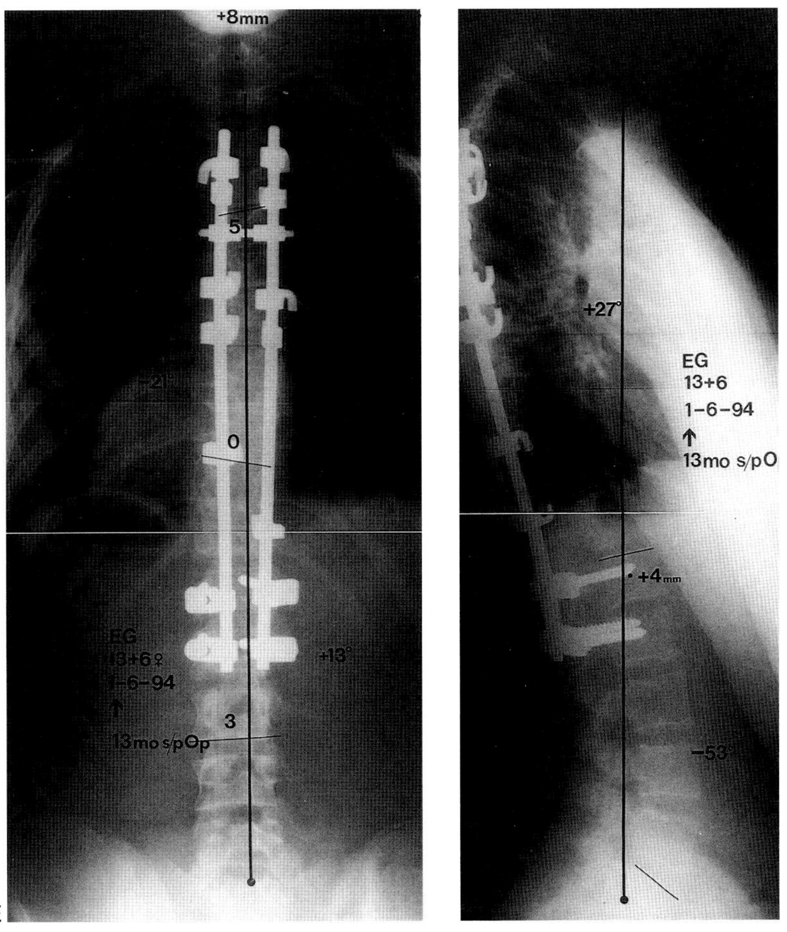

Figure 22. (*Continued.*) Thirteen-month postoperative radiographs **(E and F)**. At 24 months, she rated her function as normal (5), pain as mild (4), and appearance of trunk as excellent (5), and at 38 months she rated her result as very satisfactory.

ILLUSTRATIVE CASE FOR TECHNIQUE

Figure 21 shows clinical photographs and preoperative radiographs of a 12-year, 5-month-old girl. In the upright posterior position (Fig. 21A), the patient's left shoulder is low, right scapula prominent, and right waist crease deep, whereas the left waist crease is full. In the forward bend position (Fig. 21B), the right paravertebral prominence is apparent. To view the left paravertebral prominence would require further forward bending. Standing PA (Fig. 21C) and lateral (Fig. 21D) 36-inch deformity radiographs with regional, angular, and global translational measurements are shown.

Standing postoperative PA and lateral radiographs are shown (Fig. 22A,B). The patient was hospitalized for six days and after six weeks returned to school. Clinical photos show the patient at the three-month follow-up (Fig. 22C,D) and thirteen month follow-up; PA and lateral radiographs are also shown (Fig. 22E,F).

Acknowledgments. The author is deeply indebted to Walter E. Strippgen, Charles F. Heinig, M.D., William L. Carson, PH.D., and Terry Stahurski, M.S. Appreciation is also due to Jan Brunks, Janice Orrick, R.N., Barbara Funk, KUMC Audio Visual Services Department. AcroMed Corporation, Cleveland, Ohio paid for illustrations 17, 18, 19, and 20.

RECOMMENDED READING

1. Asher, M.A., Strippgen, W. E., Heinig, C. F., and Carson, W. L.: *Isola*[R] *Spine Implant System: Principles and Practice*. Acromed, Cleveland, 1991.
2. Asher, M. A., Strippgen, W. E., Heinig, C. F., and Carson, W. L.: Spinal instrumentation: emphasizing application during the first two decades of life. In: *The Pediatric Spine*, edited by S. Weinstein, pp. 1619–1658. Raven Press, New York, 1993.
3. Asher, M.: Isola instrumentation for scoliosis. In: *Spinal Instrumentation Techniques*, Edited by Brown, C. W. Scoliosis Research Society, Rosemont, Illinois, 1994.
4. Bernhardt, M., and Bridwell, K. H.: Segmental analysis of the sagittal plane alignment of the normal thoracic and lumbar spines and thoracolumbar junction. *Spine*, 14: 717–721, 1989.
5. Harrington, P. R.: ,Treatment of scoliosis: correction and internal fixation by spine instrumentation. *J. Bone Joint Surg.*, 44A: 591–610, 1962.
6. Harrington, P. R.: Technical details in relation to the successful use of instrumentation in scoliosis. *Orthop. Clin. North Am.*, 3: 49–67, 1972.
7. King, H. A., Moe, J. H., Bradford, D. S., and Winter, R. B.: The selection of fusion levels in thoracic idiopathic scoliosis. *J. Bone Joint Surg.*, 65A: 1302–1313, 1983.
8. Lenke, L. G., Bridwell, K. H., Baldus, C., and Blanke, K.: Preventing decompensation in King type II curves treated with Cotrel-Dubousset instrumentation. *Spine*, 17: S274–S281, 1992.
9. McCall, R., and Bronson, W.: Criteria for selective fusion in idiopathic scoliosis using Cotrel-Dubousset instrumentation. *J. Pediatr. Orthop.*, 12: 475–479, 1992.
10. Pehrsson, K., Larsson, S., Nachemson, A., and Oden, A.: Mortality and causes of death in patients with untreated scoliosis. A study of mortality, causes of death, and symptoms. *Spine* 17(9): 1091–1096, 1992.
11. Steffee, A. D.: The variable screw placement system with posterior lumbar interbody fusion. In: *Lumbar Interbody Fusion: Principles and Techniques in Spine Surgery*, edited by P. M. Liu and K. Gill. Aspen Publishers, 1989.
12. Steffee, A. D., Biscup, R. S., and Sitkowski, D. J.: Segmental spine plates with pedicle screw fixation. A new internal fixation device for disorders of the lumbar and thoracolumbar spine. *Clin. Orthop.*, 203: 45–53, 1986.
13. Stokes, I. A. F.: Three-dimensional terminology of spinal deformity. A report presented to the Scoliosis Research Society by the Scoliosis Research Society Working Group on 3-D Terminology of Spinal Deformity. *Spine*, 19: 236–248, 1994.
14. Thompson, J. P., Transfeldt, E. E., Bradford, D. S., Ogilvie, J. W., and Boachie-Adjei, O.: Decompression after Cotrel-Dubousset instrumentation of idiopathic scoliosis. *Spine*, 15: 927–931, 1990.
15. Weinstein, S. L.: Idiopathic scoliosis. Natural history. *Spine*, 11: 780–783, 1986.
16. Wood, K. B., Transfeldt, E. E., Ogilvie, J. W., Schendel, M. J., and Bradford, D. S.: Rotational changes of the vertebral-pelvic axis following Cotrel-Dubousset instrumentation. *Spine*, 16: S404–S408, 1991.

Master Techniques in Orthopaedic Surgery,
THE SPINE, edited by D. S. Bradford,
Lippincott-Raven Publishers, Philadelphia, © 1997.

24

Transpedicular Fixation

Robert F. McLain

INDICATIONS/CONTRAINDICATIONS

Segmental pedicle screw fixation has become a popular method of surgical fixation of the spinal column. The strongest portion of the vertebrae is the pedicle, which transmits all forces from the posterior elements to the vertebral body. The pedicle can withstand stressors of rotation, side bending, and extension of the spine. It is an ideal structure to lock into and control with posterior instrumentation when spinal fixation is needed.

Pedicle screw fixation provides rigid immobilization of all three columns of the spine while requiring only the presence of an intact pedicle. Several pedicle screw systems are available; whereas inherent advantages and disadvantages are found in each one, specific indications have not been clearly established in the literature. Nevertheless, successful use of each system requires appropriate preoperative indications, an appreciation of spinal biomechanics, and correct application of the device. The principal indications for pedicle screw fixation are as follows: reconstruction of spinal tumors; stabilization following osteotomies, either post-traumatic or in patients with spondyloarthropathy such as ankylosing spondylitis; isthmic and degenerative spondylolisthesis; and acquired hypermobility above or below a previously fused lumbar segment. Transpedicular lumbar devices have also been advocated for the repair and stabilization of lumbar pseudoarthrosis with persistent pain and/or hypermobility.

Trauma of the thoracolumbar spine and lumbosacral spine is an important indication for pedicular fixation: fewer functional spinal units need to be instrumented when compared with nonpedicular spinal fixation devices, preserving normal lum-

R. F. McLain, M.D.: Department of Orthopaedic Surgery, University of California Davis, Sacramento, California 95817.

Disclaimer. Currently pedicle screws are only approved by the Food and Drug Administration for the sacrum, and for fixation of L5-S1 spondylolisthesis.

bar mechanics and motion. Another indication is acquired instability or hypermobility following decompressive spinal surgery in patients with spinal stenosis. When one entire facet or half of both facets have been removed, some authors suggest that a spinal fusion is necessary to prevent spondylolisthesis. Lumbosacral fixation, a difficult problem in many spinal deformity patients, can be greatly enhanced with transpedicular fixation devices.

Sacral pedicle screws have Food and Drug Administration approval. Lumbar pedicle screws, used extensively throughout the world, are currently approved by the FDA for use in lumbosacral spondylolisthesis, and are considered a Class III device for all other applications. Successful use of transpedicular screws requires meticulous technique and preoperative planning. Specific and hands-on training in pedicle screw technique should be a prerequisite for surgeons entertaining their use in spine patients.

Contraindications to pedicle screw instrumentation include a fractured pedicle, severe osteopenia, inadequate pedicle dimensions, congenital or absent pedicles, and metal allergy (i.e., hypersensitivity to stainless steel). Poor mechanical purchase within a damaged pedicle is also a relative contraindication. Metallic implants should be avoided when infection is present.

PREOPERATIVE PLANNING

Preoperative planning is essential. First a good history is taken and a physical examination is performed. Anteroposterior (AP) and lateral radiographs of a pa-

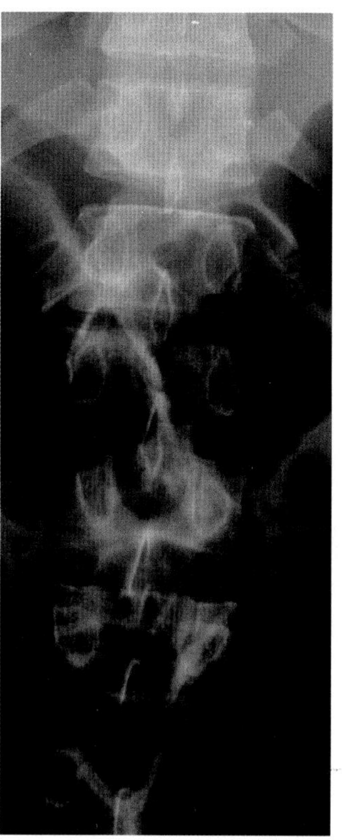

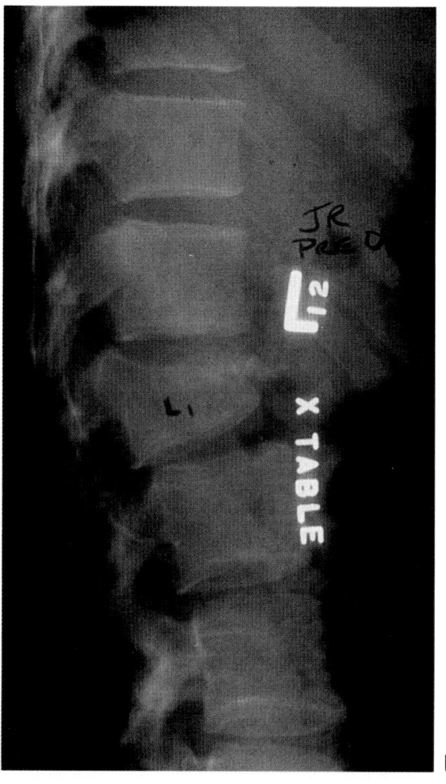

Figure 1. A 21-year-old man who was the victim of a motor vehicle accident in which he sustained an L1 burst fracture. **A:** An AP radiograph, demonstrating widening of the pedicles of L1 and a slight widening of the spinous distance between T12 and L1. **B:** A lateral radiograph demonstrating greater than 50% compression of the anterior body height with posterior displacement of the posterosuperior wall of L1 and widening of the inner spinous distance between T12 and L1.

tient with an L1 burst fracture are taken with the patient in the supine position (Fig. 1A,B). Log-rolling the patient to place the cassettes is generally the safest way to obtain the necessary views. Magnetic resonance imaging (MRI) and/or computed tomography (CT) are also mandatory (Fig. 2A,B). Myelography is rarely used but may be necessary in the event of non–spine-related medical problem(s) preventing adequate MRI or CT imaging (e.g., pacemakers, metallic devices, ocular metallic fragments, or claustrophobia).

Thrcc-dimensional thinking by the operating surgeon is essential for good preoperative planning. The spatial relationships between the neural structures and bone are critical. The surgeon must be able to conceptualize critical spacial relationships between bony and neural structures before and after pedicular fixation. How will a pedicle device help to realign, decompress, and/or stabilize the spine? How can the device take advantage of the available soft tissues and bony structures to achieve these goals? What is the relationship of the segments above and below the injured or uninstrumented segments and what might be the short- and long-term consequences of the fixation device chosen? All these questions must be answered before proceeding.

For purposes of describing the technique of pedicular fixation, I will discuss the approach to a patient with an L1 burst fracture undergoing operative treatment. The technical principles described are, in general, applicable to all cases in which pedicle screws are used.

SURGERY

L1 Burst Fracture

Patient Positioning. Patients are brought to the operating room in their own hospital bed. A Foley catheter is placed. Good venous access as well as an arterial line are essential. In spinal cord injuries, blood pressure must be monitored. To prevent progression of neural deficit and/or excess bleeding, we try to maintain

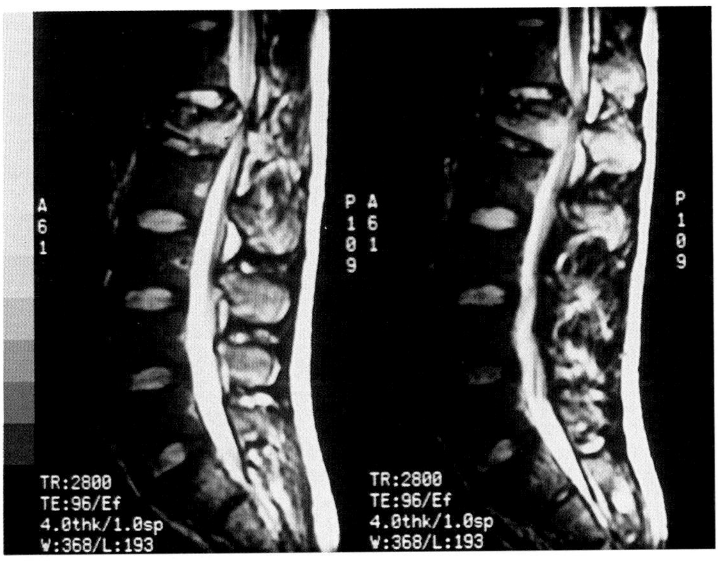

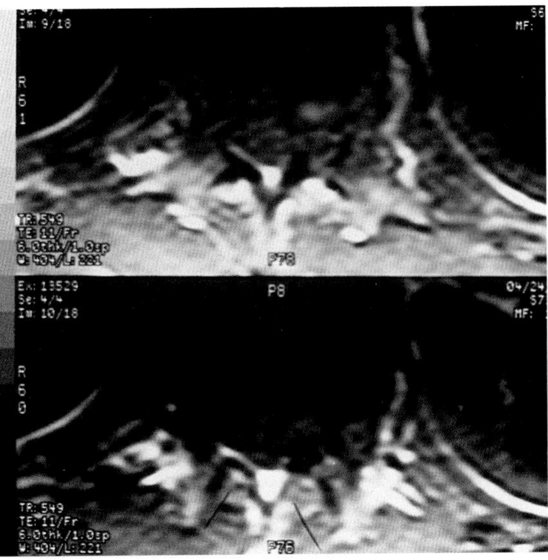

Figure 2. A: Sagittal T2 MRI demonstrating posterior displacement of the body of L1 displacing the cauda equina. The discs of T12–L1 and L1–L2 do not appear to be injured. **B:** Axial image. Posterior displacement of the middle column of L1 onto the thecal sac. Only posteriorly is epidural fat seen.

a mean pressure of 70 mm Hg, unless otherwise contraindicated. The patient is transferred supine to a turning frame, induced and intubated (Fig. 3). Spinal cord monitoring is initiated prior to turning the patient, and repeated after turning the patient prone. The pads of the frame support the chest and iliac wings, allowing gravity to spontaneously reduce the sagittal kyphosis. The operating table must allow for AP and lateral fluoroscopic or radiographic control. The patient is placed in a prone position, with the knees slightly flexed with doughnut rings under each knee and the forehead. The positioning frame can be adjusted so that the patient fits comfortably and the abdominal contents are free. Proper patient positioning and frame adjustments are done to decrease intraabdominal pressure, secondary venous congestion, and intraoperative bleeding. The lower extremities should have thigh-high hose and sequential compressive stockings in place. A fiberoptic head light with magnifying loops for the surgeon is recommended when operating on the bony spine in and around the spinal cord or cauda equina.

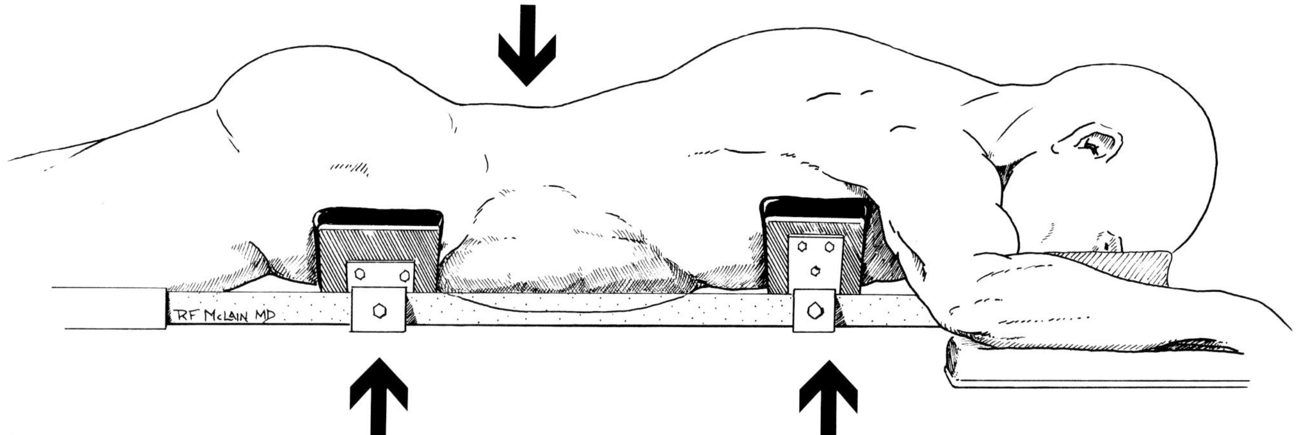

Figure 3. Positioning patient on turning frame allows surgeon to protect spinal cord during turning from supine to prone position. Pads placed under iliac crests and chest wall allow the abdomen to hang free and let gravity provide a gradual, passive reduction of the kyphotic deformity. The entire frame is radiolucent, permitting fluoroscopic visualization in both PA and lateral plains.

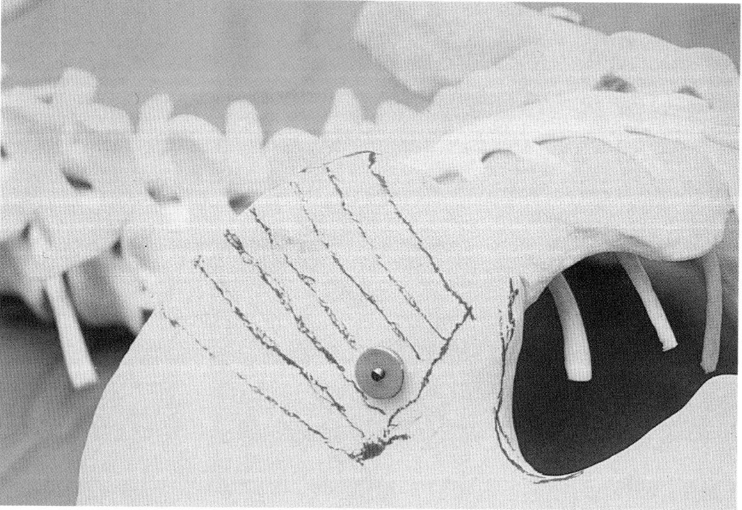

Figure 4. The iliac wing is exposed. Corticocancellous strips are taken in preparation for fusion.

Bone Graft. My preferred technique for L4-S1 is to take the bone graft through a midline incision subcutaneously above the fascia to the iliac crest. For upper lumbar fusions the graft is harvested through a separate curvilinear incision over the iliac crest. First using the hot knife, and then Cobb elevators, subperiosteal dissection is done to expose the iliac crest. Exposure is limited to about four fingers from the posterior superior iliac spine; be careful not to injure the cluneal nerves. Osteotomes are used to take our graft. First, a ½-inch straight osteotome is used to make a gutter on the superior part of the ilium from the posterior superior iliac spine to four finger breadths anteriorly, being careful to avoid the cluneal

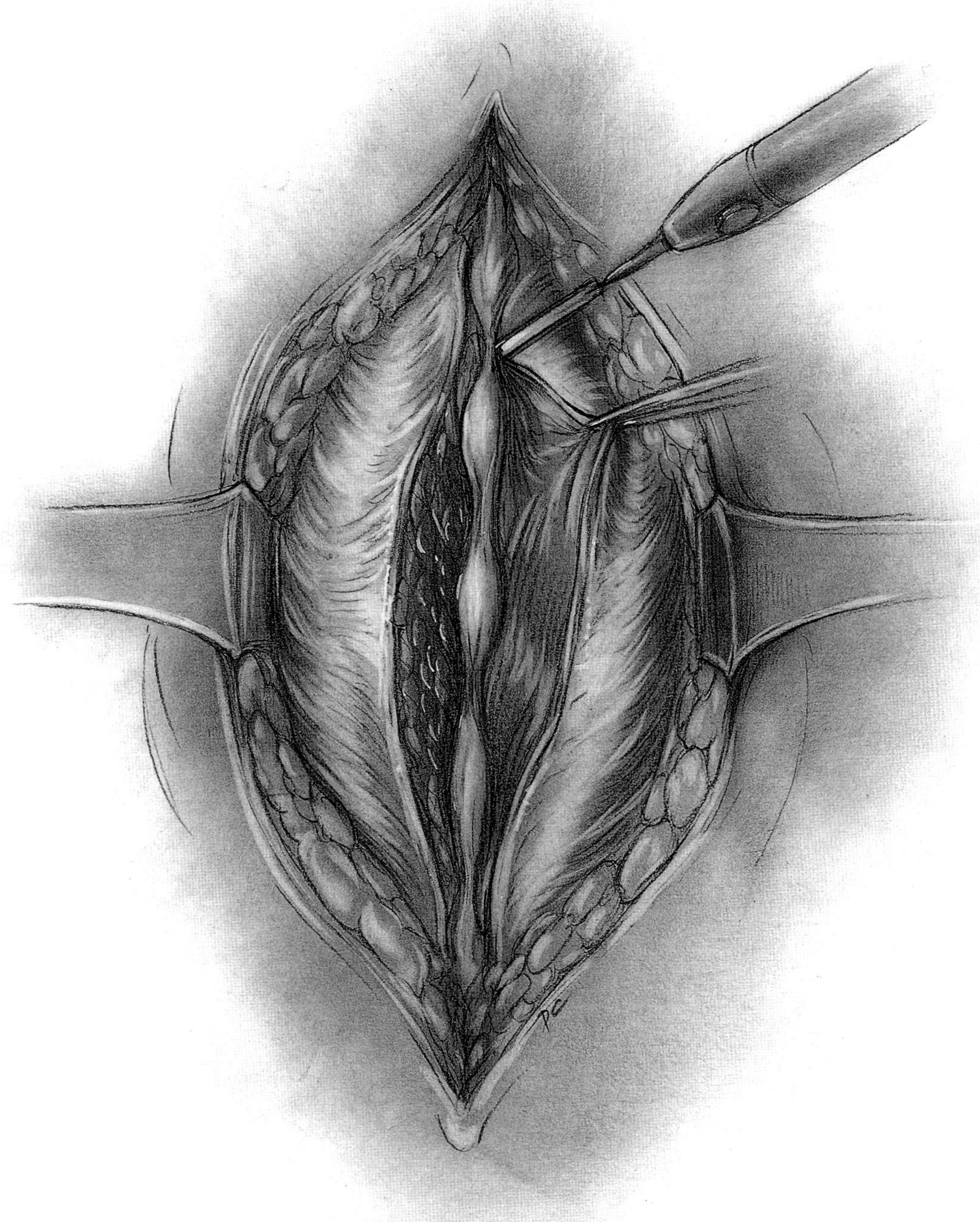

Figure 5. The surgical exposure is done midline using the electrocautery hot knife. The paraspinal muscles are stripped off the spinous processes down to the lamina.

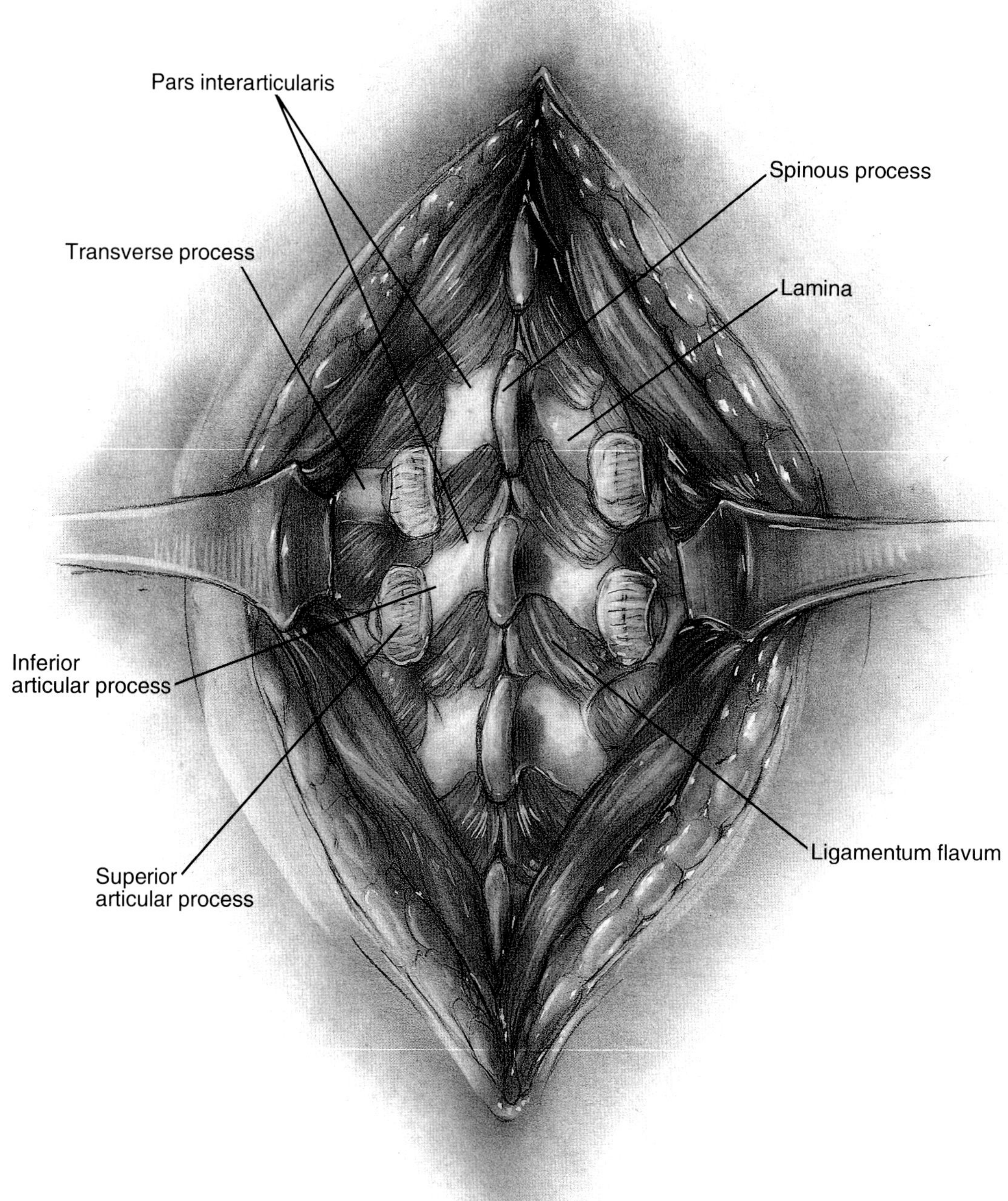

Figure 6. The thoracic and lumbar vertebrae down to the lamina out over the facet joints.

nerves. A Taylor retractor is placed between the bony crest and gluteal muscles. One-quarter-inch vertical, corticocancellous strips are made using the same osteotome. These are approximately 2½ inches in length (Fig. 4). Cancellous bone strips are taken using narrow Kapner gouges. The graft(s) are placed in lactated Ringer's solution, or blood from the wound, until we are ready to perform our fusion. The wound is irrigated thoroughly with saline. Bone wax is worked onto the remaining inner table of the iliac crest to stop any blood oozing from the cancellous bone that remains. Following further irrigation and an antibiotic rinse, the wound is closed over a medium Hemovac drain. A layered closure is performed: #0 Vicryl interrupted sutures are used to close the lumbodorsal fascia to the iliac crest; 2–0 Vicryl sutures are used for the subcutaneous layer, and a subcuticular 3–0 Dexon or Monocryl closure is used for closing the skin. The Hemovac drain (medium) is placed between the bone and gluteal muscles and is attached to a separate closed canister.

Approach to Bony Spine. I generally prefer a posterior midline approach when doing posterior transpedicular fixation of spine fractures. The skin incision is made with a #10 blade. Be generous with your skin incision to gain exposure from T10–T11 to L3–L4. Using electrocautery, the subcutaneous and paraspinal muscles are dissected off the spinous processes subperiosteally down to the spinous lamina, onto the pars interarticularis, up to the medial edge of the facet joints (Figs. 5 and 6). Using a peanut (a hemostat with a small cotton pledget) bluntly dissect the muscles from around the facet capsule, being careful not to injure the facet capsules before determining the exact fusion levels by AP and lateral C-arm fluoroscopy (Fig. 7). The facets of T12–L1 and L1–L2 are exposed. Using electrocautery the muscle insertions around the facet joint are released out onto the lateral border of the superior facets and onto the respective transverse processes. The intervening tissues between the transverse processes of the involved levels (L1 and L2) are identified and dissected free to allow space for placement of bone graft in the lateral gutters from transverse process to transverse process. This will occur later in the procedure when performing your fusion.

The vertebral laminae are thoroughly exposed out to the facet joints; remember to be careful not to damage the facet joints. The exact level(s) of instrumentation is yet to be accurately determined. For relatively stable L1 burst fracture and transpedicular fixation, I recommend instrumenting from T12 to L2, including the L1 or fractured vertebra in cases with more communition. Instrumenting the

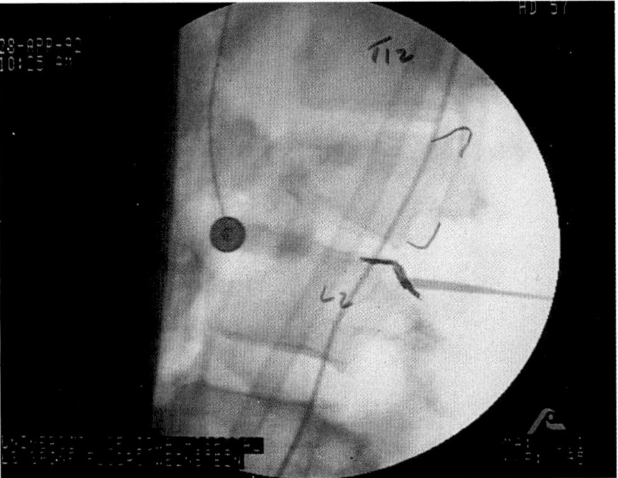

Figure 7. A lateral intraoperative image demonstrating a Penfield probe at the L2 pedicle. The L1 burst fracture is seen just above.

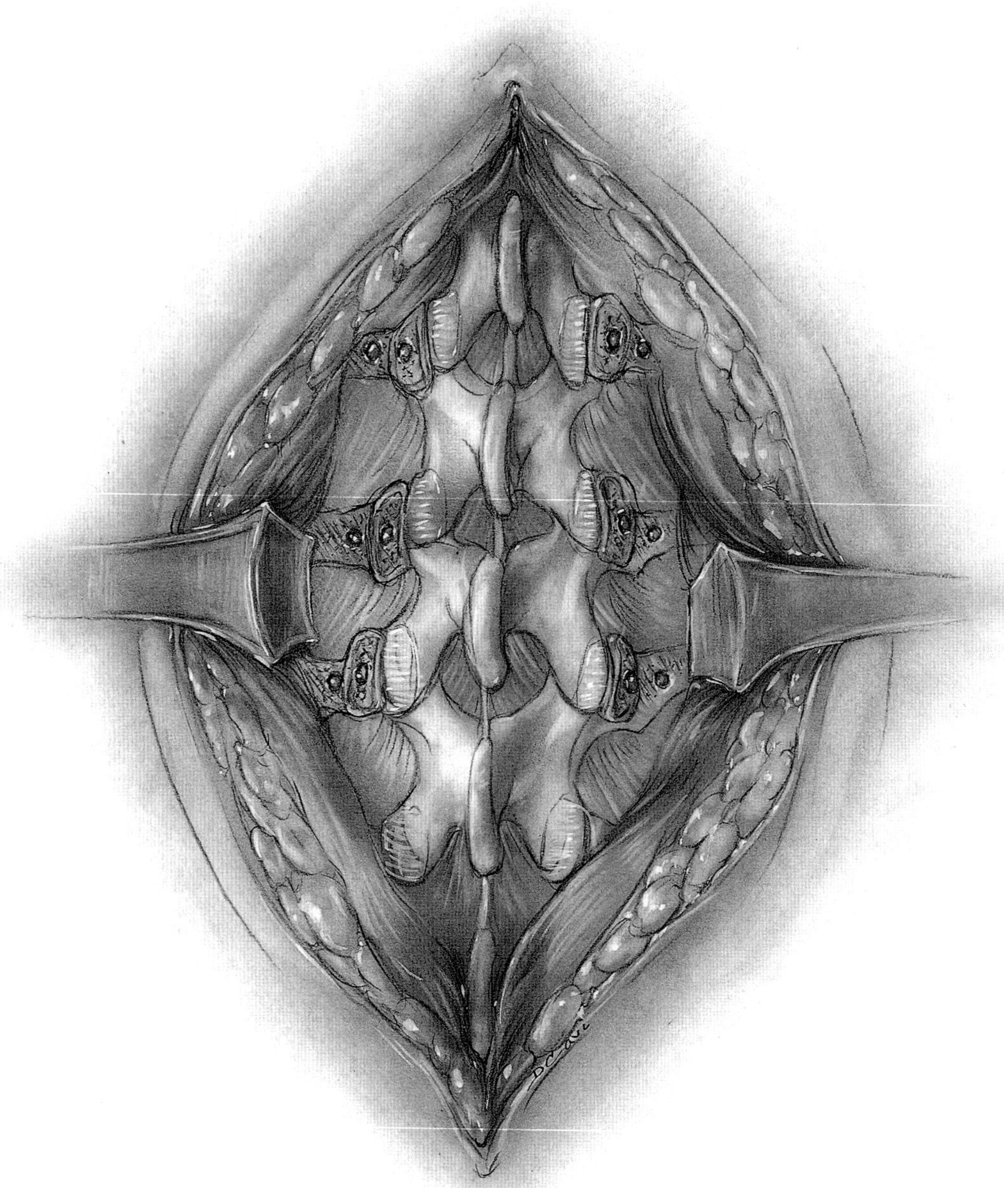

Figure 8. Identification and decortication of the lateral border of the superior facets in preparation for pedicular screw placement. Be careful not to interfere with the facet joints.

fractured vertebra, in this case L1, provides good three-point fixation and prevents the cantilever effects that may result in a junctional kyphosis. After identifying vertebral levels L1 and L2, a high-speed drill (Midas Rex, AM attachment, #8 tool) is used to bur the lateral portion of the superior facets of T12, and L2 to identify the entrance point for the pedicular screws (Fig. 8). The superior facets of L1 and L2 are to be included in the fusion and must be decorticated in preparation for screw placement (Fig. 9). In the model we demonstrate the entrance points for the T12, L1, and L2 screws. The T12 pedicle is seen on AP fluoroscopy and sits just medial to the mammillary process (Fig. 10A–C). Using a number 4 Penfield probe and the C-arm, co-axial images of each pedicle are obtained, and the center of each pedicle is identified (Fig. 11). Using a blunt awl the hole is slightly widened (Fig. 12). I prefer to use a 5.5-mm tap and no drilling of the pedicle (Fig. 13). I determine appropriate screw size and length by preoperative CT or radiograph. The lateral, plain radiograph, or lateral fluoroscopic image used intraoperatively helps me determine the depth of screw penetration, as well as cephalad or caudad angulation of my screws (Fig. 14). I try to achieve a 50% to 80% depth. The outer screw diameter may be different for each level. T12 will generally accept 5.5-mm screws, and L1 and L2 will generally accept 6.0-mm screws. L3-S1 will usually accept 7.0 mm screws. These are not absolute (8) (Fig. 15).

Once the screws are placed in T12 and L2 vertebrae on one side, the ipsilateral L1 screw is placed in the fractured vertebra. When placing screws in L1 fractured vertebra I use a Kocker clamp placed on the transverse process and/or superior facet to help me stabilize the fracture vertebral pedicle segment for screw placement. At this point I place a temporary, working, longitudinal device (rod or plate) to stabilize the spine T12 to L2 so that decompression can be performed through laminectomy and/or through the more involved lumbar pedicle. Once this is done

A
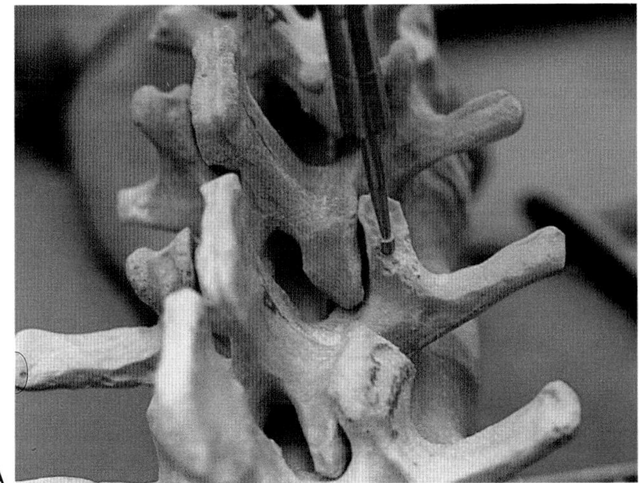

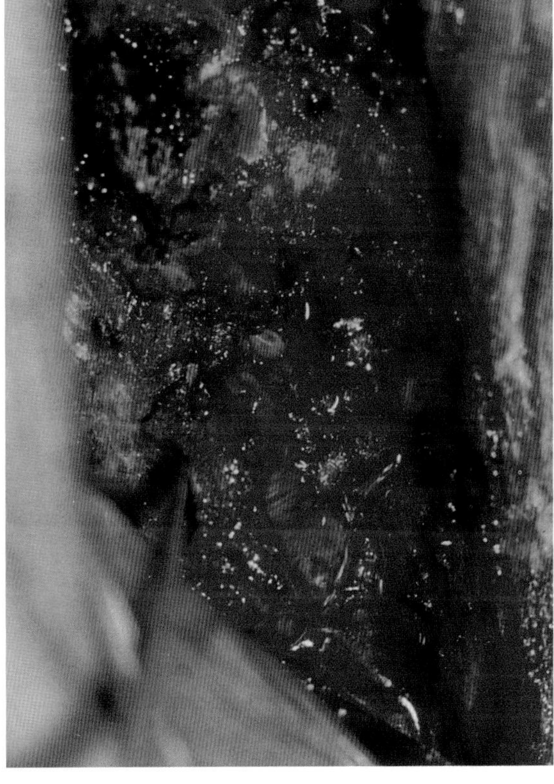
B

Figure 9. A: Decortication using a high-speed drill starts at the lateral border of the superior facet. One to 2 mm of bone are burred away down to the transverse process. **B:** Surgical view.

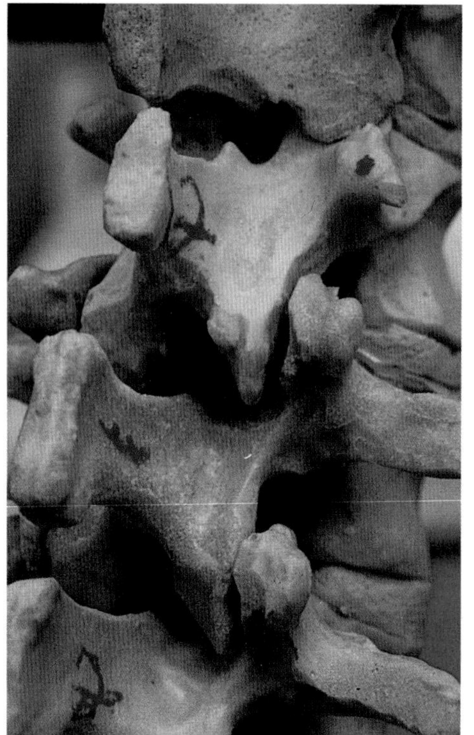

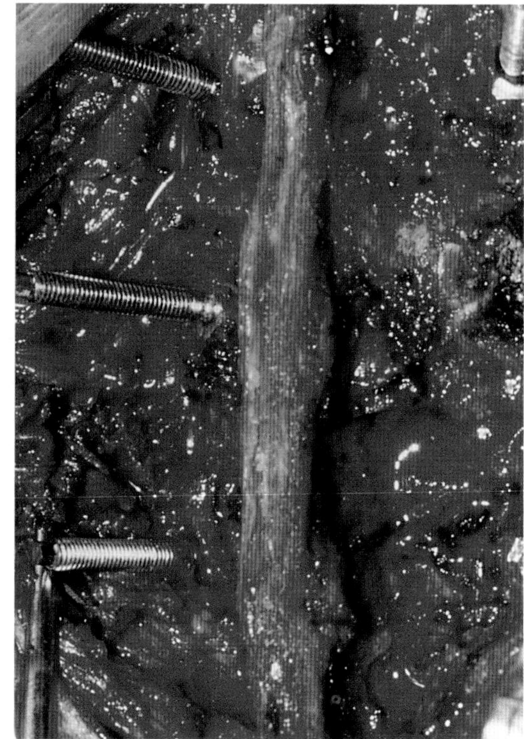

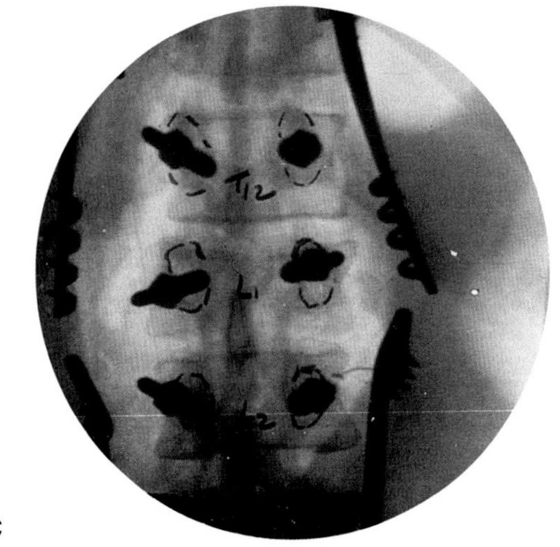

Figure 10. A: Spine model identifying the entrance point for the T12, L1, and L2 pedicle screw. **B:** Surgical view. **C:** Intraoperative fluoroscopic image showing all six pedicle screws in place. Each pedicle has been outlined, and each screw appears to be well centered at T12, L1, and L2.

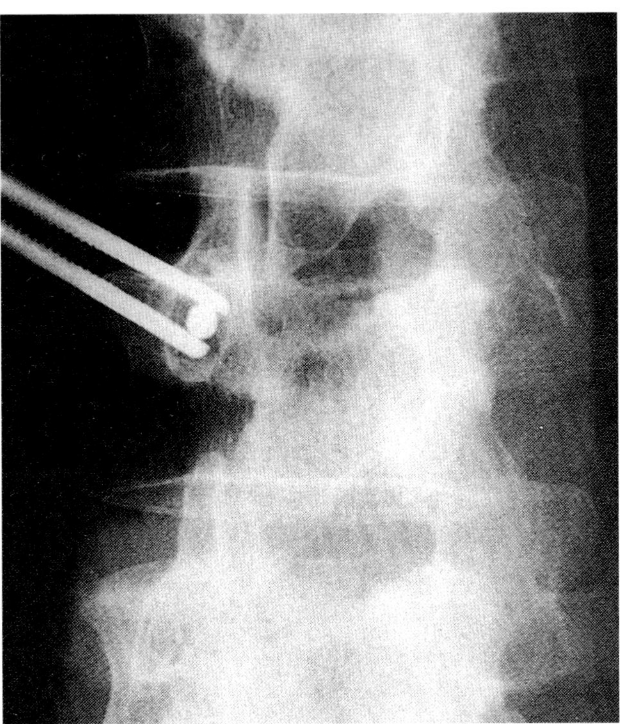

Figure 11. An intraoperative figure showing placement of a probe over center of the pedicle prior to placement of our pedicular screw.

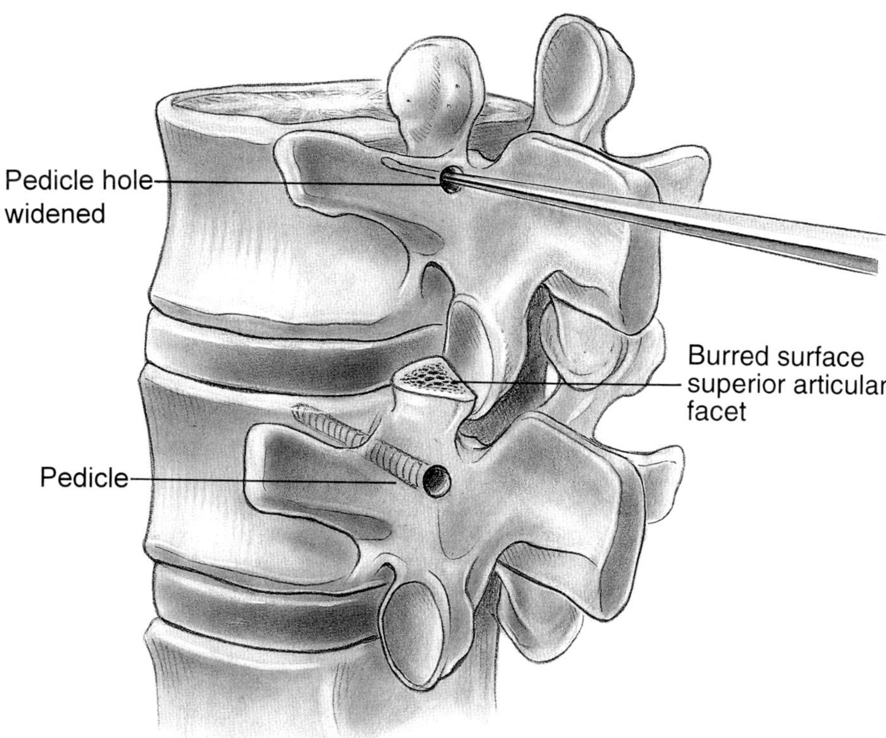

Figure 12. I prefer to use a blunt awl to probe the pedicle prior to tapping.

and I am ready to place the screws on the other side I move to the opposite side of the table. If I haven't decompressed the fracture through the pedicle I may place an additional screw in the fractured L1 level (Fig. 16). The opposite side longitudinal members are contoured to maintain sagittal contour and vertebral height and attached to the screws for rigid fixation. If, however, I plan on further surgery anteriorly, I will leave the left-sided L1 screw out, so as not to interfere with anterior decompression and strut grafting.

In cases of moderate to severe comminution the fractured vertebral body can be reinforced with a transpedicular bone graft to limit the risk of sagittal collapse. After probing the L1 pedicle, the pedicle is over drilled with a hand drill, and a specially-designed funnel is passed under fluoroscopic control into the vertebral body. In these cases I harvest part of the iliac crest graft with an acetabular reamer, producing a fine cancellous slurry that can be packed through the funnel into the anterior defect.

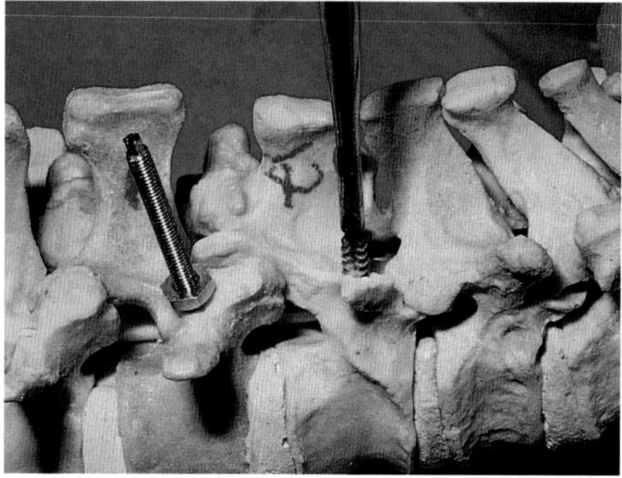

Figure 13. I prefer to tap each pedicle with a 5.5-mm tap prior to screw placement. At T12 I use 5.5-mm screws, and at L1 and L2 I try to use 6.25-mm screws.

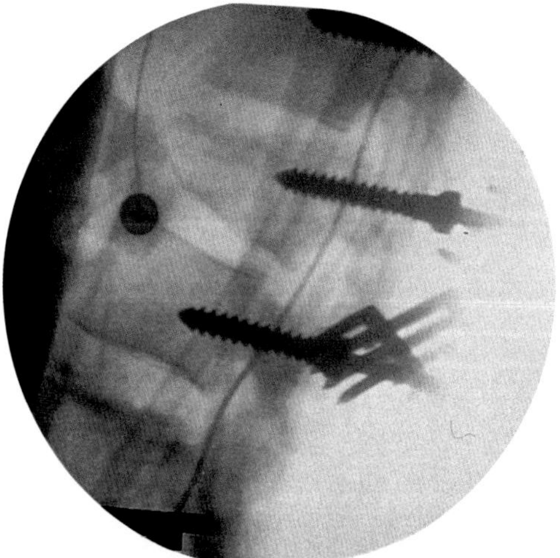

Figure 14. Intraoperative lateral fluoroscopic image allows me to check the depth of screw penetration, as well as screw inclination as it relates to the patient's kyphosis and/or lordosis.

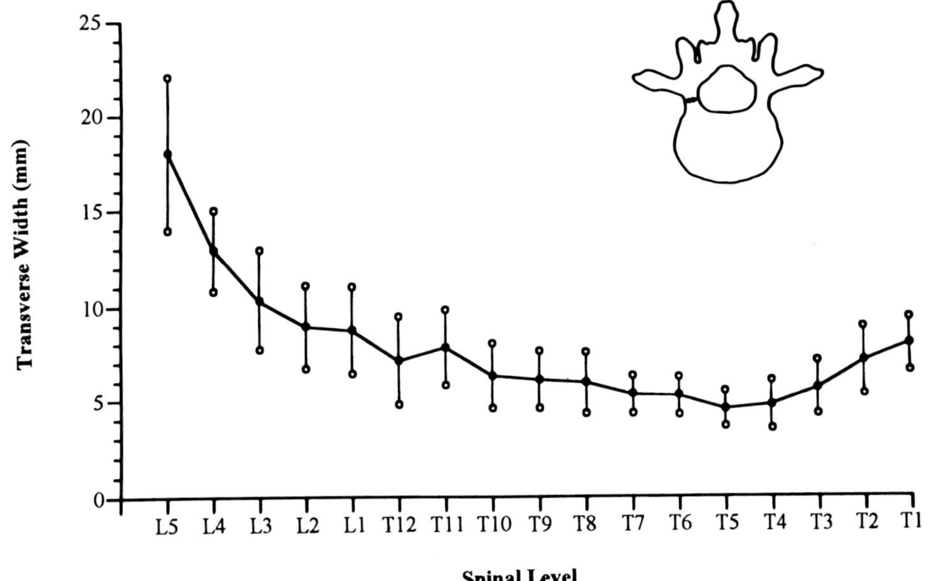

Figure 15. A graph demonstrating how the transverse width of the vertebral pedicles narrows as one goes from L5 to T5.

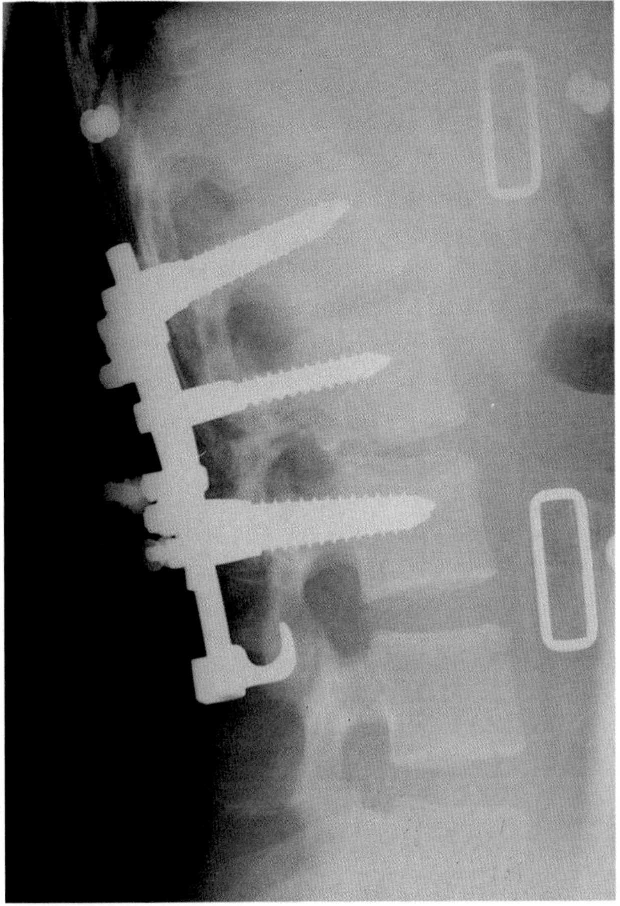

Figure 16. Lateral view of L1 fracture with pedicle screws at T12, L1, and L2. An offset laminar hook was placed unilaterally to protect the lower screw on the side that could not take an L1 screw. The offset hook reduces screw bending moments without extending the fusion into the lower lumbar spine.

When the T12 pedicles are narrow, or when the fracture occurs at T12 itself, it may not be possible to safely apply pedicle screws in the upper vertebra. In these cases I use an extended construct, running the segmental rods up to the T9-10 level where a transverso-pedicular claw provides cranial fixation. The upper and lower fixation points neutralize the fracture in optimal alignment; an intermediate hook may be used upgoing to distract the burst fracture segment or downgoing to compress the graft when an anterior strut has been placed (Fig. 17).

Severe three column disruptions may require more extensive instrumentation to provide rigid fixation and avoid screw failure. In selected cases I will place screws at two levels below the fracture (Fig. 18) or place offset sublaminar hooks to relieve the cantilever bending moment imparted to the L2 screw. While extending the construct into the thoracic spine has little effect on motion or spinal function, I still try to avoid instrumenting below L3.

Indications for anterior surgery are variable and are case/surgeon dependent. In general, injuries at or above the conus can be decompressed by an anterior approach. Middle column osteocartilaginous fragments can be difficult to decompress at the level of the spinal cord. In such cases anterior decompression is performed with or without an anterior fixation device but with autogenous tricorti-

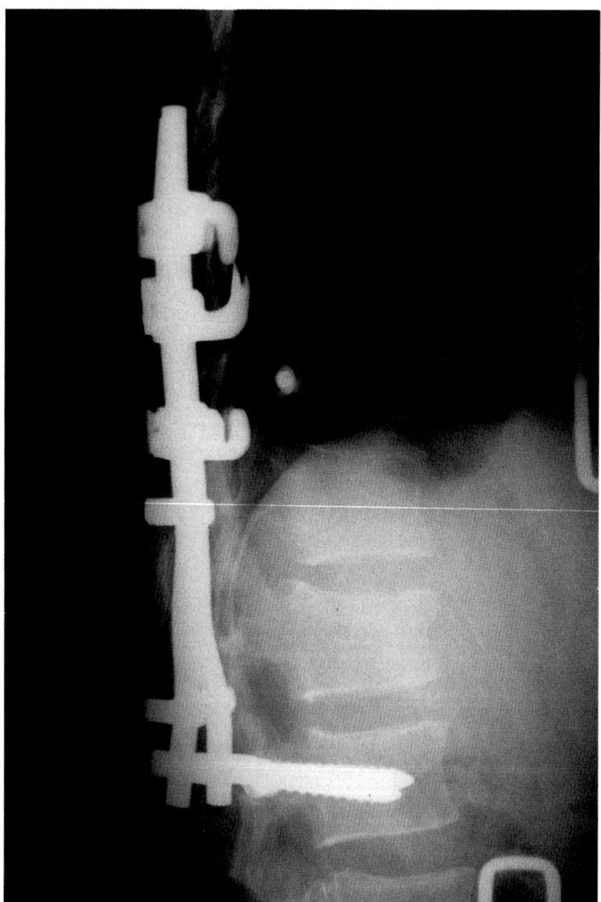

Figure 17. Lateral radiograph of L1 burst treated with pedicle screws in an extended construct. The upper transverso-pedicular claw obtains cranial purchase in the thoracic spine without the risk of pedicle screws in the smaller thoracic pedicles. The intermediate hooks have a small hook (4.0 mm) to limit canal compromise, and distract the fracture without distracting the entire spine.

cal iliac crest graft. If I do not use an anterior stabilizing device, autogenous tricortical grafting is followed by posterior fixation at the same operative setting. Another approach I sometimes employ is a transpedicular decompression from the posterior approach followed by segmental spinal fixation. This approach is often used for injuries involving the spinal cord. In any case I have found intraoperative ultrasound to be a useful tool in the operating room. If I am unsure of my decompression or, more importantly, if the patient has a neurologic deficit after the posterior procedure, I repeat the CT scan and if necessary return the patient for another procedure, in this case an anterior decompression.

Distraction appears to be most important in reduction of the fracture. Following thorough fracture decompression, decortication in preparation for bone grafting is performed. A high-speed drill or rongeur may be used for decortication. Again, I prefer a high-speed Midas Rex drill AM attachment and #8 bur. Bone graft is placed out onto and between the transverse processes of L1–L2 and T12 posteriorly. Do not interfere with the T11–T12 facets; this segment is not part of the fusion mass in a T12–L2 fusion. Bone graft is placed underneath the longitudinal device, which then holds the bone graft in place. The facet joints of T12–L1 and L1–L2 are decorticated and the cartilage removed for placement of cancellous bone graft. Again, be careful not to involve the joints of T11–T12 with either the

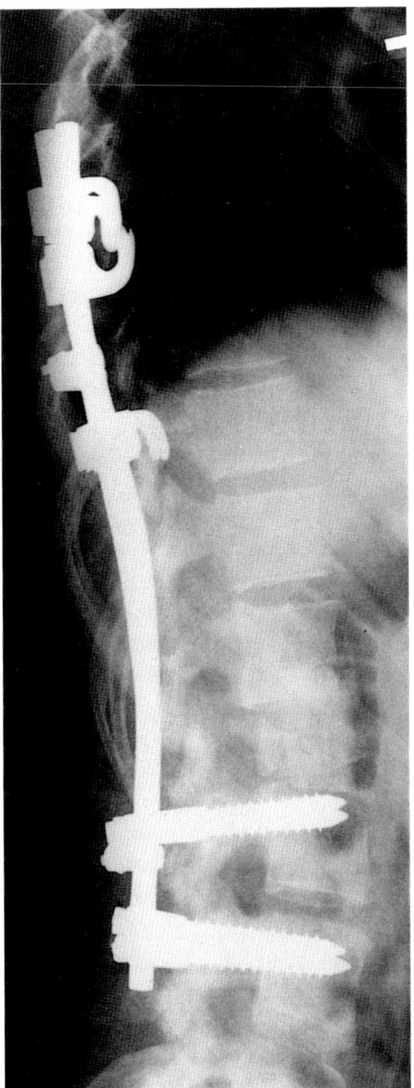

Figure 18. Severe L1 burst with incomplete cauda equina injury. Patient had anterior decompression and tricortical strut graft reconstruction, followed by an extended posterior reconstruction. Pedicle screws were applied at adjacent levels to reduce cantilever bending forces and allow early mobilization in this poly-trauma patient.

bone graft or the fixation device. After placing first the cancellous and second the corticocancellous bone graft, the longitudinal member is reattached to the screws and these are tightly affixed. The opposite plate-rod is removed and the same procedure occurs. Place the necessary locking nuts depending on the device used and trim the screws. Use lateral radiographic/fluoroscopy image for depth of screw penetration (50% to 80% range) and sagittal spine alignment (Fig. 18). Recheck all your connections, bone graft location, and hemostasis.

Spinal cord function is monitored throughout instrumentation. If unexplained changes in latency or magnitude are encountered I may ask the anesthesia team to perform a standard wake-up test. The wound is copiously irrigated with saline and neomycin and then closed. Vicryl (#1) is used to approximate the deep muscle layers and fascia; 2–0 Vicryl is used for the subcutaneous tissue, and 3–0 Dexon is used subcuticularly. If the wound is not dry, a medium Hemovac is placed in the subcutaneous tissues and attached to its own canister.

POSTOPERATIVE MANAGEMENT

The patient is log-rolled onto the usual hospital bed. The head of the bed may be elevated to 60 to 45 degrees. Once the patient's thoracolumbosacral orthosis (TLSO) is ready, the plastic shells are placed and the patient is allowed to ambulate. The shells are not necessary in bed, and the patient may move freely in the bed without the shells. Prior to ambulation, AP and lateral radiographs are taken (Fig. 19). The patient will in general be fully ambulatory within 3 to 5 days postoperatively unless neurologic problems or other concomitant overriding long bone, pelvic, or head injuries exist that preclude ambulation. The patient can expect "surgical" pain for approximately 5 to 7 days postoperatively. Some pain for up to 12 weeks should be expected. Postoperative pain is generally managed with patient-controlled analgesia. Take-home medicines usually include a nonsteroidal antiinflammatory agent as well as limited narcotic medications.

The patient wears the TLSO for approximately 6 months. This varies depending on the injury and the success of fixation (4–8 months) (Fig. 20). The patient may ambulate to tolerance and is encouraged to walk up to 2 miles per day. Riding in a car is possible, but driving is not recommended for approximately 2 months. Heavy lifting (objects over 10 to 15 pounds) should be avoided for the first 6 weeks. At 6 weeks, bicycle or treadmill activity may be added to the physical therapy program, as well as increased walking and stair climbing. Work hardening, depending on job classification, is begun at 12 to 24 weeks. Light-duty work activities are begun at 3 months and heavy-duty activities at 6 months to 1 year. Professionals sometimes, but rarely, resume working activities in 6 weeks.

The surgical devices (screws and rods or plates) are only necessary during the fusion period. Once the spine is fused the device is probably redundant. Currently, we do not recommend removing the device unless patients are younger than 20 years old. The thinking behind this is related to "stress shielding" and increased mobility at the spinal segments above and below the fused level over time. Whether this will be a necessity in the future is yet to be determined.

In this example of an L1 burst fracture, the advantages of using bone screws in the pedicle are obvious. Fewer segments need to be immobilized by instrumentation when compared with nonpedicular devices (i.e., Harrington rods). Also, with bone screws in the pedicle, we have achieved three-column fixation for a three-column problem. With fewer levels fused and better fixation, the patient can expect to be ambulatory within 1 day of surgery and have less morbidity with a small operative procedure. However, one must not forget that the advantages of these devices can be overshadowed if not used correctly. Remember, not all burst fractures require surgical treatment, and not all surgical fractures need pedicle fixation. One must weigh the risks against the benefits in each individual case and gain the patient's informed consent.

COMPLICATIONS

Posterior laminar fractures are frequently associated with dural tears.

Abnormal placement of pedicular screws may necessitate removal of the screw. If a problem exists with the placement of a screw, it is sometimes better to skip that pedicle and either extend the fusion bone level or leave that pedicle without fixation. Unilateral pedicle fixation has been shown to be effective in degenerative conditions of the lumbar spine.

An inappropriately placed screw that injures or compresses a nerve root should be removed. Remember that radiographs are generally unreliable in determining whether a screw is in or out of a pedicle. Postoperatively, CT imaging with or without myelographic enhancement may be necessary.

Failure to align the pedicle screws properly may prevent good fixation of the device. If you use a plate as the longitudinal connecting device, make sure you have good plate-to-screw contact. A stress riser at the plate-screw junction can increase the chance of breaking a screw. Washers or spacer devices will help to achieve good contact between the plate and the screw device. This, of course, varies depending on the instrumentation system being used. Failure to align rod/screw systems can interfere with solid seating of locking bolts, risking implant loosening and failure.

Loss of anterior column stability, failure to correct sagittal kyphosis, or overexuberant contouring of fixation rods can overstress the strongest of screws, leading to early bending failure and progressive kyphosis (Fig. 21). The surgeon cannot ignore the basic principles of biomechanics and depend on the device to bail him/her out. Major disruptions may often require anterior decompression, reconstruction and augmentation of implant placement. Addition of supplemental offset hooks can also protect against both screw and bone failure in unstable fractures.

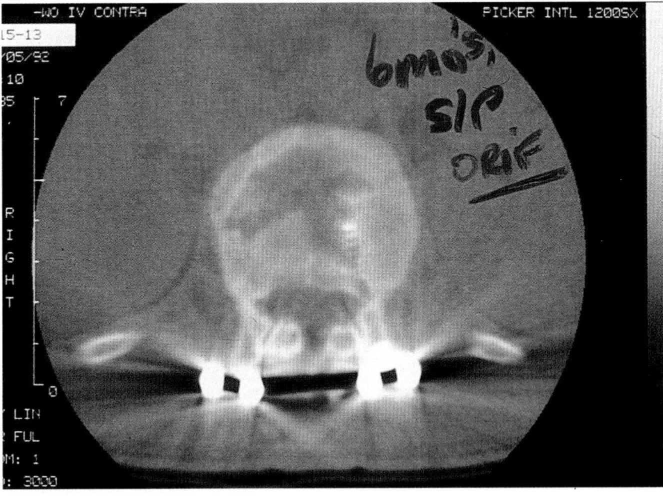

Figure 20. Axial CT image 6 months postoperatively. Note the remodeling of the middle osteoligamentous column.

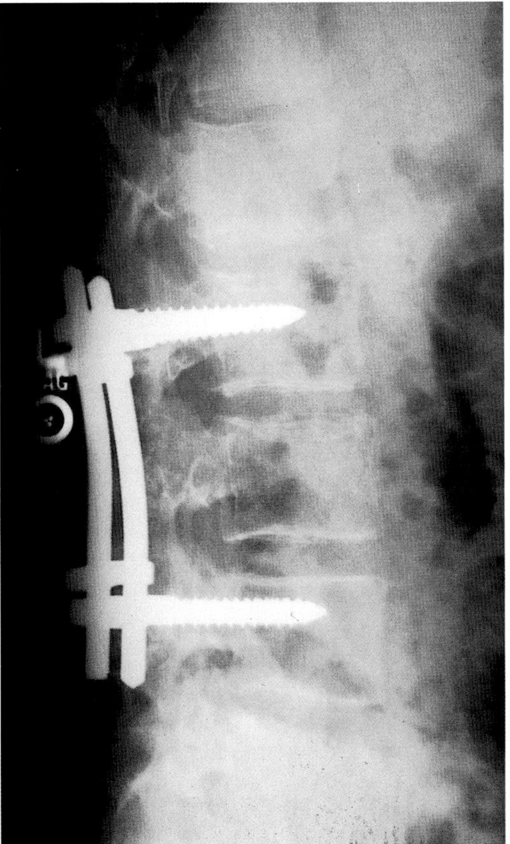

Figure 19. Lateral view of standard short segment pedicle instrumentation construct (SSPI) used in L1 burst fracture. Sagittal alignment is well restored and the anterior column is sufficiently stable to forego anterior reconstruction. Transpedicular bone grafting improves outcomes in some patients with moderate comminution.

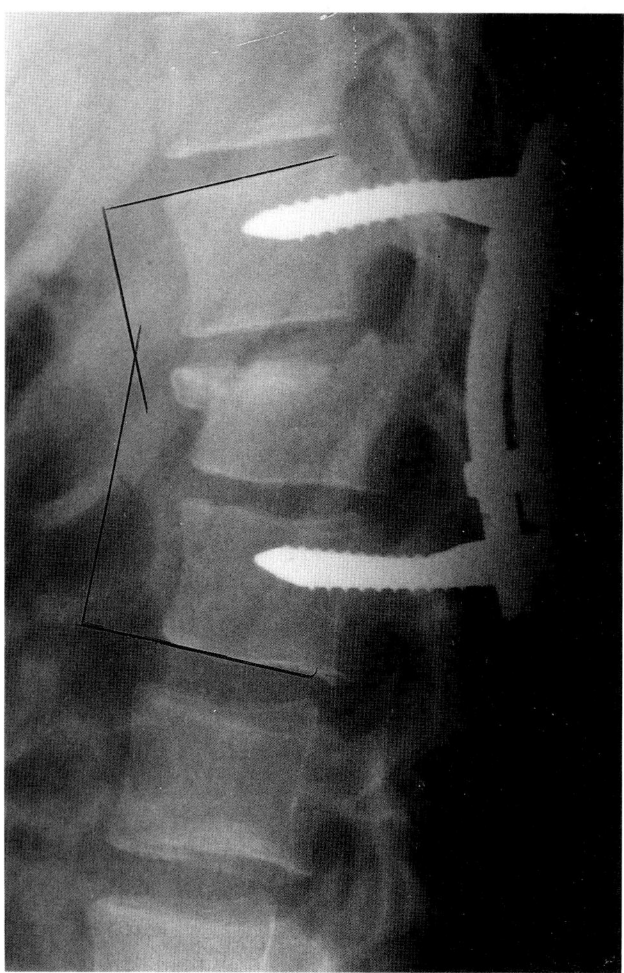

Figure 21. Screws may be bent by overzealous in-situ contouring of the fixation rods, or when the anterior spinal column is severely disrupted. Once screws begin to fail progressive bending and kyphosis often follow. Patients with bent screws may have more pain and a poorer result; intraoperative fluoroscopy can identify screws bent during contouring so that they can be immediately replaced.

RECOMMENDED READING

1. Camisa, F. P., Eismont, F. J., and Green, B. A.: Dural lacerations occurring with burst fractures and associated laminar fractures. *J. Bone Joint Surg.*, 71A: 1044–1051, 1989.
2. Chiba, M., McLain, R. F., Ysaby, S. A., Moseley, T. A., Smith, T. S., Benson, D. R.: Short segment pedicle instrumentation: biomechanical analysis of supplemental hook fixation. *Spine* 21: 288–294, 1996.
3. Fredrickson, B. E., Edwards, W. T., Rauschning, W., Bayley, J. C., and Yuan, H. A.: Vertebral burst fractures: an experimental, morphologic, radiographic study. *Spine*, 17: 1012–1021, 1992.
4. Kabins, M. B., Weinstein, J. N., Spratt, K. F., Found, E. M., et al.: Isolated L4-L5 floating fusions using the variable spinal screw placement system: unilateral vs. bilateral. *J. Spinal Disord.*, 5:39–49, 1992.
5. Krag, M. H., Fredrickson, B. E., and Yuan, H. A.: Spinal instrumentation. The Lumbar Spine, edited by J. N. Weinstein and S. W. Weisel, pp. 916–940. W.B. Saunders, Phadelphia.
6. McLain, R. F., Kabins, M., Weinstein, J. N.: VSP Stabilization of lumbar neoplasms: technical considerations and complications. *J. Spinal Disord.* 4:359–365, 1991.
7. McLain, R. F., Sparling, E., Benson, D. R.: Early failure of short-segment pedicle instrumentation for thoracolumbar fractures. *J. Bone Joint Surg.* 75A:162–167, 1993.
8. McLain, R. F., Fry, M. F., Moseley, T. A., Sharkey, N. A.: Lumbar pedicle screw salvage: pullout testing of three different pedicle screw designs. *J. Spinal Disord.*, 8:62–68, 1995.
9. McNamara, M. J., Stephens, G. C., and Spengler, D. M.: Transpedicular short segment fusions for treatment of lumbar burst fractures. *J. Spinal Disord.* 5: 183–187, 1992.
10. Weinstein, J. N., Spratt, K. F., Spengler, D. M., Brick, C., and Reid, S.: Spinal pedicle fixation: reliability and validity of roentgenogram-based assessment and surgical factors on successful screw placement. *Spine* 13: 1012–1018, 1988.
11. Weinstein, J. N., Rydevik, B. L., and Rauschning, W.: Anatomic and technical considerations of pedicle screw fixation. *Clin. Orthop.* 284: 34–46, 1992.
12. Zindrick, M. R., Wiltse, L. L., Doornik, A., Widell, E. H., et al.: Analysis of the morphometric characteristics of the thoracic and lumbar pedicles. *Spine*, 12: 160–166, 1987.

Master Techniques in Orthopaedic Surgery,
THE SPINE, edited by D. S. Bradford,
Lippincott-Raven Publishers, Philadelphia, © 1997.

25

Management of Spinal Dysraphism

Samuel F. Ciricillo and Michael S. B. Edwards

INDICATIONS/CONTRAINDICATIONS

Spinal dysraphism, including myelomeningoceles, diastematomyelia, and tethered cord syndrome, refers to a heterogeneous group of disorders of neural tube fusion that occur early in gestation. Other associated anomalies, such as hydrocephalus and Chiari II malformations, are frequently present and add to the complexity of perioperative management of these patients. The goal of early diagnosis and surgical repair of these lesions is the preservation of neurologic function. Early repair reduces the risk of ascending meningitis and ventriculitis in open neural tube defects, allows for the reconstitution of normal anatomic barriers and the flow of cerebrospinal fluid (CSF), improves blood flow and metabolism in ischemic neural tissue, and prevents progressive neurologic, orthopedic, and urologic dysfunction.

The decision to treat infants with severe neural tube defects and significant neurologic dysfunction is a difficult one that requires consultation with the family, pediatricians, neurosurgeon, geneticist, social worker, and occasionally the clergy. Contraindications to surgical repair include active, life-threatening sepsis and associated genetic syndromes with congenital anomalies that carry a uniformly fatal prognosis.

PREOPERATIVE PLANNING

Infants with open myelomeningoceles require a careful neonatal and neurologic assessment to determine the level of neurologic function prior to planned operative

S. F. Ciricillo, M.D. and M. S. B. Edwards, M.D.: Perinatal & Pediatric Specialists, Medical Group, Inc., San Francisco, California 94115.

intervention. Serial head circumference measurements are taken and cranial ultrasonography performed to evaluate for progressive hydrocephalus and the need for ventriculoperitoneal shunting. Infants are kept warm and nursed prone to avoid compression of the exposed neural elements. A moist sponge soaked in bacitracin solution and covered by Tegaderm is placed over the myelomeningocele to prevent dessication of the neural placode and is changed daily until surgery. Intravenous vancomycin and a third-generation cephalosporin are begun to prevent staphylococcal and/or gram-negative meningitis. Since the rate of infection rises significantly after 72 hours, operative intervention should be performed before 3 days or postponed for 6 weeks, when epithelialization of the placode has occurred.

Children or adults with progressive foot deformities, sensorimotor loss, hyporeflexia, or urologic symptoms should undergo careful radiologic assessment of the central nervous system and cervicothoracolumbar spine to exclude progressive hydrocephalus, Chiari malformation, hydromyelia, or tethering of the spinal cord by a diastematic bony spur, lumbosacral lipoma, fibrolipoma of the filum terminale, fibrous band, or dermal sinus tract. Plain spine radiographs may help identify coexisting vertebral body and posterior laminar arch defects such as hemivertebrae and sacral dysgenesis. Magnetic resonance imaging (MRI) remains the screening modality of choice in patients in whom an occult spinal dysraphic condition is suspected. Computed tomography (CT) may demonstrate a central bony spur not appreciated on MRI. Preoperative urologic evaluation with urodynamic studies is essential in these patients.

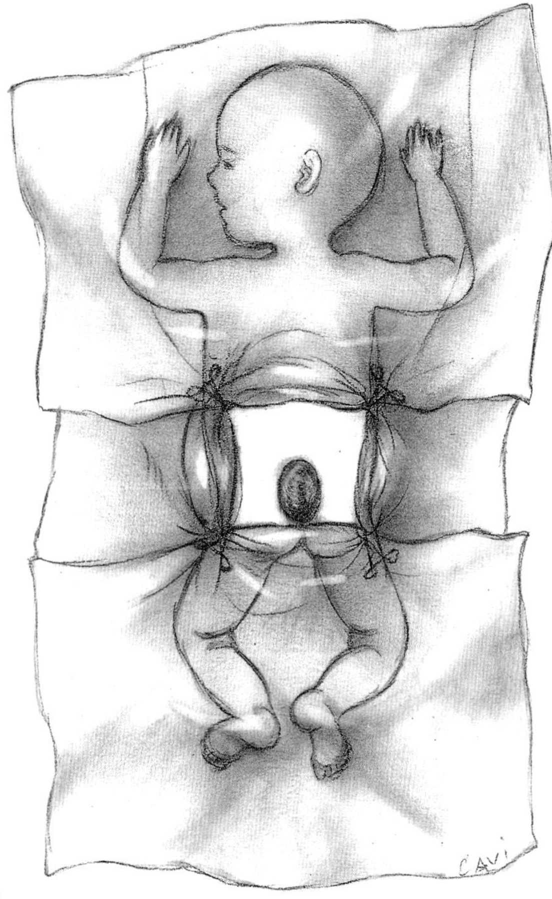

A

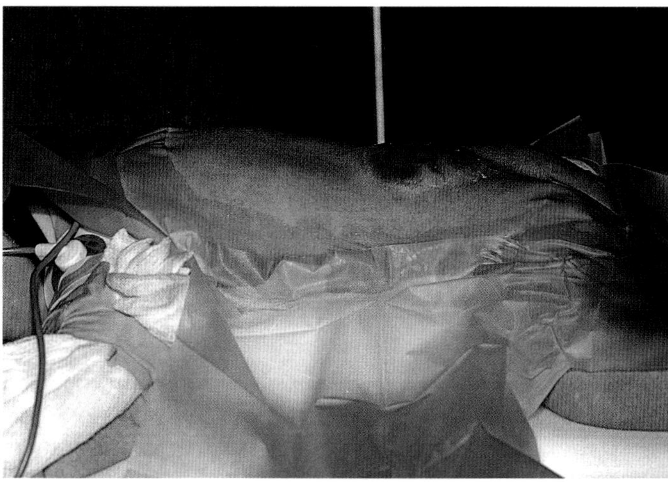

B

Figure 1. The patient is placed prone on bolsters with the arms flexed toward the head. Plastic drapes are attached across the gluteal fold and far laterally to expose the flanks in case relaxing incisions are needed for a tension-free skin closure.

SURGERY

Myelomeningocele Repair

For patients with open neural tube defects, endotracheal intubation and the establishment of good intravenous access is performed with the patient supine on a doughnut to avoid compression of the open myelomeningocele. The patient is then rolled prone onto a heating blanket to maintain body temperature throughout the procedure (Fig. 1). A sponge head-cradle may be used to suspend the infant and avoid abdominal compression, but it has the undesired effect of removing the infant from contact with the heating blanket. The head is oriented toward the anesthesiologist and the arms brought up and well padded beneath the elbows (Fig. 2). The back is lined with plastic Steri-drapes to exclude the anus and head from the surgical field (Fig. 3). The skin is scrubbed gently for 10 minutes with Betadine. Drapes are then applied as low as possible on the flanks to expose skin that may need to be undermined later to facilitate closure of the midline skin defect.

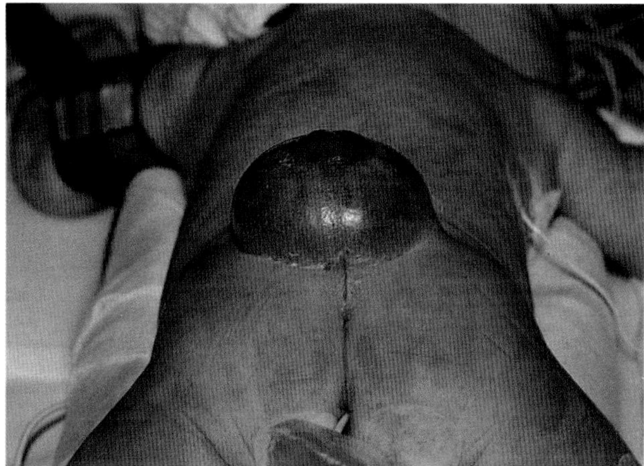

Figure 2. Operating room setup.

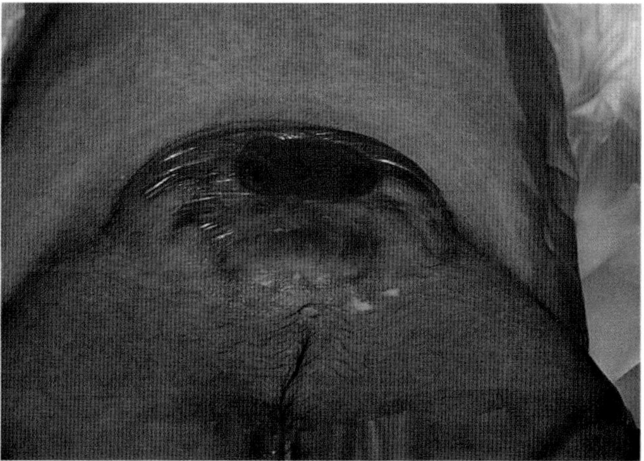

Figure 3. The myelomeningocele has been outlined with plastic drapes to avoid contamination of the surgical site.

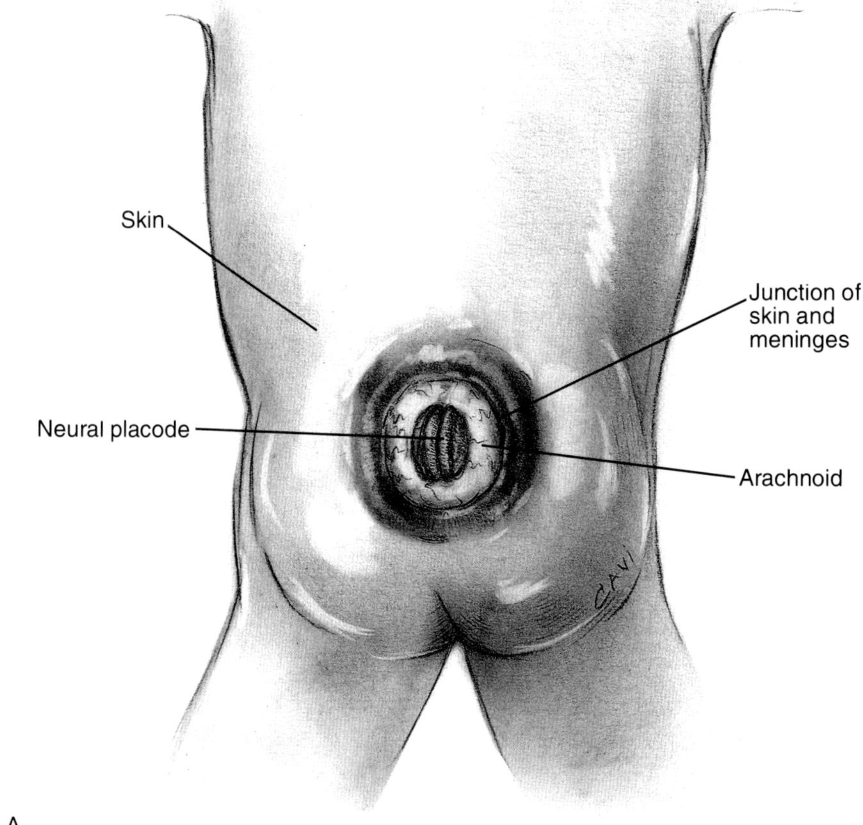

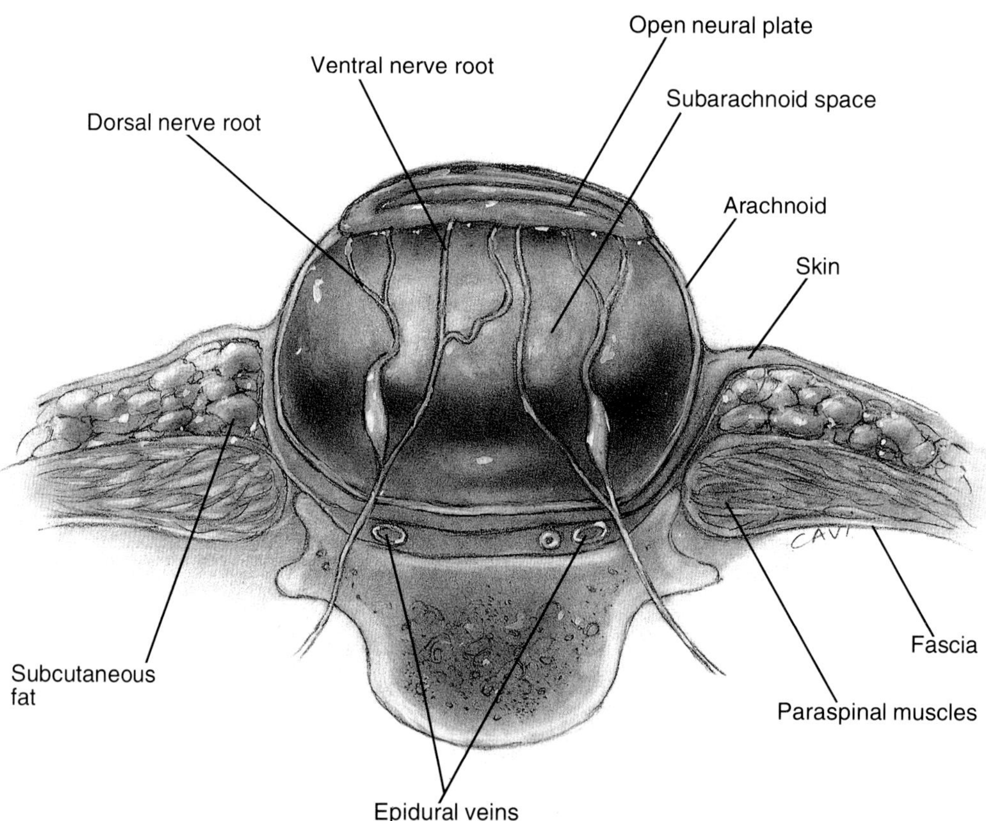

Figure 4. A: The junction of the skin with the meninges and neural placode is identified. **B:** Line drawing demonstrates the important surgical planes. Note that the nerve roots come off the ventral surface of the neural placode and are thus relatively protected.

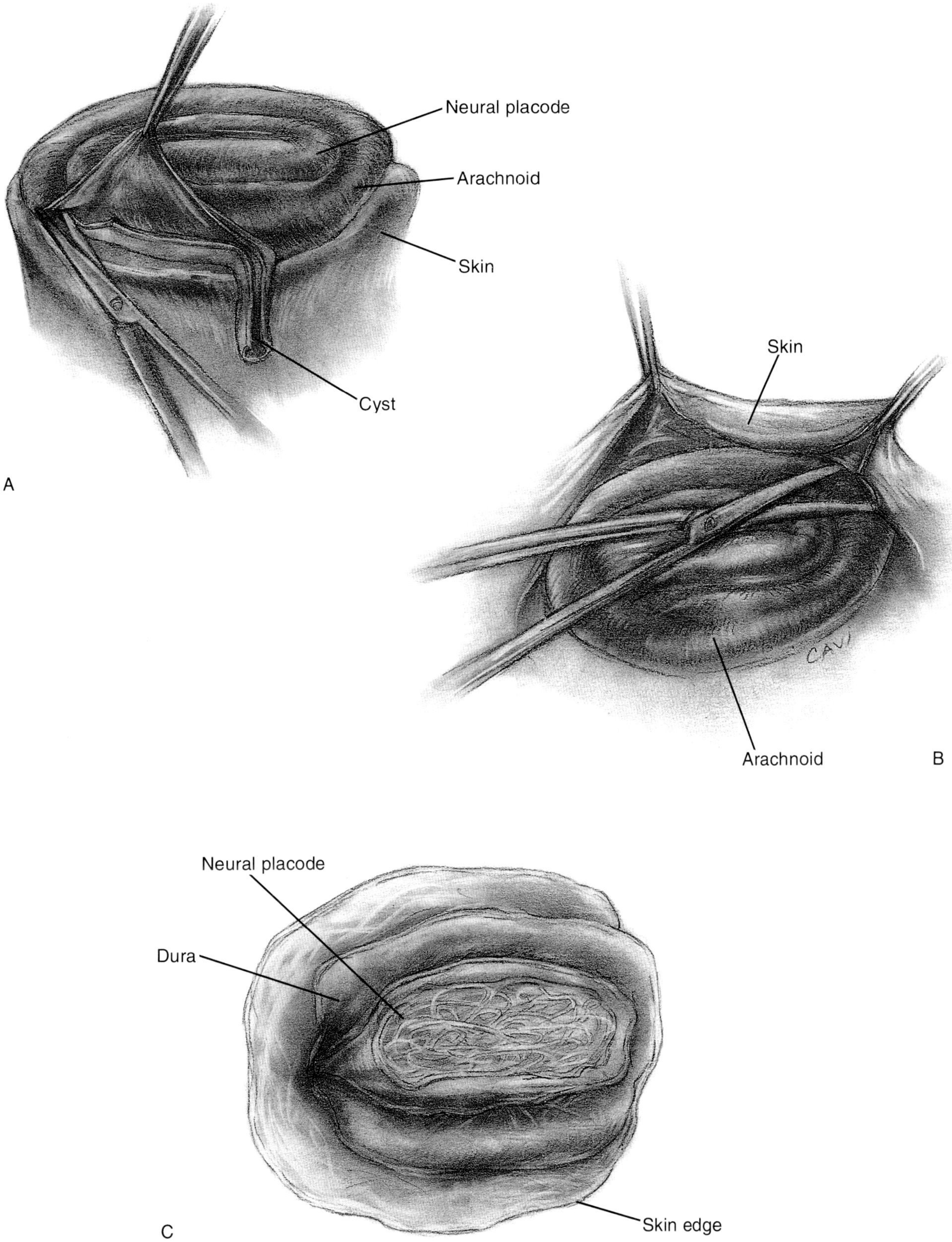

Neural placode
Arachnoid
Skin
Cyst
A
Skin
Arachnoid
B
Neural placode
Dura
Skin edge
C

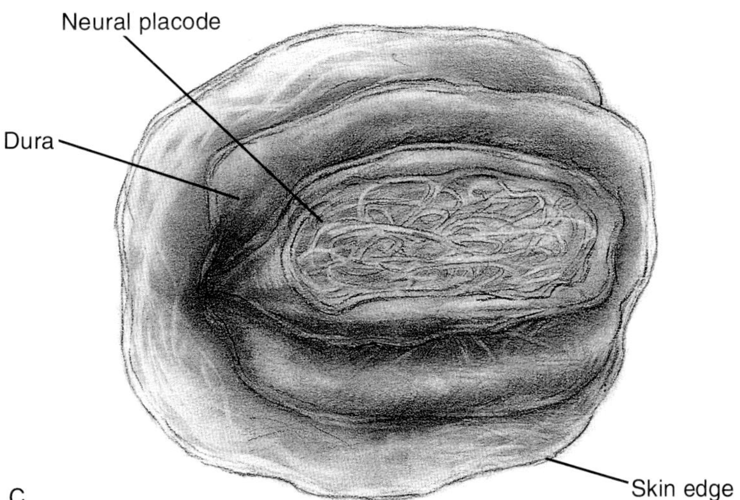

Figure 5. A,B: Fine scissors or the Shaw thermal scalpel is used to separate the neural placode from the surrounding skin. **C:** Once freed, the placode will lie against the ventral dural.

A Shaw thermal scalpel is used in all infants and children to minimize blood loss. The neural placode is dissected from its attachment with the meninges and skin (Fig. 4A) using loupes or the operating microscope for added magnification, beginning along the lateral aspects of the placode. Dissection is carried down through the meninges until the intradural compartment with CSF is reached (Fig. 4B). Dissection circumferentially around the rostral and caudal portions of the placode can then be performed safely once the level of the spinal cord and nerve roots has been identified within the dural sac (Fig. 5A,B). Care must be taken to avoid incorporation of residual epithelium with the neural placode. Any aberrant nerve roots that run blindly into the dome of the sac should be incised. Once the placode has been freed from its cutaneous attachments, it should lie freely within the ventral spinal canal (Fig. 5C). The edges of the neural placode can then be approximated with 6–0 suture to reconstitute the neural tube (Fig. 6A,B).

The dura must be dissected from its attachment with the skin as far laterally as possible to provide for a capacious dural sac (Fig. 7A,B). As the dural leaves are rolled medially, the normal epidural fat will be encountered laterally, which facilitates the dural dissection at the rostral and caudal poles of the defect. The dura is then approximated in a watertight fashion using running 5–0 or 6–0 Vicryl sutures (Fig. 8A,B). Usually more than enough dura is available for closure, but if the dura is too thin dorsally, a lyophilized dura patch can be used to ensure a watertight closure. The subarachnoid space should be irrigated with warm Bacitracin-saline solution to remove blood and lipid droplets from within the spinal canal.

To avoid a potential CSF fistula, a solid myofascial closure is next performed. Depending on the size of the midline defect, this may require the assistance of a reconstructive plastic surgeon to mobilize a myocutaneous flap. Usually, how-

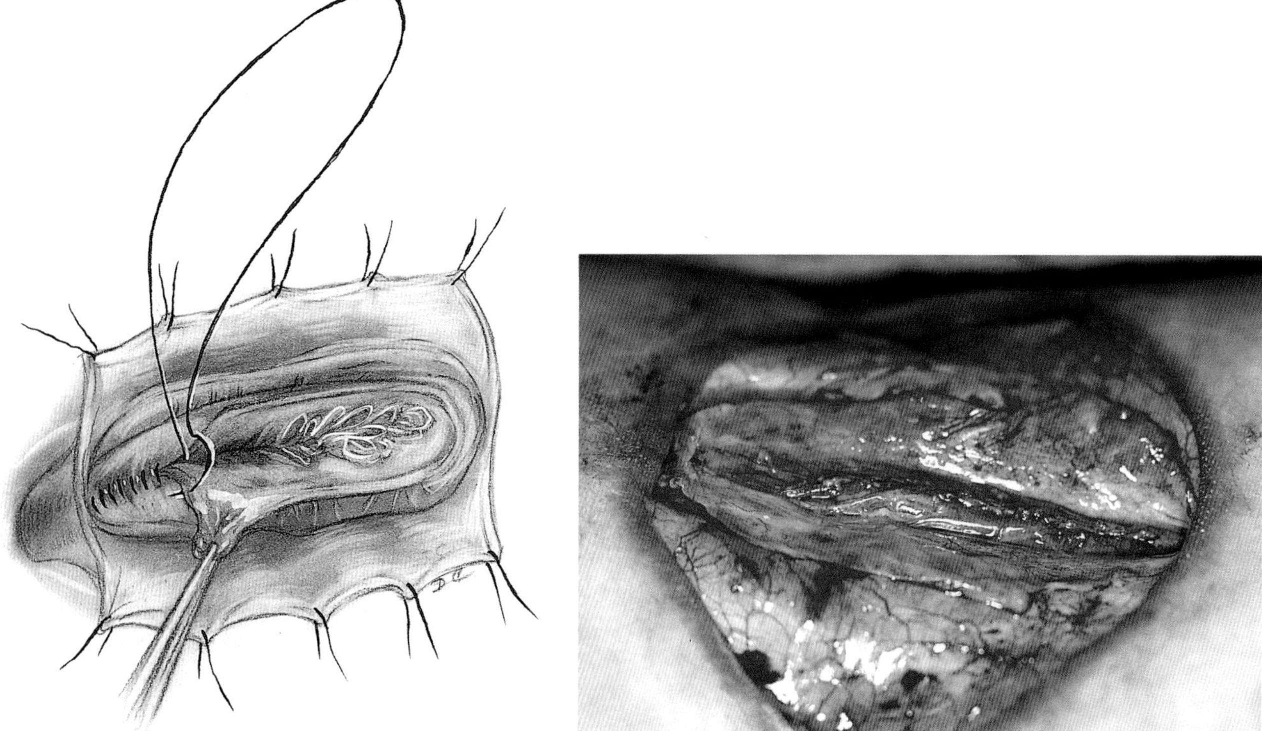

Figure 6. A,B: The neural tube is reconstituted by suturing the lateral edges of the neural placode together using a fine, absorbable suture.

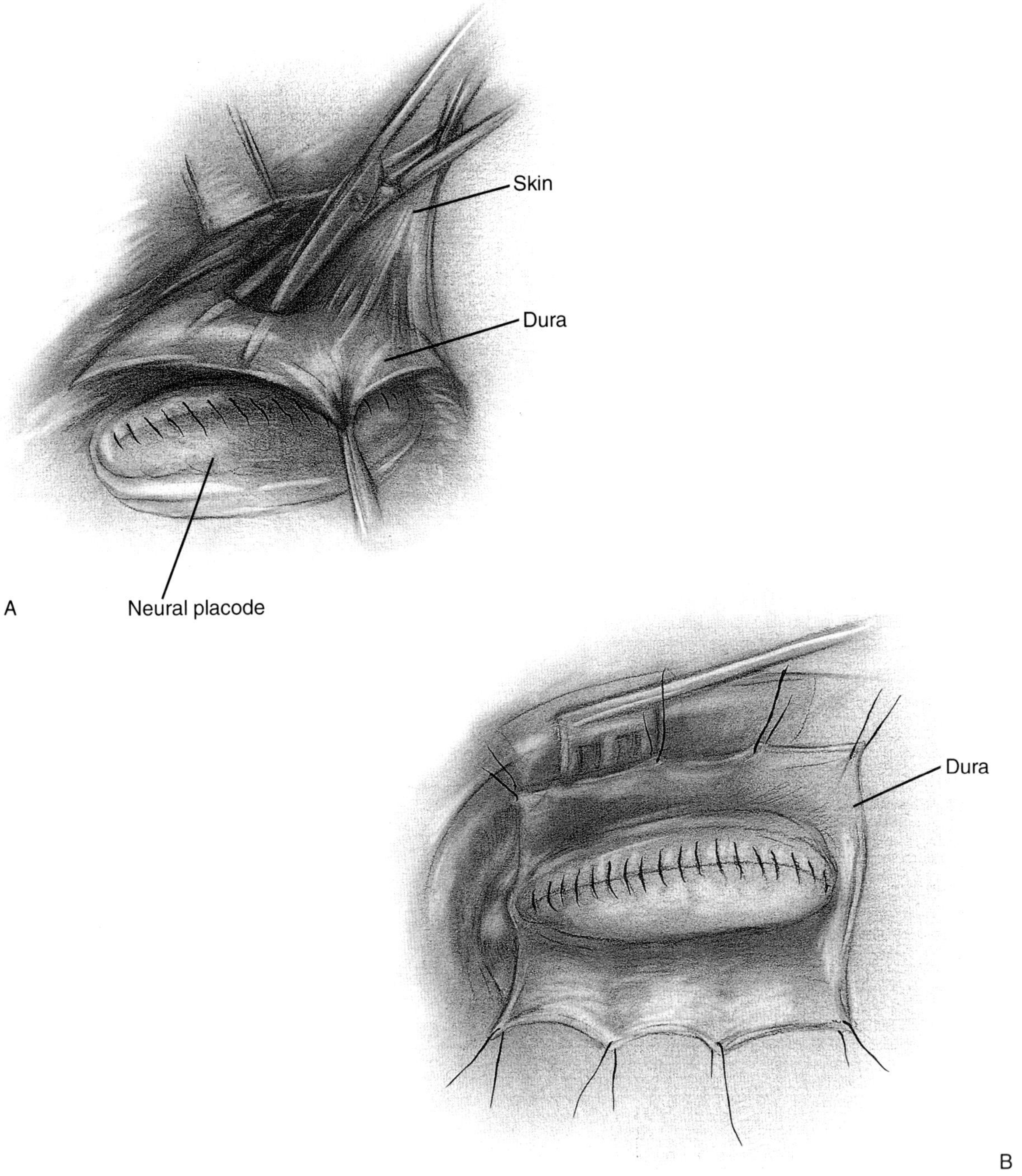

Figure 7. A,B: The dura is carefully detached from the skin as far laterally as possible to create a capacious thecal sac. Epidural fat between the dura and fascia helps keep the dissection in the correct plane.

ever, either lateral relaxing incisions (Fig. 9A) in the fascia will allow for closure in the midline without tension, or fascial "book leaves" (Fig. 10) can be fashioned to permit watertight closure above the dura using 4–0 Dexon sutures (Fig. 9B).

The subcutaneous tissue is then closed with 4–0 Dexon sutures. This may require dissection of the subcutaneous fat from the underlying fascia far laterally to allow for skin approximation without tension. The incision may be closed either longitudinally or transversely, whichever is easier. The skin edges are then apposed with 5–0 or 6–0 nylon running sutures (Fig. 11). We seal the wound with collodion to prevent fecal material and urine from contaminating the wound and to help stop CSF leaks.

Diastematomyelia Repair

In diastematomyelia, the spinal cord is split and tethered in the midline by a bony or fibrous septum or a tether of one of the hemicords at its termination, which inhibits free movement of the spinal cord. The operative setup is the same as that described above. A midline skin incision is made and the subcutaneous tissues dissected laterally. The spinous process overlying the median septum is removed with a small rongeur (Fig. 12A,A′). Extreme care must be taken, since the laminae in the region of the septum may be malformed or missing, allowing premature opening of the dura or damage to the underlying spinal cord.

Using the operative microscope and microsurgical techniques, the dura is incised longitudinally and reflected laterally with 5–0 sutures. Through the dense arachnoidal scar, the median septum can be identified and carefully dissected from the surrounding hemicords (Fig. 12B,B′). Using a diamond drill bit or small rongeur, the bony spur is removed until it is flush with the dorsal edge of the

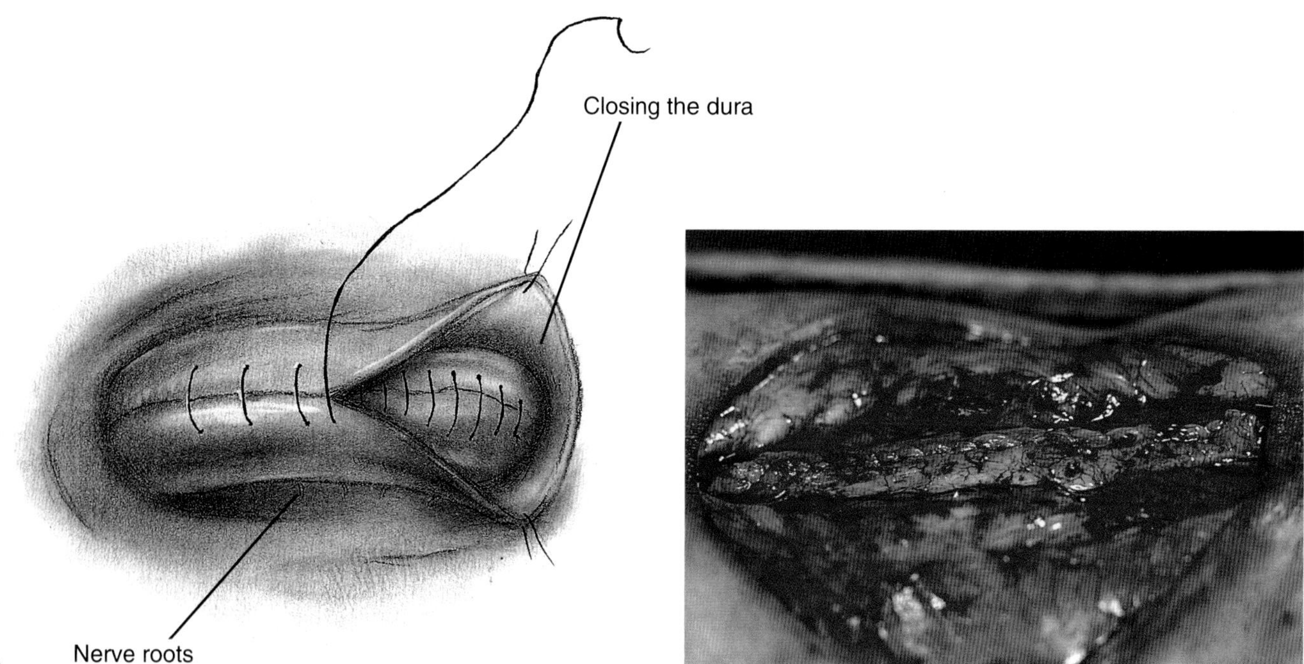

Figure 8. A,B: The dura is closed with a fine absorbable suture using a running stitch so that the closure is watertight. Fibrin glue is used to cover the dural suture line.

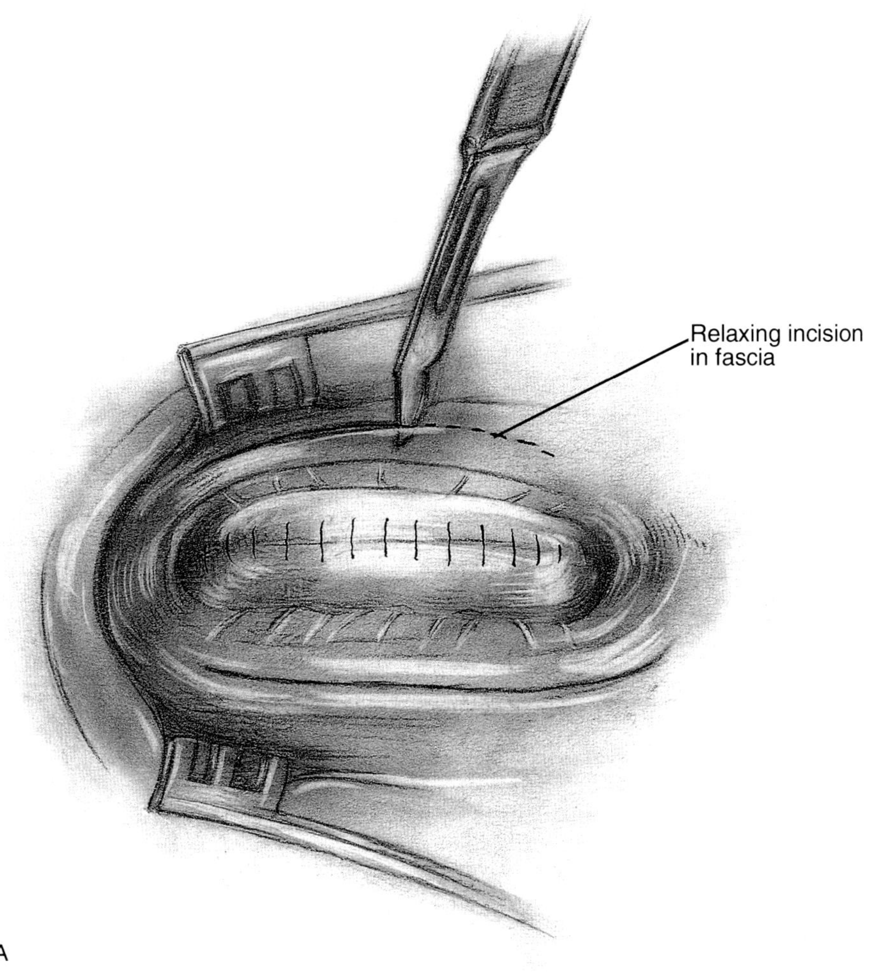

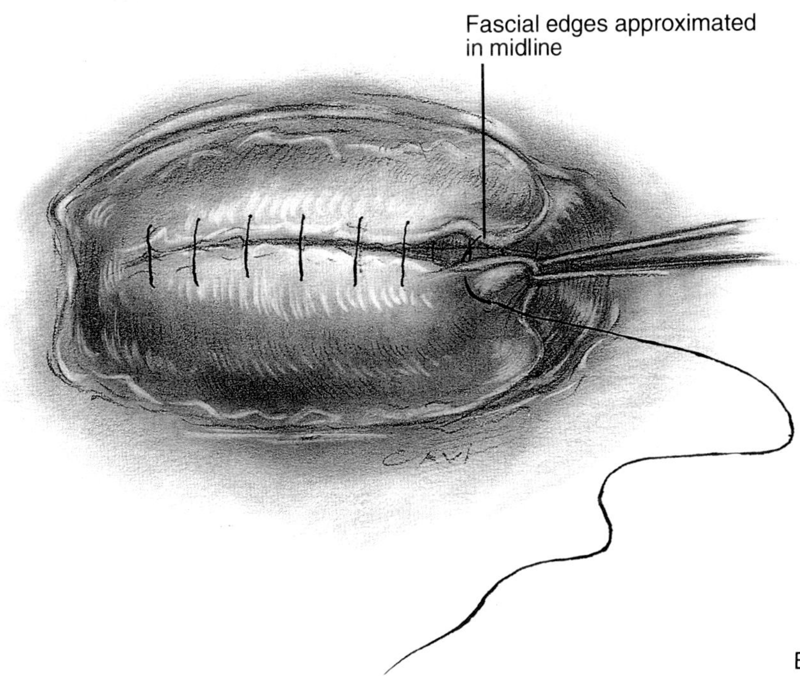

Figure 9. A: Relaxing incisions in the fascia may help mobilize the tissue so that a strong myofascial closure is obtained. **B:** Alternatively, the relaxing incisions can be used to make two fascial flaps, which can be sewn together in the midline.

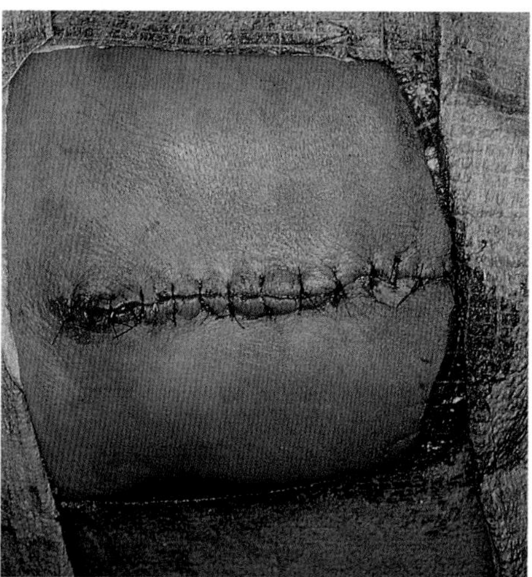

Figure 10. Principles of neural placode, dura, and fascia closure.

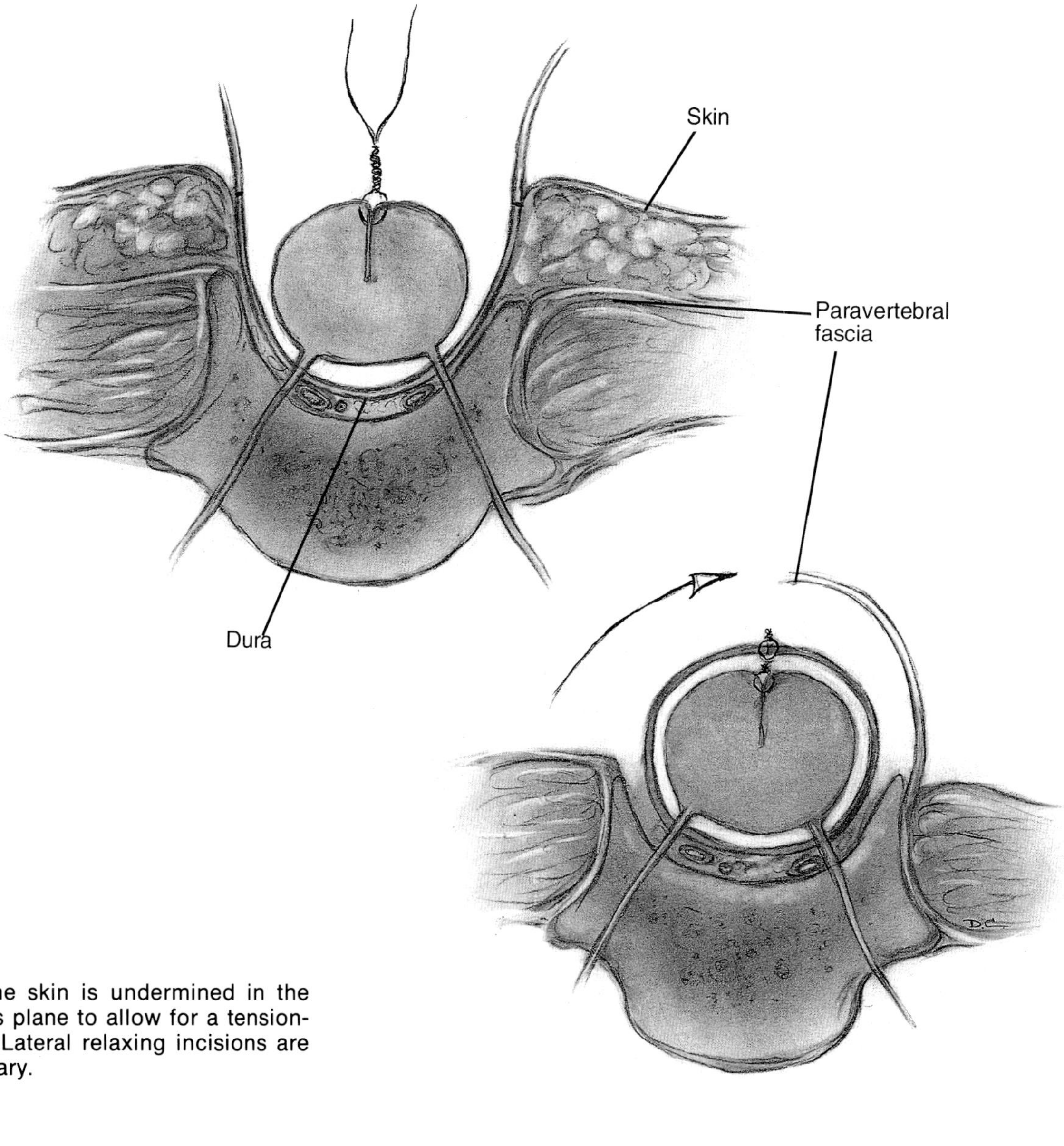

Figure 11. The skin is undermined in the subcutaneous plane to allow for a tension-free closure. Lateral relaxing incisions are rarely necessary.

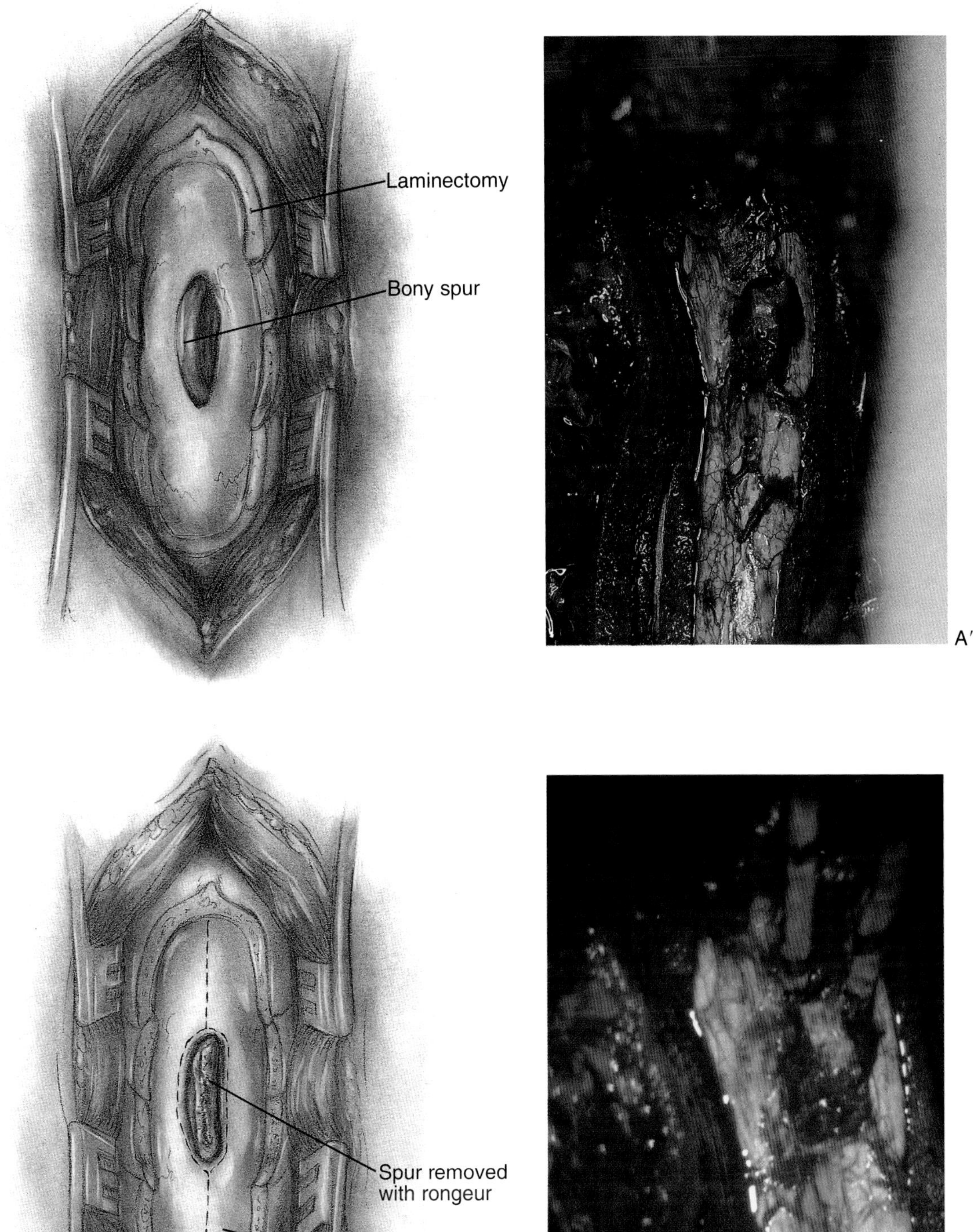

Figure 12. A,A′: A midline skin incision and laminectomy are performed, exposing the bony spur and dural sleeve. The overlying lamina may be abnormal, and care must be taken to avoid laceration of the dura. **B,B′:** After removal of the bone spur, the dura is incised around the spur.

Figure continues.

vertebral body. Large epidural vessels may be found between the spur and the dura and should be coagulated. The median dural sheath is then removed (Fig. 12C,C′) and any arachnoidal bands incised sharply to permit free mobility of the cord (Fig. 12D). The dura is then closed in a watertight fashion (Fig. 12E) and the fascia, subcutaneous tissue, and skin closed as described above.

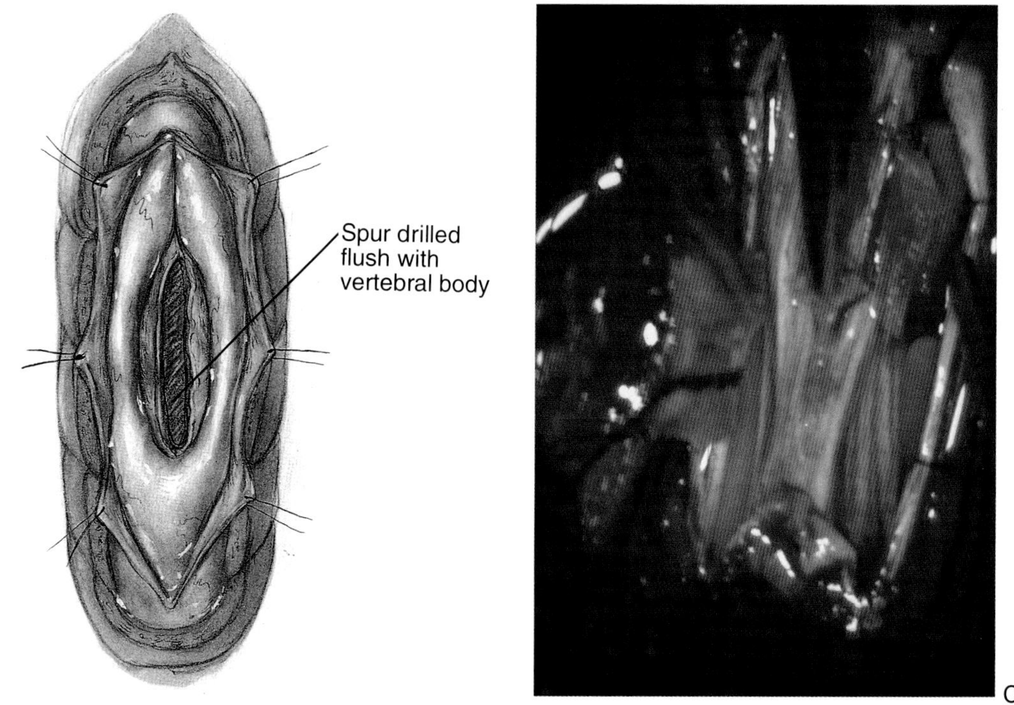

Figure 12. (*Continued.*) **C,C′:** The rest of the spur is drilled down until the dorsal aspect of the vertebral body is reached. Epidural vessels are coagulated and the remaining septal tissue excised.

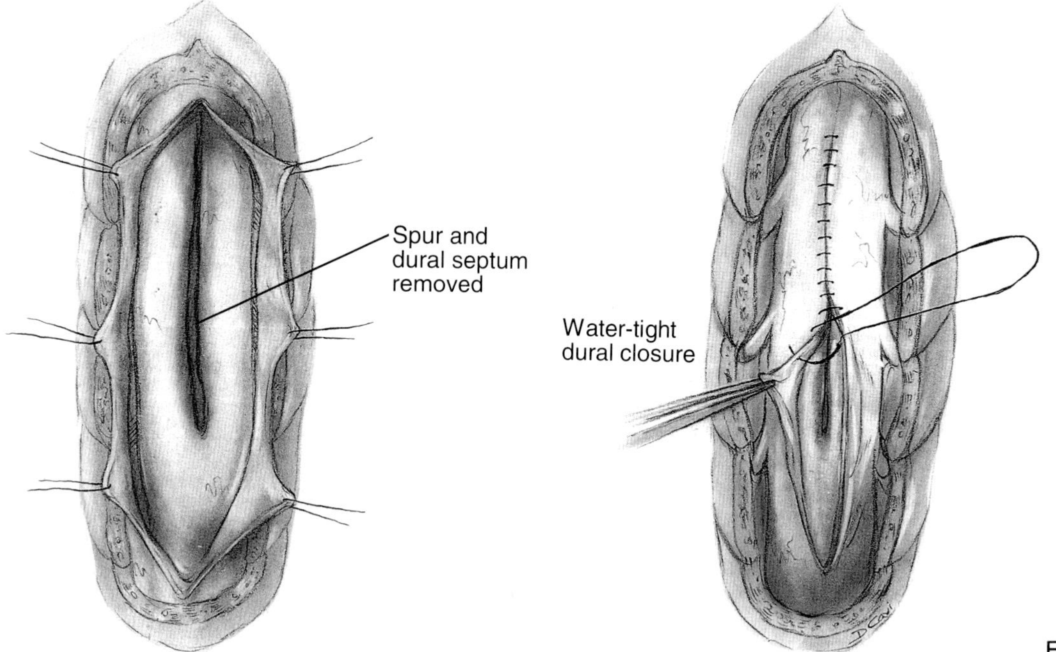

Figure 12. (*Continued.*) **D:** The spinal cord is now untethered. **E:** The dura is closed using a fine running absorbable suture.

Tethered Cord Repair

Following placement of a Foley catheter, the patient is turned prone onto bolsters, and pressure points are padded. The lumbosacral region is draped for a routine laminectomy operation. A midline incision is made and the soft tissues dissected laterally off the laminae and spinous processes using the Shaw scalpel or Bovie electrocautery. Again, care must be exercised to avoid early incision or damage to the dura and spinal cord in patients with spina bifida occulta or prior myelomeningocele repair (Fig. 13). If a dermal sinus tract or lipomyelomeningocele is present, the fibrous connective tissue band or extradural lipoma can be followed through the subcutaneous soft tissues and bone to its point of entrance through the dura (Fig. 14). The normal lamina above the tract or previous repair is removed to allow for a larger bony opening and to facilitate the identification of normal dura and spinal cord.

Using microsurgical techniques, the rostral dura is opened and the subarachnoid space entered (Fig. 15). Any arachnoidal bands are incised by sharp dissection—a #11 blade is ideal for this purpose. The bands are cut beginning rostrally and

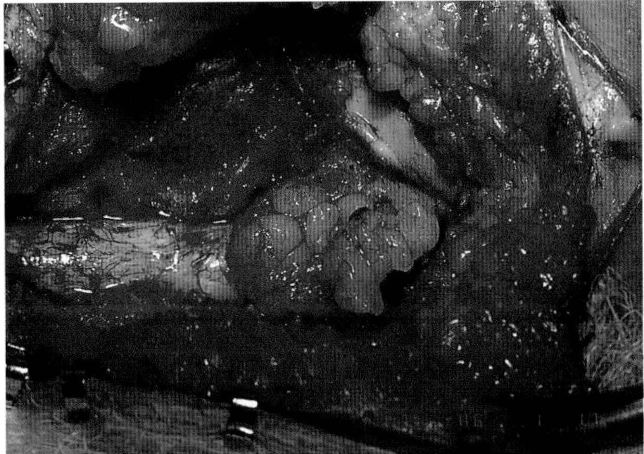

Figure 13. Following a midline skin incision and two-level laminectomy, the extradural and subcutaneous portions of the lipoma are identified.

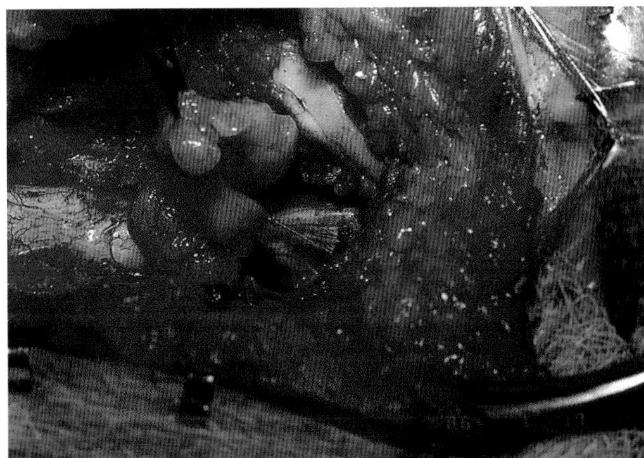

Figure 14. The extradural component of the lipoma is detached from the subcutaneous fat and transected as it penetrates the dura.

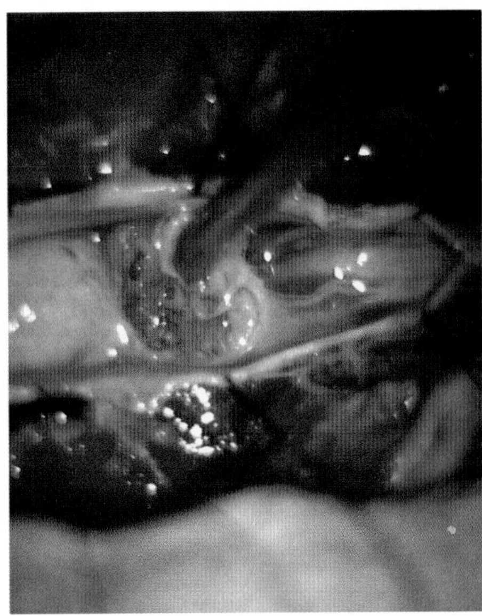

Figure 15. The dura is opened in the midline both rostral and caudal to the site where the lipoma penetrates the dura. Using the carbon dioxide laser, the lipoma can be vaporized until it is level with the neural tissue. It is not necessary to remove all of the intramedullary portion of the lipoma, since aggressive resection will result in neurologic dysfunction.

proceeding caudally, with the interface among dura, arachnoid, and cord kept clearly in view. The ventral nerve roots will be seen deep to the plane of dissection exiting through their neural foramina. Small vessels may be encountered where the neural placode is adherent to the dura and should be coagulated. Fine sutures placed along the dural edges will prevent blood from entering the CSF and give countertraction to facilitate the dissection. A fenestrated suction catheter or straight Rhoton microdissector is used to pull the cord gently away from the lateral dura to expose the arachnoid adhesions. Once the caudal pole of the thecal sac has been reached, all adhesions should have been cut and the cord should fall ventrally and superiorly into the thecal sac.

If a lipomyelomeningocele has resulted in cord tethering, the carbon dioxide laser is a useful adjunct to reduce the size of the intradural portion of the lipoma (Fig. 15). Once the lateral adhesions are removed, the superficial lipoma can be vaporized with the laser. Cottonoid patties are placed around the perimeter of the lipoma to avoid accidental coagulation of the nerve roots or spinal cord. The field should be irrigated frequently with cool saline to avoid transmission of laser-generated heat to the spinal cord. Once the cord interface is identified, vaporization should be stopped to avoid damage to the underlying neural tissue.

The filum terminale should be sought next (Fig. 16) and can be recognized as a reddish-gray band exiting the conus, which may be thicker than the caudal nerve roots. A large artery accompanies the filum and can aid in its recognition. A nerve stimulator can also help separate filum from thickened nerve roots. The filum may be significantly thickened, taut, and infiltrated with fat. Once it has been separated from the surrounding nerve roots and isolated with a cottonoid patty, the filum can be cut with the laser or with bipolar coagulation and microscissors (Fig. 17).

The dura is then closed in a watertight fashion using a dural patch graft if necessary. Fibrin glue along the suture line is used to reduce the chance of CSF leak from the wound. A tight musculofascial closure is mandatory. Muscle flaps may be necessary and may require the mobilization of paraspinal or gluteal muscle.

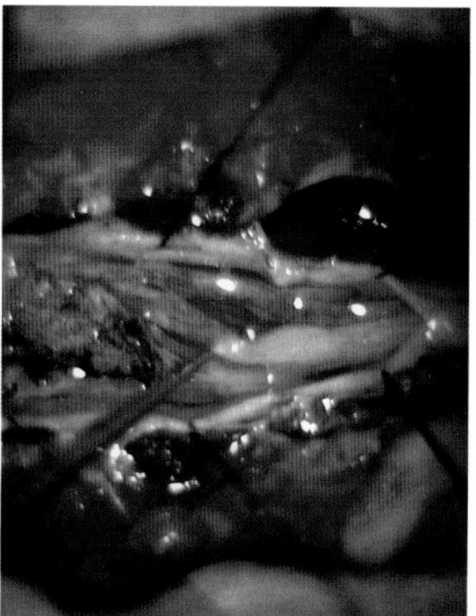

Figure 16. After the lipoma is debulked, the filum terminale is identified as a reddish-gray fibrovascular band originating from the conus medullaris. A small artery accompanies the filum and can help with its identification.

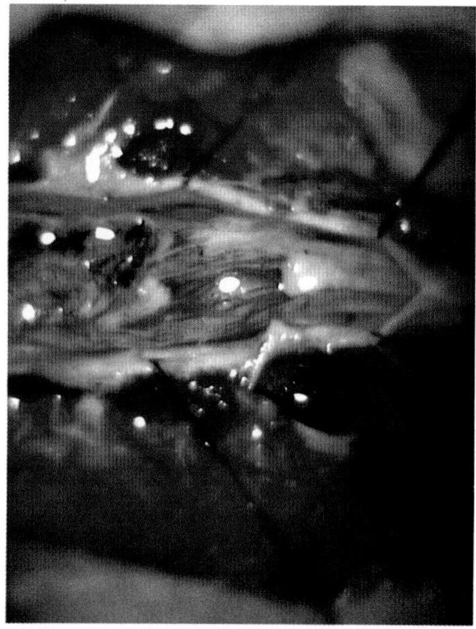

Figure 17. The filum is coagulated and transected using the carbon dioxide laser or microscissors. The spinal cord will move rostrally and lie along the ventral dura. The dura, fascia, and skin are then closed in layers.

After a tight fascial closure is completed, the remaining subcutaneous lipoma can be subtotally resected to remove the subcutaneous fatty bulge. The skin is then closed with a running 5–0 nylon suture, the wound sealed with collodion, and a sterile dressing applied.

POSTOPERATIVE MANAGEMENT

Infants with myelomeningocele repairs are nursed prone with no more than 10 degrees of head elevation for 1 to 2 weeks to allow the incision to heal without compression. Toddlers and children are positioned flat in bed, either prone, lateral, or supine, for 48-72 hours to prevent the formation of a pseudomeningocele. The head of the bed is gradually raised over the next 24-48 hours and activities liberalized if the wound remains flat. Antibiotics are continued until the Foley catheter is removed.

Patients frequently have subtle urologic dysfunction that may not be recognized preoperatively without careful urodynamic studies. Postoperative urologic reevaluation should be performed 3 to 6 months after cord release.

REHABILITATION

The vast majority of patients show no neurologic deterioration after surgery. Rarely, a clinical picture similar to spinal shock will develop following tethered cord release but will improve rapidly. Patients may require postoperative rehabilitation to loosen spastic limbs or to improve strength lost because of the cord tethering. Physical therapy is started on an inpatient basis on the fourth or fifth hospital day and continues for 3 to 6 months on an outpatient basis if necessary.

COMPLICATIONS

Increased Neurologic Deficit

Worse neurologic dysfunction following tethered cord release or myelomeningocele repair can occur from excessive traction or manipulation of the ischemic cord or nerve roots prior to untethering, from thermal damage caused by excessive laser use too near the conus medullaris, or from inadvertent transection of viable sensory or motor rootlets during lysis of arachnoidal adhesions. Careful neurologic assessment is required postoperatively to document any change in neurologic function.

Leakage of spinal fluid into the subcutaneous tissues (pseudomeningocele) or out through the skin (CSF leak) can occur in patients in whom the dural or fascial closure is inadequate or in whom hydrocephalus has developed. If wound integrity after myelomeningocele repair is compromised by an expanding CSF collection, progressive hydrocephalus is typically present and requires ventriculoperitoneal shunting to diminish CSF pressures in the lumbar thecal sac. In older children, a longer trial of bed rest and Diamox therapy to diminish CSF production may permit the subcutaneous tissues to heal without a large CSF collection. Symptomatic or enlarging pseudomeningoceles and percutaneous CSF leaks require reexploration of the lumbar wound to repair the CSF leak with sutures, fibrin glue, and Gelfoam. In older children, a temporary pseudomeningocele-to-peritoneal shunt may be the easiest and quickest way to decompress the CSF collection until scarring obliterates the subcutaneous pocket.

Meningitis

Meningitis, either aseptic or bacterial, can lead to irritability, nuchal rigidity, somnolence, and fevers in the early postoperative period. Blood and lipid droplets that enter the CSF during tethered cord release or myelomeningocele repair lead to meningeal irritation and a reactive pleocytosis that can mimic bacterial meningitis. Usually, the fevers and nuchal rigidity improve within 2 to 3 days after surgery. Persistent fevers, somnolence, or stiff neck require that CSF be obtained for cell count, glucose, protein, and culture to rule out a bacterial source. Mild aseptic meningitis can be managed with Tylenol and nonsteroidal antiinflammatory agents, whereas severe cases may require the initiation of high-dose steroid therapy. In patients in whom the etiology is uncertain, both broad-spectrum antibiotics and steroid therapy can be started until the final culture results exclude a bacterial infection.

Urinary Tract Infection

Urinary tract infections are common in the immediate postoperative period due to Foley catheterization and underlying bladder dysfunction. Any fever during the postoperative course requires microscopic urinalysis to exclude urinary tract infection.

Recurrent Spinal Cord Tethering

Despite meticulous lysis of adhesions and transection of the filum terminale, the spinal cord can become reattached to the site of the dural repair, leading to recurrent symptoms. Patients in whom this occurs should undergo repeat radiologic evaluation to exclude ventriculoperitoneal shunt malfunction, symptomatic Chiari malformation, the development of hydromyelia, cord retethering, or the persistence of another form of spinal dysraphism not previously appreciated, such as an intraspinal dermoid cyst.

ILLUSTRATIVE CASE FOR TECHNIQUE

A 3-month-old infant presented with a subcutaneous mass over the sacrum. Her neurologic and urologic examinations were normal. Magnetic resonance imaging (Fig. 18) revealed a terminal lipoma filling the thecal sac. A two-level laminectomy was performed and the dura opened. The lipoma was first detached from the lower aspect of the dural sac (Fig. 19) and reflected superiorly, exposing the underlying filum terminale (Fig. 20). After transection of the filum, the lipoma was detached proximally where it exited the conus medullaris (Figs. 21 and 22). The carbon dioxide laser was then used to vaporize residual fatty tissue, leaving only a small portion of the lipoma in the conus medullaris (Fig. 23). The dura was closed in a watertight manner and sealed with fibrin glue (Fig. 24). The baby made an uneventful recovery.

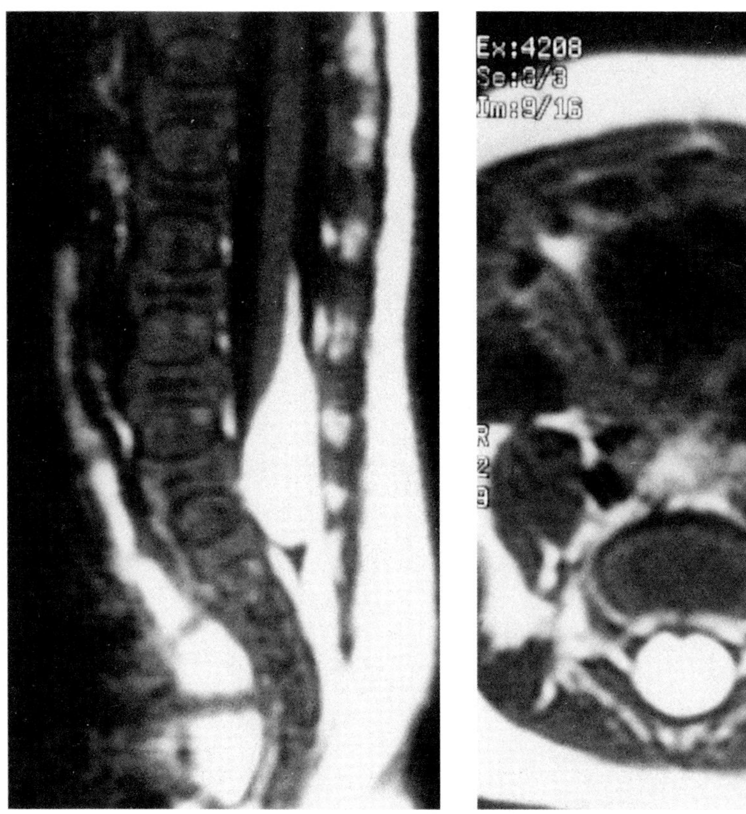

Figure 18. Magnetic resonance images of a 3-month-old infant with a subcutaneous sacral mass show a terminal lipoma that extends through the lower dural sac to attach to the subcutaneous fatty mass. Note that the conus medullaris lies at the L5 vertebral body.

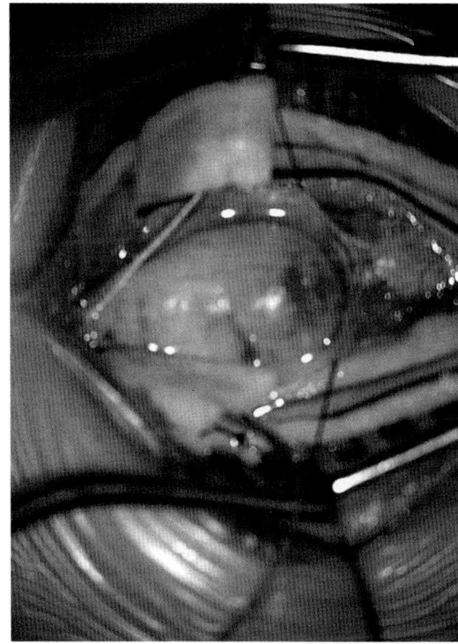

Figure 19. The dura has been opened and the intrathecal lipoma detached from its site of exit through the dural sac.

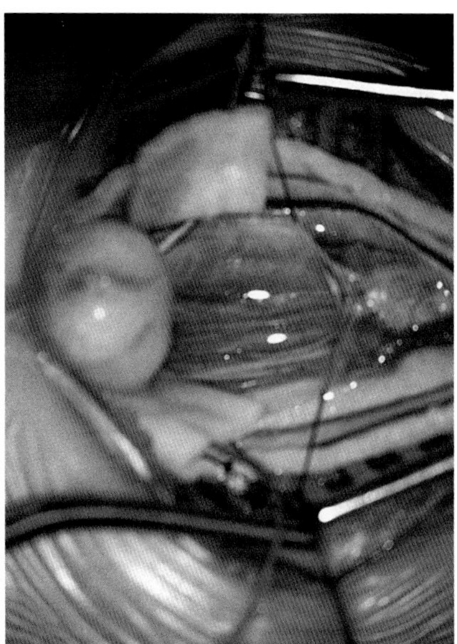

Figure 20. The lipoma is reflected superiorly, exposing the filum terminale between two sets of nerve roots. The filum was coagulated and transected.

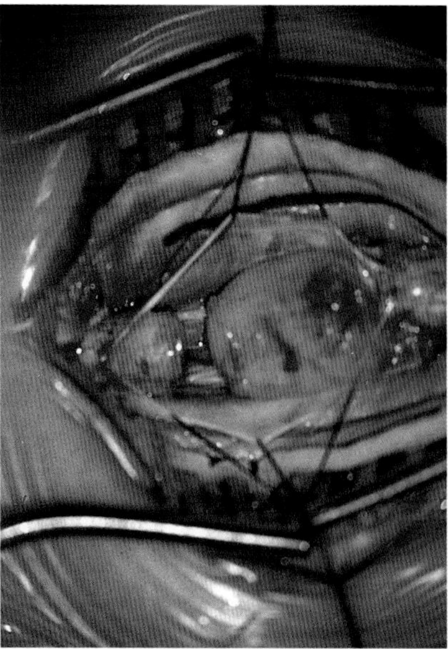

Figure 21. The carbon dioxide laser was used to transect the proximal attachment of the lipoma where it exits from the conus medullaris.

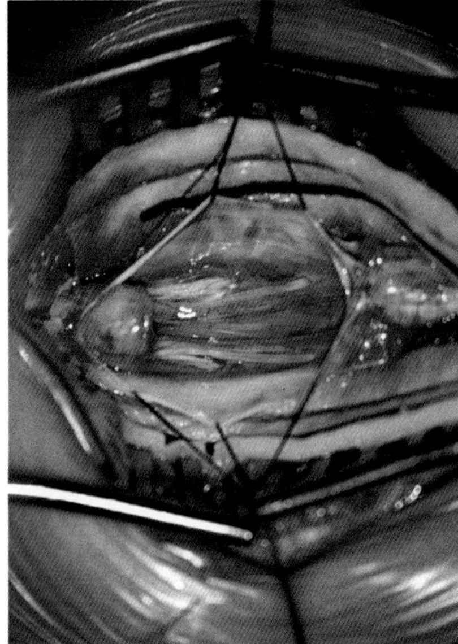

Figure 22. The bulk of the lipoma has been removed, leaving only the residual fatty tissue within the conus medullaris.

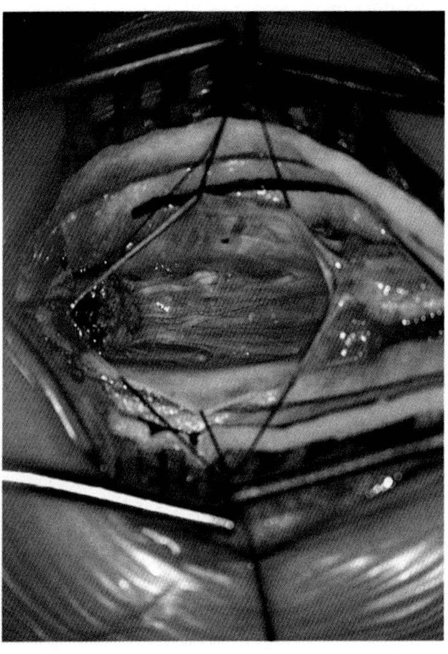

Figure 23. The residual lipoma is coagulated using the carbon dioxide laser.

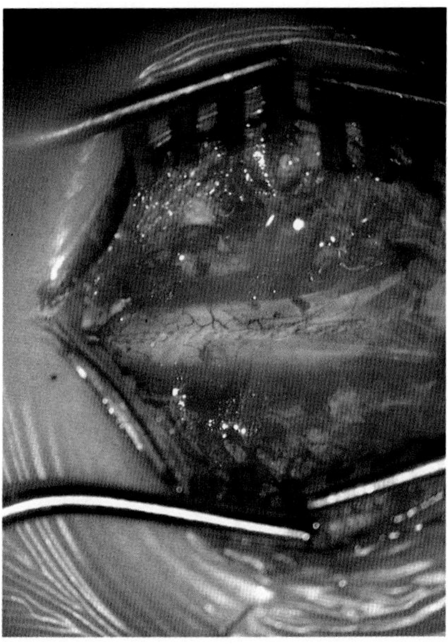

Figure 24. The dura is closed in a watertight fashion and sealed with fibrin glue to prevent leakage of CSF.

RECOMMENDED READING

1. Hendrick, E. G., Hoffman, H. J., and Humphreys, R. P.: A technique for repair of large spina bifida defects. In: *Myelomeningocele*, edited by R. L McLaurin, Grune & Stratton, New York, 1977, pp. 191–196.
2. Hoffman, J. H., Hendrick, E. B., and Humphreys, R. P.: The tethered spinal cord: its protean manifestations, diagnosis and surgical correction. *Childs Brain*, 2: 145–155, 1976.
3. Matson, D. D.: Surgical repair of myelomeningocele. *J. Neurosurg.*, 27: 180–186, 1967.
4. McLone, D. G.: Continuing concepts in the management of spina bifida. *Pediatr. Neurosurg.*, 18: 254–256, 1992.
5. McLone, D. G., and Dias, M. S.: Complications of myelomeningocele closure. *Pediatr. Neurosurg.*, 17: 267–273, 1991–92.
6. McLone, D. G., Herman, J. M., Gabrieli, A. P., and Dias, L.: Tethered cord as a cause of scoliosis in children with a myelomeningocele. *Pediatr. Neurosurg.*, 16: 8–13, 1990–91.
7. Mintz, L. J., Sarwark, J. F., Dias, L. S., and Schafer, M. F.: The natural history of congenital kyphosis in myelomeningocele. A review of 51 children. *Spine*, 16: S348–350, 1991.
8. Pang, D.: Split cord malformation: Part II: Clinical syndrome. *Neurosurgery*, 31: 481–500, 1992.
9. Pang, D., Dias, M. S., and Ahab-Barmada, M.: Split cord malformation: Part I: A unified theory of embryogenesis for double spinal cord malformations. *Neurosurgery*, 31: 451–480, 1992.
10. Raghavan, N., Barkovich, A. J., Edwards, M., and Norman, D.: MR imaging in the tethered spinal cord syndrome. *AJNR*, 152: 843–852, 1989.
11. Steinbok, P., Irvine, B., Cochrane, D. D., and Irwin, B. J.: Long-term outcome and complications of children born with meningomyelocele. *Childs Nerv. Syst.*, 8: 92–96, 1992.
12. Zide, B. M., Epstein, F. J., and Wisoff, J.: Optimal wound closure after tethered cord correction. Technical note. *J. Neurosurg.*, 74: 673–676, 1991.

Master Techniques in Orthopaedic Surgery,
THE SPINE, edited by D. S. Bradford,
Lippincott-Raven Publishers, Philadelphia, © 1997.

26

Anterior Fixation

Kiyoshi Kaneda

INDICATIONS/CONTRAINDICATIONS

Anterior surgical procedures in the thoracic and lumbar spine are generally conducted for spinal stabilization with or without spinal canal decompression. Specific indications may include deficient bone or instability anteriorly due to trauma (3), tumor (3), osteoporosis (4), infection, congenital anomaly (2), degenerative disease, or deformity (3).

Thoracolumbar Spinal Injuries

The classification of thoracic and lumbar spinal injuries has been based on the mechanism of injury to the middle part of the spinal column (3). The author uses the following classification in adding the combined type of burst fracture and flexion-distraction injury to the Denis classification: (a) wedge compression fractures; (b) burst fractures (types A–E); (c) flexion-distraction injuries; (d) combined type of burst fracture and flexion-distraction injury; (e) fracture-dislocations (flexion-rotation, flexion-distraction, shear); and (f) isolated fractures of the posterior elements. The combined burst fracture and flexion-distraction injury has not been reported in detail. The mechanism of this type of injury appears to be a combination of an axial load followed by a flexion-distraction force, disrupting both the middle and posterior columns. This type of injury is usually caused by falling from a height and landing initially on one's feet (i.e., suicide attempt) or a motor vehicle accident in which a seat-belted individual sustains an axial load in addition to the

K. Kaneda, M.D., Ph.D.: Department of Orthopaedic Surgery, Hokkaido University School of Medicine, Sapporo 060, Japan.

flexion-distraction injury when the vehicle drops from a height when driving off the road.

Indications for anterior fixation with spinal instrumentation (Kaneda device) using this classification are burst fractures of L3 or above with neurologic deficits and combined burst fracture and flexion-distraction injuries with neurologic deficits. Severe wedge compression fractures may be managed with anterior instrumentation and a strut graft following correction of kyphosis. Old fracture-dislocations with increasing kyphosis and incomplete neurologic deficits can be treated by anterior correction of kyphosis, spinal canal decompression, and fusion with instrumentation. Contraindications are ordinary wedge compression fractures, flexion-distraction injuries, fracture-dislocations, and isolated fractures of the posterior elements. These injuries should be stabilized with posterior instrumentation and fusion, if surgical intervention is required. Burst fractures of L4 or L5 with or without neurologic deficits can be managed successfully by posterior decompression and stabilization, using various types of transpedicular screw systems. Treatment of burst fractures without neurologic deficits of L3 or above depends on the severity of spinal canal compromise by the retropulsed bony fragment, the percentage of the vertebra that is collapsed, and the degree of kyphosis. In patients with severe canal compromise and/or severe vertebral collapse, anterior reconstruction should be recommended even if no neurologic complications exist.

Primary or Metastatic Spinal Tumors

In malignant spinal tumors of the thoracic and lumbar spine, subtotal or total vertebrectomy and anterior fixation with the Kaneda device are indicated if the patient has a life expectancy over 6 months, if tumor lesion is confined to one or two vertebrae, if compression of the spinal cord or the cauda equina is impending, with vertebral collapse, or if unstable pathologic fracture and severe pain exist (3). The aims of anterior surgical reconstruction for these patients are to improve their quality of life through the relief of intractable pain, to provide neurologic recovery, to reconstitute spinal stability, and to prolong the survival period, if possible. Contraindications for surgery are short life expectancy (under 6 months) due to the nature of a primary tumor (i.e., lung carcinoma, gastrointestinal tract carcinoma, etc.), radiosensitive tumors without loss of structural stability (malignant lymphoma, myeloma, plasma cell myeloma, etc.), and multiple vertebral lesions.

Osteoporotic-Posttraumatic Vertebral Collapse with Neurologic Deficit

Neurologic deficit will not normally occur immediately following compression fractures of an osteoporotic thoracic or lumbar spine. However, neural compromise due to delayed vertebral collapse after osteoporotic compression fractures of the thoracolumbar spine has been reported. Pathology of the collapsed vertebra has revealed ischemic necrosis of the osteoporotic fractured vertebra (4). Compression of the spinal cord or the cauda equina is caused by retropulsion of vertebral bony fragments into the spinal canal with unstable kyphosis. Anterior decompression by resection of the collapsed vertebra, anterior strut grafting in the vertebrectomy gap, and stabilization with anterior instrumentation are the most reasonable and direct methods of surgical intervention. In our experience, a bioactive ceramic vertebral prosthesis with surrounding autogenous bone has been useful as an anterior strut for correction of kyphosis and stabilization (3). Alternatively, an allograft strut with autogenous bone may also be used. Simple osteoporotic compression fractures usually do not require surgical treatment.

Pyogenic or Tuberculous Spondylitis

Occurring with vertebral collapse and neural compression in the thoracic and lumbar spine, pyogenic or tuberculous spondylitis is a definite indication for anterior decompression [curettage or vertebrectomy of the infected vertebra(e)] and stabilization. Anterior instrumentation will not be indicated for anterior fixation following curettage or vertebral resection in pyogenic spondylitis. The existence of the implants may disturb the healing process of pyogenic infection. On the other hand, anterior surgery by vertebrectomy for decompression, strut grafting with autogenous bone, and stabilization with the Kaneda device has resulted in successful outcomes and early ambulation without deformity or complications in treatment of unstable tuberculous spondylitis with neurologic deficit. Before application of anterior instrumentation, patients who were treated by anterior decompression and strut grafting had been kept in bed for 2 to 3 months.

Congenital Spinal Anomalies

Increasing kyphosis with or without compression of the spinal cord or the cauda equina can be an indication for surgery (1). Neural compromise will not occur without a kyphotic component such as a deformity due to failure of formation (2). Surgical correction of congenital kyphosis with incomplete decompression of the spinal cord in patients with a preoperative neurologic compromise will result in deterioration of their neurologic function. Vertebrectomy for spinal canal decompression is essential. Anterior stabilization is obtained by an anterior strut graft and instrumentation following anterior decompression. The strut graft is essential to support the anterior column and resist the normal axial loads on the anterior spine. Anterior stabilization with instrumentation but without decompression is contraindicated in the treatment of congenital spinal deformities with neurologic compromise.

Thoracolumbar Spondylosis with Neurologic Deficit

Neurologic compromise in thoracolumbar spondylosis is derived from spinal cord compression due to vertebral osteophytes and/or intervertebral disc herniations (3). This is usually associated with segmental instability and occasionally with a kyphotic deformity. An anterior approach provides the safest method for complete decompression in this region of the spine. Stability is easily obtained through anterior instrumentation. Multilevel fixation with correction of kyphosis is mandatory in some patients with multilevel lesions due to severe spondylosis.

Thoracolumbar Scoliosis

Scoliosis is another good indication for anterior instrumentation of the spine (3). Zielke instrumentation has been widely accepted for treatment of thoracolumbar scoliosis, but increasing kyphosis across the fusion area has been reported and is a cause for concern in long-term results. The two-rod semirigid system (Kaneda anterior multisegmental system) has provided a good method for deformity correction and its maintenance in sagittal alignment (3).

PREOPERATIVE PLANNING

Proper preoperative planning includes an extensive history and physical examination; the neurologic examination is especially important. Pertinent image studies [by radiograph, tomogram, myelogram, magnetic resonance imaging (MRI), computed tomography (CT), scintigram, or combinations of these] are necessary. Vertebral lesions should be looked for on these images. Destructive lesions due to infection, tumor, or osteoporotic collapse must be differentiated. Scintigram and MRI are useful in detecting multiple lesions due to metastasis or infection. Myelography provides useful information on the relation between the dural tube and the spinal canal in patients with neurologic deficit due to old burst fractures, congenital kyphosis or kyphoscoliosis, spondylosis, metastatic tumor, or osteoporotic posttraumatic vertebral collapse. Myelography may be replaced by MRI in some pathologic conditions, but it still has its value. The status of the vertebral bone should be checked on plain lateral films or by dual energy x-ray absopsiometry (DEXA) prior to anterior instrumentation surgery, because a severely osteoporotic vertebral body cannot hold the vertebral screws securely. The general medical condition must be carefully evaluated, especially in elderly patients or in those with metastatic disease. The pulmonary and cardiovascular status of the patient requires close examination prior to anterior spinal surgery.

SURGERY

Generally the spine can be approached from either the right or left side, depending on the location of the pathology (Fig. 1). If no special considerations are present, the left-sided approach to the thoracolumbar and lumbar spine is preferable for several reasons. The aorta is located on the left, anterior to the thoracolumbar and lumbar vertebral column, and this is much safer to manipulate than the vena cava. The patient is placed in the right lateral decubitus position, approaching the left portion of the spine below T9 or T10 (Fig. 1A,B). The thoracic vertebrae above T9 or T10 are approached from the right side, because the thoracic aorta is located on the left side of the thoracic vertebral column. An axillary pad is used to prevent circulatory disturbance of the upper extremity on the lower (right) side. Pressure on the peroneal nerve of the lower side should be eliminated. When the thoracic spine above T9 or T10 is exposed, a right thoracotomy approach is taken (the left lateral decubitus position). Maintenance of a secure position is essential during the surgery, even when the table is tilted, using appropriate lateral positioners and firm tape strapping. The iliac crest or the fibula must be prepped and available for bone graft harvesting, if necessary.

The thoracolumbar junction (T12 and L1 vertebrae) is usually exposed by an extrapleural-retroperitoneal approach through resection of the 10th or 11th rib. Of course, a transpleural (thoracotomy)-retroperitoneal approach can also be used for exposure of the thoracolumbar junction. The extrapleural approach is considered less invasive. The dotted line in Fig. 1 shows the skin incision for the thoracolumbar and lumbar exposures. The rib to be resected is chosen one or two levels above the area of spinal pathology. The costal cartilage of the resected rib is bisected to gain exposure to the retroperitoneal space. Either the transpleural or the extrapleural exposure is used for the thoracic and thoracolumbar segments, and the retroperitoneal exposure is used for the lumbar vertebrae. Blunt dissection can separate the retroperitoneal fat and retroperitoneal structures off the iliopsoas muscle and spine. Once the retroperitoneal space is identified, the thoracic portion of the exposure is completed, either by extrapleural dissection or via a thoracotomy. The segmental vessels of the vertebrae to be instrumented are then tied, ligated, and divided. The iliopsoas muscle is bluntly dissected off the necessary spinal segments. The lateral aspect of the vertebral bodies must be exposed for

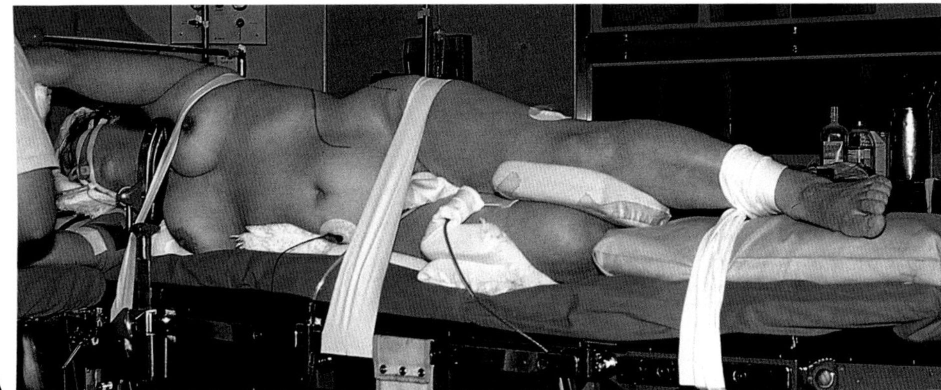
A

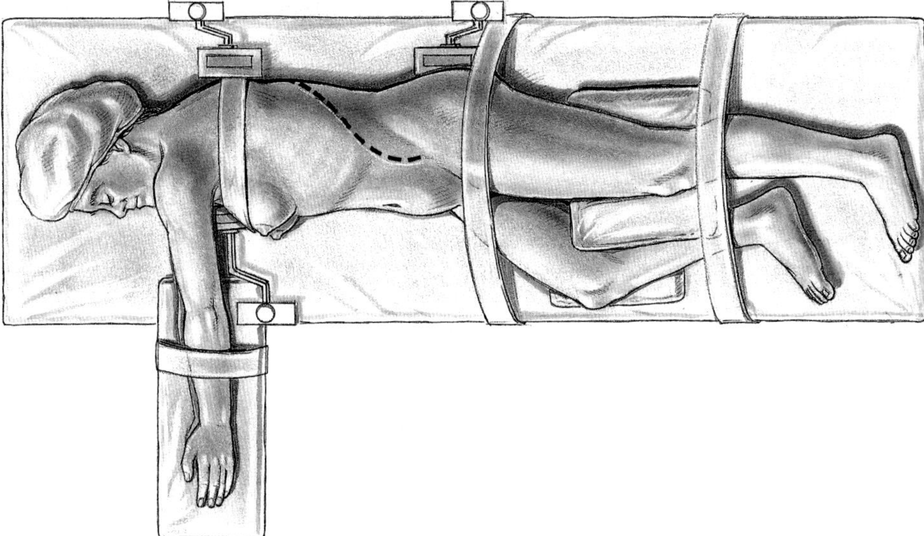
B

Figure 1. A,B: Positioning and immobilization of a patient on the surgical table.

corpectomy for anterior spinal canal decompression or application of the Kaneda device implants. The great vessels should be carefully protected during this portion of the operative procedure.

Once the area of abnormal anatomy is exposed, the discs above and below the area of bony abnormality are incised with a scalpel and excised using curettes and disc rongeurs (Fig. 2A). The abnormal vertebral body is then excised (Fig. 2B). If an indication for anterior spinal canal decompression is present, it is performed now, using the instruments with which the spinal surgeon is most familiar: osteotomes and gouges, curettes, rongeurs, high-speed pneumonic instruments, or combinations of these. The spinal canal can be safely entered through the neural foramen. The retropulsed bony or pathologic mass should be removed as completely as possible (Fig. 3A,B). In burst fractures, tumors, spondylosis, and congenital anomalies, the posterior longitudinal ligament can usually be left intact without excision during spinal canal decompression. Once spinal canal decompression is complete, appropriately sized vertebral plates are tapped into place (Fig. 4A). Care should be taken to avoid placement of the spikes into the intervertebral disc. The vertebral plates should be positioned so that a trapezoidal configuration of the Kaneda construct is created with the anterior rod of the Kaneda device longer than the posterior rod. The vertebral plates are fixed with the vertebral screws. Screw penetration of the opposite vertebral cortex is checked with the surgeon's fingertip (Fig. 4B).

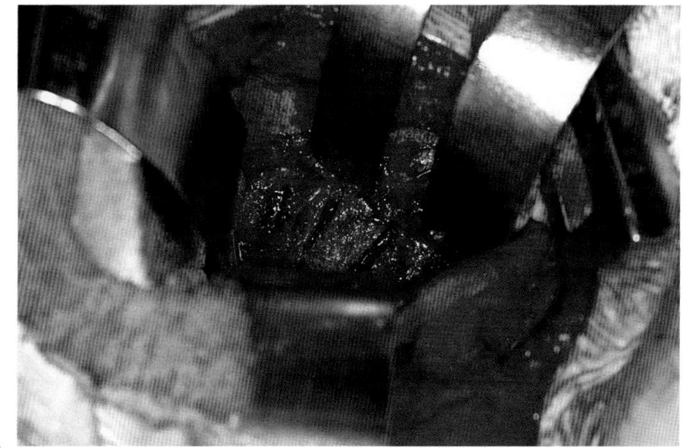

A

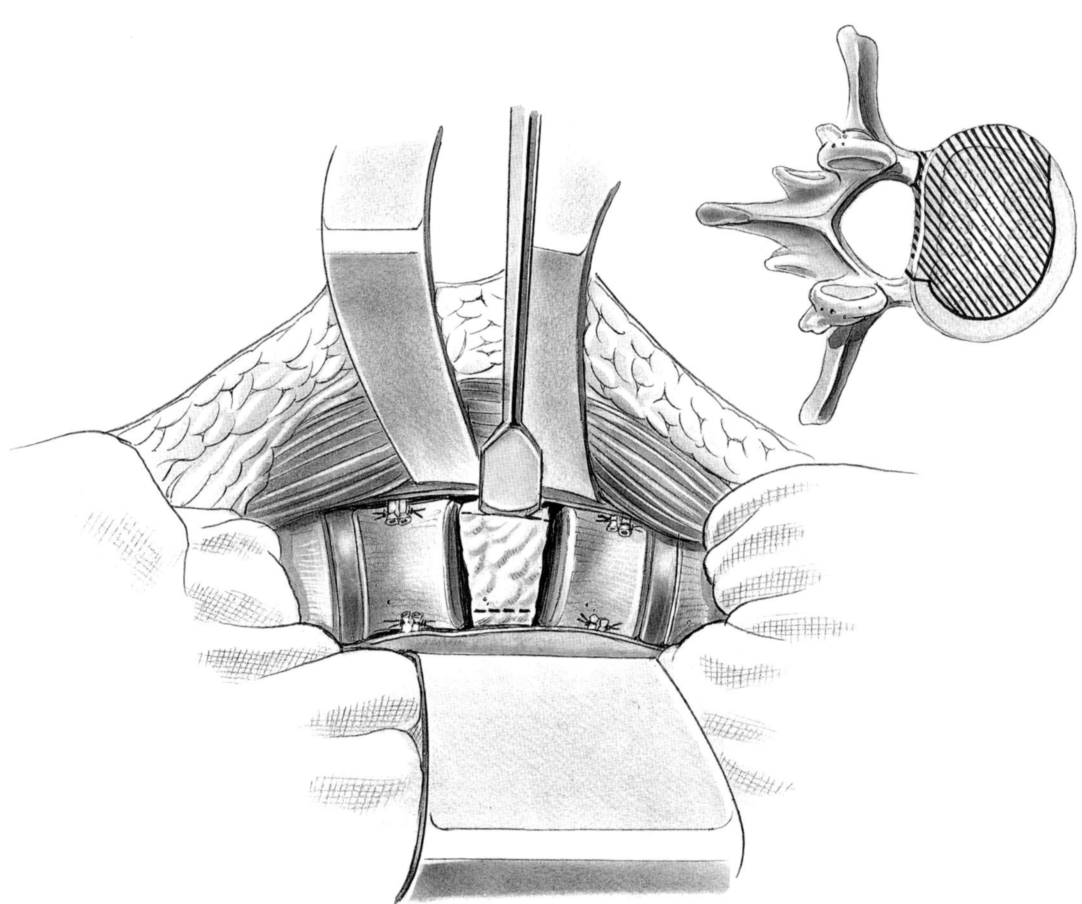

B

Figure 2. A,B: Surgical exposure of the thoracolumbar or the lumbar vertebral bodies through the extrapleural (or transpleural) retroperitoneal approach.

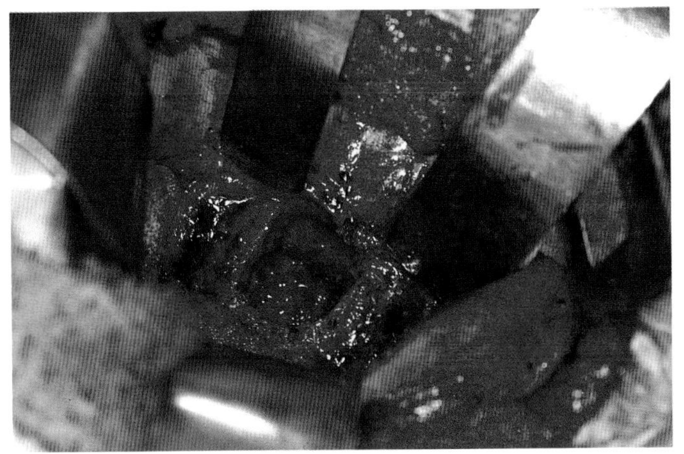

A

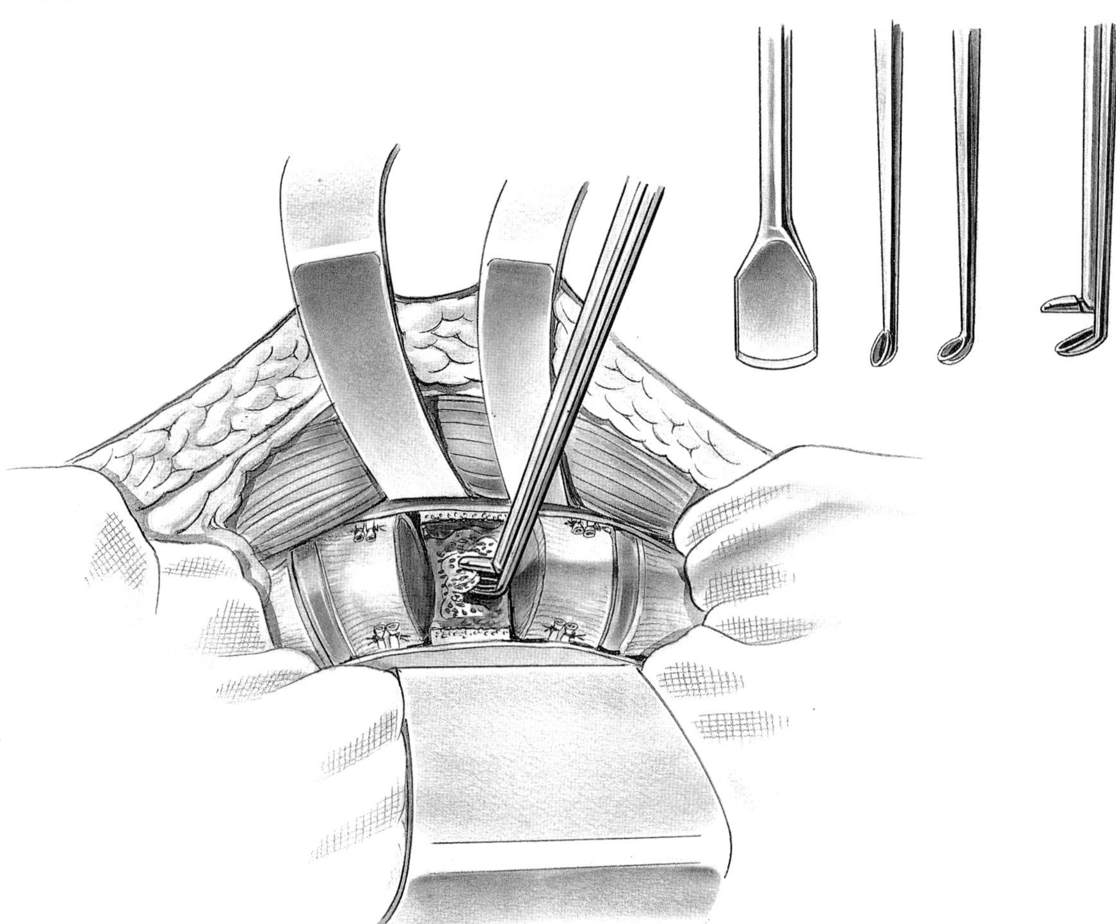

B

Figure 3. A,B: Anterior spinal canal decompression.

Once the screws are in place and the proper length is obtained, correction of the kyphotic deformity is achieved by use of a spreader between the anteriormost screws (Fig. 5A). The gap created by the vertebral resection and correction of kyphosis is then measured and an appropriate length of tricortical iliac crest graft is obtained to fill the defect (Fig. 5B). When the kyphotic deformity cannot be

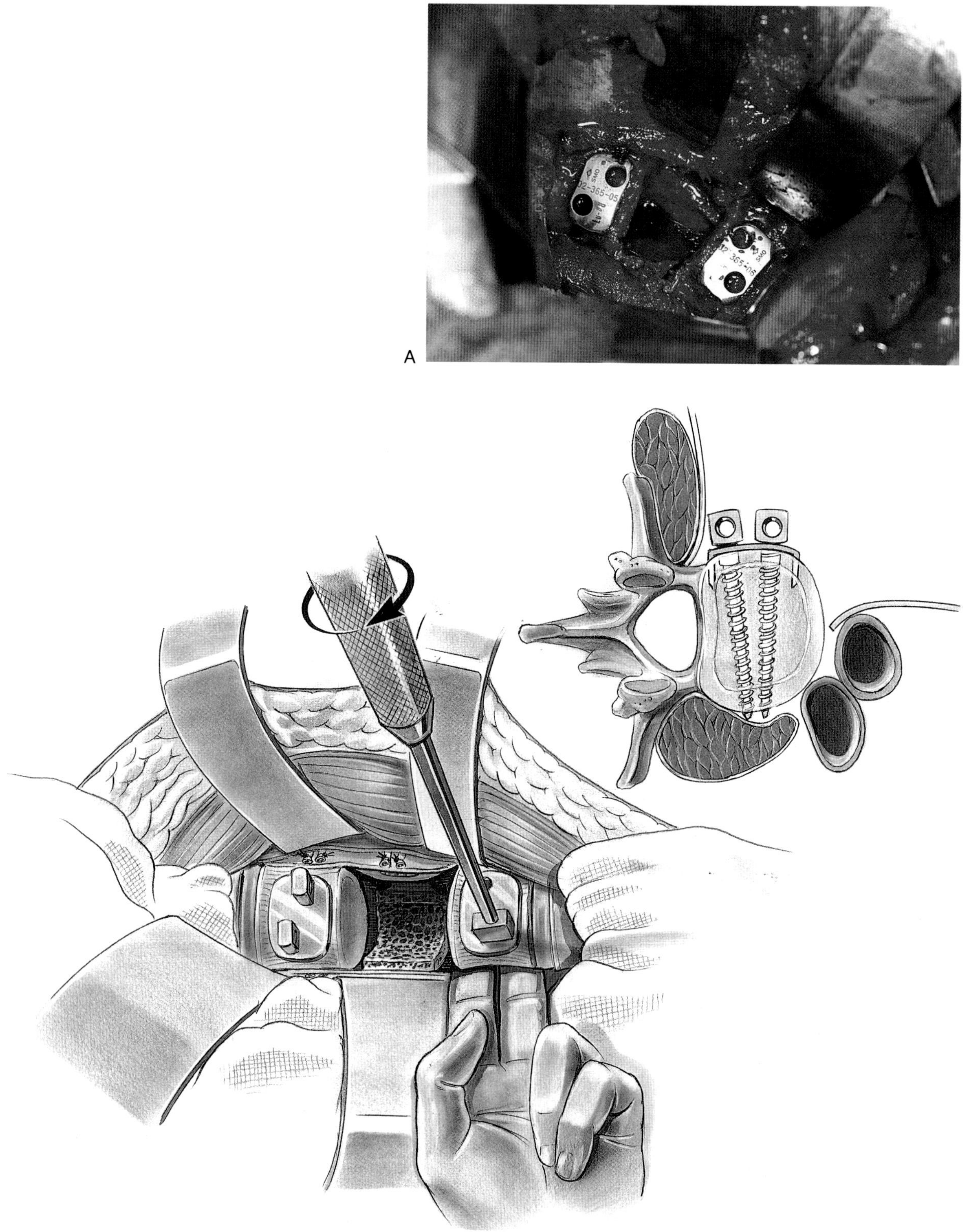

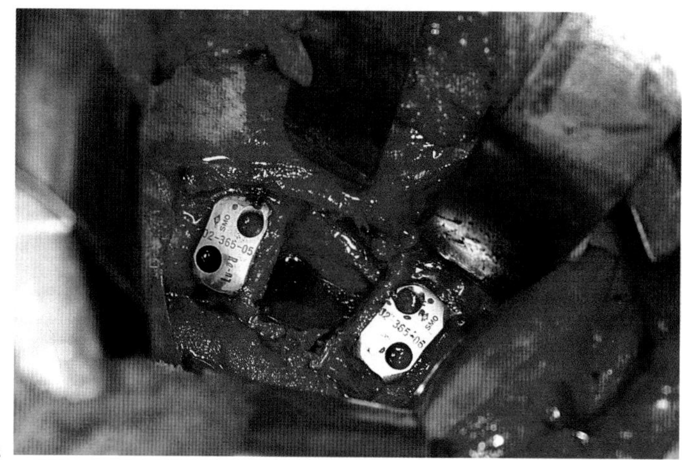

A

B

Figure 4. A,B: Placement of the vertebral plate and fixation with vertebral screws.

corrected because of tension in the contracted anterior longitudinal ligament in an old fracture case, the ligament should be divided at the disc level using an angled curette-rongeur or a knife. The iliac crest defect is reconstructed with a bioactive ceramic iliac crest spacer (1). The iliac crest strut graft should be tapped into place with the tricortical portion placed at the contralateral side of the vertebral body, opposite the side of the exposure (Fig. 6A). The area between the anterior wall of the resected vertebral body and the iliac crest strut graft should be packed with bone chip from the resected vertebral bone and pieces of rib taken at the exposure (Fig. 6B). This bone graft technique is the most important part of the anterior reconstructive stabilization. Anterior load sharing with stable strut bone is essential. If a stable strut graft is not obtained, the anterior fixation will fail despite the application of anterior instrumentation. The stability achieved with spinal instrumentation is temporary.

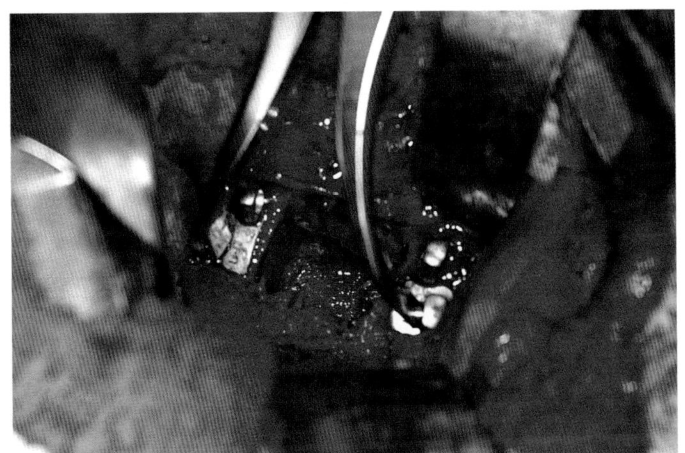

A

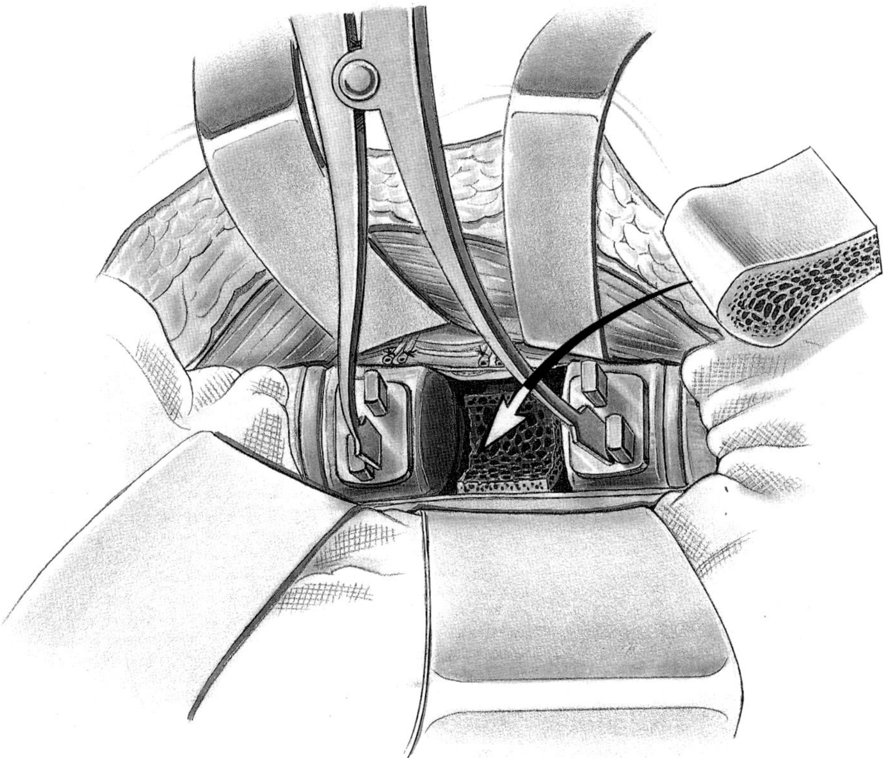

B

Figure 5. A,B: Correction of kyphosis with the spreader for anterior strut grafting.

Biologic stabilization is mandatory. If bleeding from the epidural space is present, it can be controlled with Gelfoam packed over the dura or the posterior longitudinal ligament. Once the strut graft has been placed with one piece of tricortical iliac crest, two or three pieces of rib, and bone chip from the resected vertebral bone (Fig. 7A), an appropriately sized paraspinal rod is spanned into the cephalad and caudal screwhead holes. The distal and proximal end nuts are added and compression force is applied to the graft by tightening the nuts (Fig. 7B). The rod couplers are then added to create a rectangular configuration of the biomechanical construct (Fig. 8A). After application of all the Kaneda implants, a posteroanterior radiograph is obtained to check scoliotic curvature (see Fig. 9). After confirming that the spinal alignment is correct, the nuts are completely tightened (Fig. 8B).

Closure is done in the normal fashion, suturing the diaphragm if a thoracotomy was performed. A drainage tube is placed in the retroperitoneum and a chest tube is inserted if the pleura was opened or torn.

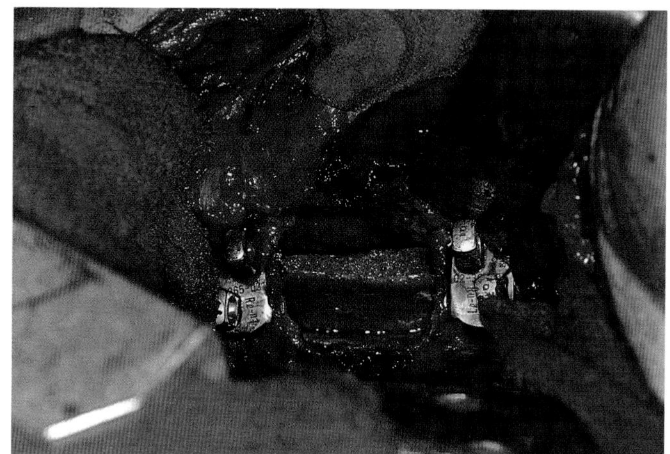

A

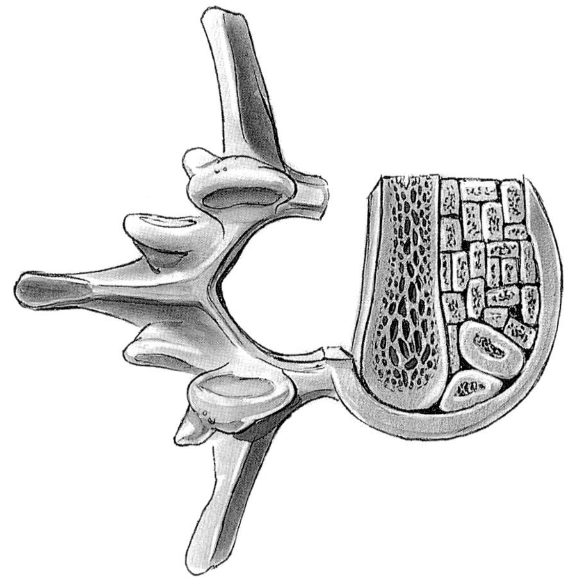

B

Figure 6. A,B: Insertion of the tricortical iliac crest and the transverse section of the bone grafts.

Note: Anterior spinal canal decompression in patients with thoracolumbar congenital anomaly (kyphoscoliosis in most patients) and thoracolumbar spondylosis is different from the one described above in thoracolumbar spinal injuries and metastatic tumors. In thoracolumbar spondylosis, vertebrectomy is not necessary, but resection of the posterior vertebral osteophytes, correction of kyphosis, and anterior fixation are necessary. In congenital thoracolumbar kyphosis or kyphoscoliosis with neurologic deficit, anterior shift of the dural tube by anterior spinal canal decompression (vertebrectomy) is mandatory. The resection gap should be replaced with stable strut bone and the Kaneda device may be available for stable anterior fixation.

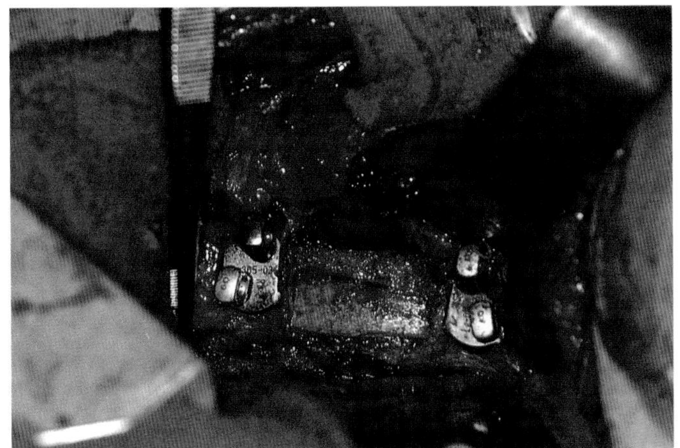
A

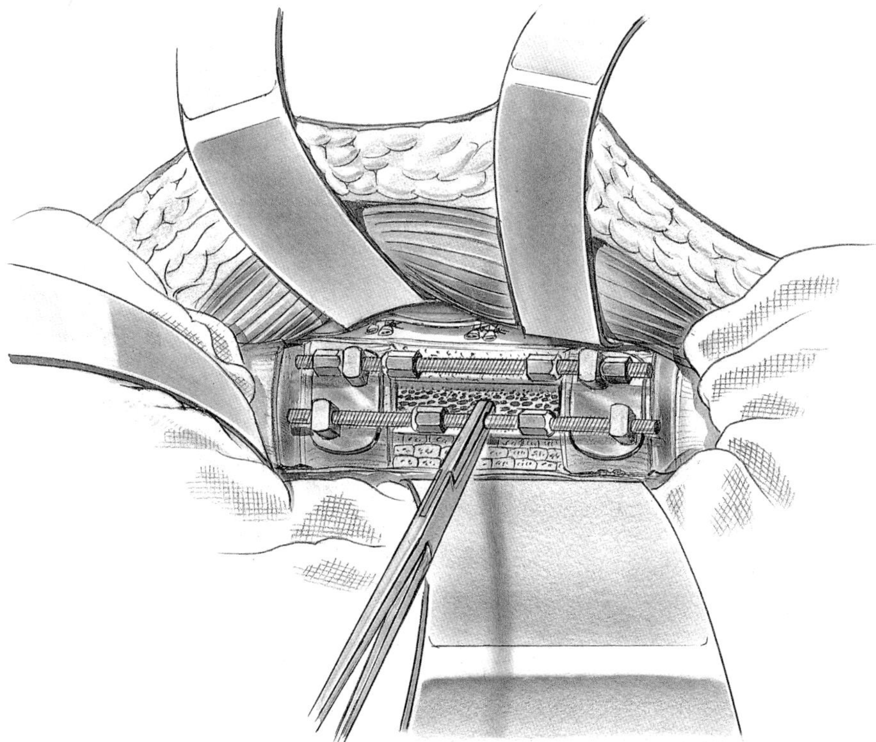
B

Figure 7. A,B: The strut graft with one piece of tricortical iliac crest, two or three pieces of rib, and bone chip from the resected vertebral bone (Fig. 6B), and insertion of the paraspinal rods with nuts.

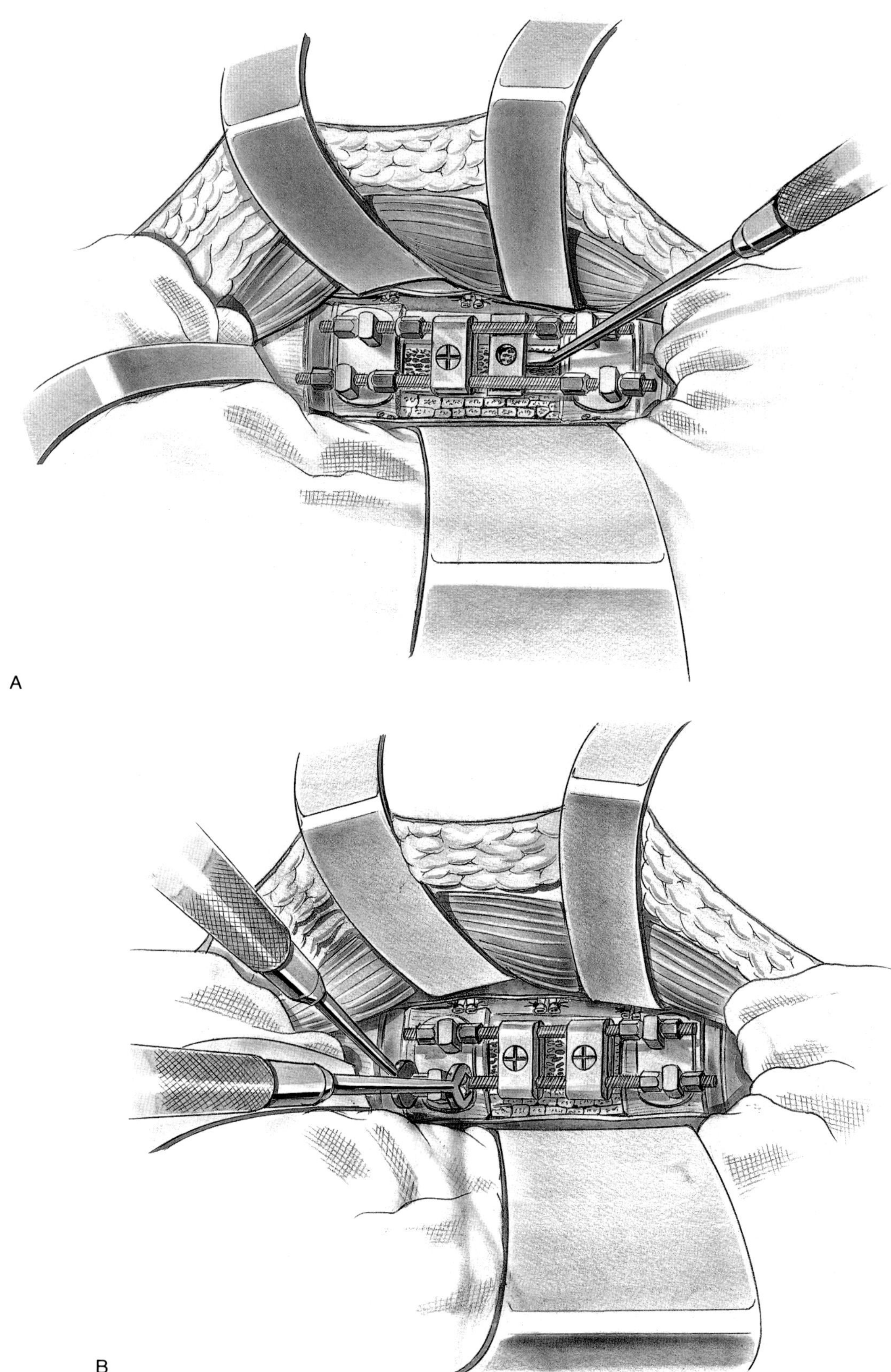

Figure 8. A,B: Application of the rod couplers to create a rectangular configuration and final tightening of the nuts after confirming the spinal alignments.

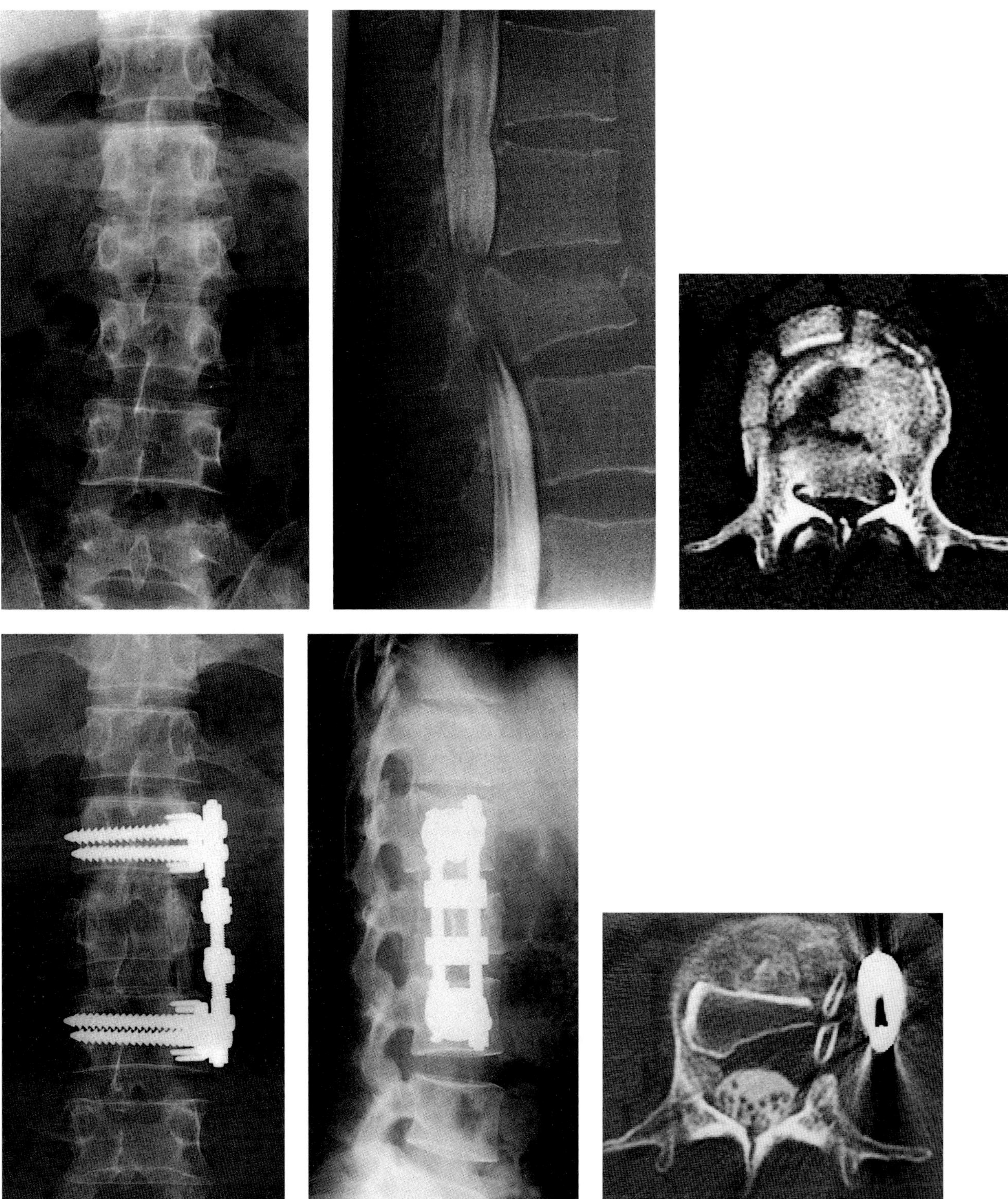

Figure 9. Case 1: Burst fracture of L2 with lesion of the cauda equina. **A:** The preoperative AP film shows widening of the interpedicular distance of L1 and lamina vertical fracture. **B:** Myelogram demonstrates massive compression of the dural tube with the retropulsed vertebral bony fragment (Denis type B burst fracture) and mild compression fracture of T12. **C:** Preoperative CT demonstrates a large bony fragment retropulsed into the spinal canal and lamina fracture. **D,E:** Five years postoperatively. These AP and lateral films show solid union of the reconstructed portion with physiologic frontal and sagittal alignment. **F:** Postoperative CT demonstrates an ideal placement of the tricortical iliac crest, two pieces of rib bone, and bone chip packing between the anterior vertebral wall and the iliac crest.

POSTOPERATIVE MANAGEMENT

Postoperatively, patients can be ambulated with a polypropylene thoracolumbosacral orthosis (TLSO) 3 to 7 days after surgery. Usually the brace is worn for approximately 20 to 24 weeks. Isometric exercise of the trunk muscle with TLSO is recommended with ambulation for protection of muscle weakness and postural back pain. Most patients, except those with severe neurologic damage and those whose jobs involve heavy lifting, can return to work in 4 to 6 weeks after surgery. Heavy workers may return to their jobs 6 months after surgery after stable fusion is verified.

RESULTS

Neurologic recovery after anterior spinal canal decompression has usually been satisfactory according to the preoperative neurologic status in our large series. Establishment of spinal stability was acceptable with correction of kyphosis. Short spinal fixation of the Kaneda device just one above and below the pathologic vertebra(e) has provided a much longer movable portion below the fusion compared with an ordinary posterior fusion with instrumentation.

COMPLICATIONS

The most important complication is pseudarthrosis, which is brought about by poor bone graft (strut graft) technique. A full thickness of tricortical iliac crest and rib should be used as a strut, and bone chip from the resected vertebral body should be packed into the resection gap (Figs. 6, 7, and 8A). In cases with poor iliac crest, a fibula can be used as a strut graft. Poor strut bone graft is easily absorbed. Instrumentation failures (vertebral screw breakage) come from pseudarthrosis or poor bone graft in the early stage. There was no instrumentation failure with a solid fusion. All instrumentation failures with pseudarthrosis were repaired by posterior instrumentation with fusion. Loosening of the implants (screw pull-out) can occur in the osteoporotic poor bone. Bone cementing in the screw holes was used in several osteoporotic patients. After application of the ceramic iliac spacer for reconstruction of iliac crest defect, postoperative complaints (pain, deformity) at the iliac crest have almost been resolved (1). Neurologic deterioration following anterior spinal canal decompression has not been observed. No vascular complications and no retrograde ejaculation problems have been reported in our large series of more than 500 patients. (Anterior instrumentation is not used for L5 pathology.) If the implants are located very close to the aorta, they should be covered with a Teflon sheet. The implants have never required removal in any patients including those with instrumentation failures.

ILLUSTRATIVE CASES FOR TECHNIQUE

Case 1

This 44-year-old man was injured in a fall from a height. At the time of admission on the day of injury, he suffered from paresis of the lower extremities due to a burst fracture of L2. He was treated conservatively for 2 days and transferred to our hospital. Anteroposterior (AP) film showed elongation of the interpedicular distance and collapse of the vertebral body (Fig. 9A). Myelography clearly demonstrated compression of the cauda equina with the retropulsed vertebral fragment (type-B by Denis; Fig. 9B). CT scan showed a large bony fragment in the spinal

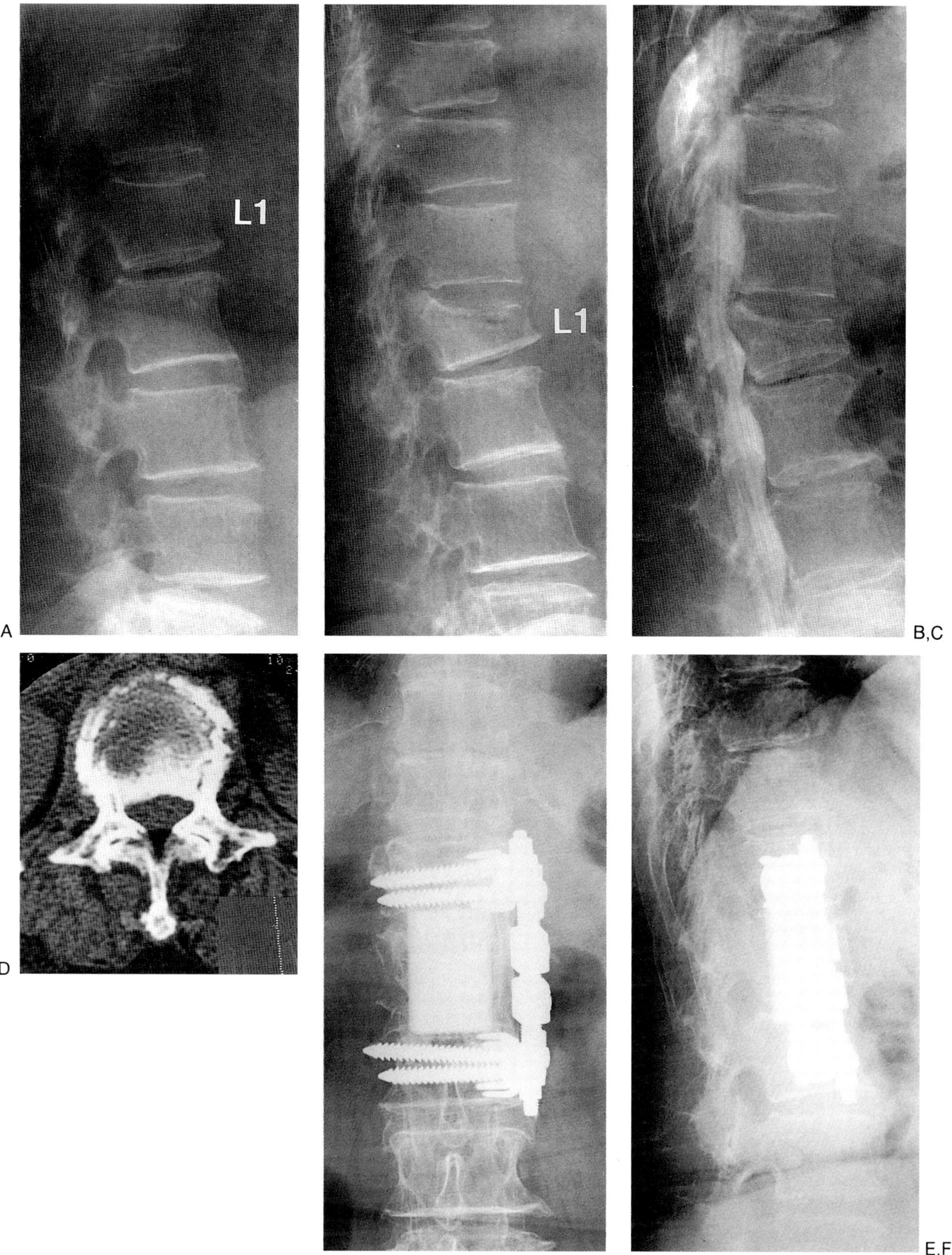

Figure 10. Case 2: Osteoporotic posttraumatic vertebral collapse of L1 with lesion of the conus medullaris. **A:** A mild compression fracture of L1 on the day of injury. **B:** Three months after injury, osteoporotic collapse of L1 fractured body. **C:** Myelogram: the retropulsed bony fragment of the superior-posterior corner of L1 vertebral body compresses the dural tube. **D:** Preoperative CT demonstrates the massive retropulsion of the vertebral bone into the spinal canal. **E,F:** Postoperative follow-up at 3 years and 10 months of the patient at 74 years old. These two AP and lateral films show firm bonding (fusion) of the A-W glass ceramic vertebral prosthesis to the upper T12 and lower L2 vertebral bodies. This was also confirmed by tomogram.

canal (Fig. 9C). Anterior spinal canal decompression was conducted by the anterolateral approach from the left side in the right lateral decubitus position. At 5 years after operation, the reconstructed spine was stable with alignment. Spinal canal decompression was complete (Fig. 9D,E). The postoperative CT-myelogram shows complete spinal canal decompression. This view shows no compression to the dural tube, ideal placement of the tricortical iliac crest and two pieces of autogenous rib as strut graft, and bone chip graft with the resected vertebral body into the cavity between the anterior vertebral wall and the tricortical iliac crest. The implants shown here are portions of the two paravertebral rods and the rod coupler (Fig. 9F).

Case 2

This 71-year-old woman fell on her buttocks while walking. Her radiograph showed a mild compression fracture of the L1 vertebral body on the day of injury (Fig. 10A). She was followed up conservatively without any type of bracing. Three months later she complained of increasing back pain, weakness of the lower extremities, and disturbance in walking and urination. At that time her thoracolumbar film showed the osteoporotic posttraumatic collapse of the L1 vertebral body with instability (Fig. 10B). Myelogram showed compression of the dural tube with a retropulsed bony mass into the spinal canal (Fig. 10C). A CT scan demonstrated retropulsion of the bone from the vertebral body (Fig. 10D). She was free from symptoms in the supine position, but neurologic symptoms appeared after standing and walking for more than 10 minutes. Anterior decompression by vertebrectomy was performed through the extrapleural and retroperitoneal approach by resection of the 11th rib. Due to osteoporosis, the iliac crest was not used. A bioactive ceramic (A-W glass ceramic) vertebral prosthesis was used as a strut with two pieces of autogenous rib (4). The patient started ambulation 4 days after surgery with TLSO. Postoperatively her neurologic symptoms have disappeared. At the most recent postoperative follow-up of 3 years and 10 months, the reconstructed portion of the spine showed stable union with a normal alignment. She is now 74 years old and free from symptoms (Fig. 10E,F).

RECOMMENDED READING

1. Asano, S., Kaneda, K., Abumi, K., Satoh, S., Hashimoto, T., and Fujiya, M.: Reconstruction of an iliac crest defect with a bioactive ceramic prosthesis. *Eur. Spine J.*, 3: 39–44, 1994.
2. Kaneda, K.: Spinal cord compression secondary to spinal deformity. In: *The Pediatric Spine*, edited by D. S. Bradford and R. M. Hensinger, pp. 286–306. George Thieme Verlag, Stuttgart, 1985.
3. Kaneda, K.: Kaneda anterior spinal instrumentation for the thoracic and lumbar spine. In: *Spinal Instrumentation*, edited by H. S. An and J. M. Cotler, pp. 413–433. Williams and Wilkins, Baltimore Maryland, 1992.
4. Kaneda, K., Asano, S., Hashimoto, T., Satoh, S., and Fujiya, M.: The treatment of osteoporotic-posttraumatic vertebral collapse using the Kaneda device and a bioactive ceramic vertebral prosthesis. *Spine*, 17S: S295–S303, 1992.

Subject Index

Subject Index

NOTE: *f* following page numbers indicates figures, *t* indicates tables.

D

M

U

ISBN 0-7817-0033-7

9 780781 700337